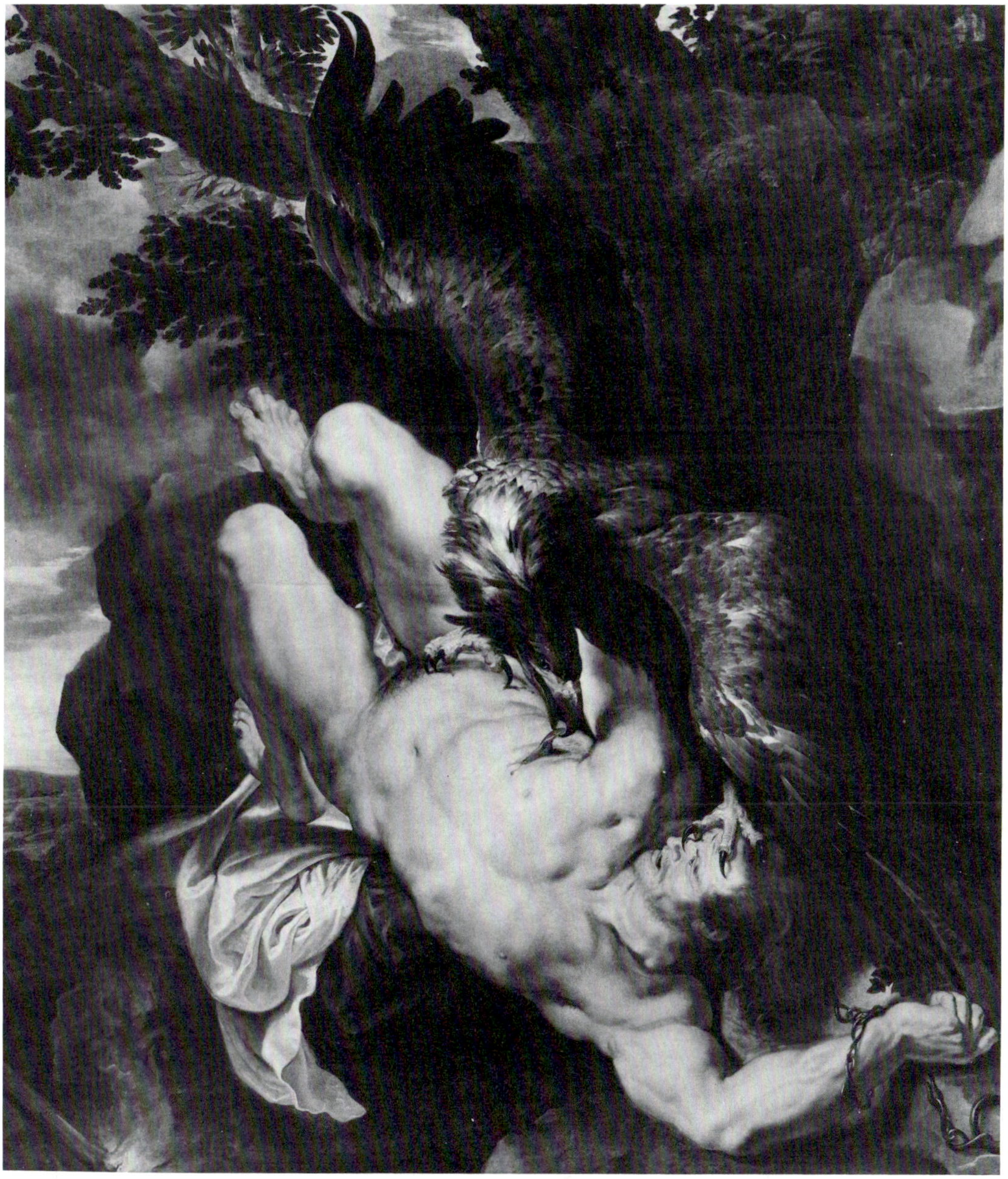

Prometheus Bound by Pieter Paul Rubens. Purchased: The W.P. Wilstad Collection. (Photograph by the Philadelphia Museum of Art.)

Clinical Radiology of the Liver

Diagnostic Radiology Series

editors
Louis Kreel
Queen Mary's Hospital for the East End
and London Hospital Medical College
London, England

Morton A. Meyers
School of Medicine-Health Sciences Center
State University of New York at Stony Brook
Stony Brook, New York

Volume 1 Clinical Radiology of the Liver (in two parts)
edited by Hans Herlinger, Anders Lunderquist, and Sidney Wallace

Volume 2 Radiology in Inflammatory Bowel Disease
edited by Clive I. Bartram

Clinical Radiology of the Liver

in two parts

Part B

edited by

Hans Herlinger
Hospital of the University of Pennsylvania
Philadelphia, Pennsylvania

Anders Lunderquist
University Hospital
Lund, Sweden

Sidney Wallace
University of Texas Cancer Center
M.D. Anderson Hospital and Tumor Institute
Houston, Texas

Marcel Dekker, Inc. New York • Basel

Library of Congress Cataloging in Publication Data
(Revised for vol. 1 pt. B)
Main entry under title:

Clinical radiology of the liver.

(Diagnostic radiology series; v. 1)
Includes bibliographical references and index.
1. Liver—Radiography. 2. Liver—Diseases—Diagnosis.
I. Herlinger, Hans, [date]. II. Lunderquist, Anders,
[date]. III. Wallace, Sidney, [date].
IV. Series. [DNLM: 1. Liver—Radiography.
2. Technology, Radiologic. W1 DI258JR v.1 / WI 700 C641]
RC847.C54 1982 616.3'6207572 82-14878
ISBN 0-8247-1069-X (PT.A)
ISBN 0-8247-1739-2 (PT.B)

MARCEL DEKKER, INC.
270 Madison Avenue, New York, New York 10016

Current printing (last digit):
10 9 8 7 6 5 4 3 2 1

PRINTED IN THE UNITED STATES OF AMERICA

Series Introduction

The change in radiodiagnosis in the last ten years could not have been predicted even by a modern Nostradamus. Those who were conversant with computers saw the future in terms of the more rapid handling of data acquired from conventional radiography or to its use in administration in radiology departments. It took genius to use computers to invent totally new equipment, vastly more efficient in the utilization of x-rays, producing images of exquisite anatomical detail. Suddenly, computed tomography became the gold standard for contrast and spatial resolution.

Ultrasonography was not long in accepting the challenge. The lower cost, the possibility of real time images and the ease of manipulating the equipment were soon apparent but more importantly the modality uses a harmless form of non-ionizing energy.

Obstetrics soon yielded, followed shortly by the gallbladder and liver, and then, surprisingly, the neonatal brain. Ultrasonography produced a different kind of detail but with high accuracy and specificity. Even the diagnosis of thyroid and testicular disease became feasible.

The slow but inexorable march of nuclear medicine has been equally noteworthy if less dramatic. Diagnostic procedures in bone, lungs, kidneys, and the heart are providing invaluable information. New pharmaceuticals constantly expand the possible clinical uses of this discipline.

No sooner had these modalities reached maturity when radiology was faced with yet newer imaging methods, nuclear magnetic resonance and digital radiography. Shortly these techniques will also be added to our diagnostic armamentarium.

While imaging was thus progressing, remorselessly and relentlessly from the administrative and financial viewpoint, angiography took on new dimensions, becoming therapeutic rather than diagnostic; angioplasty was born, balloon catheters became commonplace, bleeding was not only diagnosed but staunched, nor were radiologists slow to exploit the many other situations where needles, catheters, dilators and prostheses could be manipulated. Jaundice, gallstones, renal stones, abscesses, biopsies all became familiar as radiological problems for total patient management from diagnosis to treatment, from palliation to cure.

This may sound too dramatic a presentation of the last decade in radiology, but it is, if anything, an understatement when the individual patient is considered. How else is one to compare angioplasty with a bypass, percutaneous abscess drainage with laparotomy or needle biopsy with open operation?

Equally important is the totally new emphasis which has emerged, the problem-solving role of radiology as opposed to the mere demonstration of pathology. The diagnostic procedure is not merely a record of the previously known pathology, but must serve a definite role in patient management. Criteria for efficacy have been developed and applied to radiological procedures.

Hence, a new radiological series. The new diagnostic modalities will be assessed not only in their own right, but in relation to the newer techniques, not only as interesting physical signs, but as a contribution to patient management, not only as diagnostic procedures, but also in fulfilling a therapeutic role. In all, the patient must be paramount, rather than the technology.

Detection of tumors requires a special mention because of their common occurrence and unrelenting nature. The principle of using the least invasive and most accurate method is particularly important but diagnosis as such takes on a new meaning. In patients with tumor, the primary diagnosis is not the only important aspect, but staging the disease is crucial for management, as is the subsequent monitoring of treatment and planning radiotherapy when applicable. The detection of residual disease and any recurrence at the earliest possible time is equally important. Furthermore the diagnostic radiologist is now directly involved in the treatment of patients with malignant disease by undertaking tumor embolization, intra-arterial catheter localization for cytotoxic infusion, and even the introduction of radioactive material into tumors.

The modern radiologist is in the true sense a clinician, requiring technical expertise, diagnostic skills, a therapeutic and management commitment, and a thorough knowledge of anatomy and pathology. It is hoped that this series will fulfil the need of the modern radiologist.

Louis Kreel
Morton A. Meyers

Foreword

Clinical Radiology of the Liver represents the most comprehensive, in-depth review yet published of the various diagnostic and interventional radiological procedures available for the study and treatment of liver disease. It is somewhat surprising that even though the liver represents the body's largest gland, liver pathology has eluded conventional diagnostic methods. In an attempt to unravel its secrets, many techniques have been introduced only to ultimately fall by the wayside. This frustration at not being able to diagnose abnormalities of the liver is not new.

> From time to time, tests for determining the functional activity of the liver have been advanced, but few have withstood critical investigation, and we have made scarcely any progress in our endeavors to correlate definite disorder of function with definite alterations of structure. This is attributable, in part, to the complexity of the processes involved; but it is due also, in part at least, to the fact that the functions of the liver are not altered specifically by what we recognize grossly as definite diseased processes; . . . (*Modern Medicine Its Theory and Practice* by William Osler, M.D., 1908)

The more recent technological advances in liver imaging have occurred at a breathtaking pace and there does not appear to be an end in sight. Around the corner, one can see dynamic computed tomography, computed sonography, positron emission tomography, and in vivo chemical analyses and imaging with nuclear magnetic resonance. Since many of the newer tests are complementary rather than competitive, they tend to be added to already existing diagnostic methods. One cannot help but sympathize with our medical and surgical colleagues who find the technological explosion exciting, but at the same time confusing, redundant and always expensive. The radiologist can serve a very important role by the orderly and knowledgeable guidance of patients through this diagnostic maze so that work-ups are thoughtful, expeditious, and cost-effective. By the careful, objective reporting of the merits and shortcomings of these newer diagnostic and interventional methods, the editors as well as their contributors from both sides of the Atlantic have come a long way in accomplishing these goals.

In an attempt to present a correlative approach, the editors have solicited views from physiologists, gastroenterologists, and surgeons. These contributors are very successful in defining the expectations these disciplines have of radiologic methods.

The role of the radiologist has been expanded to include interventional therapeutic procedures such as catheter biliary decompression, intra-arterial administration of cytotoxic drugs, as well as intra-arterial hepatic embolization of neoplasms, and bleeding due to trauma. The description of the technique at the beginning of each chapter is particularly helpful in the section on special procedures.

The editors and contributors are to be congratulated on bringing a sense of cohesiveness and rationality to a very difficult area. This work represents a major advance in the practice and science of radiology.

Stanley Baum, M.D.
Eugene P. Pendergrass Professor
and Chairman of Radiology
University of Pennsylvania
School of Medicine

Preface

According to Greek mythology, Prometheus stole fire from Heaven and gave it to Man. In vengeance, Zeus had Prometheus chained to a crag on Mt. Causasus, where an eagle fed daily on his liver, every part of which, once consumed, grew back only to be devoured again. The frontispiece—a reproduction of the Rubens painting at the Museum of Art in Philadelphia—depicts what must be the first-ever percutaneous approach to the liver and represents an early awareness of the remarkable fact of its regenerative capacity. Ancient descriptions have regarded the liver as the source of bravery, desire, love, and passion. These references, and especially those pertaining to the immortality of the liver, are a few of the more than 500 functions attributed to this complex, vital organ.

It is the purpose of the editors to present a team approach to the liver in health and disease. The milieu for this understanding is created by the combined views of the physiologist, the internist, and the surgeon interrelating with those of the radiologist to maintain a proper perspective. The radiologist is an essential member of this team, contributing to both diagnosis and management. The editors have gathered the opinions of a number of radiologists from divergent environments around the world who, because of their needs and circumstances, employ different modalities. In the process, we have allowed and, in fact, encouraged overlap, especially when different opinions exist. From this consensus, readers must develop their own plan of action in patient management.

It was difficult to decide how far to extend our consideration into related and adjacent structures. We have excluded biliary pathology not directly linked with hepatic disease and we have kept away from the pancreas as much as possible. On the other hand, we have incorporated a more far-reaching chapter on the radiology of ascites and one on extrahepatic manifestations of liver disease. A large number of illustrations are included, many of them depicting identical pathologies in different chapters, and this has been done for the convenience of the reader.

The diagnostic radiologic armamentarium is now so substantial that choices must be made between available modalities. The diagnostic approach must be tailored to the specific problem, avoiding redundant tests that will not influence management. We also caution the radiologist to keep in contact with reality, that of good and reasonable care and the judicious employment of available personnel, talents, and facilities. An examination should be performed only if the information sought is likely to alter management. To increase the yield of such investigation, it is necessary to be familiar with the natural history of the disease in order to define the sites and extent of involvement. A thorough knowledge of the therapeutic alternatives, as well as the side effects, may assist in the decision as to the method and depth of the search.

There is undoubtedly a strong emphasis on arteriography, perhaps reflecting the inclination and bias of the editors. Until recently, angiography was the only standard against which all other procedures were measured. The interventional radiologists, equipped to perform invasive procedures, have become increasingly involved in patient management. They must be aware of the possible complications and must be prepared to handle acute problems. Consultative support is as essential to the radiologist as it is to all other physicians who require assistance outside their immediate realm.

Our intention in this text has been one of problem solving with emphasis on the radiologist's participation in this endeavor. Any success in this task is largely due to our contributors, and to them we wish to express our sincere appreciation.

Hans Herlinger
Anders Lunderquist
Sidney Wallace

Contributors

Tryggve Aakhus, M.D. Professor and Chairman, Department of Radiology, Rikshospitalet, University of Oslo, Oslo, Norway.

David J. Allison, M.D., M.B., M.R.C.S., L.R.C.P., F.R.C.R., Consultant, Department of Diagnostic Radiology, Hammersmith Hospital and Royal Postgraduate Medical School, London, England

Stig Bengmark, M.D., Ph.D. (Surg.) Chairman, Department of Surgery, University of Lund, Lund, Sweden

Erik Boijsen, M.D. Professor and Chairman, Department of Radiology, University Hospital, Lund, Sweden

Vincent P. Chuang, M.D. Professor, Department of Diagnostic Radiology, University of Texas System Cancer Center, M.D. Anderson Hospital and Tumor Institute, Houston, Texas

W. Peter Cockshott, M.D., M.R.C.P. (L), F.R.C.P. (Ed. & C.), F.R.C.R., F.A.C.R. Professor, Department of Radiology, McMaster University Medical Center, Hamilton, Ontario, Canada

Ivar Enge, M.D. Professor and Chairman, Department of Radiology, University Clinic, Aker Hospital, Oslo, Norway

Edmund A. Franken, Jr., M.D. Professor and Head, Department of Radiology, University of Iowa Hospitals and Clinics, Iowa City, Iowa

Roy L. Gordon, M.D. Senior Lecturer, Department of Radiology, Hebrew University; Acting Chief, Department of Radiology, Hadassah University Hospital, Jerusalem, Israel

Hans Herlinger, M.D., F.R.C.R. Professor, Department of Radiology, Hospital of the University of Pennsylvania, Philadelphia, Pennsylvania

Louis Kreel,* M.D., F.R.C.P., F.F.R., F.R.C.R., Senior Lecturer, Department of Radiology, London Hospital Medical College, London, England.

Herbert Y. Kressel, M.D. Professor, Department of Radiology, Hospital of the University of Pennsylvania, Philadelphia, Pennsylvania

John W. Laws, M.B., F.R.C.P., F.R.C.R. Director, Department of Radiology, King's College Hospital, London, England

Monty S. Losowsky, M.D., F.R.C.P. Professor of Medicine, University of Leeds, Leeds, England

Anders Lunderquist, M.D. Associate Professor, Department of Diagnostic Radiology, University Hospital, Lund, Sweden

Heather B. Nunnerley, M.B., F.R.C.R. Consultant Radiologist, Department of Radiology, King's College Hospital, London, England

Ernest J. Ring, M.D. Professor, Department of Radiology, Chief, Vascular Radiology, Hospital of the University of Pennsylvania, Philadelphia, Pennsylvania

Aslam R. Siddiqui, M.D. Associate Professor, Department of Radiology, Indiana University School of Medicine, Indianapolis, Indiana

Wilbur L. Smith, M.D. Professor, Department of Radiology, University of Iowa Hospitals and Clinics, Iowa City, Iowa

Sidney Wallace, M.D. Professor and Head, Department of Clinical Diagnostic Radiology, University of Texas System Cancer Center, M.D. Anderson Hospital and Tumor Institute, Houston, Texas

**Present affiliation:* Director of Radiology, Newham Health District, Queen Mary's Hospital for the East End, London, England

Contents

Contents of Part A

CLINICAL APPLICATIONS

22

The Physician's Viewpoint

Monty S. Losowsky
University of Leeds
Leeds England

Presentation to the Physician

The physician may be presented with the patient in a number of different ways. In the first place the patient may attend because of a *symptom*, for example, dyspepsia. In contrast, the physician may find a *physical sign*, for example, enlargement of the liver or spleen, either incidentally when the patient has attended complaining of something quite different or at a routine medical examination. A third way in which a physician may be presented with a patient is because of some *abnormal radiological or pathological finding*. For example, calcification beneath the diaphragm may be revealed on chest x-ray. A further way in which the patient may present is if a particular *disease is suspected* either because of a family history such as Gaucher's disease, or following an epidemiological survey as with screening for the hepatitis virus B surface antigen in a locality.

The Physician's Approach

The first consideration for the physician is to *decide the course of action*. This transcends the necessity for making a specific diagnosis. For example, in a patient with severe gastrointestinal bleeding blood transfusion and other methods of resuscitation must be undertaken prior to consideration of the cause of the bleeding. In other circumstances it may be decided that a clinical problem should not be pursued. For example, a minor degree of splenomegaly in an elderly person may be felt not to warrant further investigation.

In deciding on long-term management the physician requires a number of items of information. In the first place a *diagnosis* is usually desirable. For example, does the patient have cirrhosis of the liver? A second major consideration is the *progress* of the disease. A patient may have chronic liver disease; is this in an active phase? A third item of information, applicable to some diseases but not others, is that knowledge may be required of the *extent* of the disease. If a patient has a primary hepatocellular carcinoma, is this confined to one lobe of the liver, and is there evidence of extension beyond the liver? A further consideration involves a wider understanding of pathophysiological mechanisms involved in the disease process so as to *seek, identify, and manage complications*. For example, in a patient with chronic liver disease portal hypertension may develop and this may be manifested by a variety of consequences. There may be splenomegaly and effects on the formed elements of the blood (anemia, leukopenia, and thrombocytopenia), esophageal varices and gastrointestinal bleeding, or there may be ascites. In chronic liver disease there may be other pathophysiological consequences, such as defective synthesis of bile salts, which may lead to intestinal malabsorption and consequent malnutrition and this may be manifested as vitamin D-deficiency osteomalacia. Chronic liver disease may, however, affect bone and vitamin D in other ways, and the forms and manifestations of bone disease may be complex and multifactorial.

The Physician's Problems

Having determined a course of action and decided that investigation is desirable, there are still a number of uncertainties. In the first place the physician must consider the *consequences of each investigation* used. There are no known complications for the identification of a mass in the liver by ultrasound. Needling of the mass does, however, introduce an element of risk and this risk must vary with the likelihood of different diagnoses. If there were to be a likelihood that the mass is a hydatid cyst, further investigation would be indicated to exclude this, as far as possible, prior to a consideration of needling. Similarly, the demonstration of dilated intrahepatic bile ducts by ultrasound is without risk, whereas percutaneous transhepatic cholangiography, even by modern techniques, must be regarded as involving some risk to the patient. A second important consideration in the United Kingdom is that *the consultant physician is legally responsible* for all that is done to the patient and thus must take responsibility for sanctioning any invasive procedure.

Very often in clinical medicine the diagnosis is not certain and the physician must decide on the degree of certainty required. For example, a diagnosis of systemic lupus erythamatosus as the cause of splenomegaly may remain a matter of opinion. There may, however, be occasions when it is felt that, to make the diagnosis, invasive and even operative procedures, perhaps carrying a significant element of risk, must be undertaken to enable necessary management to be initiated. Decisions of this sort need to be taken by the physician and in this a major consideration is *the consequences that result from being wrong*. If in a patient with mitral stenosis it is thought possible that splenomegaly may be due to subacute bacterial endocarditis, then, even if this diagnosis is felt to be unlikely, it may be considered necessary to treat the patient for this because of the severe consequences of delay. Investigation may thus be directed at narrowing the options for diagnosis in some circumstances, some diagnoses being intrinsically more certain than others on the basis of the evidence obtainable in a relatively noninvasive program of investigation.

A further problem to the physician is the *possibility of multiple diagnoses*. This becomes more common the older the patient and, for example, gallstones may be found but may not be responsible for the patient's symptoms. As a further example, in a patient with chronic liver disease, exacerbation of the jaundice may be part of the natural history of the disorder but may be due to coincident gallstones, which are more common than would otherwise be expected. Whether to investigate for the presence of gallstones, and how often this should be done in a patient with fluctuating jaundice in association with chronic liver disease, is a problem for the physician.

A final problem in diagnosis is to what extent the physician should pursue the *possibility of extreme rarities*. The decision about this may depend on the effectiveness of available treatment, as for example, pursuing the diagnosis of Wilson's disease (hepatolenticular degeneration) is extremely worthwhile in view of the effectiveness of treatment. A further consideration may be the necessity for giving genetic advice, as in a patient with a lipid storage disorder. Another consideration is the practicality of obtaining a specific diagnosis, such as in the different varieties of glycogen storage disease. Yet another consideration must be the *expense* involved.

Cholestasis

Cholestasis may be regarded as jaundice of the obstructive type. A more correct definition would be "defective delivery of bile to the duodenum." Clearly, those hereditary hyperbilirubinemias associated with excess of unconjugated bilirubin in the serum would be excluded. By the strict terms of the definition the hereditary hyperbilirubinemias associated with mainly conjugated hyperbilirubinemia should be excluded, but I propose to include them since they form part of the differential diagnosis of obstructive jaundice.

Clinical Features (1)

The initial symptoms are almost invariably jaundice or itching or both. A history of pale stools and dark urine is elicited on questioning.

Prolonged obstructive jaundice leads to a syndrome which includes (1) skin xanthomas, particularly xanthelasma, (2) melanin pigmentation of the skin, and (3) steatorrhea and consequent nutritional effects, particularly deficiencies of the fat-soluble vitamins which may present with a bleeding tendency due to vitamin K deficiency, and osteomalacia due to vitamin D deficiency, and weight loss, (4) osteoporosis, (5) the development of secondary biliary cirrhosis, and (6) in some cases with the development of renal failure without structural renal disease.

Causes

The causes of cholestasis (Fig. 1) may broadly be divided into the *intrahepatic* and the *extrahepatic*. Intrahepatic obstruction may be further subdivided into lesions affecting the *major tributaries* of the common hepatic duct near the hilum of the liver and lesions

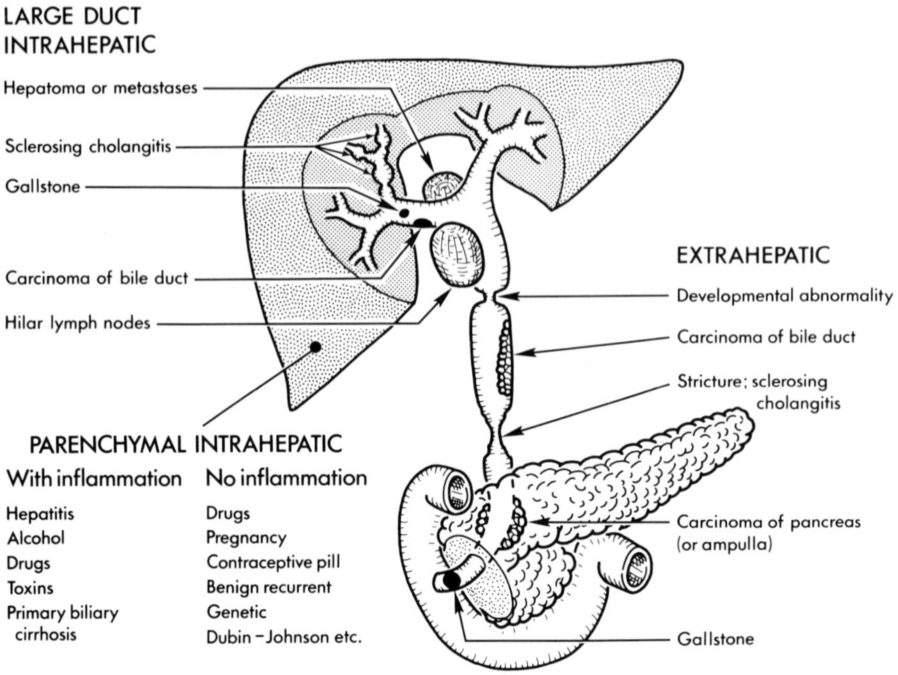

Figure 1 Causes of cholestasis.

affecting the *smaller tributaries* and the hepatic parenchyma. This latter group may be further subdivided:

1. Conditions with a *primary inflammatory reaction*, which include viral hepatitis (which sometimes presents with solely cholestatic features), alcoholic hepatitis (which similarly may be cholestatic in presentation), certain sorts of jaundice due to drugs (2) or to nonpharmaceutical toxins, and the very different condition of primary biliary cirrhosis to be considered below.
2. Conditions *without an inflammatory reaction*. Such lesions may be due to certain drugs, and occur in the condition of benign recurrent intrahepatic cholestasis and the probably related condition of recurrent cholestasis of pregnancy, which, in turn, is probably related to the cholestatic syndrome in a minority of females taking the contraceptive pill.

There are a number of *hereditary conditions* giving rise to hyperbilirubinemia of the conjugated type and hence to features suggesting cholestatic jaundice, and these include the Dubin-Johnson syndrome and other related hereditary hyperbilirubinemias and also much rarer genetic forms of cholestatic jaundice.

There are a number of other conditions which come into the differential diagnosis of cholestasis. Included are a form of conjugated hyperbilirubinemia sometimes seen after major surgery or after severe trauma; a form of conjugated hyperbilirubinemia sometimes seen with severe infections not involving the liver and biliary system, particularly in urinary tract infections in children; the pericholangitis syndrome seen in some patients with ulcerative colitis; and a rare form of conjugated hyperbilirubinemia sometimes seen in certain patients with lymphomas not directly infiltrating the liver.

In *pediatric practice* obstruction involving the extrahepatic and main intrahepatic ducts may be due to atresia or ductal agenesis or alternatively may be due to a choledochal cyst. In pediatric practice cholestasis without obstruction in the major biliary system may, of course, be due to hereditary hyperbilirubinemias mentioned above and in addition to a range of cholestatic disorders in young children, including neonatal hepatitis, $alpha_1$-antitrypsin deficiency, galactosemia, hereditary fructose intolerance, and other extremely rare disorders.

General Approach

The general approach to a patient suspected of having cholestasis is initial confirmation by serum bilirubin estimation since there are other, albeit rare, causes of yellowness of the skin. Biochemistry may suggest that despite the clinical impression of cholestasis, the condition is more likely to be due to parenchymal disease of the liver. In this case biochemical tests provide quantitation and allow assessment of progress which may avoid the need for further investigation. In due course a clinical decision must be taken as to whether some form of imaging should be undertaken or whether some other investigation, such as a liver biopsy, should take precedence.

Primary Biliary Cirrhosis (3)

Primary biliary cirrhosis is a rare, but not very rare, disorder of the liver in which the primary lesion is an inflammation of the small intrahepatic bile ducts, causing insidious progressive obstruction to bile flow. The term "primary biliary cirrhosis" is not a good one since the early stages of the disease do not conform with the definition of cirrhosis. The term "chronic, nonsuppurative, destructive, intrahepatic cholangitis" encompasses many of the important features of the disorder. The condition is pathologically relentlessly progressive, the initial destructive cholangitis being followed by proliferation of atypical bile ductules and then by scarring, septum formation, and eventually cirrhosis. Particularly in the early stages, granulomas are frequent in the portal tracts and occasionally occur in organs other than the liver.

The pathogenesis is quite unknown, but current views favor an immunological mechanism as the cause of damage.

Clinical Features

The disease is very much more common in females and indeed is a rarity in the male. It is much commoner at or after middle age. Pruritus is one of the dominant features, not infrequently preceding the jaundice by months or even years. Few patients escape this distressing symptom. The jaundice may come on relatively suddenly or extremely slowly and in due course other features, such as clubbing of the fingers, melanin pigmentation of the skin, and xanthelasma, follow.

Portal hypertension is frequently late but may be early in the course of the disease. Other features of chronic liver disease, such as liver palms, spider nevi, ascites, and hepatic encephalopathy, occur in the later stages.

Associated Features

Other disorders occur in patients with primary biliary cirrhosis, with a frequency which suggests that they are more than coincidence. These include thyroid disease, scleroderma with the CRST syndrome (calcinosis, Raynaud's phenomenon, sclerodactyly, and telangiectasia), the sicca complex, renal tubular acidosis, hypertrophic pulmonary osteoarthropathy, and peptic ulcer. Despite the frequent granulomas, sarcoidosis is not an association.

Features of the late syndrome of cholestasis, as described above, all occur in primary biliary cirrhosis. Particular mention should be made of osteomalacia, since in recent years it has become clear that this is common in primary biliary cirrhosis, usually with no suggestive features by conventional biochemical or radiological assessment.

Portal Hypertension and Its Causes (4)

Portal hypertension is not a disease; it is a patho-physiological manifestation that can arise in the course of a number of different disease processes. Portal hypertension may be due to prehepatic, hepatic, or posthepatic causes (Fig. 2).

Prehepatic

Obstruction of the splenic vein leads to hypertension in the splenic portion of the portal venous system; obstruction of the portal vein leads to hypertension in all parts of the system distal to the obstruction.

Causes of thrombosis of portal or splenic veins include carcinoma of the pancreas or pancreatitis, surgery in the region of the posterior abdominal wall, shunt surgery, primary

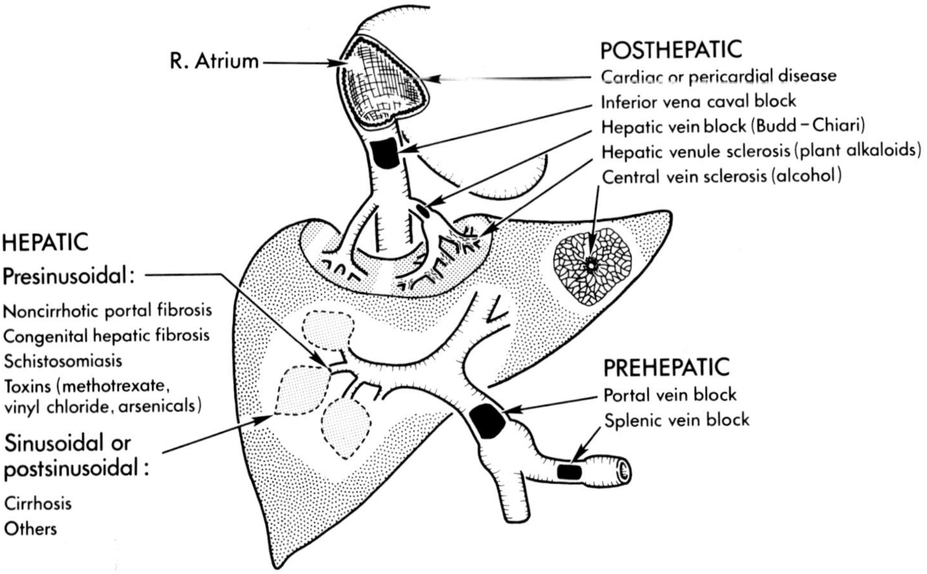

Figure 2 Causes of portal hypertension.

or secondary carcinoma near the hilum of the liver as a complication of cirrhosis of the liver, severe trauma to the abdomen, umbilical sepsis in the neonate, and diseases predisposing to venous thrombosis, such as the myeloproliferative disorders and paroxysmal nocturnal hemoglobinuria.

Hepatic

Hepatic causes of portal hypertension may be divided into the presinusoidal and those which are sinusoidal and/or postsinusoidal.

Presinusoidal Causes

A presinusoidal cause is the condition often known as *noncirrhotic portal fibrosis* or idiopathic portal hypertension, which is relatively common in underdeveloped countries. At least some cases may be due to multiple small thromboses in fine branches of the portal venous system within the liver. A rather similar lesion may be due to certain drugs and toxins, including alcohol, methotrexate, exposure to vinyl chloride monomer during the production of plastics, and prolonged arsenic ingestion, whether as medication or as contamination in drinking water. Infestation with *Schistosoma mansoni* or *S. japonicum* gives rise to fibrosis in the portal areas secondary to granulomas forming around parasites.

Congenital hepatic fibrosis, occurring in members of families affected with congenital polycystic disease of the kidneys and polycystic disease of the liver, gives rise to extensive fibrosis and to presinusoidal portal hypertension without the formation of nodules or the disturbance of the lobular architecture of the liver which characterize cirrhosis.

A number of other, rare, benign conditions within the liver can cause presinusoidal hypertension. *Nodular regenerative hyperplasia* is a condition in which there are small nodules of hepatocytes scattered throughout the liver, with only minimal fibrosis, most cases but not all being associated with polyarthritis of the rheumatoid type. *Partial nodular transformation* is a condition in which relatively few large nodules occur, near the hilum of the liver, surrounded by fibrous tissue, and cause compression of main portal vein branches. *Benign liver tumors* (or other space-occupying lesions such as hydatid cysts) occurring in this region may cause similar effects. *Focal nodular hyperplasia* is a condition with a single large nodule or multiple nodules usually peripherally located and thus unlikely to cause portal hypertension. These conditions cannot always be clearly separated one from another.

Infiltration of portal zone areas throughout the liver may occur in lymphomas, myeloproliferative disorders, and granulomatous hepatitis, and presinusoidal portal hypertension may result.

Sinusoidal and/or Postsinusoidal Causes

In disease directly affecting the hepatic parenchymal cells, particularly when there is disturbance of the architecture of the liver, the mechanism of portal hypertension tends to be a mixture of sinusoidal and postsinusoidal.

In *cirrhosis of the liver*, there are multiple mechanisms of portal hypertension, including (1) sinusoidal block due to disturbance of the architecture of the liver cell plates, fibrosis, and nodule formation; (2) postsinusoidal block due to pressure by regenerating nodules on the small hepatic venules; and (3) abnormal shunts between hepatic arterioles and small portal vein radicles.

In most parts of the world cirrhosis of the liver is by far the commonest cause of sinusoidal/postsinusoidal hepatic portal hypertension and, indeed, is by far the commonest cause of portal hypertension of any variety. There are, however, many other causes of hepatic portal hypertension of the sinusoidal or postsinusoidal variety; these include *chronic active hepatitis*, gross *fatty liver*, *acute viral hepatitis*, *alcoholic hepatitis*, and *metastatic carcinoma*.

Posthepatic

Posthepatic portal hypertension may be due to obstruction in any part of the venous drainage of the liver from the central veins within the nodules through to the inferior vena cava and beyond.

In patients with *alcoholism* there may be portal hypertension even at the stage when there is no gross histological disturbance of the liver. If special stains are used, some patients are seen to have a sclerosing hyaline process surrounding the central veins of the liver lobules, and the clinical concomitant of this is portal hypertension.

Sclerosis of the small hepatic veins, giving rise to *veno-occlusive disease*, may be due to plant alkaloids, particularly in association with the taking of ''bush tea'' in certain parts of the world.

Obstruction of the major hepatic veins is usually termed the *Budd-Chiari syndrome*. Many such cases are of unknown cause but when a cause is found it may be a tumor within the liver or a tumor of the posterior abdominal wall. The condition is sometimes due to a thrombotic tendency found in association, for example, with myeloproliferative disease or with the taking of oral contraceptives.

A condition that presents similarly to obstruction of hepatic veins and which, for reasons that are not obvious, may sometimes cause symptoms only in the second or third decade is a *diaphragm in the inferior vena cava*, presumed to be of congenital origin. Other forms of obstruction to the inferior vena cava such as thrombosis or external pressure may present similarly.

Disease of the heart or pericardium causing chronic increase of pressure within the inferior cava, such as *constrictive pericarditis*, may produce the same effects and give rise to portal hypertension.

Portal Hypertension Due to Increased Blood Flow

It may be speculated that some part of the portal hypertension in association with chronic liver disease may be due to increased blood flow, perhaps partly due to increased splenic flow associated with the splenomegaly and perhaps due to intrahepatic shunting between hepatic artery, portal vein, and hepatic vein, as mentioned above.

There are some rare patients in whom portal hypertension is due to increased portal vein flow associated with an arteriovenous fistula, as between the hepatic artery and the portal vein.

A degree of portal hypertension, rarely severe, occurs with many causes of *splenomegaly*, perhaps due to increased blood flow through the enlarged spleen. This may be part of the explanation of portal hypertension seen, for example, in patients with myeloproliferative disorders.

Effects of Portal Hypertension (Fig. 3)

Variceal Bleeding (5)

The importance of gastrointestinal, submucosal collateral vessels resulting from portal hypertension is their tendency to bleed into the lumen of the gastrointestinal tract. The overwhelming majority of such bleeds arise from esophageal varices, the next most common site being from gastric varices. Varices in other sites occur occasionally and bleed rarely.

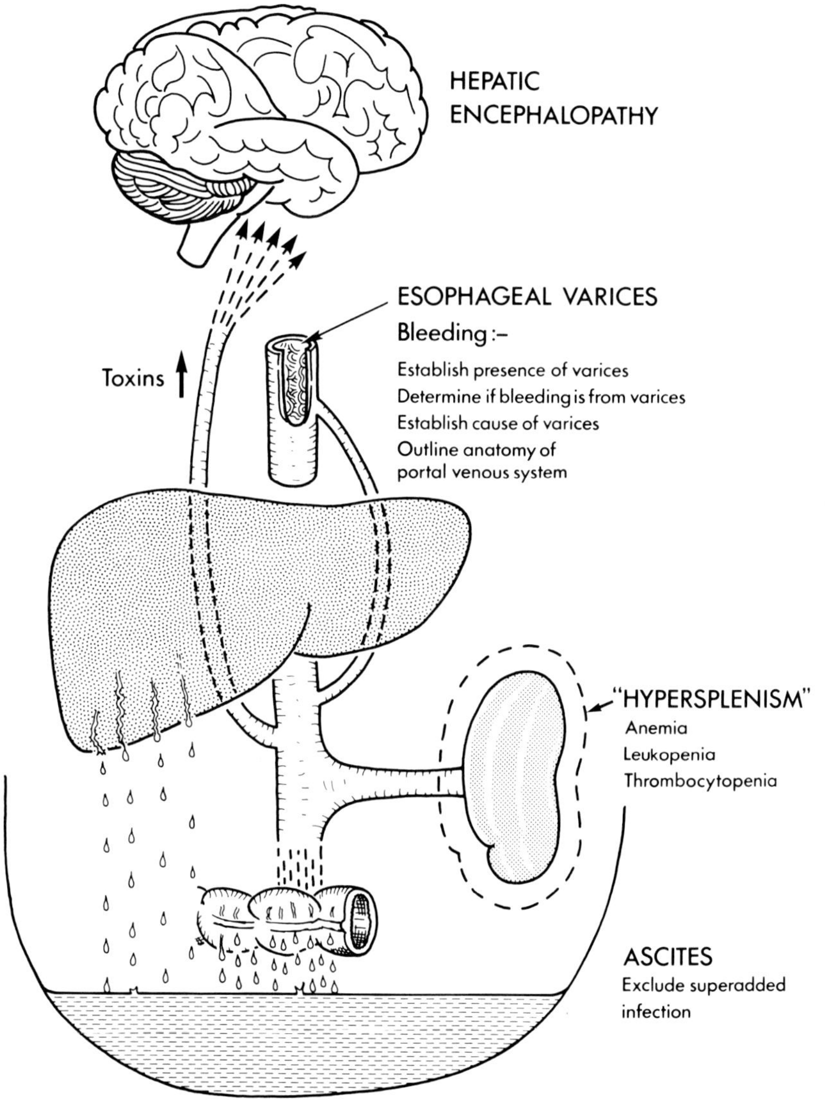

Figure 3 Effects of portal hypertension.

Bleeding from *esophageal* or *gastric varices* usually presents as frank hematemesis or frank melena. If the bleeding is particularly rapid, relatively unchanged blood may appear per rectum. Occasionally, prolonged occult bleeding leading to anemia may be attributed to gastroesophageal varices.

The *differential diagnosis* of bleeding from gastroesophageal varices must be seen in the context of the much more frequent occurrence of bleeding for other reasons. Frequent causes are acute or chronic *gastric* or *duodenal* ulcer and the relatively neglected cause of the *Mallory-Weiss* lesion, consisting of a tear at or around the cardia, which in our experience is considerably more frequent than bleeding from esophageal varices, as found in an unselected series (6).

Major hematemesis or *melena*, particularly in a patient suspected of having chronic liver disease, is a medical emergency. In the presence of chronic liver disease mortality is high and admission to hospital is mandatory. After initial resuscitation the duties are (1) to establish the presence of esophageal varices, (2) to determine whether the varices are the cause of bleeding, (3) to establish the cause of the esophageal varices, and (4) to obtain the necessary information about the anatomy of the portal venous system, its tributaries, and the systemic venous system to allow consideration of appropriate surgery.

For practical purposes the presence of esophageal varices may be taken to indicate portal hypertension, although there are occasional other causes described in the literature.

In the presence of esophageal varices it is not uncommon for upper gastrointestinal bleeding to arise from elsewhere; indeed, in some studies a majority of bleeds have been from sources other than the varices. Endoscopy is a very effective way of demonstrating the source of bleeding (6) and is now widely available in the Western world. Thus endoscopy is now the common method by which the presence of esophageal varices, or indeed gastric varices, is established. Radiological methods are also, of course, effective in demonstrating the presence of varices but less so in demonstrating that they are the source of bleeding.

In the *acute situation* it may not be possible to undertake definitive investigations to establish the cause of portal hypertension. For example, liver biopsy is not performed as an emergency procedure. In many cases, however, the underlying disease process is already known or strongly suspected from the history, and in the United States and the United Kingdom chronic liver disease is by far the commonest cause of portal hypertension.

In the *definitive therapy* for bleeding from esophageal or gastric varices, some form of surgical shunt therapy is often considered and if so, in order to assess the types of surgery that are possible, some anatomical demonstration of the portal venous system and its tributaries is necessary. An alternative possibility is local obliteration of the esophageal veins by sclerotherapy via an esophagoscope. A similar procedure is not available for gastric varices. Percutaneous transhepatic sclerosis of esophageal varices is an alternative procedure. A recent study has shown that continued propranolol markedly reduces the incidence of recurrent gastrointestinal bleeding in patients with cirrhosis. The relative indications and contraindications for these various modes of treatment as applied to individual patients require further study.

Hypersplenism (7)

The concept of hypersplenism is that an enlarged spleen may be associated with an increase in splenic function, resulting in a decreased concentration of the formed elements of the peripheral blood. The presentation of hypersplenism may be any one of *anemia*, *leukopenia*, or *thrombocytopenia*; any two of them; or all three. If the concept is correct, reduction of the size of the spleen or its removal should reverse the anemia, leukopenia, and thrombocytopenia.

Even in the presence of splenomegaly, the incidence of blood changes suggesting hypersplenism in chronic liver disease varies from study to study and with the type of liver disease. Moreover, in those patients with features suggesting hypersplenism, attempts to define the mechanism of splenic influence on the blood show no consistent differences between those with and without the blood features of hypersplenism (8).

Thus in the present state of understanding, the use of the term "hypersplenism" in relation to patients with chronic liver disease is not very meaningful. Reduction of the portal pressure by surgical portosystemic shunting does, however, cause a reduction in the size of the spleen and concomitantly there is often, but by no means always, an improvement in the features of hypersplenism. Splenectomy, similarly, may lead to an improvement in features of hypersplenism. Since, however, our understanding of the role of the spleen in the causation of the altered blood picture is sadly imperfect, the risks of abdominal surgery in patients with chronic liver disease are not inconsiderable, and the benefits of shunting or splenectomy are inconsistent, surgery of this type should be contemplated only if the anemia, leukopenia, or thrombocytopenia produces severe and threatening clinical effects.

Ascites (5)

Ascites must ultimately be attributed to a shift in the balance of hydrostatic and osmotic forces across the peritoneal membrane. Equally, the increased total body content of salt and water must ultimately be due to increased retention of salt and water by the kidneys.

Ascites is common in severe liver disease in which there is an increase in the portal venous pressure (and hence in the splanchnic capillary pressure) and a decrease in the plasma albumin concentration (and hence in the plasma colloid osmotic pressure). Ascites is rare with portal hypertension due to prehepatic causes unless there is also a cause for a fall in the plasma albumin concentration, such as a major gastrointestinal hemorrhage. It is tempting to assume, perhaps rather simplistically, that the combination of increased splanchnic capillary pressure and decreased plasma colloid osmotic pressure, both of which are factors tending to favor the accumulation of fluid within the peritoneal cavity, are the primary features that cause the ascites (9), while the excessive retention of salt and water by the kidneys is a reaction to this loss of fluid from the circulating volume. The precise sequence of events is, however, by no means well understood and the alternative order of events, that the increased renal retention of salt and water comes first and causes the loss of fluid from the circulation into the peritoneal cavity, receives support from some investigations (10).

Ascites must, of course, be differentiated from other causes of generalized abdominal distention.

Ascites due to liver disease must be differentiated from ascites due to other causes, most commonly intra-abdominal malignancy, chronic cardiac or pericardial disease, chronic renal disease, pancreatic disease, and chronic infection of the peritoneal cavity, such as tuberculous peritonitis.

Major collections of ascitic fluid may be associated with *pleural effusions*, usually right sided.

Bacterial infection of ascitic fluid may occur without obvious cause and may be remarkably asymptomatic, not showing the severe pain and rigidity of bacterial peritonitis and sometimes with remarkably little abdominal pain or fever to signal the presence of infection.

Thus bacterial infection of the ascitic fluid may present simply as resistance of the ascites to therapy or worsening of the clinical features of the liver disease.

Encephalopathy (5)

This is a reversible disturbance of cerebral function occurring in association with chronic liver disease and occasionally with portal hypertension in the absence of liver disease.

The effect on the brain appears to be due to toxins formed in the gut and normally removed by the liver. The toxins may reach the brain if the liver function is reduced, so that detoxification of the blood passing through is inadequate or if the blood is shunted past the functioning hepatic parenchymal cells either intrahepatically or extrahepatically, by natural collaterals or by surgical shunts.

The main *clinical features* are a progressive interference with consciousness from mild drowsiness through to deep coma, psychiatric changes initially consisting of intellectual blunting and personality alteration, and neurological manifestations including dysarthria, interference with motor function, and a characteristic but not pathognomonic tremor of the outstretched hands.

Development of encephalopathy may merely reflect progression of the liver disease, but encephalopathy may be *precipitated by a number of factors*, which should be assiduously sought. Constipation, gastrointestinal bleeding, and occult infection are frequent causes. Encephalopathy may be precipitated by a rise in the blood urea secondary to defective renal function, renal infection, or dehydration. Sedatives, opiates, antidepressants, or diuretics may precipitate encephalopathy.

Remote Complications of Liver Disease

Radiology plays a major part in the recognition and assessment of a variety of remote complications in patients with liver disease.

Bone disorders include osteomalacia and osteoporosis. In addition, the condition of hypertrophic pulmonary osteoarthropathy occurs in some forms of liver disease, particularly in primary biliary cirrhosis and also in association with hepatocellular carcinoma.

Gallstones are, of course, a well-known complication of chronic liver disease.

Abnormalities in the *chest and mediastinum* are well described, including pleural collections of fluid, expansion of the azygos system, and variceal venous masses which may be seen behind the heart or at the hilum of the lung and are often mistaken for other lesions.

Renal failure is a not uncommon complication of liver disease, and the assessment of the kidneys assumes importance in the exclusion of complicating anatomical kidney disease.

Various forms of *arthritis* accompany certain types of liver disease, and particular mention may be made of the peripheral polyarthritis occurring in patients with hemochromatosis.

References

1. Read AE: Biliary tract disorders: medical cholestasis. *Br J Hosp Med 23*:490, 1979.
2. Sherlock S: Progress report—hepatic reactions to drugs. *Gut 20*:634, 1979.
3. Losowsky MS: Primary biliary cirrhosis. *Medicine (3rd series)*:884, 1979.
4. Resnick RH: Portal hypertension and its complications—an overview. *J Clin Gastroenterol 2*:259, 1980.
5. Losowsky MS: Chronic liver failure. *Br J Hosp Med 23*:448,1979.
6. Foster DN, Miloszewski KJA, Losowsky, MS: Stigmata of recent haemorrhage in diagnosis and prognosis of upper gastrointestinal bleeding. *Br Med J 1*:1173, 1978.
7. Richmond J: The spleen—hypersplenism. *Br J Hosp Med 24*:405, 1980.
8. Toghill PJ and Green S: Splenic influences on the blood in chronic liver disease. *Q J Med 48*:613, 1979.
9. Atkinson M and Losowsky MS: The mechanism of ascites formation in chronic liver disease. *Q J Med 18*:153, 1961.
10. Taggart GJ and Conn HC: Ascites: its causes, complications and correction. In *Problems in Liver Disease*, Davidson CS (Ed). G. Thieme, Stuttgart, 1979, pp 25–41.

23

The Surgeon's Viewpoint

Stig Bengmark
University of Lund
Lund, Sweden

Introduction

Indications and use of liver surgery are increasing. Approximately one in four of all malignant disease processes in the body will sooner or later affect the liver. This makes tumor involvement of the liver as frequent as malignancy in other parts of the abdomen, such as the stomach, pancreas, and colon. Although still rather rare in Western countries, primary cancer of the liver and of the bile ducts is, like cancer of the pancreas, rapidly increasing in incidence. In the Orient and in Africa, primary cancer of the liver constitutes the most common tumor.

The liver presents a fertile ground for malignant growth. Tumors grow five to seven times faster in the liver than in most other organs of the body. This is why the prospect for survival is extremely poor for patients with untreated hepatic tumor disease (Fig. 1). It is thus a challenge to physicians, surgeons, and radiologists to detect, and if possible have treated radically, early manifestations of liver cancer. But it must be recognized that, in the author's experience, we have been successful so far in no more than 10% of cases. This must mean that palliative management still remains the most commonly applied form of treatment. Malignant disease is not the only indication for active liver surgery. Since surgery of the liver has been shown to have a low preoperative and postoperative mortality and morbidity (1,2), the surgical approach has been frequently applied to traumatic lesions, intrahepatic biliary stones, abscesses, cysts, strictures, and to hemobilia.

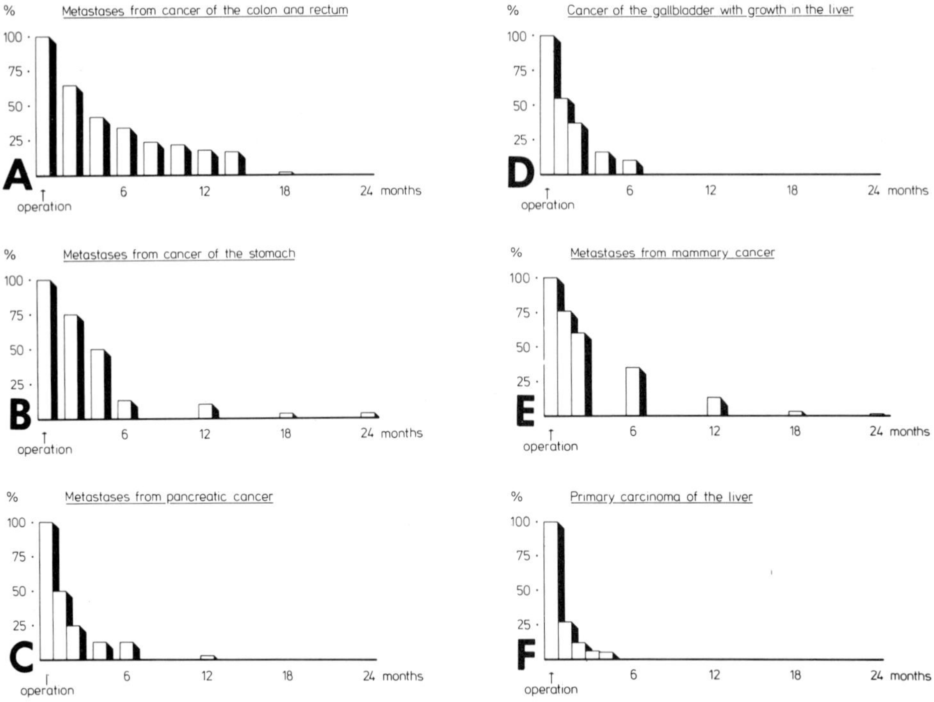

Figure 1 Diagram showing survival in months of nontreated cases of secondary liver tumors with the primary carcinoma in the colon or rectum (A), stomach (B), pancreas (C), gallbladder (D), breast (E), and in patients with primary liver carcinoma (F).

A More Conservative Attitude to Surgery in Liver Trauma

The liver, like the spleen, is frequently traumatized. For the localization and the demonstration of the extent of any such injury, aortography and selective angiography are outstanding (3–10) although computerized tomography (CT) can now take their place to a considerable extent. Until quite recently, the presence of blood in the abdomen was considered an indication for surgery. The author believes that laparotomy should not be performed early if shock can be controlled without it (10). It has often been found that bleeding had already stopped at the time of laparotomy and that the surgical evacuation of a blood clot could cause bleeding to resume and so create a situation the surgeon may not always be able to handle. In the nonoperated patient, however, blood in the abdomen does not constitute a major problem. Once shock has been controlled, ample time exists for a radiological workup. In due course the blood can be evacuated, although even this is not often required. We have been able to follow patients whose liver injury had been documented by angiography and who had been treated conservatively. Complete healing of these injuries has been demonstrated as well as the resorption of blood accumulated around the liver (see Chap. 27).

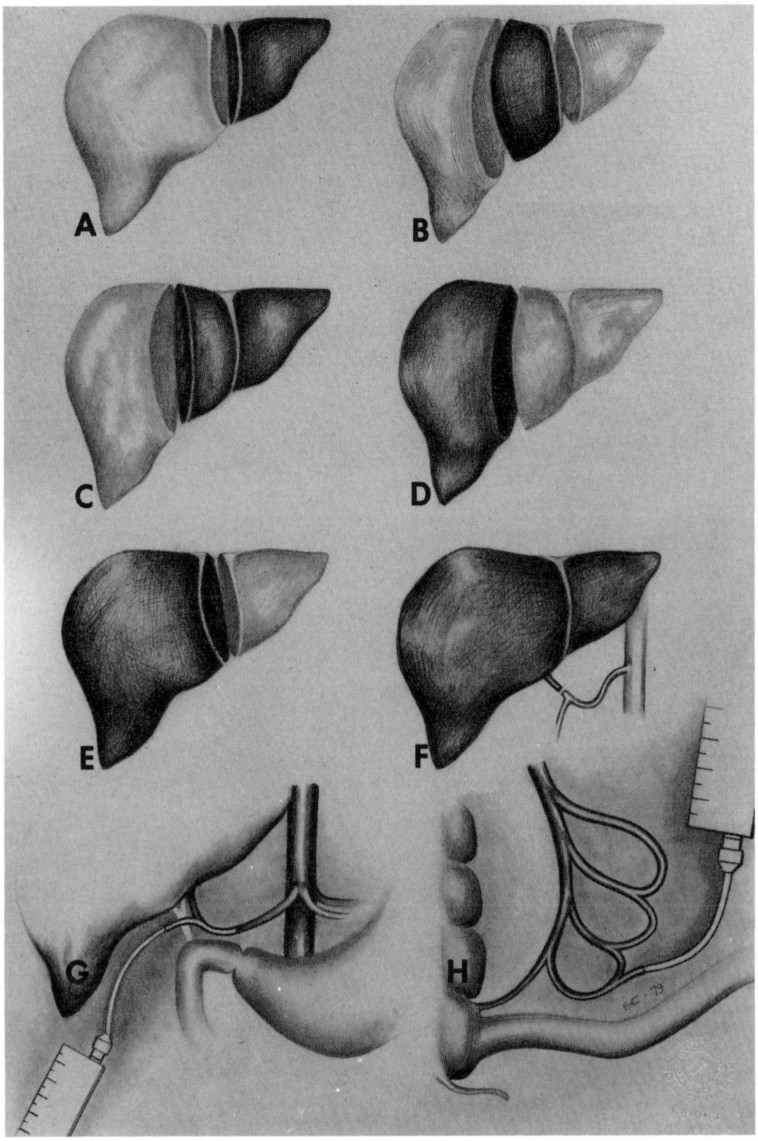

Figure 2 The surgical armamentarium in liver tumors and intrahepatic bile duct tumors. (A–E) Various forms of liver resection; dark areas, resected part of the liver; light parts, remaining part of the liver. (F–H) Nonresection methods. (A) Left lateral segmentectomy; (B) left medial segmentectomy; (C) left lobectomy; (D) right lobectomy; (E) extended right lobectomy; (F) hepatic dearterialization; (G) intra-arterial infusion of oncolytic drugs; (H) intraportal infusion of oncolytic drugs.

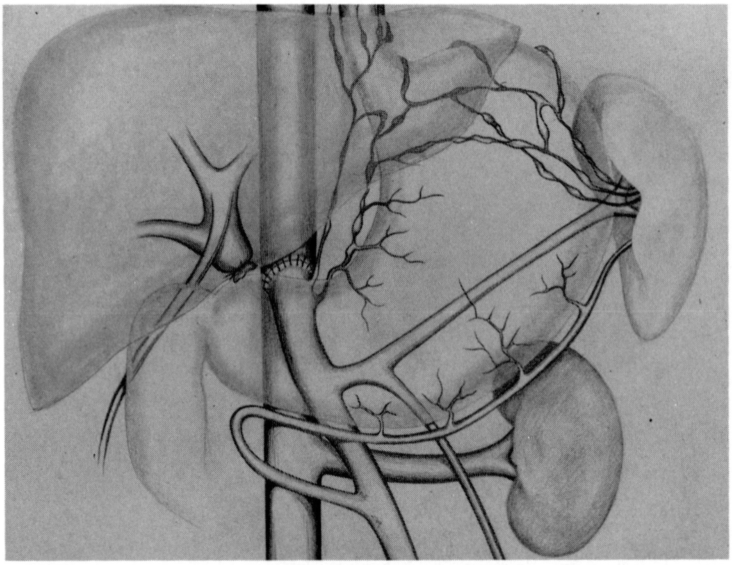

(A)

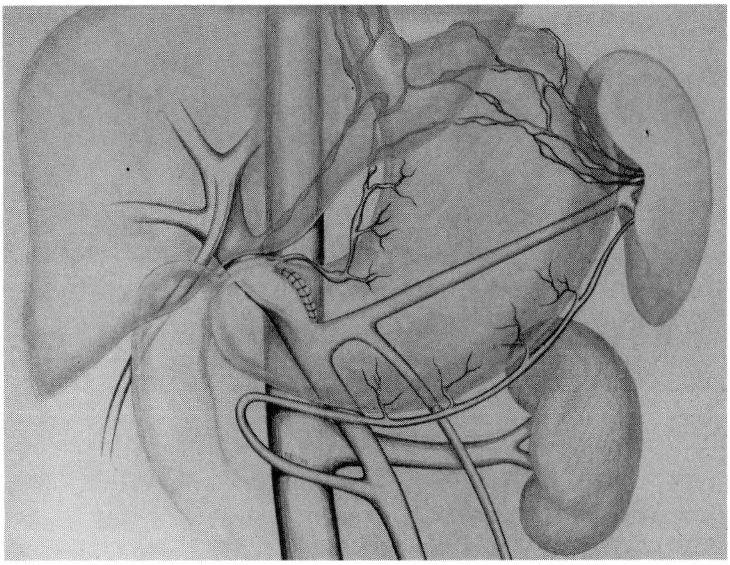

(B)

Figure 3 The four traditional portosystemic shunts: (A) end-to-side portocaval shunt, (B) side-to-side portocaval shunt, (C) splenorenal shunt, (D) mesocaval shunt.

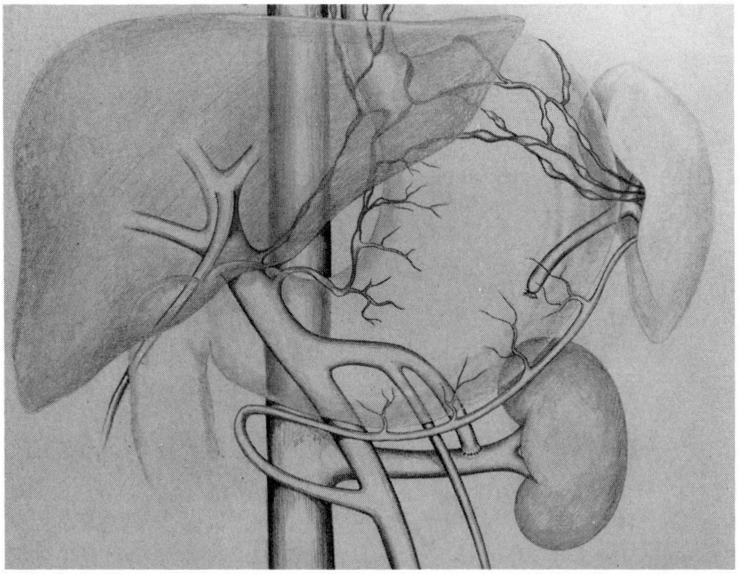

(C)

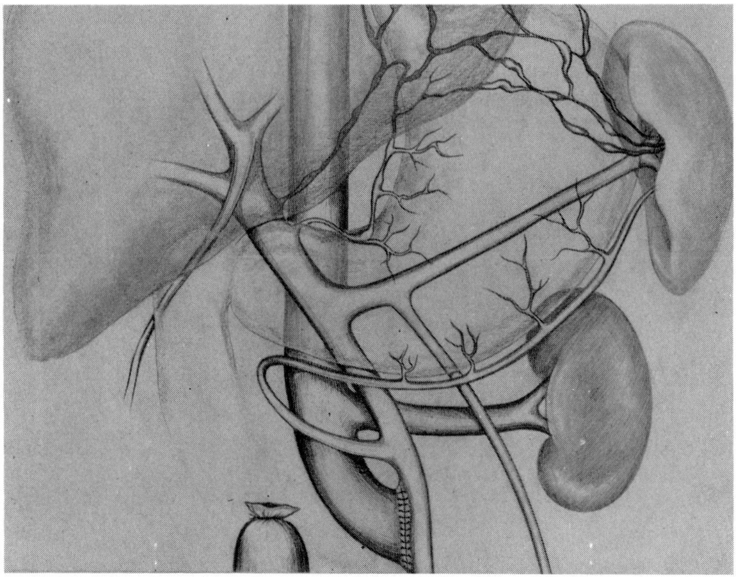

(D)

Figure 3 (continued)

Methods of Liver Surgery

The surgical arsenal can be divided into two groups: (1) procedures primarily designed for liver tumors, but often also used for benign conditions (Fig. 2); and (2) operative procedures designed for portal hypertension and its complications, mainly bleeding esophageal varices (Figs. 3–5). Resections vary from 20% (segmentectomies) to 80% of

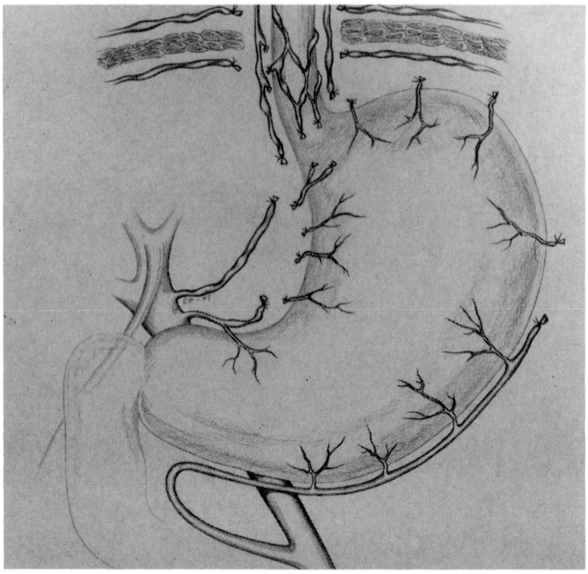

(A)

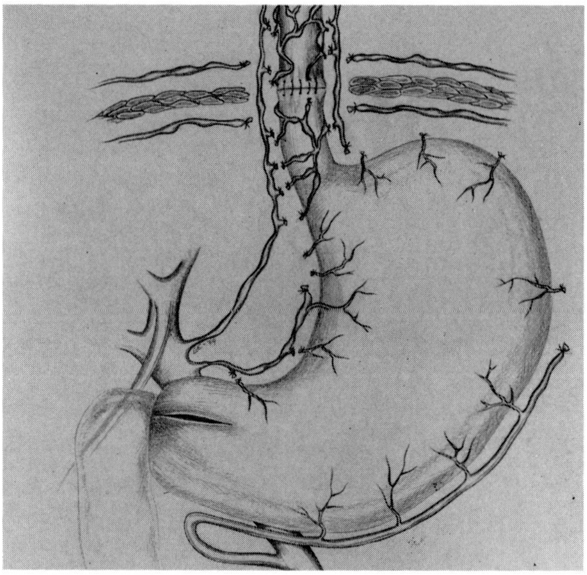

(B)

Figure 4 The devascularization operations introduced by (A) Hassab and (B) Sugiura (usually include splenectomy).

the liver mass (extended right lobectomy). In expert hands, these operations can today be performed almost without mortality and with very low postoperative morbidity. Special reference is made to medial segmentectomy (11,12). At this operation the medial segment of the left lobe is removed (Fig. 2B), mostly to obtain access to the hilus of the liver, an essential first step to resection of a cancer at the junction of the hepatic ducts.

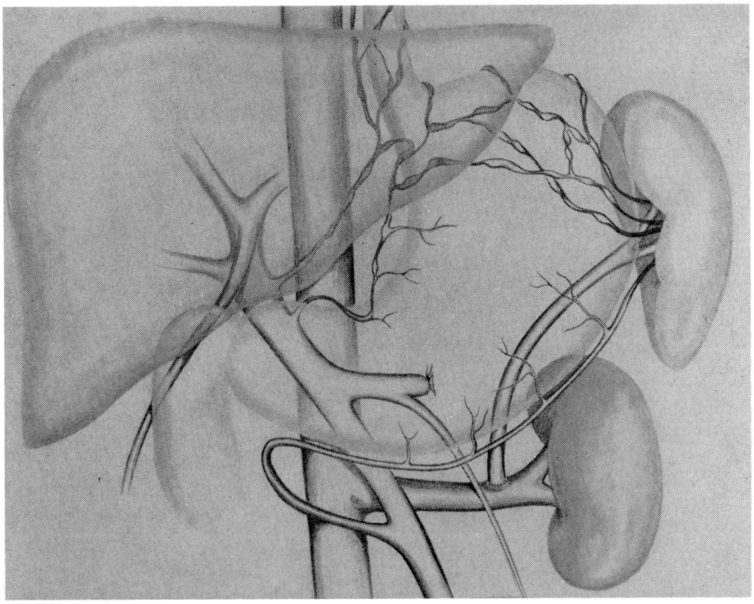

(A)

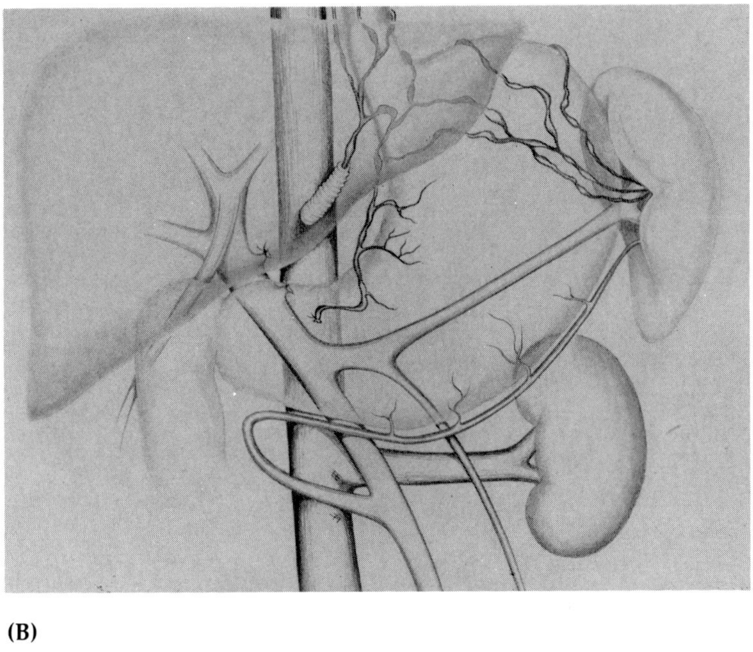

(B)

Figure 5

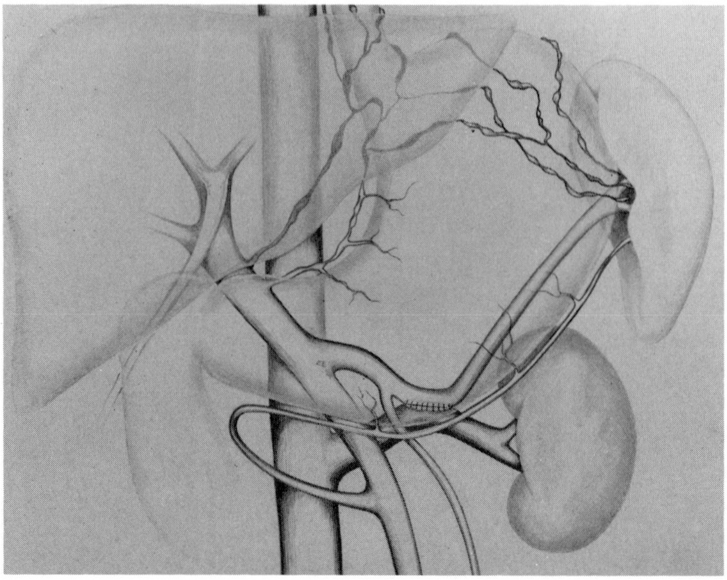

(C)

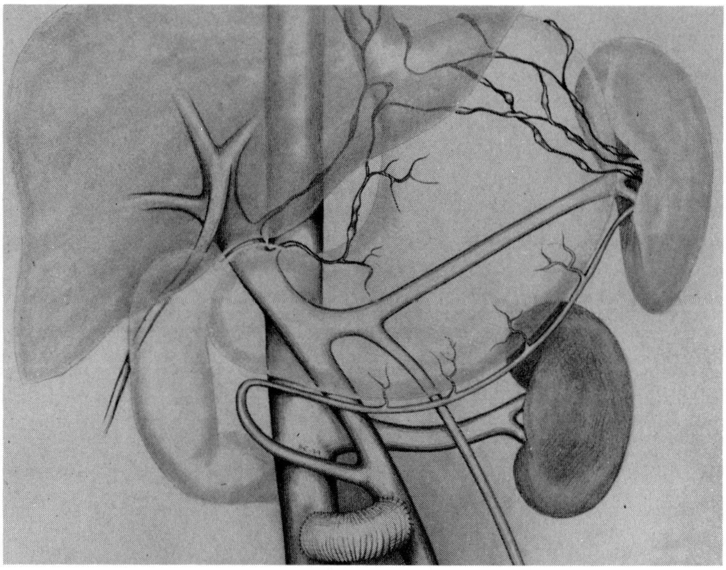

(D)

Figure 5 Some modern selective portosystemic shunts: (A) distal splenorenal shunt, (B) coronarteriocaval shunt, (C) side-to-side splenorenal shunt, (D) interposition-mesocaval shunt.

Radiology in Surgery Planning

Diagnosis and Distribution of the Disease Process

Most important for the outcome of treatment is the early diagnosis of disease, particularly in malignancy. This must mean that a referral to effective radiology should not be deferred to the appearance of clear-cut symptoms.

The plain films of the abdomen provide very limited information regarding the liver. Where liver disease is postulated, it should be routinely supplemented by ultrasonography or computerized tomography. Arteriography will probably remain an important radiological method. Transhepatic portal venography will continue to be valuable, especially in the workup of patients with endocrine tumors or with portal hypertension. This investigation should be combined with the selective collection of blood for chemical assay or with manometry. Splenoportography is only rarely used any more. In most cases, information it provided can be obtained from the venous phase of an arterioportogram. The peroperative cholangiogram may lose in importance in the coming years, to be replaced by preoperative cholangiography plus choledochoscopy during operation (for a review, see Ref. 13). Hopefully, a good and reliable method for hepatic lymphography will become available in future.

Surgical Anatomy

It is important for the surgeon to be shown the exact biliary and vascular anatomy of the liver before the surgical intervention takes place. From where derives the arterial supply to the right lobe of the liver? From where derives the arterial supply to the left lobe? Are there any aberrant vessels? Is the portal vein obstructed? Is portal flow hepatopetal or hepatofugal? What is the morphological potential for special shunt surgery? These are some of the questions that can be answered by the radiologist.

Radiology in Liver Tumors

Hepatic angiography is essential although, for a complete diagnosis, the hepatic portion of the vena cava and a catheterization of the hepatic veins should be included in the study. To be managed successfully, it is crucial that liver tumors be detected at a stage when liver resection is still feasible. Angiography is often left until too late. Noninvasive modalities such as ultrasound or CT scanning are therefore most welcome, as these techniques can be used more widely and on indications that need not be precise. They are also valuable in the follow-up patients operated for cancer of abdominal organs.

For the planning of a resection it is essential to know if one of the two lobes of the liver is free from disease. This is sometimes very difficult to determine even by angiography, especially with the left lobe. It is of less value to know the arterial segmental distribution within a lobe, as lobectomy is a routine procedure in most of the cases. It is important, however, to identify the area where hepatic veins connect with the vena cava and to relate this to the distribution of the tumor. Even if the tumor mass is not large, an unfavorable location may render liver resection almost impossible.

Resective surgery is usually restricted to patients with fewer than three tumors in only one of the two lobes. In the author's experience, the presence of more than three tumors, even if concentrated in only one lobe, will render the results of liver resection unfavorable. The exception is carcinoid disease, where the aim is the reduction of the tumor mass (14–17). In these patients segmental resection and the enucleation of tumors can be performed in both lobes and at the same laparotomy.

Liver Dearterialization in Carcinoid Disease

Fifteen years ago dearterialization of the liver was introduced (18–21) and has since become a most effective treatment of carcinoid disease (22).

In most other malignant diseases, the procedure would probably be ineffective by itself although more successful if combined with oncolytic treatment. In our experience, as well as that of other writers, liver dearterialization has only a short-lasting effect. After a few days new arteries begin to grow into the liver from adjacent organs and blood flow through the hepatic artery bed resumes (23).

A disadvantage of hepatic dearterialization, as originally designed, is that it permanently occludes the hepatic artery, which can then no longer be used for a subsequent infusion of cytostatics. This has led to the development of temporary dearterialization, where the hepatic artery is occluded for several hours (24). We hope that this will in future be achieved by nonsurgical radiological techniques.

Portal Hypertension

Radiological Workup

In portal hypertension arteriography is essential to exclude hepatic or other malignancy, map the extent and anatomic variation in the nutritive supply to the liver, and give detailed information on the portal venous system.

Arterioportography can serve as a basis for estimating the feasibility of an intended method of shunt surgery (25). A mapping of the portal vein, its tributaries and collaterals, and its flow pattern and pressure, is most effectively and easily done by the percutaneous transhepatic route. We no longer use splenoportography in the routine workup of these patients.

Surgery in Portal Hypertension

All surgical treatment in portal hypertension is purely symptomatic. The aim is to limit as far as possible the harmful consequences of the complications of the disease: bleeding esophageal varices, ascites, jaundice, and neuropsychiatric disorders. Attention has mostly been given to bleeding from esophageal varices.

The traditional portosystemic shunts (Fig. 3) succeed in decompressing the portal system and, with continued patency, will prevent further bleeding from the esophageal varices. The decreased death rate from variceal bleeding, however, has been obtained at the cost of diminished liver perfusion and an increased incidence of death from liver insufficiency. Thus there has been no significant gain in patient survival.

Selective decompression shunts have, therefore, been developed. The distal splenorenal shunt described by Warren et al. (26) aims to decompress the esophagogastrosplenic sector of the portal bed after isolating it from the main portion of the portal system (Fig. 5A). This preserves the elevated portal and superior mesenteric venous pressure necessary for continued liver perfusion. However, follow-up of patients 2 years after surgery showed flow diminution or flow reversal in the portal vein with flow diversion toward the splenorenal shunt (27). In our opinion, it is against biological principles to disconnect two venous systems which have a pressure gradient between them. New collaterals will rapidly cause equalization of pressures. However, in only a few of the patients followed up did encephalopathy develop.

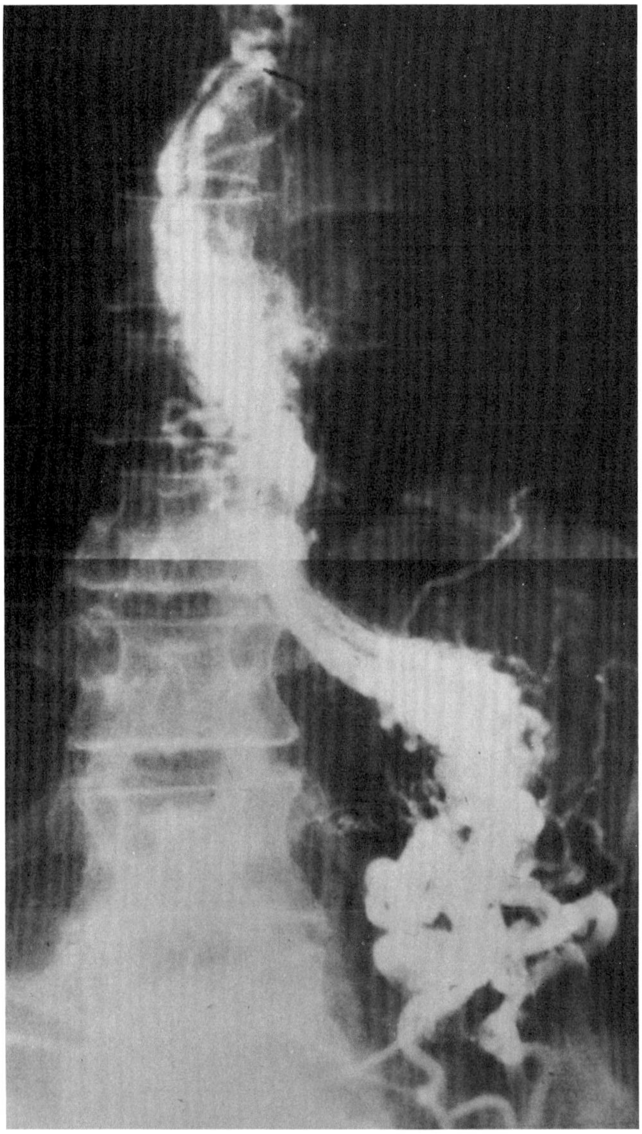

Figure 6A Transhepatic portogram showing esophageal varices before sclerosing.

Dissatisfaction with the results of shunt surgery is now widespread, and devascularization procedures are gaining ground (28–31). A detailed review of available selective procedures is presented in Ref. 32.

Sclerosing of Esophageal Varices

Esophageal varices can be obliterated transhepatically by means of catheters in the portal vein or by injection in the course of esophageal endoscopy. The two methods differ significantly. In the transhepatic method, the aim is to occlude venous collaterals by the

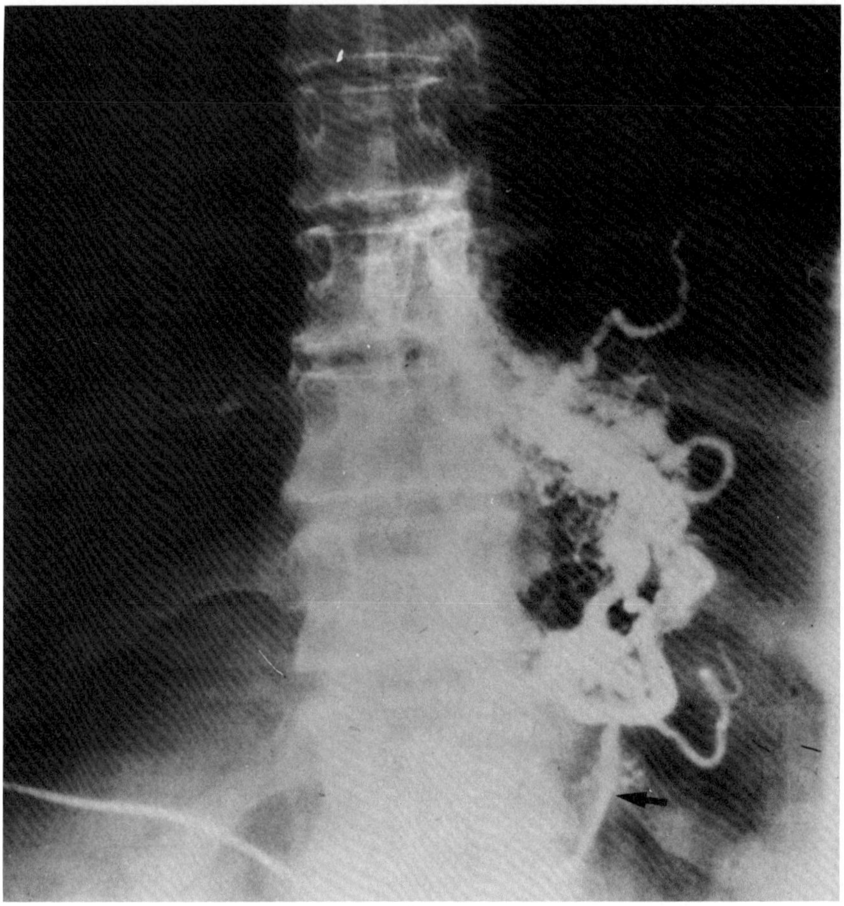

Figure 6B In less than 2 months new collaterals had developed; catheter now in a short gastric vein.

deposition of a blocking agent within them (33). In the transesophageal method a sclerosing agent is injected under the mucosa, not necessarily into the varicosities, to produce secondary occlusion through edema and fibrosis (34).

When the first attempts at treating patients by transhepatic occlusion of varices were published in 1974 (33), the results seemed promising. Since then it has become clear that permanent occlusion cannot be obtained by this method (35,36). Within a few days or weeks of the injection new collaterals are formed and high-pressure variceal channels once again extend into the esophagus (Fig. 6). To be managed effectively, therefore, transhepatic variceal occlusion should be regarded merely as a temporizing measure and must be followed within a very short time interval by elective shunt surgery. Transesophageal sclerotherapy can be carried out repeatedly and may be used to replace shunt surgery.

Expansion of Therapeutic Radiology

There are good reasons why surgeons should increasingly look to radiology for assistance in the management of patients with liver disease. Advances in the treatment of liver disease by radiological means cover a number of areas: percutaneous intubation and drainage of the common duct in obstructive jaundice (37), percutaneous extraction of retained stones (38–41), percutaneous introduction of stents in common duct obstruction (42,43), selective introduction of catheters for the administration of cytostatics (44), placement of catheters for the temporary occlusion of the hepatic artery (45), arterial embolization of primary liver tumors (46), sclerosing of the coronary or short gastric veins in bleeding from esophageal varices (47), occlusion of the splenic artery in hypersplenism (48), and percutaneous drainage of abscesses and cysts (49).

It is easy to forecast and in the interest of patients to hope that the scope and range of therapeutic radiology will continue to expand.

References

1. Wilson SM and Adson MA: Surgical treatment of hepatic metastases from colorectal cancers. *Arch Surg 111*:330, 1976.
2. Foster JH: Survival after liver resection for secondary tumors. *Am J Surg 135*:389, 1978.
3. Boijsen E, Judkins MP, Simay A: Angiographic diagnosis of hepatic rupture. *Radiology 86*:66, 1966.
4. Boijsen E, Kaude J, Tylen U: Angiography in hepatic rupture. *Acta Radiol (Diagn.) 11*:363, 1971.
5. Trunkey DD, Shires GT, McClelland R: Management of liver trauma in 811 consecutive patients. *Ann Surg 179*:722, 1974.
6. Wilson Defore W, Mattox K, Jordan GL, Beall AC: Management of 1,590 consecutive cases of liver trauma. *Arch Surg 111*:493, 1976.
7. Schorn L and Coln D: Hepatic angiographic changes after trauma. *Am J Surg 134*:754, 1977.
8. Levin A, Gover P, Nance FC: Surgical restraint in the management of hepatic injury: a review of charity hospital experience. *J Trauma 18*:399, 1978.
9. Blumgart LH, Druruy JK, Wood CB: Hepatic resection for trauma, tumour and biliary obstruction. *Br J Surg 66*:762, 1979.
10. Anderson R, Bengmark S, Goransson G: Operative or non-operative treatment of liver trauma. 1980 (to be published).
11. Launois B, Campion J, Brissot P, Gosselin M: Carcinoma of the hepatic hilus; surgical management and the case for resection. *Ann Surg 190*:151, 1979.
12. Evander A and Bengmark S: Evaluation of aggressive surgery for carcinoma of the extrahepatic bile ducts. *Ann Surg 191*:23, 1980.
13. Goransson AM: Cholegraphy, its applicability and reliability in connection with gallstone operations. Thesis, *Acta Chir Scand (Suppl) 496*, 1980.
14. Wilson H and Butterick OD: Massive liver resection for control of severe vasomotor reactions secondary to malignant carcinoid. *Ann Surg 149*:641, 1959.
15. Bersohn I and Bleloch J: Right hemipatectomy in secondary carcinoid of the liver: clinical course and liver function tests. *S Afr Med J 1*:27174, 1967.
16. Stephen JL and Graham-Smith DG: Treatment of carcinoid syndrome by local removal of hepatic metastases. *Proc R Soc Med 65*:444, 1972.
17. Davis Z, Moertel CG, McIlrath DC: The malignant carcinoid syndrome. *Surg Gynecol Obstet 137*:637, 1973.
18. Aune S and Schistad G: Carcinoid liver metastases treated with hepatic dearterialization. *Ann Surg 180*:305, 1974.

19. McDermott WV and Hensle TW: Metastatic carcinoid to the liver treated by hepatic dearterialization. *Ann Surg 180*:305, 1974.
20. Idema AAJ, Niermeyer P, Oldhoff J: Hepatic dearterialisation for carcinoid syndrome due to liver metastases. *Arch Chir Neerl 29*:2, 1977.
21. Khoury GA, Divine T, Bolt DE: Complete liver dearterialization and the carcinoid syndrome. *Br J Surg 66*:253, 1979.
22. Allison DJ, Modlin IM, Jenkins WJ: Treatment of carcinoid liver metastases by hepatic artery embolization. *Lancet 2*:1323, 1977.
23. Bengmark S and Rosengren C: Angiographic study of the collateral circulation to the liver after ligation of the hepatic artery in man. *Am J Surg 119*:620, 1970.
24. El-Domeiri A and Kamal M: Intermittent occlusion of the hepatic artery and infusion chemotherapy for carcinoma of the liver. *Am J Surg 135*:771, 1978.
25. Sherlock S: Progress report portal circulation and portal hypertension. *Gut 19*:70, 1978.
26. Warren WD, Zeppa R, Fomon JJ: Selective trans-splenic decompression of gastroesophageal varices by distal splenorenal shunt. *Ann J Surg 166*:437, 1967.
27. Widrich WC, Robbins AH, Johnson WC, Nasbeth DC: Long-term follow-up of distal splenorenal shunts. *Radiology 134*:341, 1980.
28. Hassab MA: Gastro-esophageal decongestion and splenectomy: a method of prevention and treatment of bleeding from esophageal varices, associated with bilharzial hepatic fibrosis. *J Int Coll Surg 41*:232, 1964.
29. Hassab M: Gastroesophageal decongestion and splenectomy in the treatment of esophageal varices in bilharzial cirrhosis. Further studies with a report on 355 operations. *Surgery 61*:169, 1967.
30. Sugiura M and Futagawa S: A new technique for treating esophageal varices. *J Thorac Cardiovasc Surg 66*:677, 1973.
31. Sugiura M and Futagawa S: Further evaluation of the Sugiura procedure in the treatment of esophageal varices. *Arch Surg 112*:1317, 1977.
32. Bengmark S, Borjesson B, Joelsson B: Developments in management of portal hypertension, a plea for selective symptomatic treatment *Surg Annu 12*:317, 1980.
33. Lunderquist A and Vang J: Transhepatic catheterization and obliteration of the coronary vein in patients with portal hypertension and esophageal varices. *N Engl J Med 291*:646, 1974.
34. Paquet K-J and Oberhammer E: Sclerotherapy of bleeding oesophageal varices by means of endoscopy. *Endoscopy 10*:7, 1978.
35. Lunderquist A, Simert G, Tylen U, Vang J: Follow-up of patients with portal hypertension and esophageal varices treated with percutaneous obliteration of gastric coronary vein. *Radiology 122*:59, 1977.
36. Lunderquist A, Borjesson B, Owman T, Bengmark S: Isobutyl 2-cyanoacrylate (Bucrylate) in obliteration of gastric coronary vein and esophageal varices. *Am J Roentgenol 130*:1, 1978.
37. Hoevels J, Lunderquist A, Ihse I: Percutaneous transhepatic intubation of bile ducts for combined internal/external drainage in preoperative and palliative treatment of obstructive jaundice. *Gastrointest Radiol 3*:23, 1978.
38. Bean WJ and Mahorner HR: Removal of residual biliary stones through T-tube tract. *South Med J 65*:377, 1972.
39. Domellof L and Karlsson K-I: Non-surgical, postoperative exploration of the extrahepatic bile ducts under fluoroscopic control. *Acta Chir Scand 139*:449, 1973.
40. Burhenne HJ: Nonoperative roentgenologic instrumentation techniques of the postoperative biliary tract. *Am J Surg 128*:111, 1974.
41. Burhenne HJ: Complications of nonoperative extraction of retained common duct stones. *Am J Surg 131*:260, 1976.
42. Burcharth F, Jensen LI, Olesen K: Endoprosthesis for internal drainage of the biliary tract. Technique and results in 48 cases. *Gastroenterology 77*:133, 1979.

43. Hoevels J and Ihse I: Percutaneous transhepatic insertion of a permanent endoprosthesis in obstructive lesions of the extrahepatic bile ducts. *Gastrointest Radiol 4*:367, 1979.
44. Sundqvist K, Hafstrom L, Jonsson P-R, Ryden S, Forsberg L, Lunderquist A: Treatment of liver cancer with regional inter-arterial 5-FU infusion. *Am J Surg 136*:328, 1978.
45. Bengmark S and Fredlund P: Palliative treatment of primary and secondary malignant liver neoplasms. In *Liver Surgery*, Calne RY and della Rovere Q (Eds). Piccin, Padova, Italy. (In press.)
46. Wheeler PG, Melia W, Dubbins P, Jones BM, Nunnerley H, Johnson P, Williams R: Non-operative arterial embolization in the management of primary liver tumors. *Br Med J 2*:242, 1979.
47. Bengmark S, Borjesson B, Hoevels J, Joelsson B, Lunderquist A, Owman T: Obliteration of oesophageal varices by PTP—a follow-up of 43 patients. *Ann Surg 190*:92, 1979.
48. Owman T, Lunderquist A, Alwmark A, Borjesson B: Embolization of the spleen for treatment of splenomegaly and hypersplenism in patients with portal hypertension. *Invest Radiol 14*:457, 1979.
49. Andersen BN, Kancke S, Damgaard Nielsen SA, Schmidt A: The diagnosis of pancreatic cyst by endoscopic retrograde pancreatography and ultrasonic screening. *Ann Surg 185*:286, 1977.

24

Radiology in Jaundice

Ernest J. Ring and Hans Herlinger
Hospital of the University of Pennsylvania
Philadelphia, Pennsylvania

Roy L. Gordon
Hebrew University and Hadassah Hospital
Jerusalem, Israel

Introduction

The rapid development of new imaging techniques affords the clinician a wide variety of approaches for the evaluation of the jaundiced patient. Precisely because of this breadth of choice, and to avoid the unnecessary duplication of frequently overlapping methods, it is important to develop a rational, economical, and practical system of evaluation. Inevitably, preference for a particular method may be biased, especially by the local availability of diagnostic equipment or by a physician with a particular interest and expertise in one technique rather than another. As experience is gained with the new imaging modalities and expertise in each technique is disseminated, algorithmic approaches can be developed and tested in practice. We suggest here a practical sequence of imaging examinations for the evaluation of the jaundiced patient. The validity of specific imaging techniques already described in detail in earlier chapters is reviewed briefly and a few additional diagnostic modalities are discussed. Inevitably, technologic advances are being made in several of these modalities, and these will continually affect their relative values.

Indications for Radiology

Radiology is indicated primarily to make the therapeutically important differentiation between jaundice due to obstruction of bile flow which may be amenable to surgical treatment or percutaneous drainage, and hepatocellular or intrahepatic cholestatic jaundice which inappropriate surgery may exacerbate. In addition to providing evidence of biliary obstruction as such, accurate information regarding the exact site, extent, and where possible, the etiology of the obstructing lesion is of obvious management importance. If the obstructive jaundice is caused by a metastatic neoplasm, further radiologic examination may be required to establish the location of the primary tumor. The intimate interrelationship between biliary and pancreatic pathology will often demand evaluation of the state of the pancreas.

Available Diagnostic Modalities

Clinical

In the diagnostic workup of the jaundiced patient the history of the disease, the physical examination, and observation over a period of time are of relevance. With the help of laboratory tests it becomes possible to reduce the wide range of potential causes of jaundice to a probable diagnosis of cholestasis. As described in Chapter 22, cholestasis can be of two types:

1. *Intrahepatic* without macroscopically demonstrable biliary obstruction
2. Due to *mechanical obstruction* of extrahepatic or major intrahepatic bile ducts

The latter condition may benefit from surgical or radiological intervention; in the former condition, surgery is contraindicated. This important distinction can be extremely difficult to make and cannot be based on biochemical tests alone. Nevertheless, the experienced physician has been able to predict the correct diagnosis in 70% of cases (1).

Needle Biopsy for Histology

Many centers consider cholestatic jaundice to be a contraindication to the use of needle biopsy, but notable exceptions to this view exist (2). Other contraindications include an abnormal prothrombin ratio and platelet count, and the possible presence of a hydatid cyst or a hemangioma.

The method now in general use is the Menghini "1-second technique"; the needle has an outer diameter of 1.0, 1.2, or 1.4 mm and a depth limiter can be employed (3). Among 3000 liver biopsies undertaken for a variety of indications, there were only two fatalities, both of which occurred before the Menghini needle was available (2).

Biopsy specimen histology is of value in a wide range of focal and generalized liver pathologies. It will help to differentiate jaundice due to viral hepatitis from that caused by alcohol or drugs. There are a number of reports of its use in cholestatic jaundice. No fatality and only one case of bile peritonitis requiring surgery occurred with 127 needle biopsies in 125 patients with mechanical bile duct obstruction (4). Histology was considered diagnostic in 83% of the patients.

Transjugular biopsy (see Chap. 21) may be a safer although more complicated form of needle biopsy of the liver and can be used in patients with bleeding dyscrasias or massive ascites (Fig. 1). A flexible transjugular liver biopsy needle which can be introduced through an F9 or F10 catheter is now available (5).

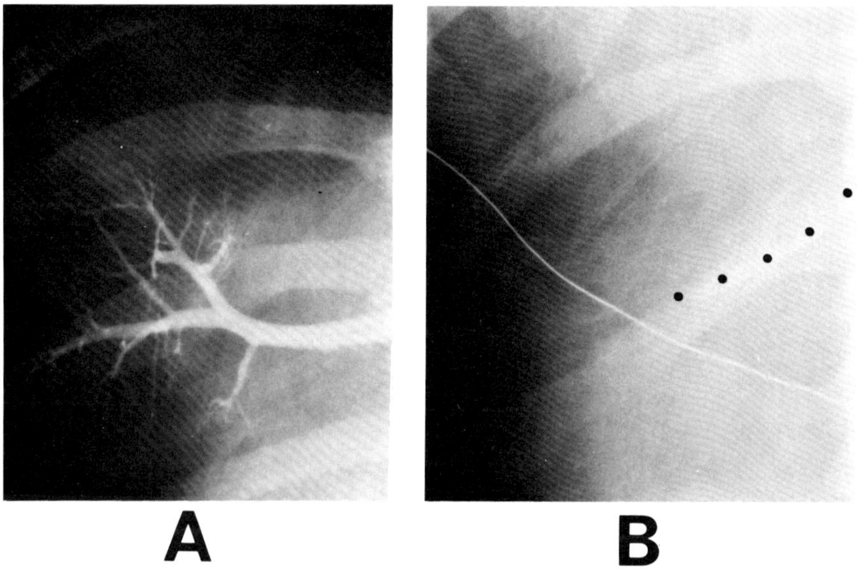

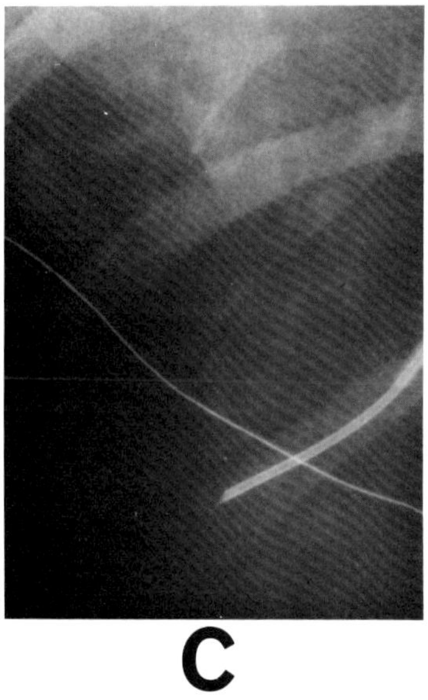

Figure 1 Transjugular liver biopsy. (A) A Teflon catheter is introduced through the right internal jugular vein and advanced under fluoroscopic guidance into a hepatic vein. Contrast is injected. (B) Position of the catheter (dots) in the hepatic vein radicle. (C) A thin-walled needle is passed through the catheter into the liver parenchyma to obtain a "core" biopsy.

Ultrasound (US)

The technique and applications of ultrasonography have been described in Chapter 9. To a greater degree than in most other modalities, the diagnostic reliability of the method must vary with the skill of the operator, the commitment and experience of the diagnostician, and the ever-improving quality of the apparatus.

When used in the diagnosis of cholestatic jaundice it is necessary to outline intrahepatic and extrahepatic bile ducts to determine whether they are of normal caliber or dilated. If dilated, jaundice is deemed to be due to obstruction and surgical; if nondilated, to be nonobstructive, intrahepatic, and medical. Whenever possible, information is also provided regarding the level and causative pathology of any obstruction and the general state of the liver parenchyma. Common duct (CD) diameter imaging and measurement are best done with the patient right anterior oblique, using the liver itself as the acoustic window (6).

There is no exact millimeter number at which CD diameter normality ends and dilatation begins. Diameters between 6 and 8 mm (measured at the widest point of the CD) constitute an indeterminate group in which most patients will be nonobstructed yet a significant number will have surgical jaundice. Even among patients with readings below 6 mm there will be some with obstruction, usually incomplete and recent and due to duct stones.

For practical purposes an arbitrary normality limit is selected. The lower the chosen level, the more sensitive the examination, and the fewer the false negative cases, although this at the expense of including false positives (7,8).

It is also important to image intrahepatic bile ducts to determine if they are dilated. When both intrahepatic and extrahepatic bile ducts are demonstrated, the diagnosis of biliary obstruction by US can reach an accuracy level of 97% (8). Bile ducts that were dilated before surgery usually continue to be dilated even after an obstruction has been relieved. Bile ducts of normal caliber before cholecystectomy remain normal (9). A partially obstructed CD may be dilated, especially distally, this without intrahepatic dilation (10).

Only very few publications clearly state the criteria for diagnostic adequacy, and they report a partial failure rate of at least 10% (7,11). Others, without detailing criteria for examination success, have claimed a much lower rate of nondiagnostic examinations (12,13). In less expert hands and in the day-to-day clinical practice, the frequency of nondiagnostic studies is likely to be considerably higher.

Although a positive diagnosis of biliary dilatation made by a competent US department is highly reliable, the sonographic determination of the level, extent, and cause of obstruction is less adequate, varying from as high as 56% (12) to as low as 7.7% (14). Using dynamic sonography, the level of obstruction could be determined in 79.5% of patients, the cause in 57% (11). The recognition of stones in a dilated CD can be difficult in the most experienced hands (8). A diagnosis of stones in a nondilated CD remains as unsatisfactory as ever; in only 1 of 16 cases could a correct diagnosis be made (8).

Computed Tomography (CT)

Technique, indications, and results of CT used in a wide range of liver pathologies have been described in Chapter 11.

Intrahepatic bile ducts of normal diameter are not usually shown by a CT at the present time. When dilated, they are readily identified, especially against contrast-enhanced liver parenchyma. This could be correctly observed in 22 of 25 examinations of patients with obstructive jaundice (15). A possible differential diagnostic problem seems to be caused by metastatic liver disease (15). An extrahepatic common duct of normal diameter could be demonstrated in 30% of patients after contrast enhancement of the hepatic artery, portal vein, and pancreatic capillary bed (16).

The accuracy of CT diagnosis of biliary obstruction is similar to that claimed for US, about 90% (17). However, CT is more consistently able to demonstrate the site and cause of obstruction, especially if due to tumor (18). The identification of CD stones, particularly in the absence of intrahepatic biliary dilatation, is less adequate (19).

Bile duct dilatation confined to a segment of the liver has been demonstrated both by US and CT, this usually in the absence of jaundice; a significant elevation of serum alkaline phosphatase is usually present (20).

Needle Aspiration or Brushing for Cytology

Needle aspiration biopsy through a 21- to 23-gauge needle introduced percutaneously into a tumor is a safe and highly sensitive method, which has not given any false positive results (21). In the context of jaundice diagnosis, the needle is best guided by ultrasound, as in the case of a pancreatic tumor, or by fluoroscopy when a transhepatic biliary drainage catheter is in position and/or biliary contrast medium is still present (Fig. 2A). Cholangiocarcinoma cytology material can also be obtained by advancing a flexible needle through a transhepatic catheter. A 22-gauge needle with internal cutting edge is now available. If introduced by rotary motion, fragments of tissue can be obtained which are suitable for histology as well as cytology (22) (Fig. 2B). Thousands of examinations have been done with very few complications; there are only two reports of malignant seeding of the needle tract (23,24); tumor seeding along a needle/catheter tract is shown in Figure 2C.

Percutaneous brush biopsy in cases of suspected extrahepatic or major intrahepatic bile duct carcinoma can be performed in the course of a transhepatic drainage procedure (Fig. 3). Brushes can be passed through 5 or 6F catheters and several passes can be made. This is a useful and complication-free method which may be of value in the diagnosis of a cholangiocarcinoma (25).

Intravenous Cholangiography (IVC)

The biliary excretion of contrast medium molecules by the hepatocyte relies on a rate-limited, active transport mechanism which competes with bilirubin. Successful bile duct visualization therefore relates to serum bilirubin levels, being 40% at levels 2–3 mg per 100 ml, 31.8% at 3–4 mg per 100 ml, and only 9.3% when in excess of 4 mg per 100 ml (26). Employing an overnight drip infusion technique (27) for the administration of iodipamide (Cholografin), bile duct opacification improves somewhat in jaundiced patients. Newer contrast media, such as iodoxamate or iotroxamate, have shown a higher transport maximum through the liver cell, but this does not seem to have led to better bile duct opacification when bilirubin levels are elevated (28).

IVC was recently reevaluated in a group of 45 jaundiced patients in whom it was compared with US; IVC failed to visualize the CD in 11 (24.5%) and missed CD stones in 9 of 14 (64%). IVC is particularly unreliable in the demonstration of the ampullary area of the CD, an important site for stone and tumor obstruction. In addition to its low accuracy in the presence of jaundice, IVC is time consuming and causes a high radiation dose to the patient. Toxic effects are not inconsiderable, and include anaphylactoid reactions, hypotension, renal failure, and also hepatotoxicity (29).

IVC may be of occasional value in a mildly jaundiced patient with a falling bilirubin level, where the possibility of calculus occlusion of a nondilated CD could not be excluded by US. In the general investigation of jaundice, however, the use of IVC has been virtually abandoned.

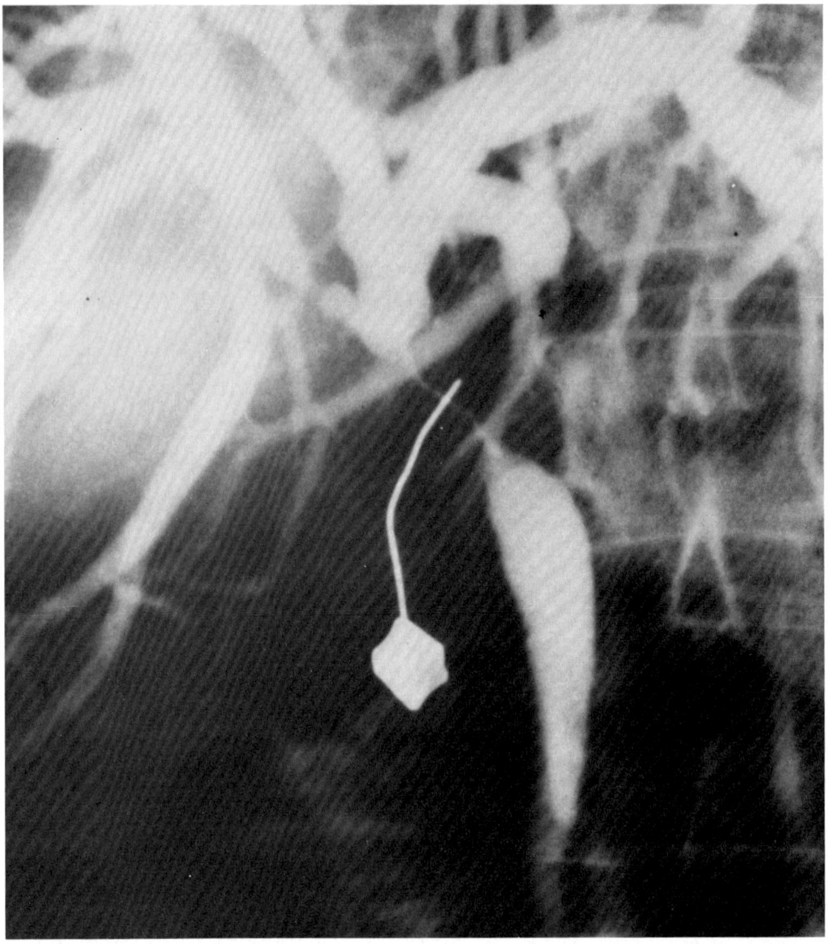

Figure 2A Percutaneous biopsy of a mass obstructing the common hepatic duct. After transhepatic cholangiography demonstrated a lesion in the proximal duct, a thin needle percutaneous biopsy was performed.

Percutaneous Transhepatic Cholangiography (PTC)

This important modality has been described in Chapter 18. With the use of the fine needle, complications have decreased remarkably, and it is now possible to perform a large number of needle passes per examination. This has led to an almost 100% success rate when intrahepatic bile ducts are dilated and to an 85% success rate with nondilated ducts (30). Sepsis, the most frequent complication, can be largely avoided.

In a group of 25 patients with suspected obstructive jaundice PTC was successful in all of 19 in whom obstruction was later confirmed, but failed in 1 patient with hepatocellular jaundice, thus giving an overall accuracy of 96%; the site and cause of obstruction are demonstrated in all the patients with surgical jaundice (31). It is important,

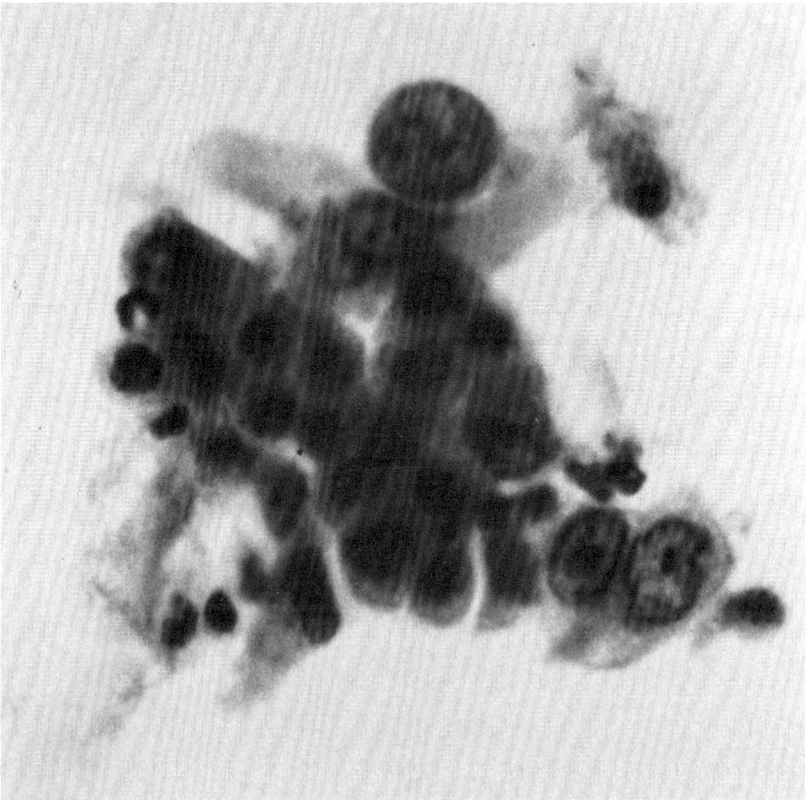

Figure 2B Class V cytology confirmed that the obstructing lesion was an adenocarcinoma.

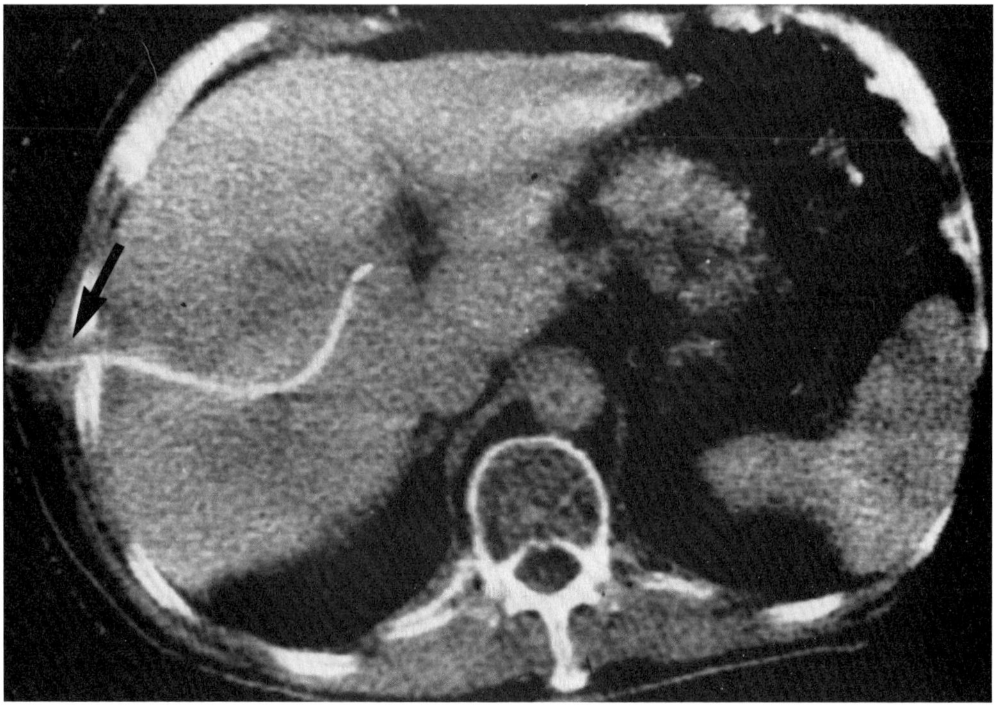

Figure 2C Chest wall tumor (arrow) shown by CT close to the catheter after 16 months of biliary drainage through an obstructing cholangiocarcinoma. Histology consistent with metastatic cholangiocarcinoma. (From Oleaga JA, Ring EJ, Freiman DB, MacClean GK, Rosen RJ: Extension of neoplasm along the tract of a transhepatic tube. *Am J Roentgenol 135*:841, 1980.)

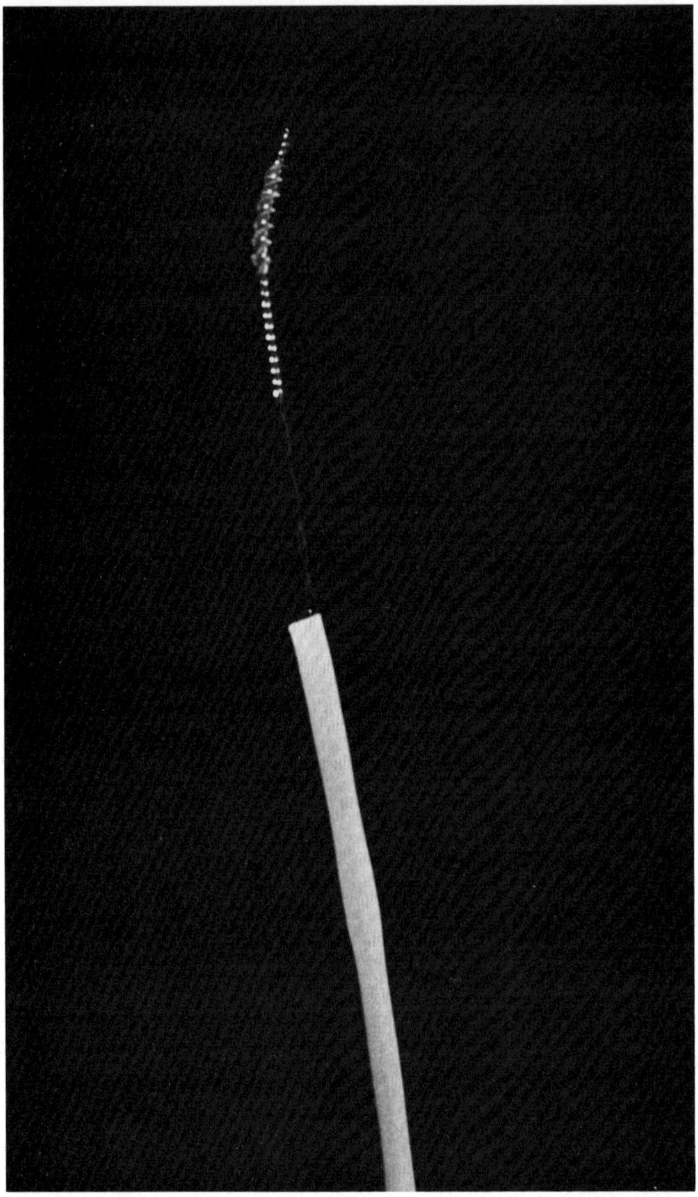

Figure 3A Brush biopsy of a bile duct obstruction. A specially constructed guide wire with nylon bristles can pass through the lumen of standard-size angiographic catheters.

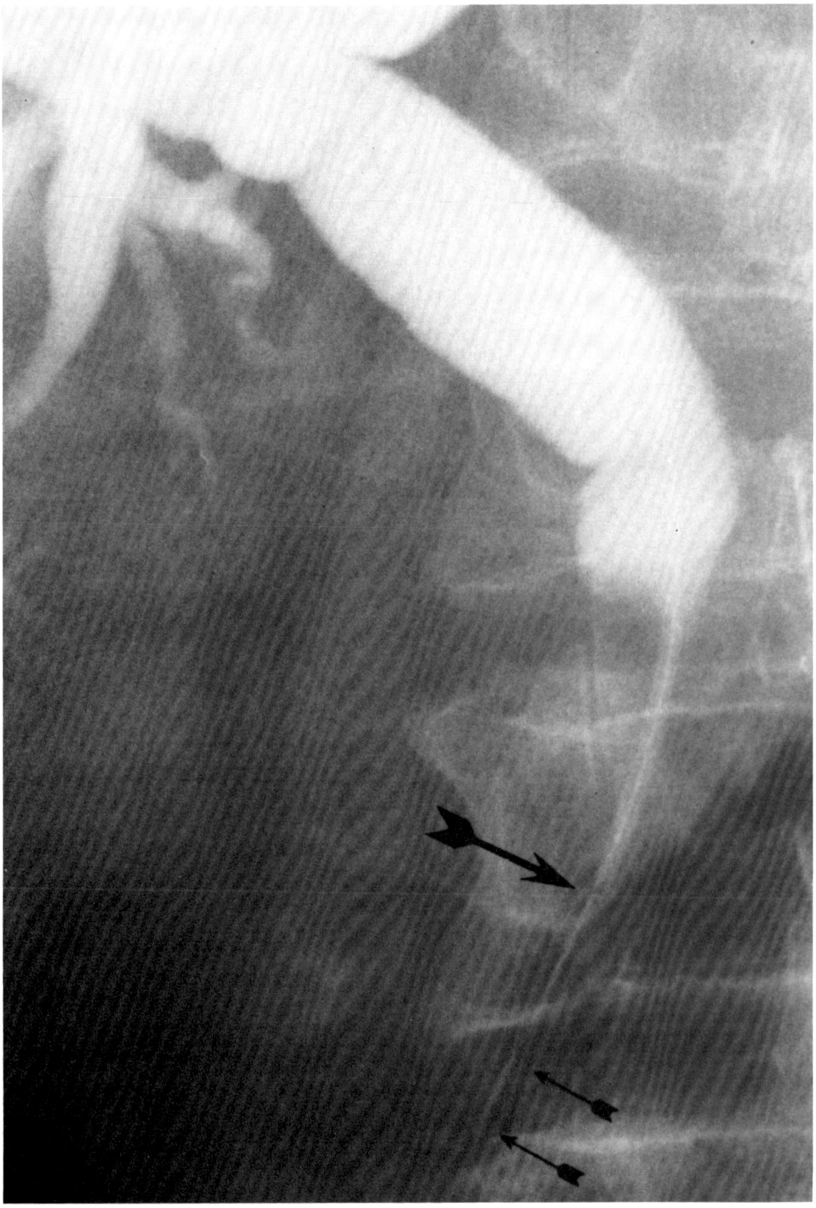

Figure 3B During the course of a percutaneous biliary drainage procedure the brush (small arrows) is passed through the sheath catheter (large arrow) to obtain a biopsy specimen.

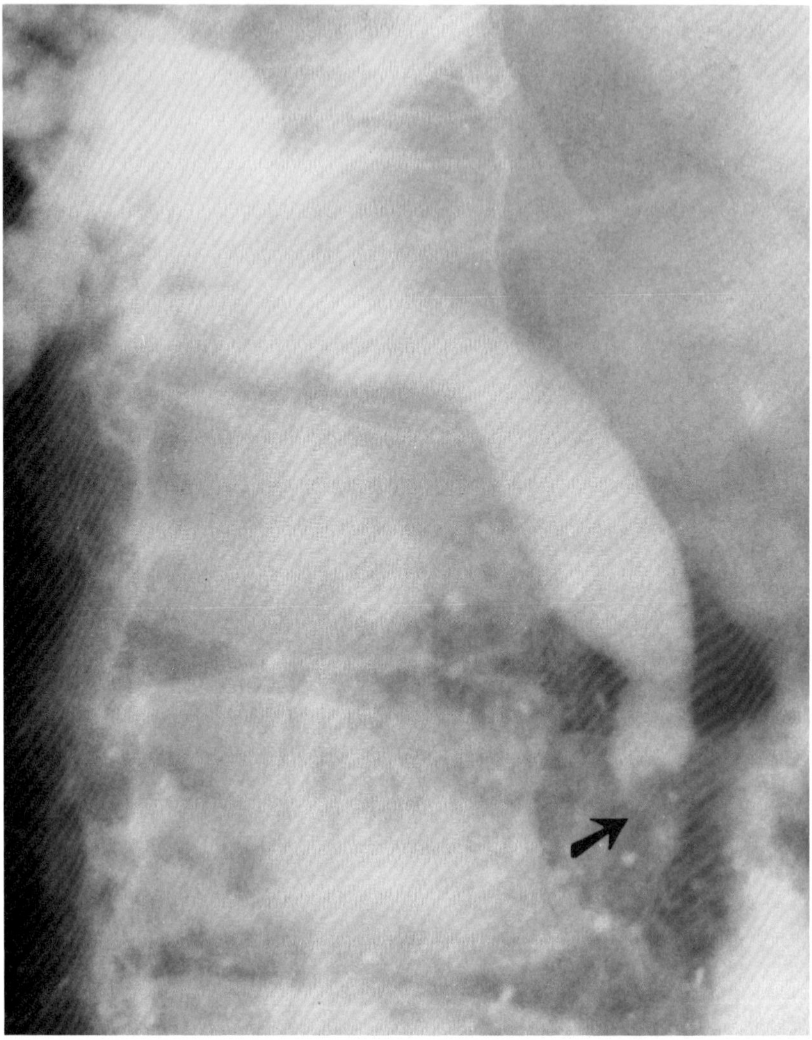

Figure 4A A common duct stone lodged above an obstructing pancreatic malignancy. A transhepatic cholangiogram reveals a stone in the distal common bile duct (arrow).

when using PTC or any other imaging modality, to pay attention to the CD distal to a partially obstructing stone in order not to miss the possible presence of an underlying tumor, the real cause of obstruction, with the stone merely a secondary phenomenon (32) (Fig. 4).

Endoscopic Retrograde Cholangiopancreatography (ERCP)

A description of this method is found in Chapter 18. The success rate in this more complex examination depends significantly on the skill and experience of the operator. Intentional selective cannulation of the CBD has been achieved in 81% and of the pancreatic duct in 92%. Experience also reduces examination time and the incidence of complications.

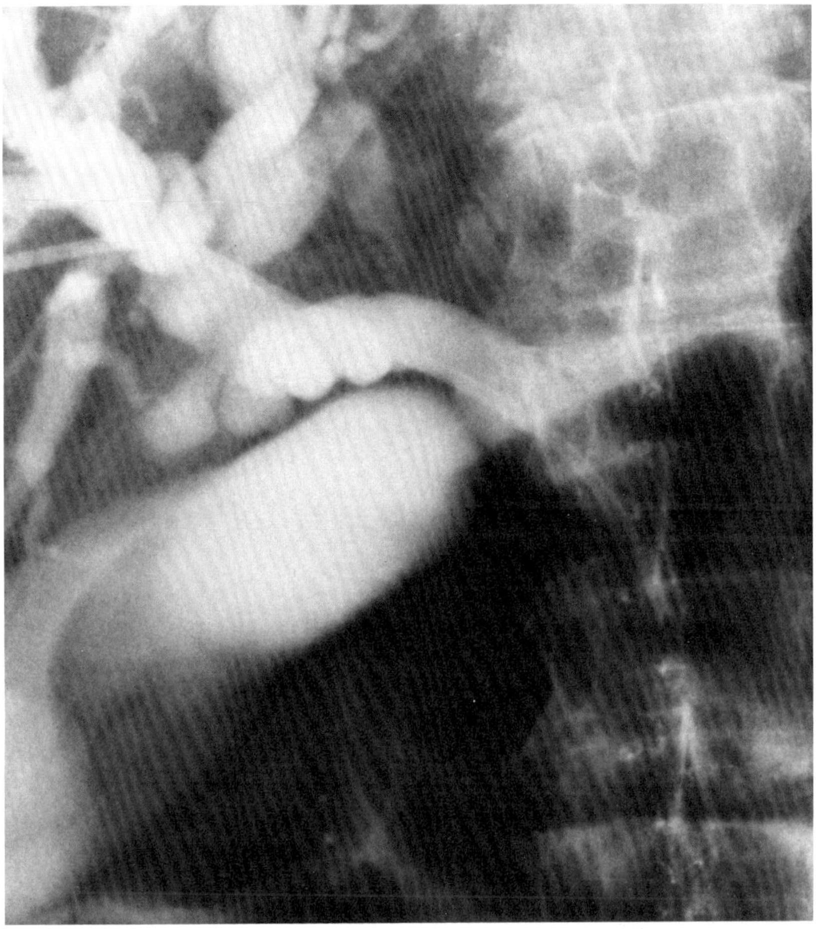

Figure 4B A catheter introduced transhepatically dislodged the stone into an intrahepatic duct.

In the course of ERCP the papilla can be inspected and biopsied, brush biopsies can be obtained from either duct system, and secretions can be aspirated for cytology.

Angiography

We no longer use angiography for the primary diagnosis of the cause or site of biliary obstruction. The angiographic diagnosis of an extrahepatic cholangiocarcinoma is difficult, as the tumor tends to be scirrhous and of low vascularity. There may be arterial encasement at the porta hepatis or focal encasement of the portal vein above the level usually found in pancreatic carcinoma; rarely is there evidence of fine neovascularity (33).

Carcinoma of the ampullary area can produce clear-cut angiographic changes, but more often such alterations are very subtle, and at times vascular abnormality is lacking

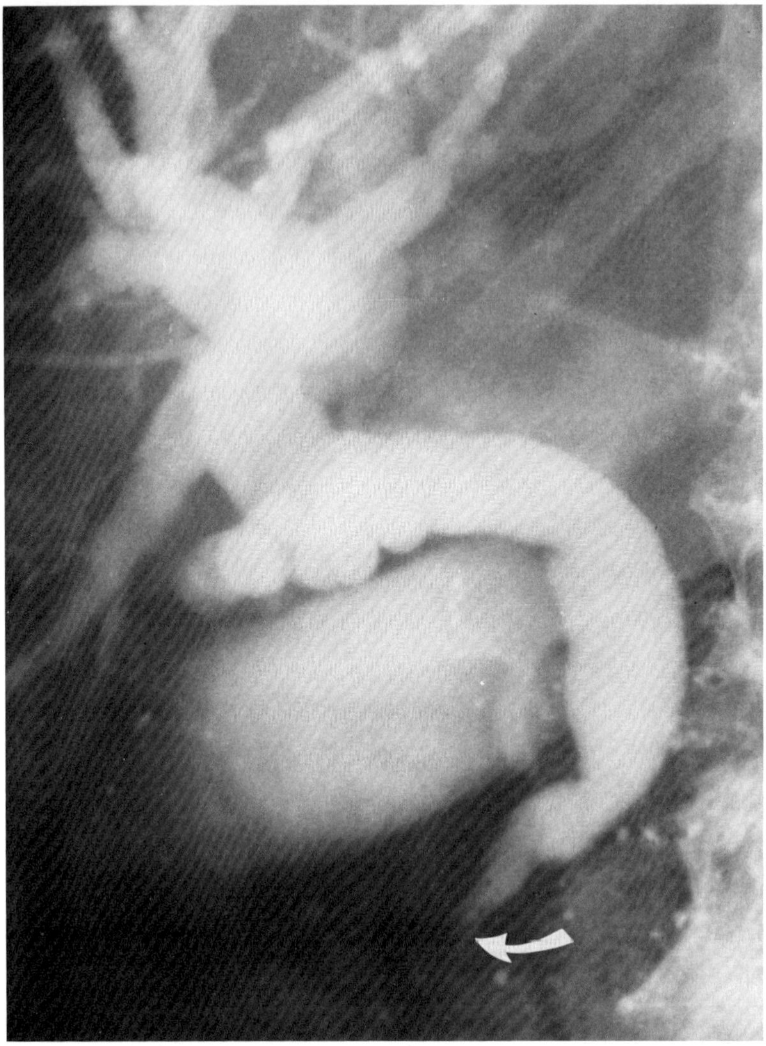

Figure 4C The duct distal to the stone shows a tapered obstruction (arrow). At surgery a periampullary pancreatic carcinoma was found.

altogether (Fig. 5). Other diagnostic modalities—US, CT, PTC, and ERCP, especially if associated with needle or brush biopsy—are adequate for most diagnostic purposes, and diagnostic angiography will be reserved for occasional problem solving.

Tumor resectability determination has been considered an important function of angiography in patients whose obstructive jaundice has been shown to be due to pancreatic or bile duct malignancy. Where CT has unequivocally demonstrated an associated lymph node enlargement, retroperitoneal or at the porta hepatis, or the obliteration of fat planes in tissues behind the pancreas, nonresectability has been considered to exist (34). However, further work is needed to substantiate this association fully. The presence of liver metastases, shown by US, CT, or scintigraphy, contraindicates resective surgery.

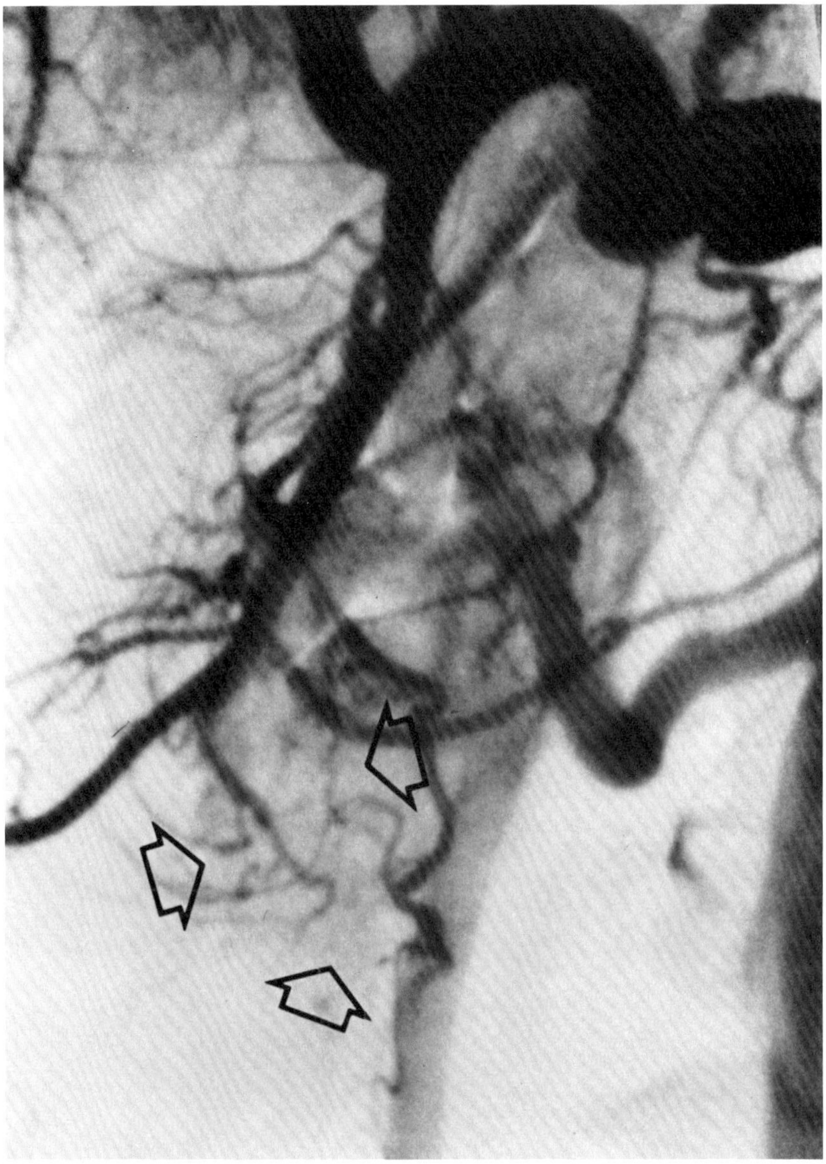

Figure 5A Angiography should no longer be used in the primary diagnosis of periampullary carcinoma. Subtle arteriographic changes—small vessel encasement (arrows)—with a 1.5-cm carcinoma of the ampulla.

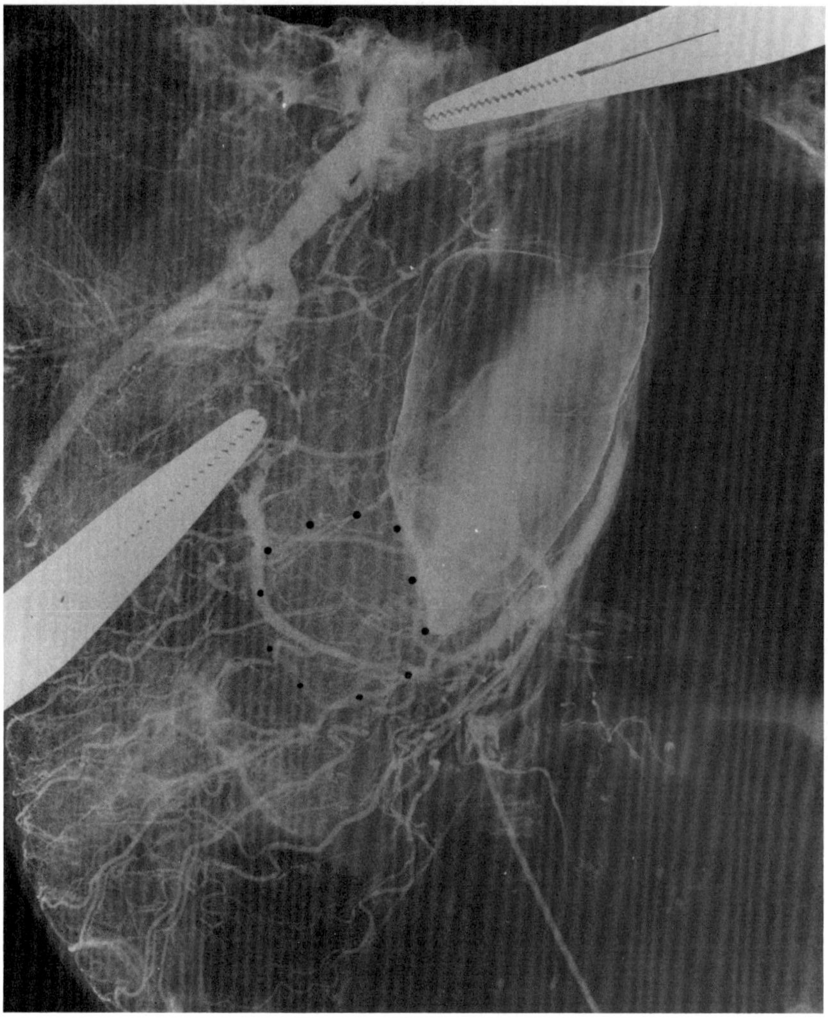

Figure 5B Resected papillary carcinoma, injected specimen with the dilated common bile duct outlined by double contrast. The tumor is indicated by dots. No vascular abnormality is seen.

In many cases angiography will still be required before surgery (35). Involvement of the portal vein or its main tributaries (36) or of extrapancreatic arteries (37) virtually rules out resectability. (For further details, see Chap. 14.)

Scintigraphy

With the introduction in 1975 of ^{99m}Tc-dimethyliminodiacetic acid (HIDA), functional biliary tract imaging with nuclear techniques has become readily available and widely used. Newer derivatives, such as DISIDA, allow visualization of bile ducts in patients with bilirubin levels as high as 30 mg per 100 ml (38). The procedure is simple, fast, without morbidity, and requires only equipment available in any nuclear medicine department.

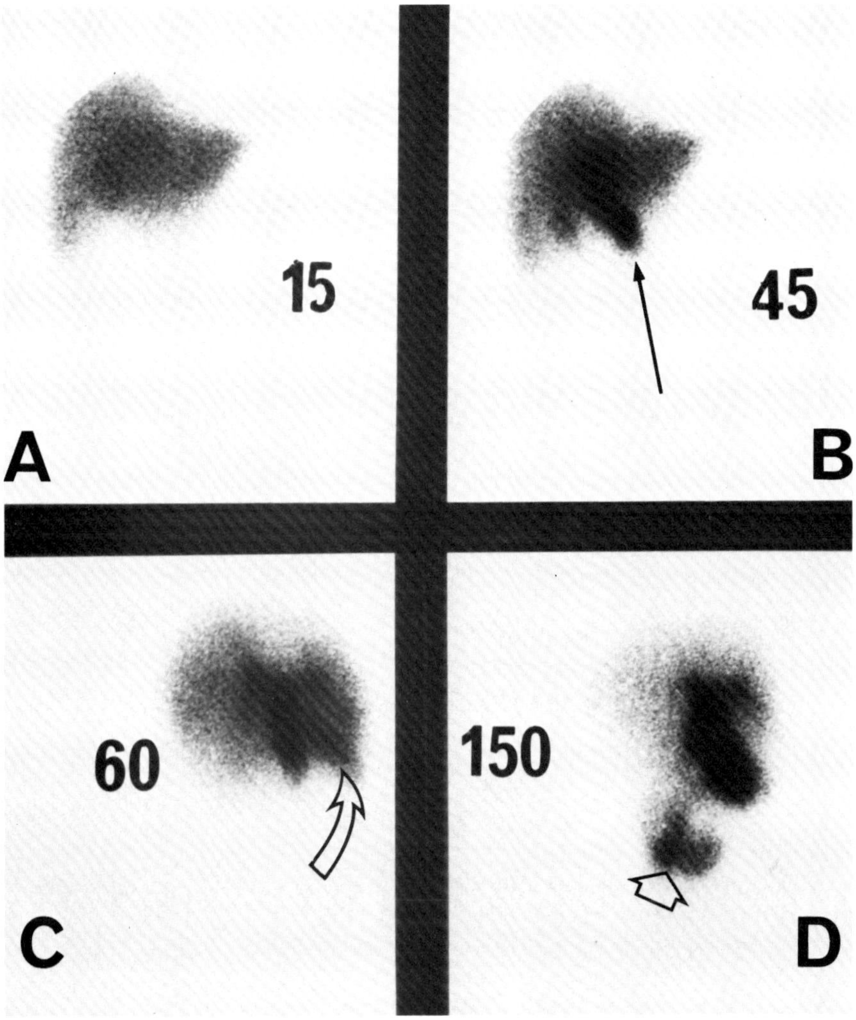

Figure 6 Obstructive jaundice, cholescintigraphy using a ^{99m}Tc-IDA analog. (A,B) Anterior scan. At 45 min a delayed visualization of the dilated common bile duct (arrow). (C) Lateral scan at 60 min. The gallbladder is now seen (open arrow), anterior to the dilated common duct. As yet no activity is shown in small bowel. (D) Lateral scan at 150 min. A very much delayed appearance of activity in small bowel (arrowhead). Transhepatic cholangiography later demonstrated calculus obstruction of the common bile duct. (Courtesy of Dr. Abass Alavi, University of Pennsylvania, Philadelphia.)

Although minimal common duct dilatation may not be appreciated by this method, a more pronounced dilated state of extrahepatic bile ducts may be clearly demonstrated. Complete common duct obstruction presents with prompt hepatic uptake of the agent and with nonvisualization of bile ducts and absence of flow into the bowel. Intrahepatic cholestasis will probably produce the same pattern. In partial obstruction, dilated intrahepatic and extrahepatic ducts may become visible, but transit into gut will be delayed (Fig. 6).

It is therefore possible, by cholescintigraphy, to obtain functional information on bile flow (38), to show ductal obstruction even before dilatation, or to show bile duct dilatation without obstruction, as after biliary surgery.

Radiologic Management Sequence

In a patient with a probable clinical diagnosis of cholestasis in whom sequential laboratory tests and observation over a period of time have indicated the likelihood of a mechanical extrahepatic or major intrahepatic bile duct obstruction, further imaging will have to be performed. It is possible to separate these imaging procedures into four distinct stages (see Table 1), at each of which it may be decided that an end point has been reached.

Stage I: The initial screening test

Stage II: The direct opacification of the biliary system (with needle or brush biopsy, as indicated)

Stage III: Percutaneous transhepatic biliary drainage, if considered indicated

Stage IV: Evaluation of tumor resectability

Table 1 Diagnosis and Management Sequence for the Jaundiced Patient.

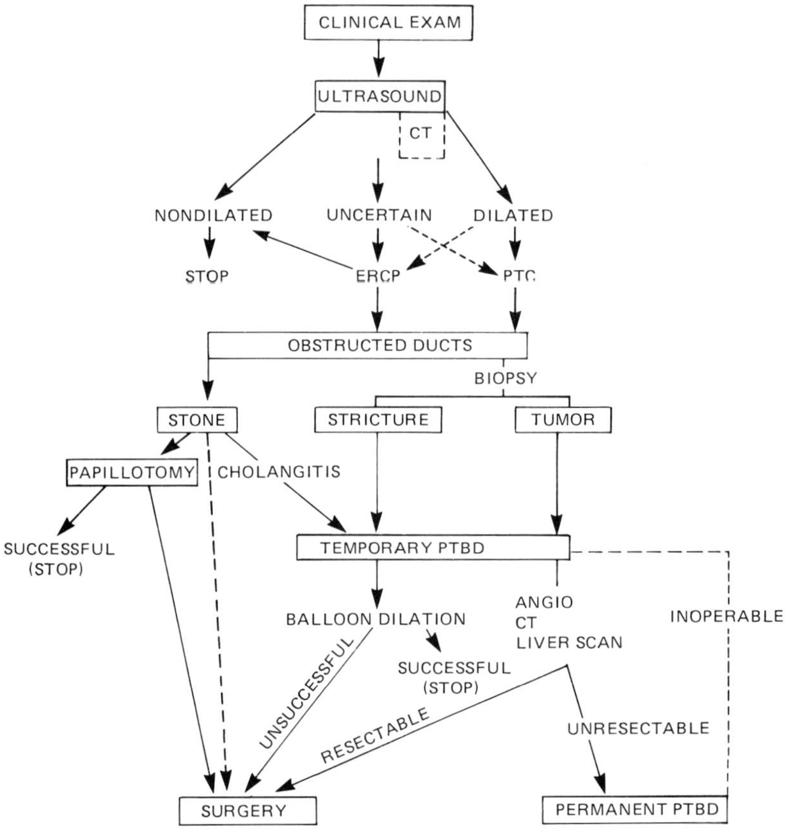

Stage I, Initial Screening Test

Ultrasonography (US) is the preferred initial study; CT is used if US has failed or has given an inaccurate reading.

Advantages of US over CT US is much less costly, can deal with more patients; no ionizing radiations are involved, there is no need for intravenous contrast; scan sections can be adjusted to the long axis of ductal structures; and a special transducer is available to facilitate needle biopsy.

CT advantages over US Gas or bone do not obscure structures; there is no need for direct contact with the abdominal wall; excessive fat is helpful; and it is more reliable than US in outlining obstructing masses.

The result of the screening test together with the clinical background of each patient will determine whether an end point has been reached or stage II imaging should be undertaken.

End point reached If US (or CT) has shown a nondilated bile duct system, many centers would proceed to a Menghini needle liver biopsy. With the clinical impression not sufficiently in support of mechanical obstruction and/or with biopsy histology not typical of surgical cholestastis, no further imaging is needed.

Stage II imaging follows (1) If a nondilated ductal system was found by US (or CT) and there is strong clinical indication of major duct obstruction, possibly supported by Menghini needle biopsy histology. (2) If ductal dilatation was shown by US (or CT), in which case a Menghini needle biopsy would not be advisable.

Stage II, Direct Cholangiography (PTC or ERCP)

Advantages of PTC over ERCP It is simple to perform, quicker, more widely available; is usually successful in every case with intrahepatic duct dilatation; can be followed by transhepatic biliary drainage procedures; and can be used in patients who have had gastric surgery.

Advantages of ERCP over PTC Ability to biopsy the region of the papilla of Vater; stomach and duodenum can be inspected in passing; pancreatic ducts can be opacified; and endoscopic sphincterotomy can be performed.

Both methods can be combined with needle or brush biopsy for cytology. There is no difference in their low complication rate or in the success rate of opacifying a nondilated ductal system. In patients who were shown to have nondilated bile ducts, the choice between PTC and ERCP will be strongly influenced by local custom and expertise. We prefer to use PTC except where associated pancreatic disease is likely or where PTC is contraindicated. In our experience, patients have expressed a greater acceptance of PTC than of ERCP.

In patients known to have dilated bile ducts, PTC is the method of choice. In cases of complete obstruction, opacification of the proximal portion of the biliary tree is generally of greater practical value than would be the demonstration of the distal part by ERCP.

Why should the US (or CT) demonstration of biliary obstruction be followed by direct cholangiography? The suggestion has been made (6) that invasive PTC could be restricted to cases with obstruction at the porta hepatis, to those with distal obstruction in whom the cause has not been adequately identified, or when sclerosing cholangitis was suspected. In our opinion, direct cholangiography should almost always be done in jaundice before surgery is considered. In the case of stone obstruction it will identify their number and distribution (possibly intrahepatic), will exclude an associated tumor, and will precede a preoperative catheter drainage procedure in debilitated patients with more severe jaundice. PTC done before surgery can replace operative cholangiography, as it will produce more adequate images and will allow surgical planning. In the case of an obstructing tumor, direct cholangiography will indicate the exact extent of involvement of the common duct and will serve as a prelude to transhepatic drainage. In cases with proximal obstruction, continuity between the left and the right hepatic bile ducts can be demonstrated, an essential requirement before hepatojejunostomy.

Why do stage I screening if direct cholangiography is to follow in most cases? The continued use of US (or CT) has been questioned (3) since PTC can be performed with a high rate of success and a minimum of complication. We do not agree. Stage I screening will help to identify some patients with medical cholestasis. It can be used to determine whether Menghini needle biopsy of the liver may be undertaken. It will influence the choice between PTC and ERCP. It will affect PTC technique and lead to a greater number of needle passes being made in patients whose intrahepatic bile ducts have been shown to be nondilated.

Following direct cholangiography there are four possible further alternatives:

1. A nondilated and nonobstructed biliary tree has already been demonstrated. *End point reached.*
2. Minimal biliary dilatation, common duct incompletely obstructed by stone, shown by ERCP; proceed to sphincterotomy. If shown by PTC without evidence of cholangitis, the patient should be referred to endoscopic sphincterotomy. If cholangitis is present, temporary external biliary drainage should be established.
3. Bile ducts dilated, calculus obstruction, high bilirubin levels. Only the younger patient in fair general condition and without cholangitis should proceed to early surgery. Older patients, those in poor condition, and all those with infection will proceed to *stage III*.
4. Patients with dilated bile ducts due to obstruction by tumor, stricture or extrinsic compression will proceed to *stage III*.

Stage III, Percutaneous Transhepatic Biliary Drainage

Technique, methods, and indications have been described in Chapter 20. Patients will be offered one of three drainage methods, selected in accordance with stage II findings and associated circumstances.

Temporary external drainage will be instituted before calculus surgery in some patients, as already indicated. In the presence of *obstruction and cholangitis*, the combination of drainage and antibiotic therapy will control infection that cannot be managed by antibiotics alone (Fig. 7). In patients with iatrogenic strictures and bile leaks, longer-term external percutaneous drainage is valuable in two ways: (1) it provides an immediate solution to the problem of drainage of bile, and the drainage can be maintained for as long as considered useful; and (2) by diverting the bile from the leaking segment, resolution of the acute edema and inflammation in this area is made possible. Reconstructive surgery can be performed electively at a later stage when the ducts are in the best condition for successful repair.

Definitive biliary drainage can be applied to malignant or nonmalignant conditions that are not amenable to corrective surgery. *Strictures* high in the porta hepatis and

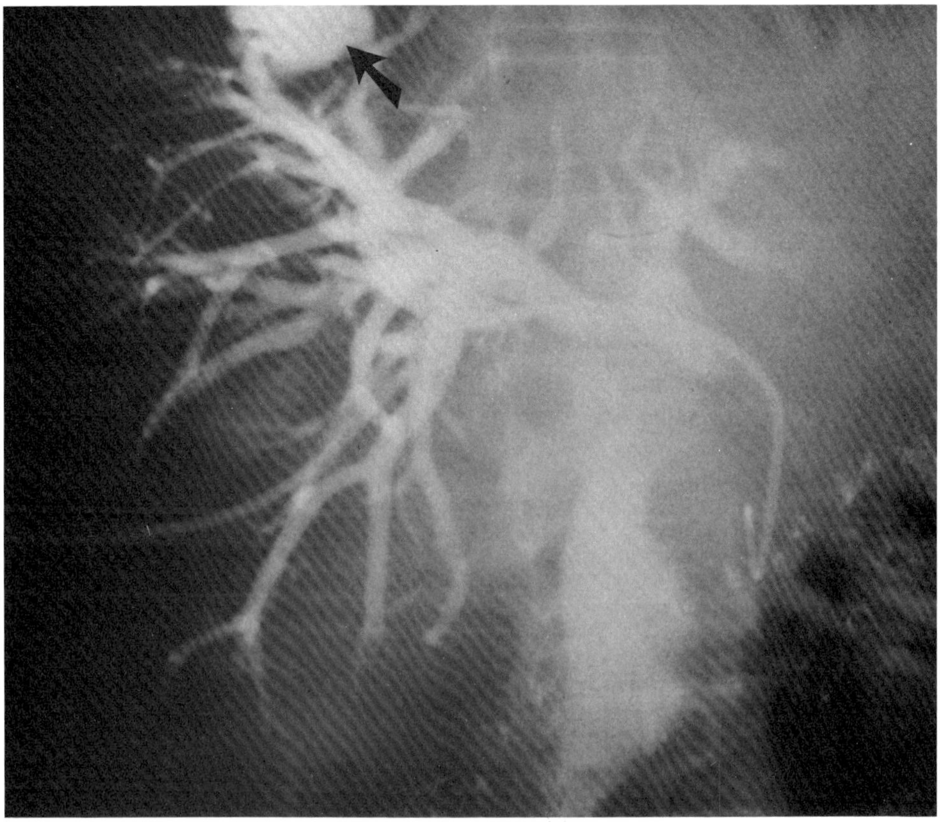

Figure 7 Temporary external drainage for sepsis and acute suppurative cholangitis. A percutaneous drainage catheter was positioned in the common duct above a distal obstruction. The aspirated bile was purulent. An abscess is seen (arrow) communicating with an intrahepatic duct.

obstructions in *sclerosing cholangitis* can be managed by transhepatically placed catheters.

In *obstructing metastatic disease* or in cases of *primary pancreatic* or *bile duct carcinoma* already known to have metastasized or spread retroperitoneally, internal drainage by transhepatic catheter is an attractive nonoperative alternative to a palliative surgical bypass. Clear advantages of percutaneous drainage are the elimination of surgery and anesthesia, shorter hospitalization time, reduction in morbidity and mortality, and a reduced cost. The method of biliary drainage may be by internal-external catheter or by an internally placed stent.

Potentially definitive biliary drainage is important in patients with obstruction due to carcinoma in whom resective surgery is considered a possibility; transhepatic drainage by the internal-external method is established to improve the patient's status before surgery, this while proceeding to stage IV, the determination of resectability. The drainage procedure may convert a patient at first considered unfit for resective surgery on general health grounds into one whose resectability status needs to be determined.

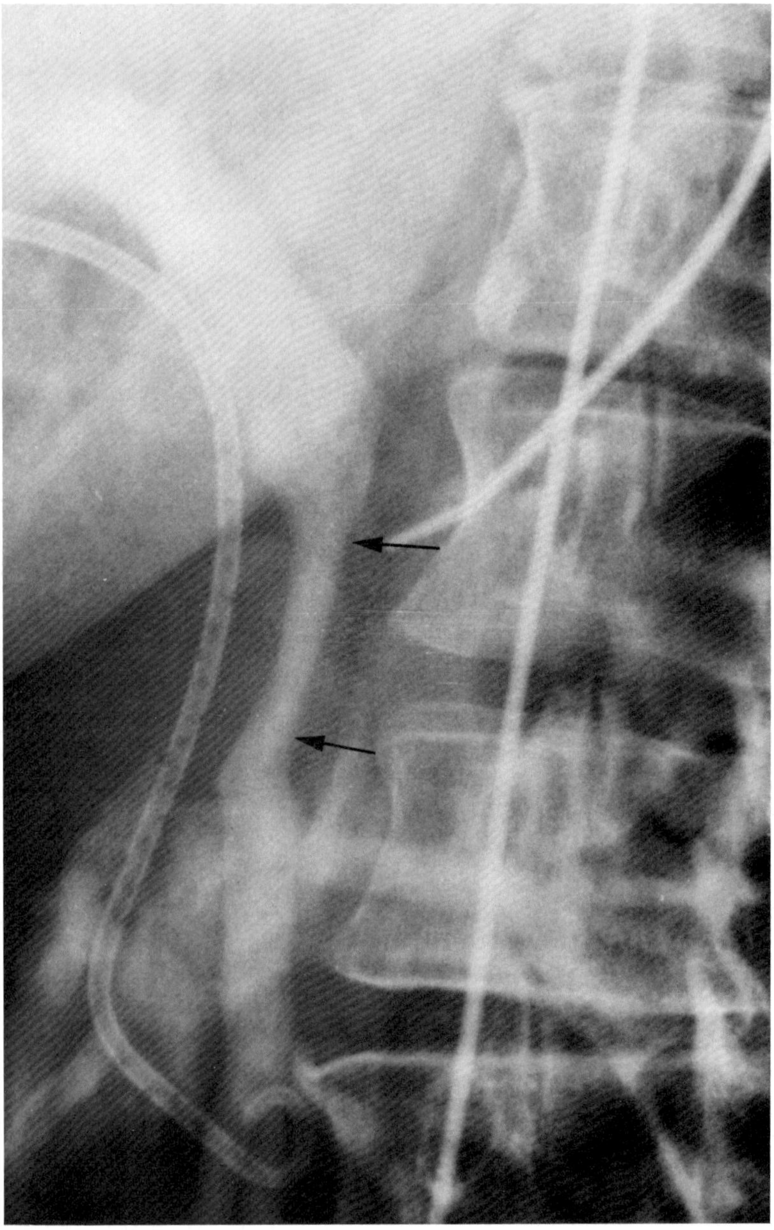

Figure 8A Use of angiography to stage pancreatic carcinoma. A superior mesenteric arteriogram performed 24 hr after percutaneous transhepatic biliary drainage shows encasement of the mesenteric vein (arrows), indicating an unresectable tumor.

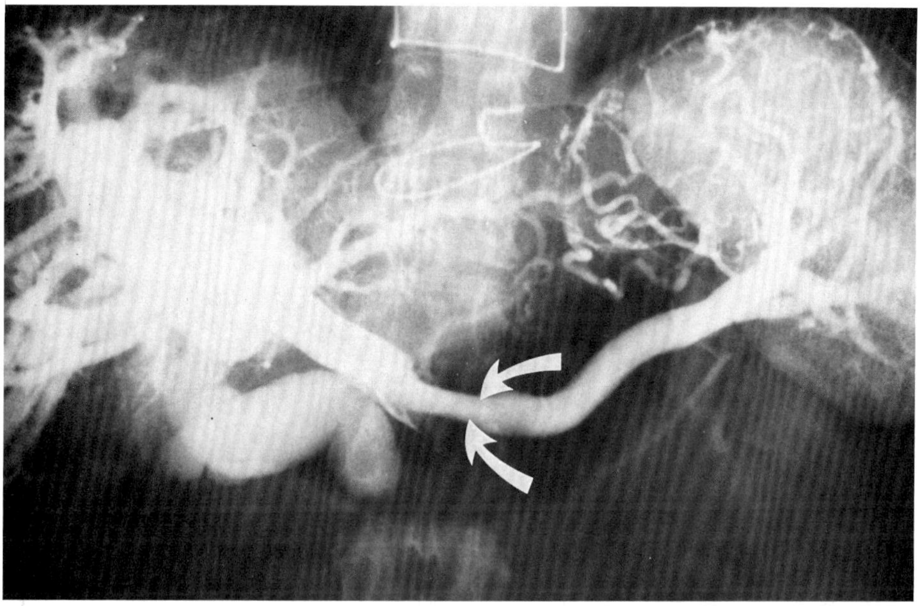

Figure 8B If a portal vein branch is entered during attempts at catheterization of the bile duct, the sheath can be advanced through the portal vein into the mesenteric and splenic vein. Venography performed in this fashion readily assesses the patency of the major venous structures. Shown here is encasement of the splenic vein (arrows).

There will be a group of patients psychologically unable to accept a diagnosis of nonresectability based on any form of indirect evidence; in these patients it would be futile to proceed to stage IV, and an exploratory laparotomy will be indicated, preferably after biliary drainage has been instituted.

Stage IV, Evaluation of Tumor Resectability

The great majority of obstructing tumors being nonresectable makes it particularly important to identify those which allow salvage. Where nonresectability has not already been determined in a stage I procedure, angiography will have to be undertaken at this stage, often while transhepatic biliary drainage proceeds. An example is illustrated in Figure 8.

Other Interventional Procedures

Dilatation of Benign Strictures

Initial experience using the transhepatic route for both drainage and dilatation of benign biliary strictures has been encouraging (39). Strictures can be dilated using vascular, balloon-tipped catheters that are used for angioplasty (Fig. 9) or using bougie-type catheters. The balloon catheter is positioned in the narrowed duct employing standard techniques previously described. Inflation of the balloon causes dilatation of the stenosed

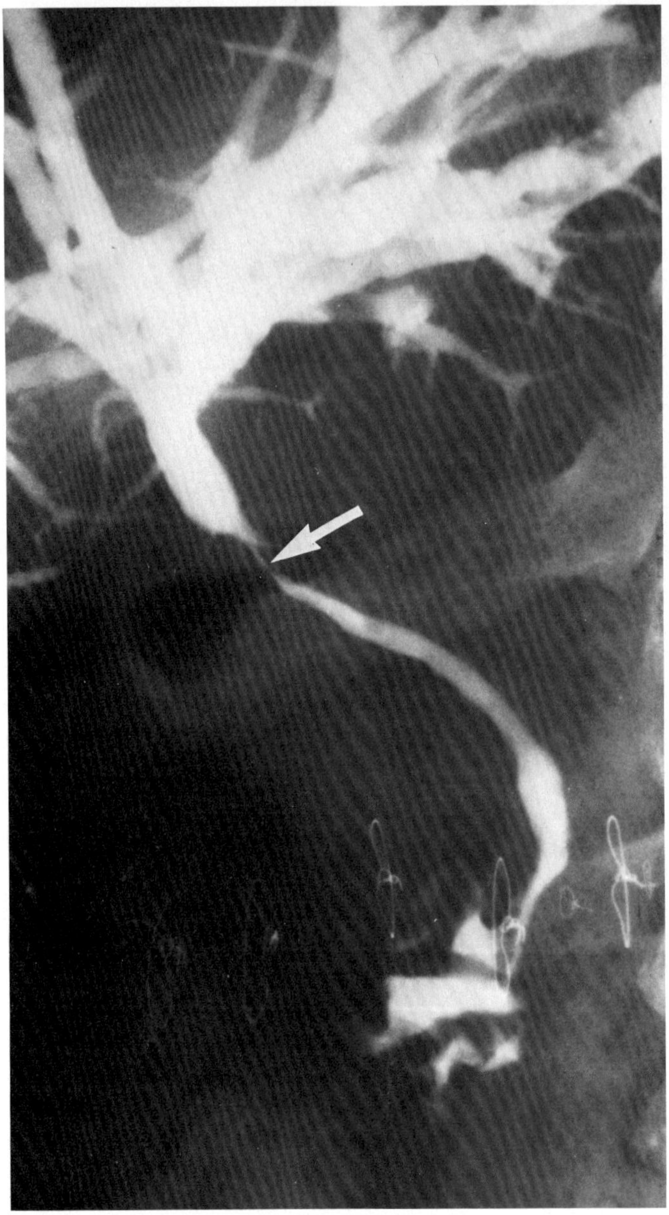

Figure 9A Percutaneous dilatation of a benign postoperative stricture. A 59-year-old man developed cholangitis and jaundice following cholecystectomy. A percutaneous transhepatic cholangiogram demonstrates a stricture of the common bile duct (arrow).

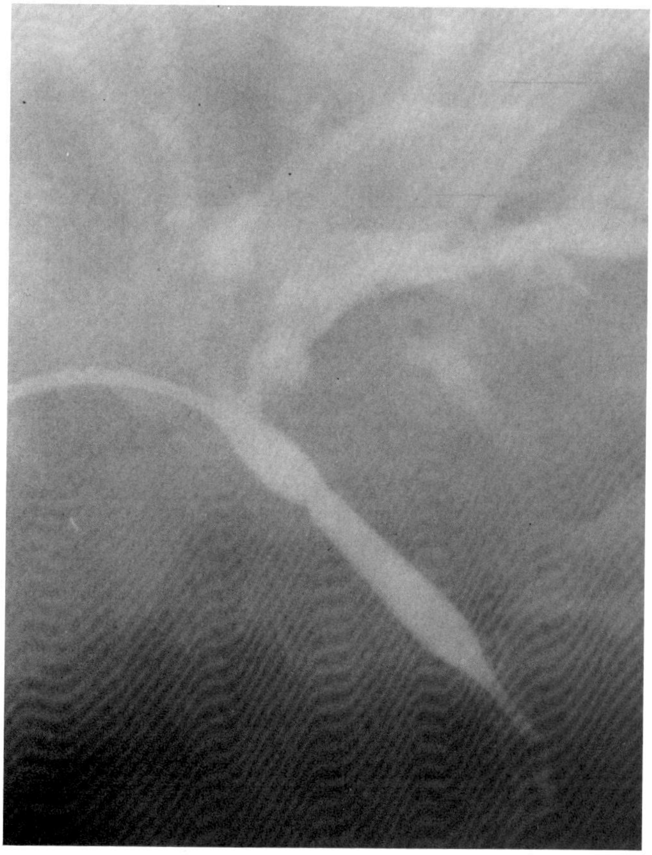

Figure 9B A percutaneously inserted balloon catheter was used to dilate the stricture.

segment, allowing antegrade drainage into the duodenum. The transhepatic drainage catheter is maintained in position above the dilated stricture to allow for progressive dilatations at intervals over many weeks. We have been able to open tight strictures by this means and patency has been maintained for over 2 years. Because of the well-known tendency of strictures to reform in the biliary tract, the long-term value of this treatment is yet to be established.

Removal of Stones

In special cases, obstruction caused by a common bile duct stone can be treated by removing the stone by the percutaneous transhepatic route. At the University of Pennsylvania a gallstone causing obstruction immediately after cholecystectomy was moved from the distal common bile duct into the duodenum using a transhepatically inserted biliary stone basket, thus relieving the obstruction (40) (Fig. 10). Later, Dotter reported crushing a gallstone with a basket inserted through the liver (41). The potential of this method is likely to be more widely exploited in the future as experience is gained with the transhepatic route.

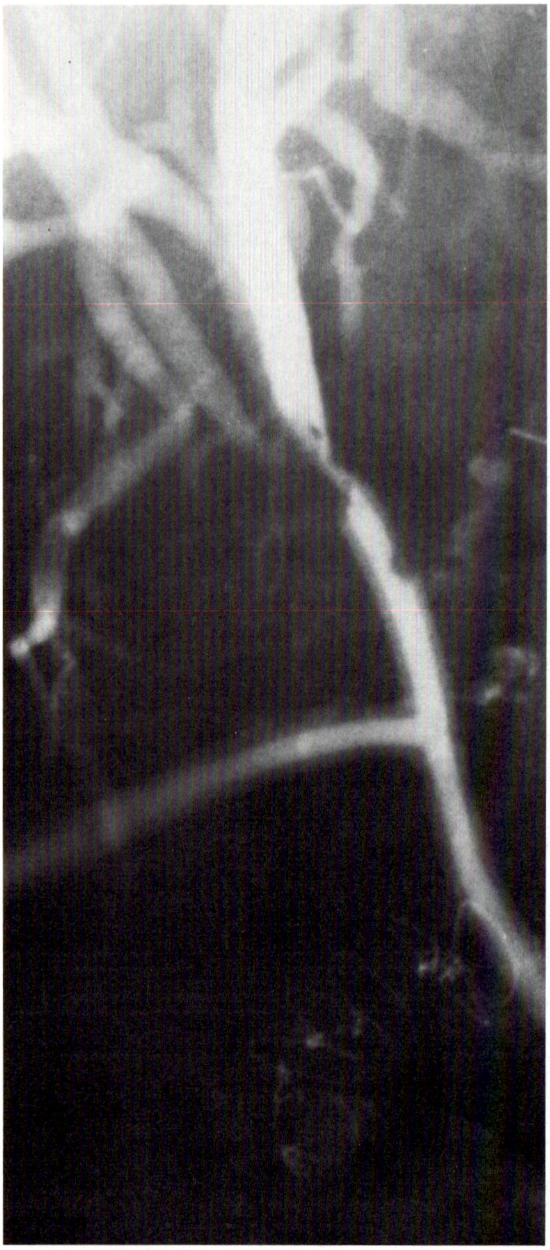

Figure 12B Six months later the patient developed cholangitis. A repeat cholangiogram shows an irregular obstruction of the duct above the proximal limb of the T tube, due to tumor extension.

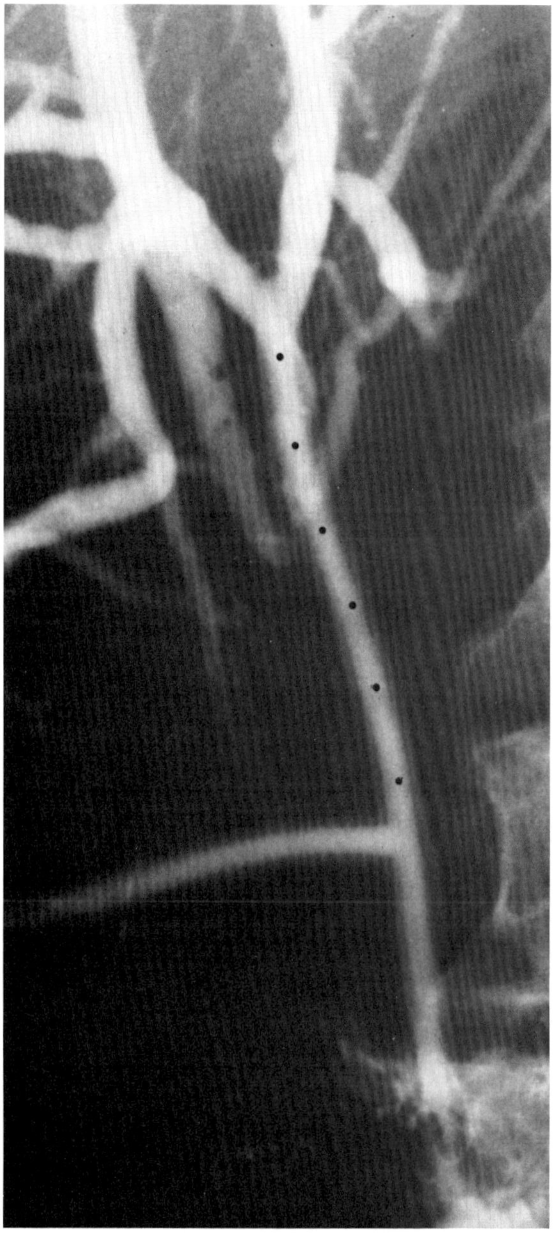

Figure 12C The T tube was removed and a new, longer limb tube introduced through the tract. The upper limb of the new tube (dots) now extends through the obstructing lesion to provide a conduit for bile flow.

References

1.. Schenker S, Balint J, Schiff L: Differential diagnosis of jaundice: report of a prospective study of 61 proved cases. *Am J Dig Dis 7*:449, 1962.
2. Conn HO: Liver biopsy in extrahepatic biliary obstruction and in other ''contraindicated'' disorders. Editorial. *Gastroenterology 68*:817, 1975.
3. Menghini G and Ghergo GF: Needle biopsy of the liver. In *Gastroenterology*, Vol. 3, 3rd ed, Bockus HL (Ed). W. B. Saunders, Philadelphia, 1976.
4. Morris JS, Gallo GA, Scheuer PJ, Sherlock S: Percutaneous liver biopsy in patients with large bile duct obstruction. *Gastroenterology 68*:750, 1975.
5. Allison D: Personal communication, 1980.
6. Behan M and Kazam E: Sonography of the common bile duct: value of the right anterior oblique view. *Am J Roentgenol 130*:701, 1978.
7. Sample WF, Sarti DA, Goldstein LI, Weinter M, Kadell BM: Gray-scale ultrasonography of the jaundiced patient. *Radiology 128*:719, 1978.
8. Kazam E, Schneider M, Rubensfein WA: The role of ultrasound and CT. In *Multiple Imaging Procedures, Abdomen*. Alavi A and Arger PH (Eds). Grune & Stratton, New York, 1980.
9. Mueller PR, Ferrucci JT Jr, Simeone JF, Wittenberg J, Sonnenberg E, Polansky A, Isler RJ: Postcholecystectomy bile duct dilatation: myth or reality? *Am J Roentgenol 136*:355, 1981.
10. Zeman RK, Dorfman GS, Burrell MI, Stein S, Berg GR, Gold JA: Disparate dilatation of the intrahepatic and extrahepatic bile ducts in surgical jaundice. *Radiology 138*:129, 1981.
11. Haubek A, Pedersen JH, Burcharth F, Gammelgaard J, Hancke S, Willumsen L: Dynamic sonography in the evaluation of jaundice. *Am J Roentgenol 136*:1071, 1981.
12. Vallon AG, Lees WR, Cotton PB: Gray-scale ultrasonography in cholestatic jaundice. *Gut 20*:51, 1979.
13. Wheeler PG, Theodossi A, Pickford R, Laws, J, Knill-Jones RP, Williams R: Noninvasive techniques in the diagnosis of jaundice—ultrasound and computer. *Gut 20*:196, 1979.
14. Morris AI, Fawcitt RA, Food R, Forbes WSC, Isherwood I, Marsh MN: Computed tomography, ultrasound and cholestatic jaundice. *Gut 19*:685, 1978.
15. Havrilla TR, Haaga JR, Alfidi RJ, Reich NE: Computed tomography and obstructive biliary disease. *Am J Roentgenol 128*:765, 1977.
16. Foley WD, Wilson CR, Quirox FA, Lawson TL: Demonstration of the normal extrahepatic biliary tract with computed tomography. *J Comput Assist Tomogr 4*:48, 1980.
17. Goldberg HI, Filly RA, Korobkin M, Moss AA, Kressel HY, Callen PW: Capability of CT body scanning and ultrasonography to demonstrate the status of the biliary ductal system in patients with jaundice. *Radiology 129*:731, 1978.
18. Levitt, RG, Sagel SS, Stanley RJ: Accuracy of computed tomography of the liver and biliary tract. *Radiology 124*:123, 1977.
19. Shanser JD, Korobkin M, Goldberg HI, Rohlfing BM: Computed tomographic diagnosis of obstructive jaundice in the absence of intrahepatic ductal dilatation. *Am J Roentgenol 131*:389, 1978.
20. Whalen JP: Radiology of the abdomen: impact of new imaging methods. *Am J Roentgenol 133*:587, 1979.
21. Ferrucci JT Jr, Wittenberg J, Mueller PR, Simeone JF, Harbin WP, Taft PD, Kirkpatrick RH: Diagnosis of abdominal malignancy by radiologic fine-needle aspiration biopsy. *Am J Roentgenol 134*:323, 1980.
22. Mueller PR, Wittenberg J, Ferrucci JT Jr: Fine needle aspiration of abdominal masses. *Semin Roentgenol 16*:52, 1981.
23. Ferrucci JT Jr, Wittenberg J, Margolies MN, Carey RW: Malignant seeding of the tract after thin needle aspiration biopsy. *Radiology 130*:345, 1979.

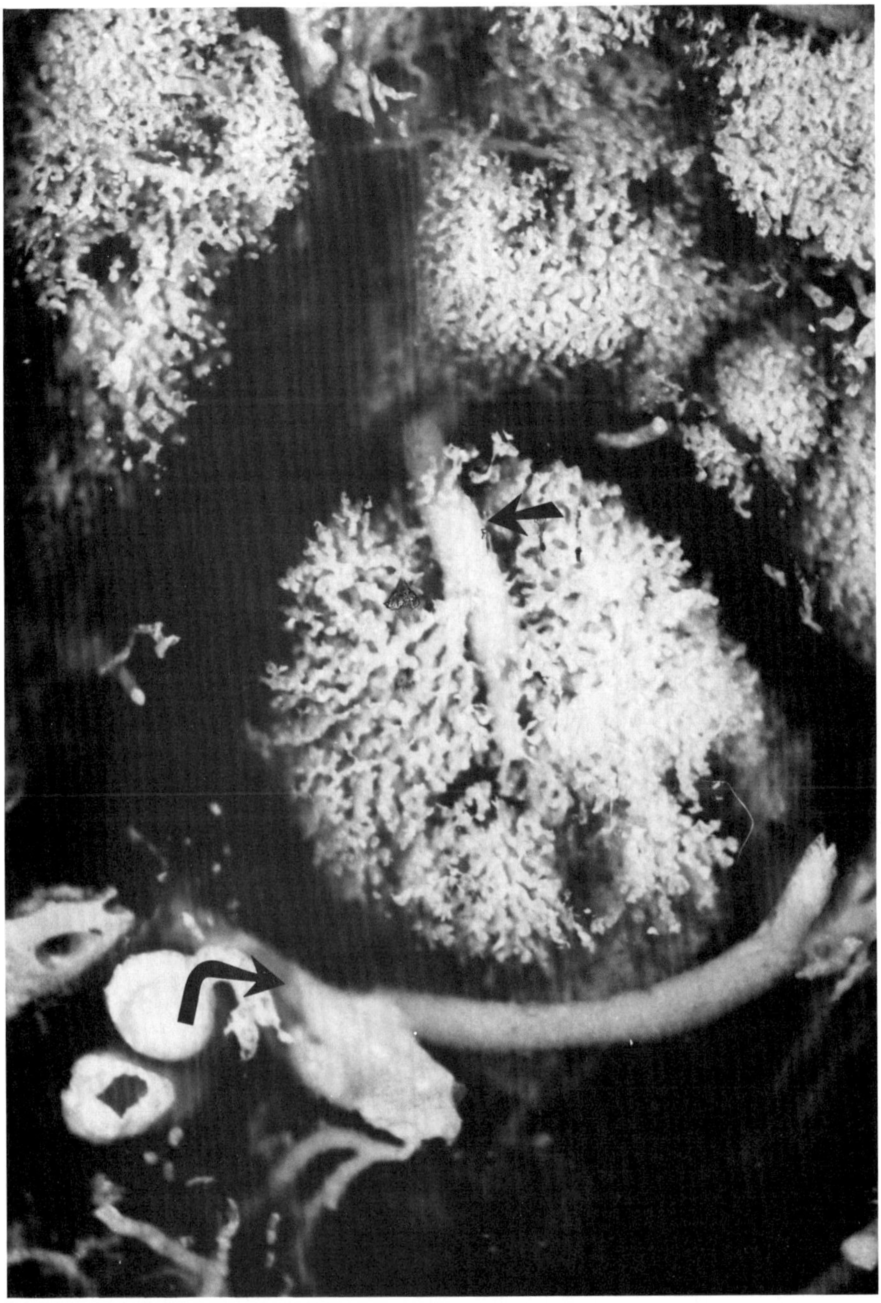

(B)

Figure 2 (continued)

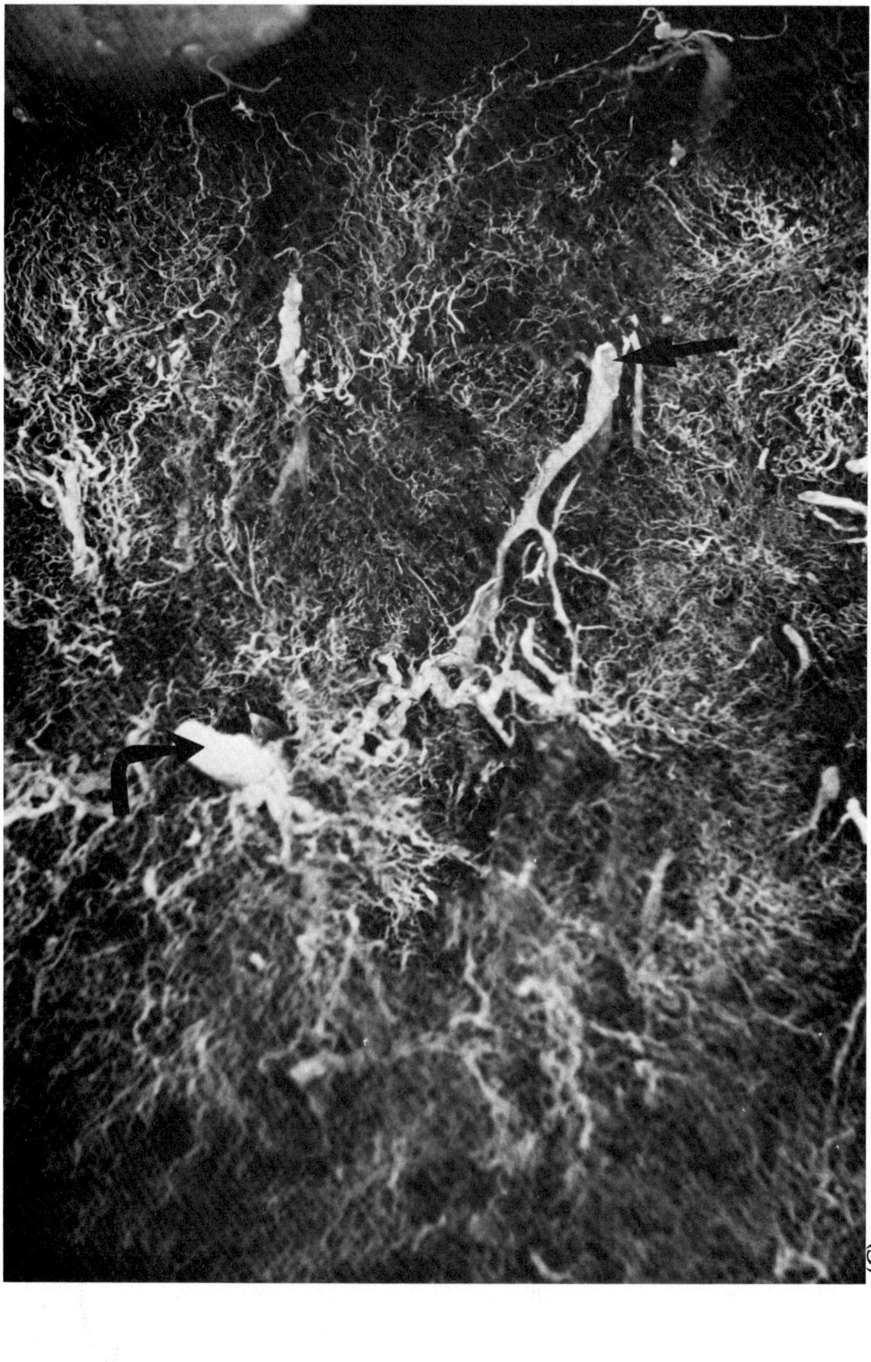

(C)

Figure 2 (continued)

Table 1 Normal Values and Pressure and Changes in Representative Conditions

	WHVP	FHVP	HIVC	CSP	RA	LIVC	LRV
Normal Value (mmHg):	4–11	5–8	5–8	5–7	5	5–10	10–16
PV thrombosis	NC	NC	NC	NC	NC	NC	NC
Schistosomiasis	NC	NC	NC	NC	NC	NC	NC
Cirrhosis	↑	NC	NC	↑	NC	NC	NC
Cirrhosis, contracted liver	↑	NC	NC	↑	NC	↑	↑
Cirrhosis, ascites	↑↑	↑	↑	↑	NC	↑	↑
Noncirrhotic ascites	↑	↑	↑	NC	NC	↑	↑
IVC web	↑	↑	↑	NC	NC	↑	↑
Constrictive pericarditis	↑	↑	↑	NC	↑	↑	↑

[a]Pressure recordings in portal hypertension: WHVP, wedged hepatic vein pressure; FHVP, free hepatic vein pressure; HIVC, high inferior vena caval pressure; CSP, corrected sinusoidal pressure; RA, right atrial pressure; LIVC, low inferior vena caval pressure; LRV, left renal vein pressure.
[b]↑, increase; NC, no change.

hepatoma and other abnormalities of visceral organs can be excluded. The patency of the portal system and the presence of varices can be observed in the venous phase.

Hepatic venography can be performed with the catheter tip either wedged or free in the hepatic vein. Wedged hepatic venography demonstrates the degree of hepatic sinusoidal distortion and the direction of the portal venous flow. Free hepatic venography shows an overall view of the segmental and lobar hepatic vein distribution in cirrhosis but does not assess the portal venous flow direction (7). Inferior vena cavography is performed to evaluate an abnormality in the cava or right atrium, especially if a marked pressure difference exists between the high and low inferior vena cava or between the free hepatic vein and the right atrium or inferior vena cava (2). A left renal venogram can reveal a developmental anomaly, important if a distant splenorenal shunt is contemplated (8).

Manometric recordings are routinely obtained with a catheter wedged in a hepatic vein, free in a hepatic vein, high in the inferior vena cava, low in the inferior vena cava, in the right atrium, and in the left renal vein. The normal values and the pressure changes in certain representative conditions are listed in Table 1.

Causes of Portal Hypertension

Portal hypertension can be caused by a great variety of diseases. Classification is best done according to the site of vascular obstruction, distinguishing prehepatic, intrahepatic, and posthepatic types (Table 2). The intrahepatic portal hypertension is further divided into presinusoidal, sinusoidal, and postsinusoidal. However, many diseases in their advanced form often cause more than one level of involvement (e.g., metastatic neoplasm may lead to presinusoidal as well as postsinusoidal portal hypertension).

Table 2 Classification of Portal Hypertension

Prehepatic	Portal vein thrombosis	
	Splenic vein thrombosis	
	Extrinsic compression of portal system	
Intrahepatic	Biliary cirrhosis	Presinusoidal
	Portal fibrosis	
	Schistosomiasis	
	Congenital hepatic fibrosis	
	Neoplasm, primary or malignant	
	Arteriovenous fistula	
	Fatty liver	Sinusoidal
	Sickle cell disease and sinus thrombosis	
	Hepatitis	
	Postnecrotic cirrhosis	
	Laennec's cirrhosis	
	Alcoholic cirrhosis	Postsinusoidal
	Hepatic vein obstruction	
	Veno-occlusive disease	
	Neoplasms	
Posthepatic	Congestive heart failure	
	Constrictive pericarditis	
	Inferior vena cava obstruction (Web)	
	Rheumatic heart disease	

Prehepatic

Portal vein or splenic vein thrombosis is the most common form of prehepatic portal hypertension.

Portal vein thrombosis frequently accompanies liver cirrhosis. Its etiology often remains uncertain, although neonatal omphalitis is a frequently suspected causative condition. Portosystemic collaterals, including esophageal and gastric varices, may be present and are regularly seen when the portal vein thrombosis is combined with liver cirrhosis. Portal vein thrombosis produces an extensive network of venous channels in the hepatoduodenal ligament, the so-called cavernous transformation of the portal vein (Fig. 3). It has been suggested that these collaterals represent the dilated vasa vasorum of the portal vein; however, it is more likely that they are dilated right gastric and common bile duct veins (Fig. 4).

Splenic vein thrombosis is most often caused by a pancreatic carcinoma or pancreatitis. Extrinsic compression of the splenic vein from a pseudocyst can also cause splenic vein occlusion (Fig. 5) with possible reversal to patency when the pseudocyst has been drained. Bridging collaterals to the lower pressure portal venous system are usually

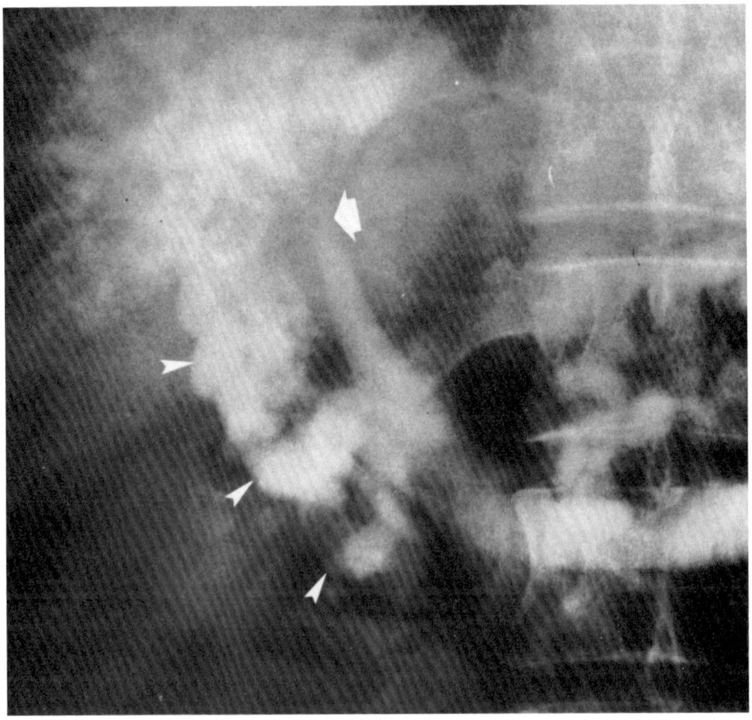

Figure 3 Splenoportogram in a patient with portal vein thrombosis (arrow). Wide collaterals reach the liver in the hepatoduodenal ligament (arrowheads).

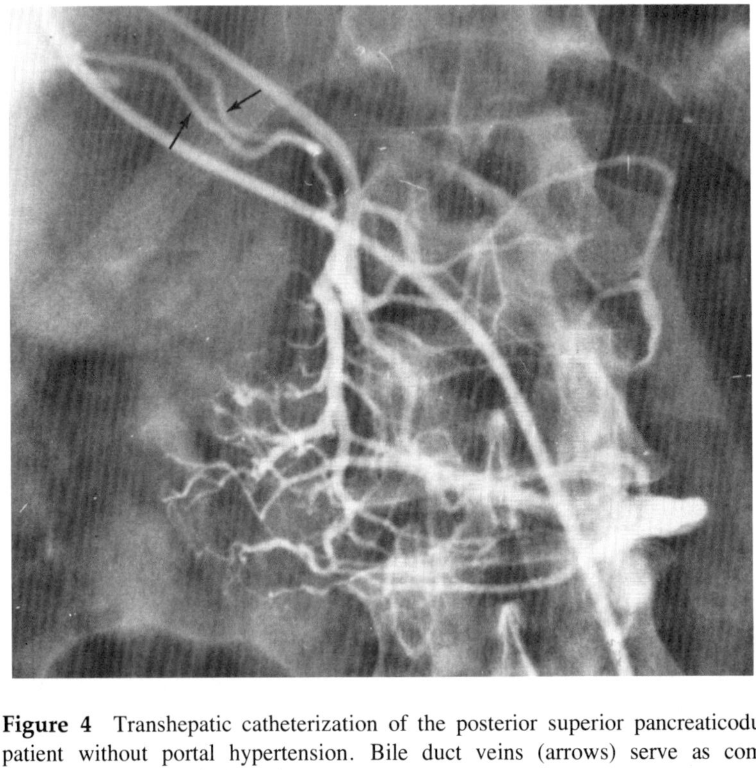

Figure 4 Transhepatic catheterization of the posterior superior pancreaticoduodenal vein in a patient without portal hypertension. Bile duct veins (arrows) serve as communication with intrahepatic portal vein branches.

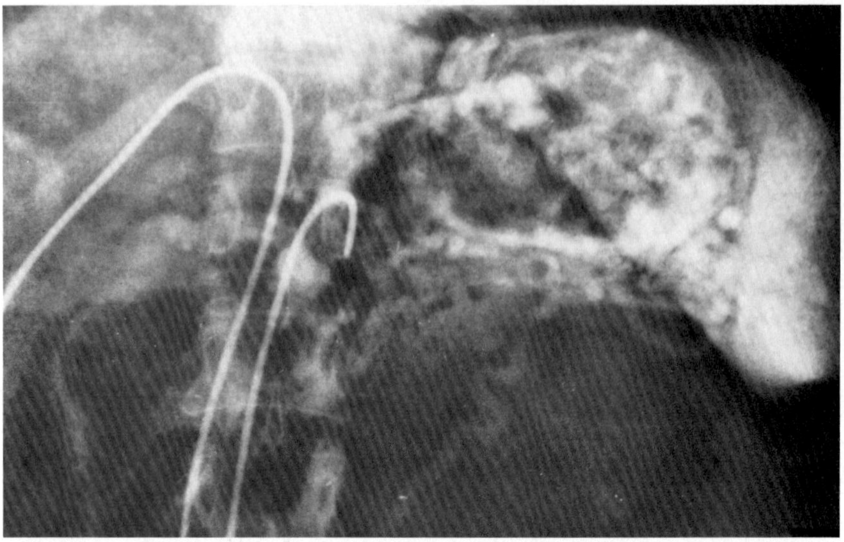

(A)

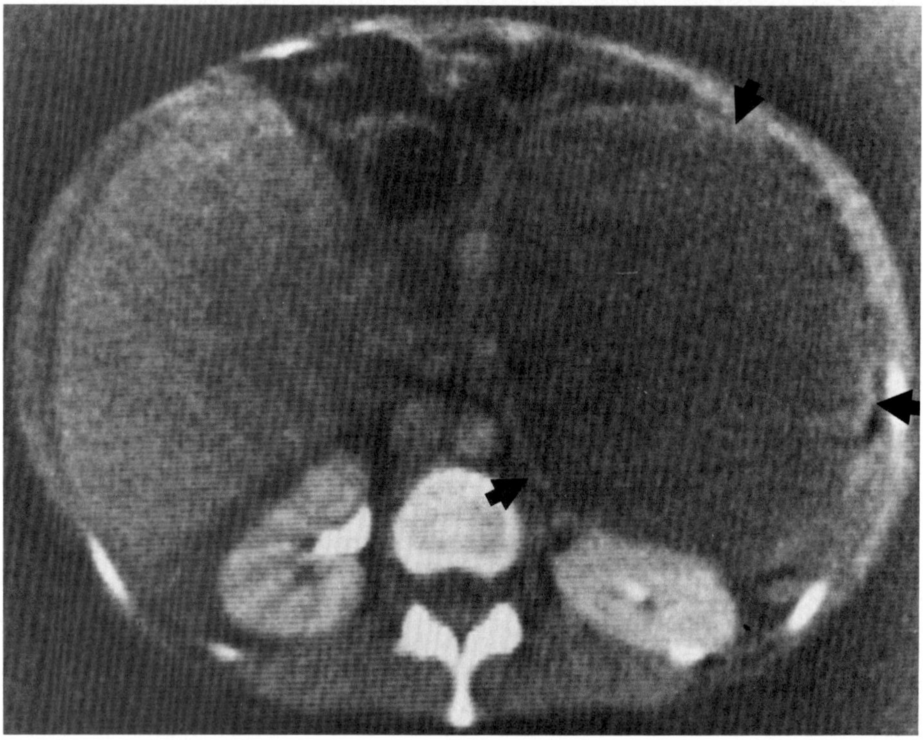

(B)

Figure 5 Pseudocyst of pancreas. (A) Venous phase of celiac arteriogram. Splenic and portal veins are occluded due to a large mass in the left upper quadrant. Massive collateral veins (varices) are seen around the pancreas and stomach. (B) CT scan of the abdomen. A large pseudocyst is shown (arrows). During an exploratory laparotomy, the pseudocyst was drained and the splenic and portal veins opened immediately.

formed over the short gastric veins to the left gastric vein, and over the left gastroepiploic to the right gastroepiploic and superior mesenteric veins. A lack of splenic and portal vein opacification and the presence of multiple collateral veins around the spleen after splenic artery injection of a high dose of contrast medium are indicative of splenic and/or portal vein thrombosis (Fig. 6).

Superior mesenteric arteriography with injection of a vasodilator substance assists in the evaluation of the mesenteric and portal veins. When thrombosis of the entire portal venous system occurs, the hepatic artery frequently increases in size and the liver becomes hypervascular, to compensate for the decreased portal flow (Fig. 7). In all these circumstances the wedged hepatic venous pressure is normal and the splenic pulp pressure markedly elevated (9).

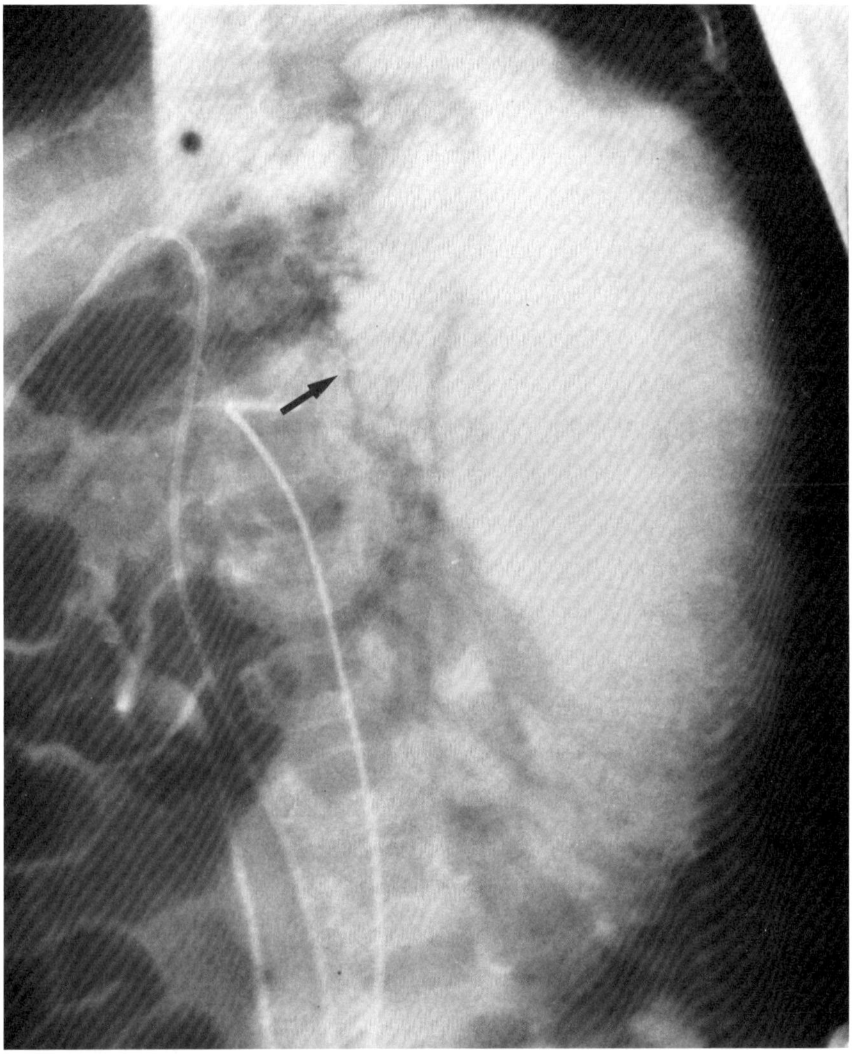

Figure 6A Panportal venous system thrombosis. Splenic arteriogram, venous phase. Splenomegaly and splenic vein thrombosis. Note varicose veins in the splenic hilus (arrow).

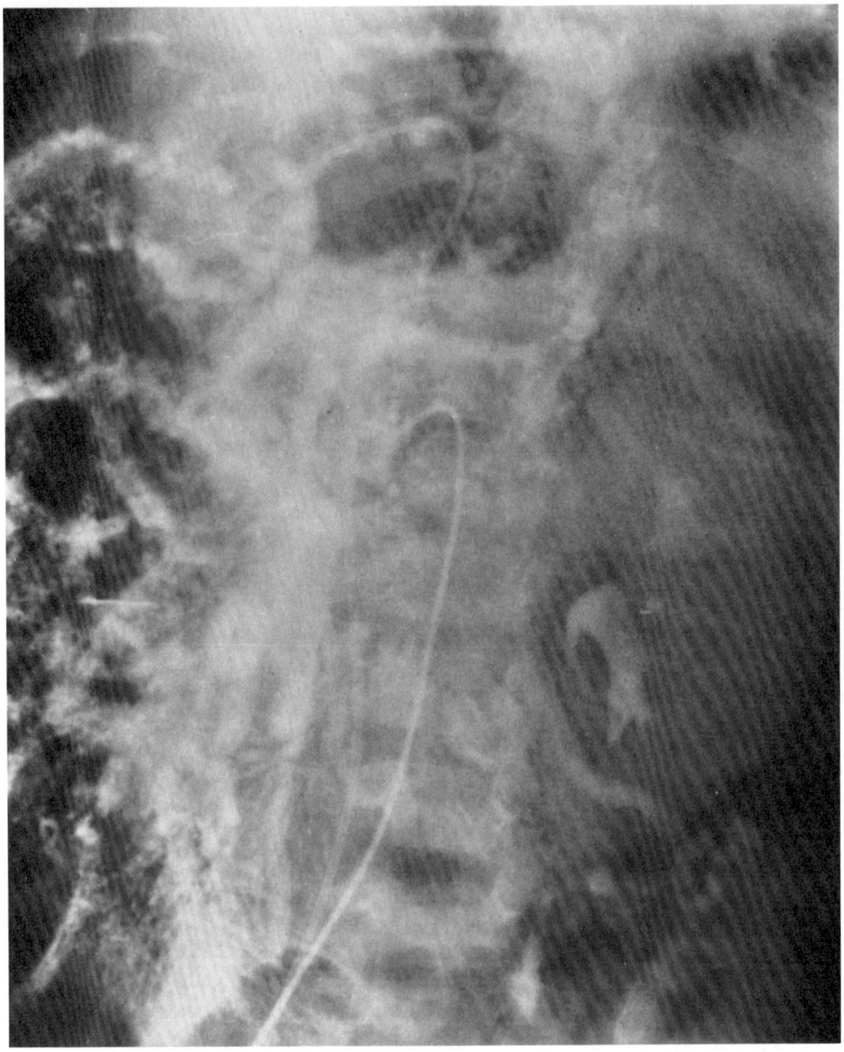

Figure 6B Superior mesenteric arteriogram, venous phase. Superior mesenteric and portal vein thrombosis; mainstems not outlined. Diffuse varicose veins of the intestine and mesentery.

Increased portal inflow can be a cause of portal hypertension. This could be the result of a congenital or acquired arteriovenous fistula in the portal area. Congenital arteriovenous fistulae are usually related to hereditary hemorrhagic telangiectasia (10); the acquired form is a result of trauma or the rupture of an aneurysm (11,12). Splenic aneurysms have been shown to occur frequently in portal hypertension (13).

A rare type of portal hypertension is due to increased portal inflow in the absence of an arteriovenous fistula, called *hyperkinetic portal hypertension* (14). Marked

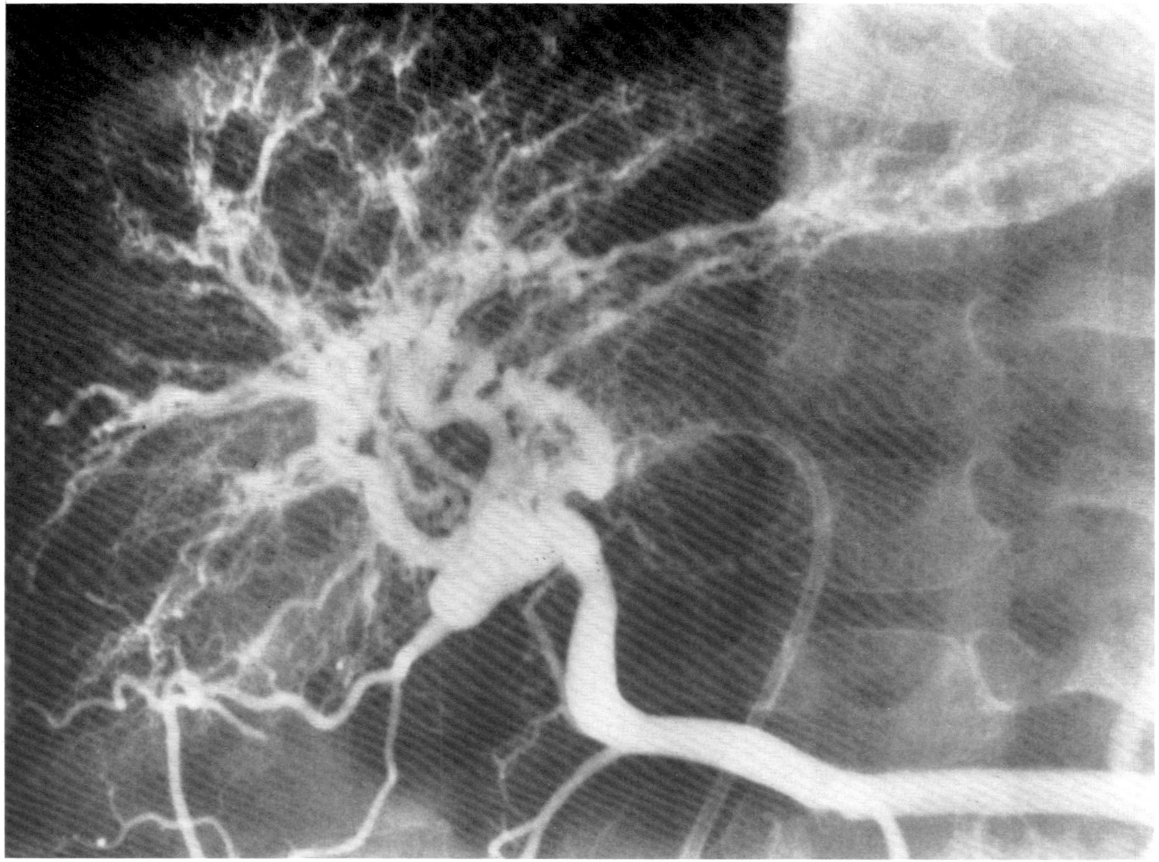

Figure 7 Panportal thrombosis. Hepatic arteriogram, arterial phase. Marked increase in hepatic arterial flow, producing apparent duplication of the tortuous hepatic artery branches.

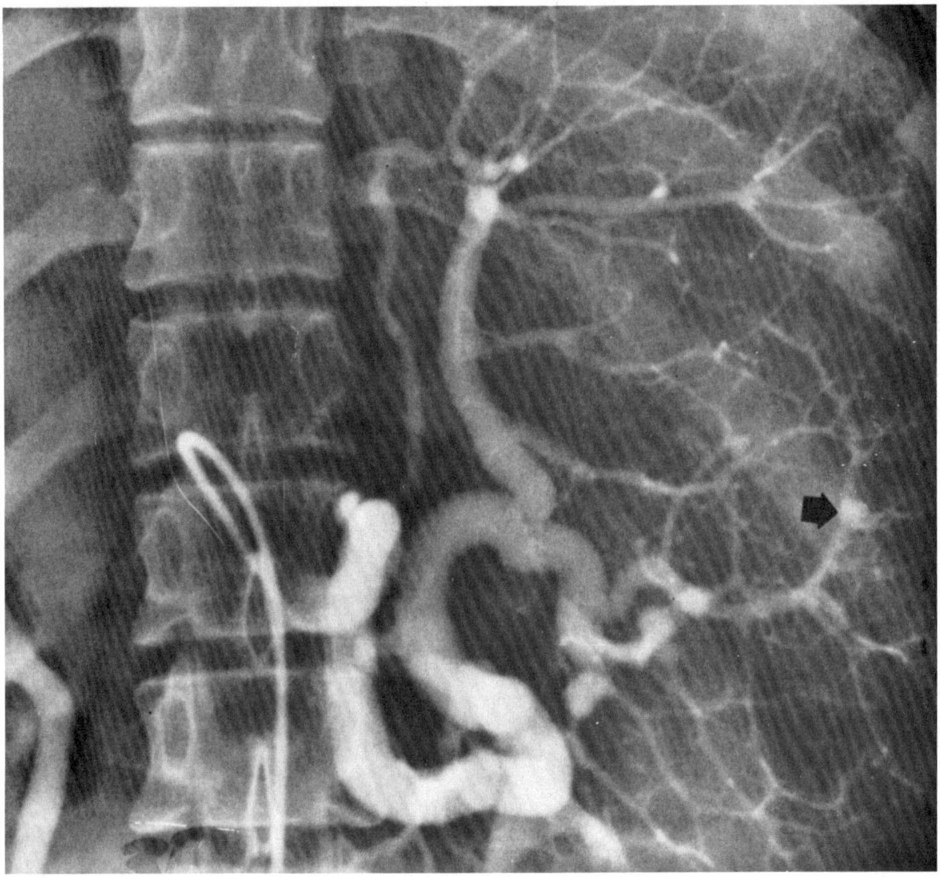

Figure 8A Hyperkinetic portal hypertension due to increased flow from hypersplenism. Tortuous and enlarged splenic artery. A splenic aneurysm (arrow) is present.

splenomegaly, with increased flow in both the splenic artery and vein, are the typical feature (Fig. 8A,B). The liver is initially normal in size and the hepatic arterial flow is normal. Eventually, the persistently elevated portal flow leads to increased vascular resistance in the liver, and thus portal hypertension. However, the hemodynamic data in this entity are still incomplete. In two patients with hyperkinetic portal hypertension the WHVP remained unchanged after a 30-min splenic artery infusion of 0.2–0.4 unit of vasopressin. Splenectomy is performed in these patients if increased portal inflow leads to variceal bleeding or hypersplenism. Despite splenectomy, some patients eventually progress to portal vein thrombosis and cirrhosis of the liver (Fig. 8C); the clinical features of such a condition are then indistinguishable from the idiopathic portal hypertension.

Intrahepatic (Cirrhosis)

Cirrhosis of the liver is the most common cause of portal hypertension. Cirrhosis is a diffuse process characterized by fibrosis, cell death, and the formation of structurally

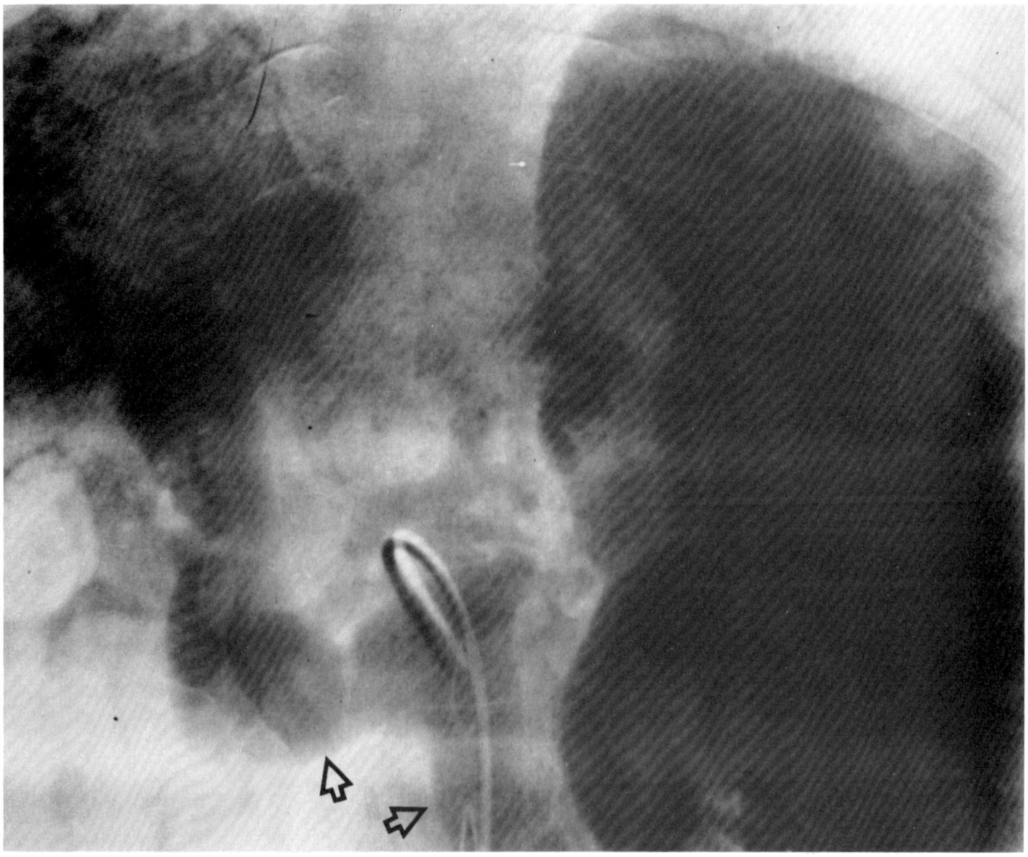

Figure 8B Splenic vein tortuous, enlarged and patent (arrows). Splenectomy was performed later.

abnormal nodules (15). The various causes of cirrhosis are listed in Table 2. According to the site of involvement, cirrhosis of the liver is classified as presinusoidal, sinusoidal, and postsinusoidal. Some types of cirrhosis begin in one specific site but, as the disease process advances, portal blockage will extend to involve further sites. Cirrhosis is usually a progressively destructive disease.

Presinusoidal block is typically caused by schistosomiasis, biliary cirrhosis, and congenital hepatic fibrosis. On a worldwide basis, schistosomiasis is the most common condition. Hemodynamically, presinusoidal cirrhosis resembles the obstruction of the main stem of the portal vein (16). Various types of cirrhosis which typically cause sinusoidal block may extend to presinusoidal or postsinusoidal levels. Both primary and metastatic neoplasms may do this. Angiographic findings are similar in different types of cirrhosis. Presinusoidal and postsinusoidal blockages are best differentiated by wedged hepatic venous pressure measurement rather than by hepatic angiography.

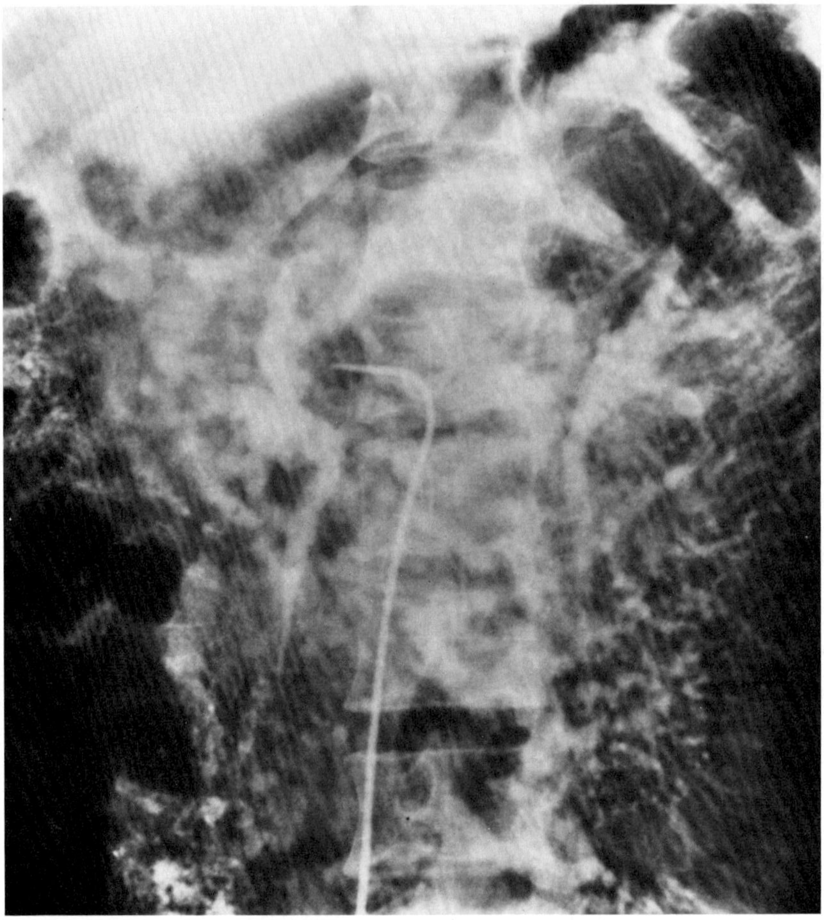

Figure 8C The patient returned 5 years postoperatively with massive gastrointestinal hemorrhage and a superior mesenteric arteriogram was done. The venous phase shows thrombosis of superior mesenteric and portal veins. Diffuse mesenteric varices are present, which caused the gastrointestinal bleed. Only conservative management is possible, as no vein of adequate size is available for a venous shunting procedure.

Angiographic Features of Cirrhosis

In the early phase of cirrhosis (stage I), with portal pressure slightly elevated, the portal and hepatic arterial flow maintain their normal level and direction. No portosystemic collateral shunting is present. The only detectable abnormality is minimal distortion of hepatic sinusoids seen at wedged hepatic venography and a mildly elevated WHVP and portal vein pressure (PVP) (Fig. 9).

When the cirrhosis progresses (stage II), fibrosis and obstruction of central veins and sinusoids further elevate the portal venous pressure. A portion of the portal flow is diverted through portosystemic collaterals, while the remaining portion continues through

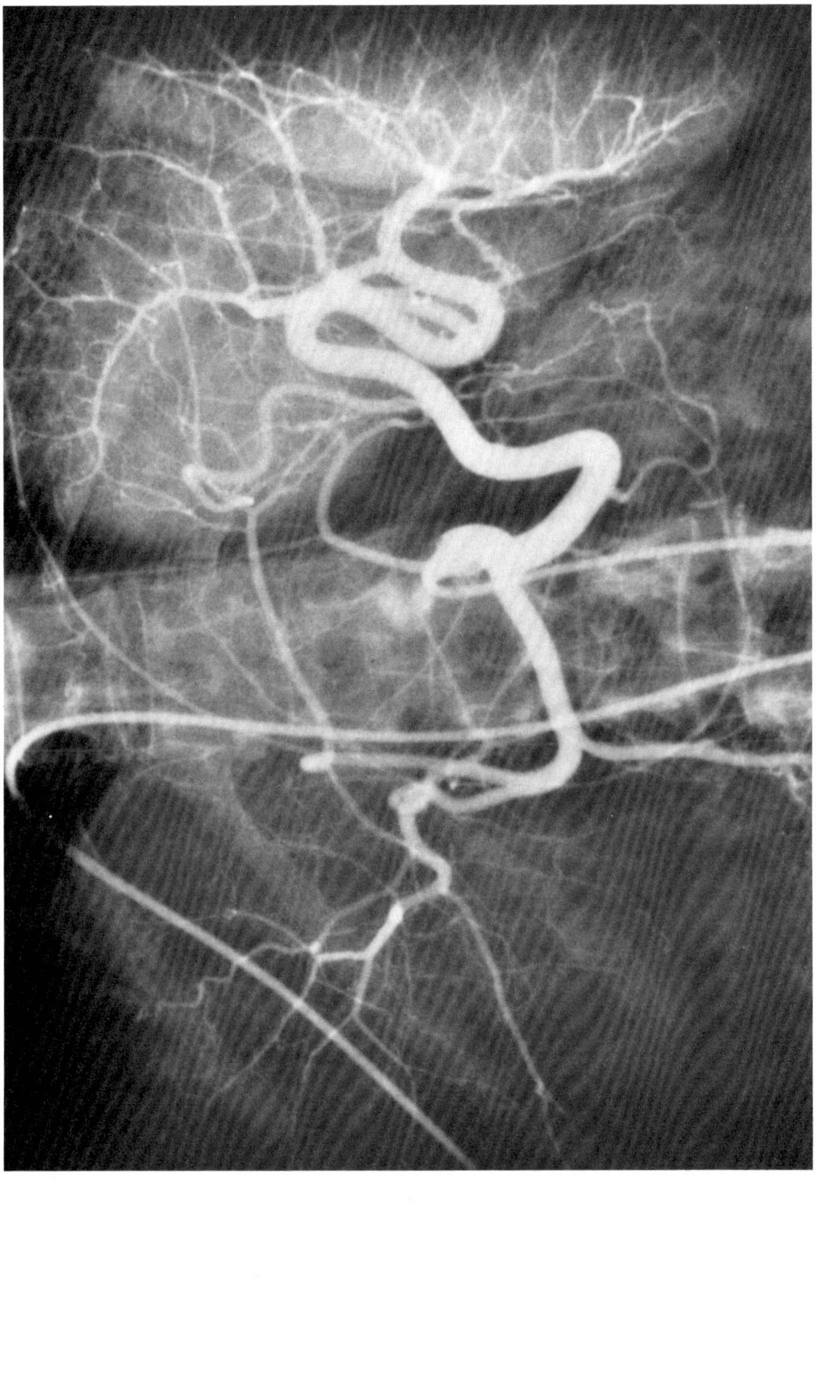

Figure 9A

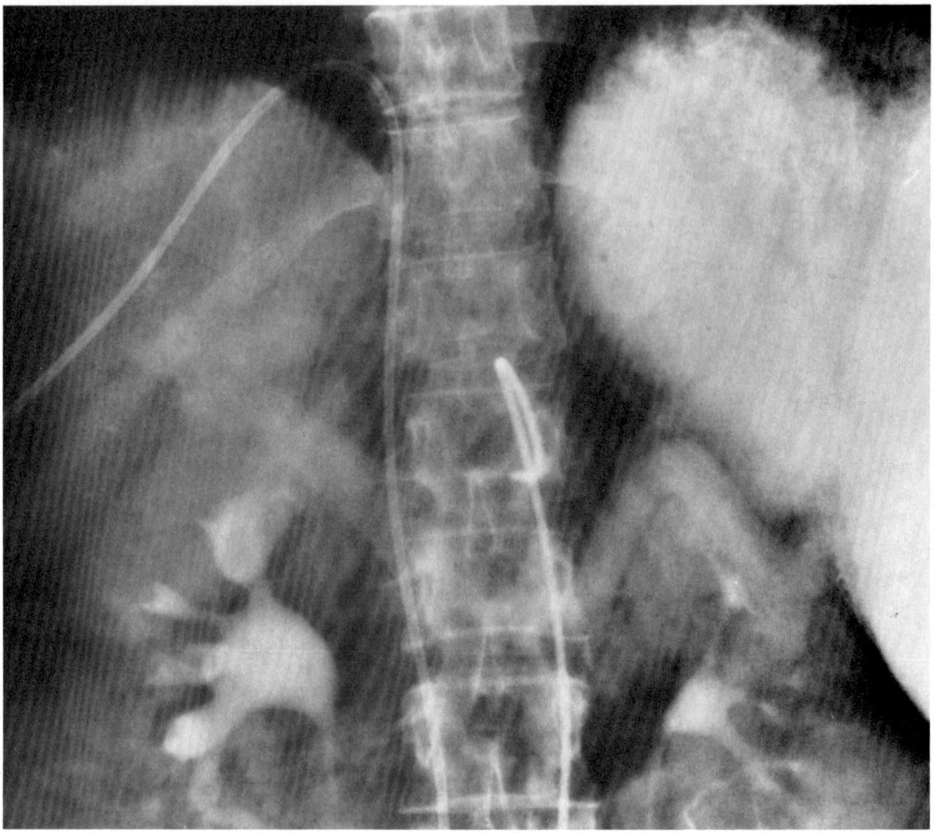

(B)

Figure 9 Stage I cirrhosis. (A) Celiac arteriogram, arterial phase. Normal hepatic arteries and slightly enlarged spleen. (B) Celiac arteriogram, venous phase. Normal splenic and portal vein with hepatopetal flow. No varices. (C) Superior mesenteric arteriogram, venous phase; 40 mg of priscoline used. Normal hepatopetal flow of superior mesenteric and portal veins. (D) Wedged hepatic venogram. Contrast medium injection, 2 cc/sec for 4 sec. Nonhomogenous sinusoidogram with moderate distortion. The corrected sinusoidal pressure was 9.5 mmHg, which is slightly elevated.

the hepatic sinusoids. The portal flow thus becomes bidirectional. The majority of patients with portal hypertension belong to this group (Figs. 10, 11).

In the end stage of cirrhosis (stage III), the resistance in the distorted hepatic sinusoids surpasses the combined hepatic arterial and portal venous pressure, and the flow in the portal vein reverses away from the liver toward the systemic venous circulation (i.e., hepatofugal portal flow). The hepatic artery becomes the only blood supply to the liver and its flow is drained by both hepatic and portal veins (Fig. 12).

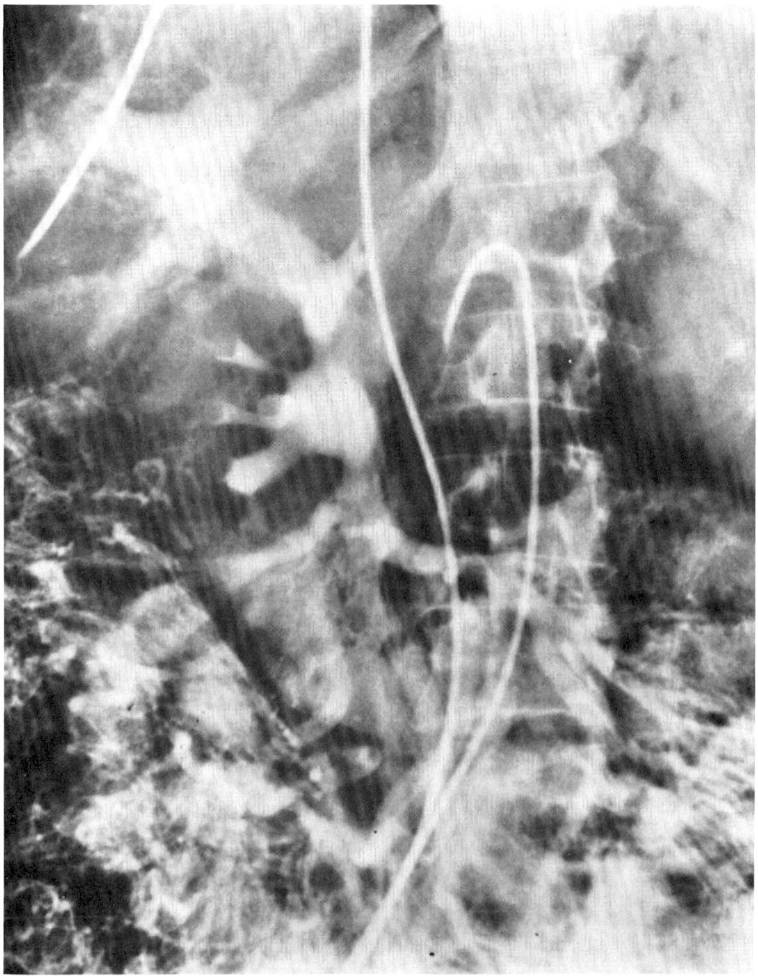

(C)

Figure 9 (continued)

In stages II and III, when the portal flow partially or totally shunts away from the liver, the hepatic arterial inflow increases to compensate for the lost portal flow. However, the total hepatic flow volume can never reach that found in normality.

In Table 3 the arteriographic features of cirrhosis are summarized. They correlate well with the pathophysiological and hemodynamic changes of cirrhosis. Hypervascularity and apparent duplication of the hepatic artery result from increased flow to compensate for the decreased portal supply. There is no real increase in the number of artery branches but an increase in the size of the concomitant arteries, sufficient to render

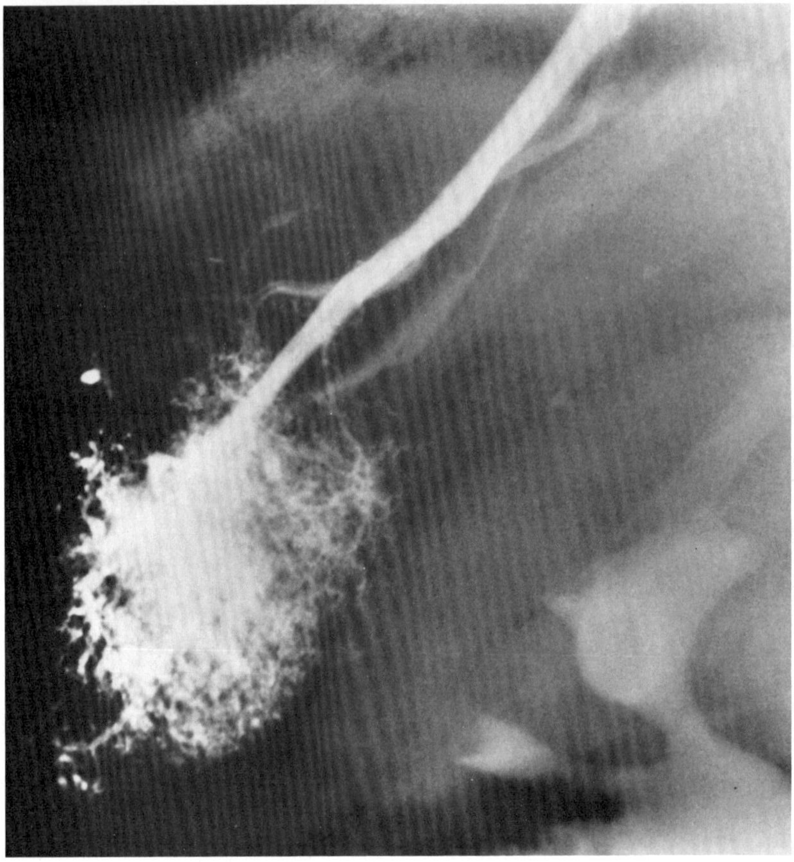

(D)

Figure 9 (continued)

them angiographically visible (17) (Fig. 13). In early cirrhosis, the liver size remains normal or may be increased from fatty infiltration. In advanced cirrhosis the liver is contracted and the elongated and "duplicated" hepatic arterial branches become very tortuous, giving the so-called "corkscrew" appearance. Regenerating nodules frequently show increased parenchymal staining, and when they intermingle with areas of fibrosis, cause the hepatogram to become nonhomogeneous. Splenomegaly and ascites are commonly associated features. The incidence of hepatoma in cirrhotic patients is known to be higher than in the normal population.

Venographic Staging of Cirrhosis

The direction of portal flow is the basis for the angiographic classification of cirrhosis. This can best be evaluated by the injection of contrast medium into the hepatic sinusoids

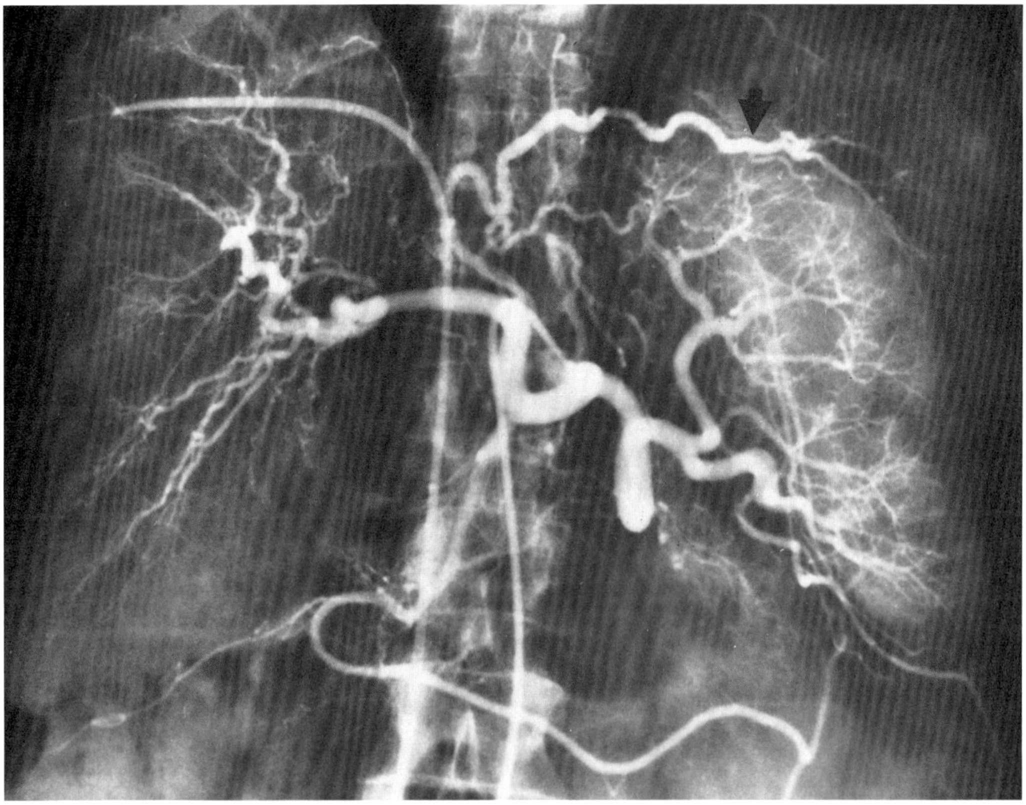

(A)

Figure 10 Stage IIA cirrhosis. (A) Celiac arteriogram, arterial phase. Tortuous (corkscew) appearance and increased number of hepatic branches. The lateral segment of the left lobe extends beyond the lateral margin of the spleen (the arrow points to the left hepatic artery). (B) Celiac arteriogram, venous phase. Bidirectional portal flow. The splenic vein and portal vein are patent, affirming the hepatopetal flow. The coronary vein (closed arrows), esophageal varices, and inferior mesenteric vein (open arrow) are also opacified, which signifies the hepatofugal flow. There are also unnamed varices in the inferior aspect of both the spleen and liver. The liver is separated from the abdominal wall due to ascites. (C) Superior mesenteric arteriogram, arterial phase; 40 mg of tolazoline used. Normal superior mesenteric artery and its intestinal branches. (D) Superior mesenteric arteriogram, venous phase. Bidirectional portal flow is shown by the demonstration of the portal vein and varices (arrows). (E) Following 0.2 unit/min vasopressin infusion of the superior mesenteric artery for 20 min, marked constriction of intestinal branches of SMA and regurgitation of contrast medium into the abdominal aorta. (F) The venous phase shows decreased opacification (decreased flow) of both the portal vein and varices (arrow). (G) Wedged hepatic venogram. Mottled sinusoidogram and opacification of the portal vein (dots) for approximately 3 sec. The corrected sinusoid pressure was 15 mmHg, which decreased to 13 mmHg following vasopressin infusion.

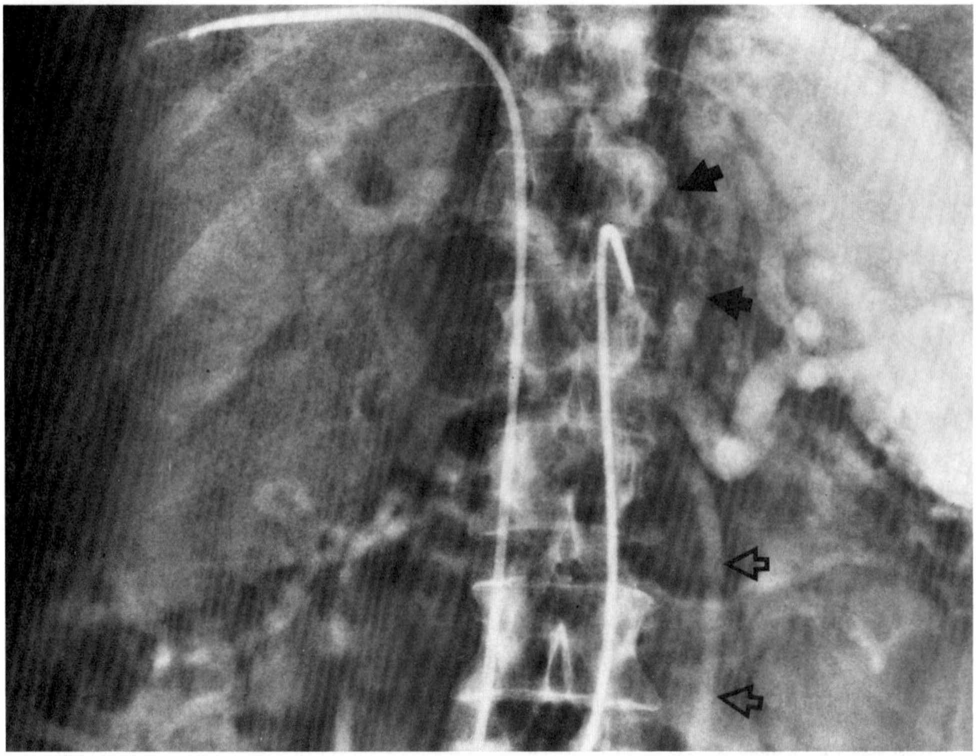

(B)

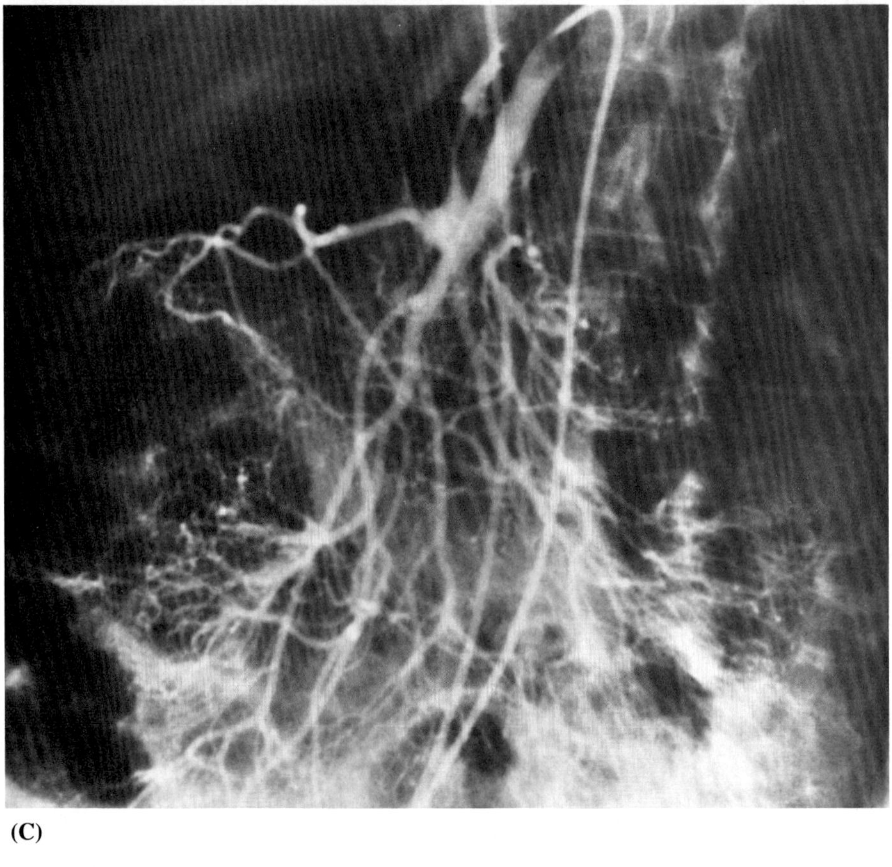

(C)

Figure 10 (continued)

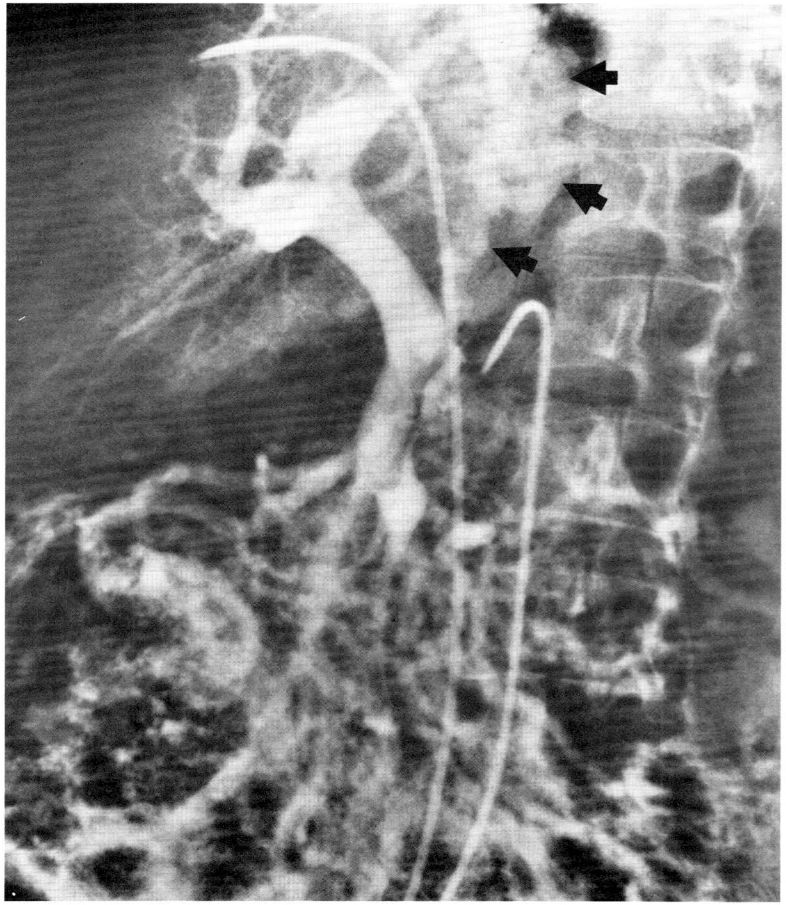

(D)

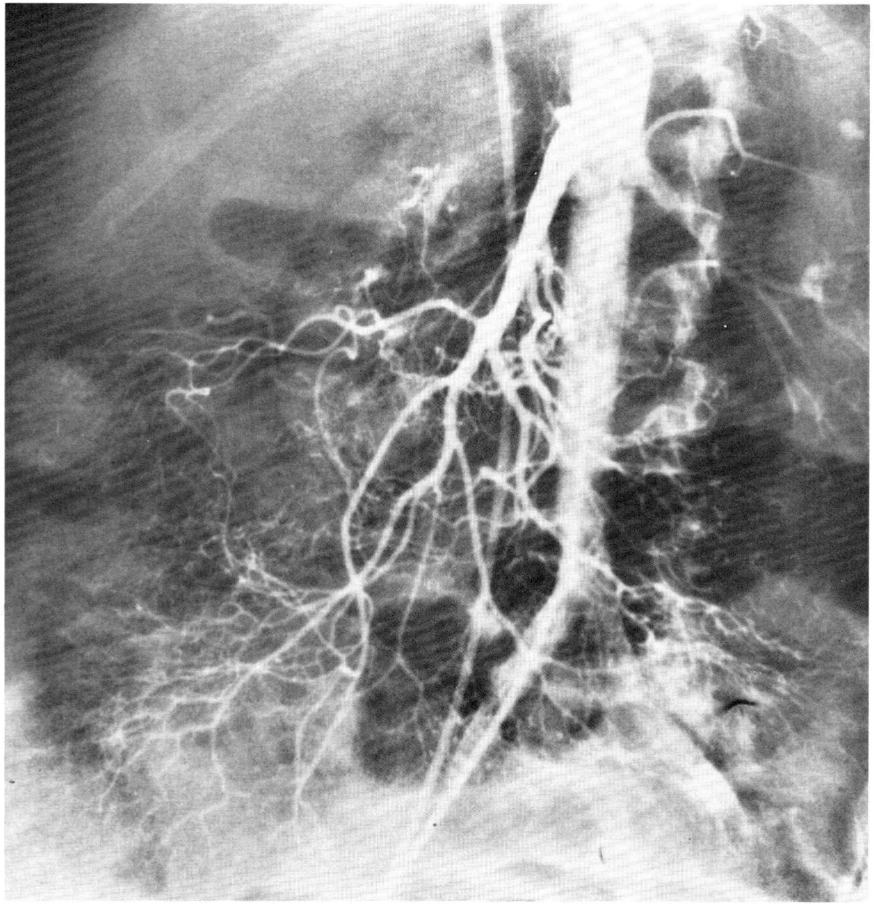

(E)

Figure 10 (continued)

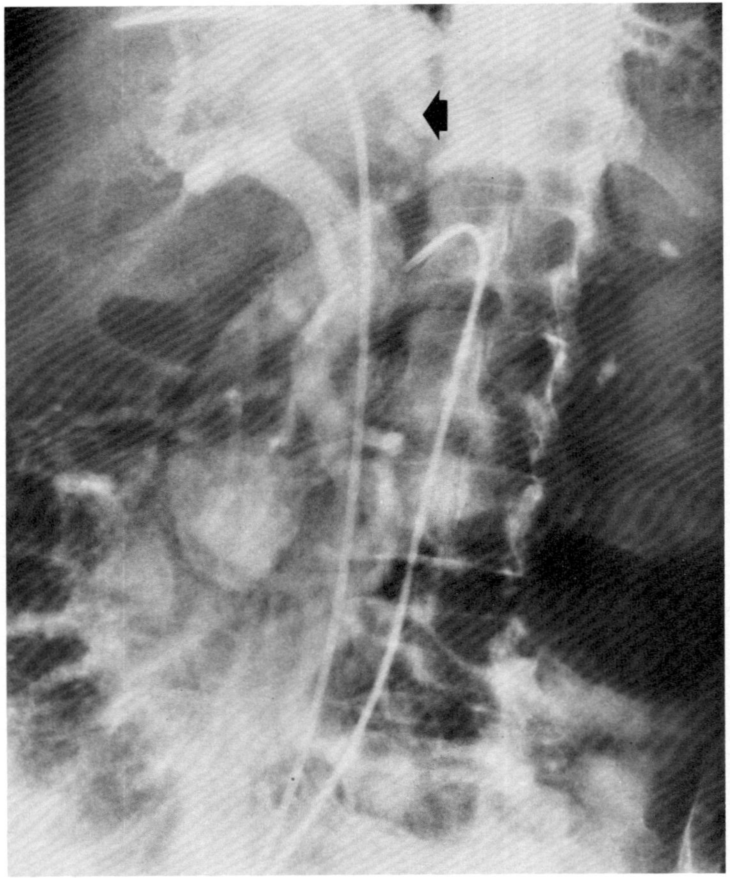

(F)

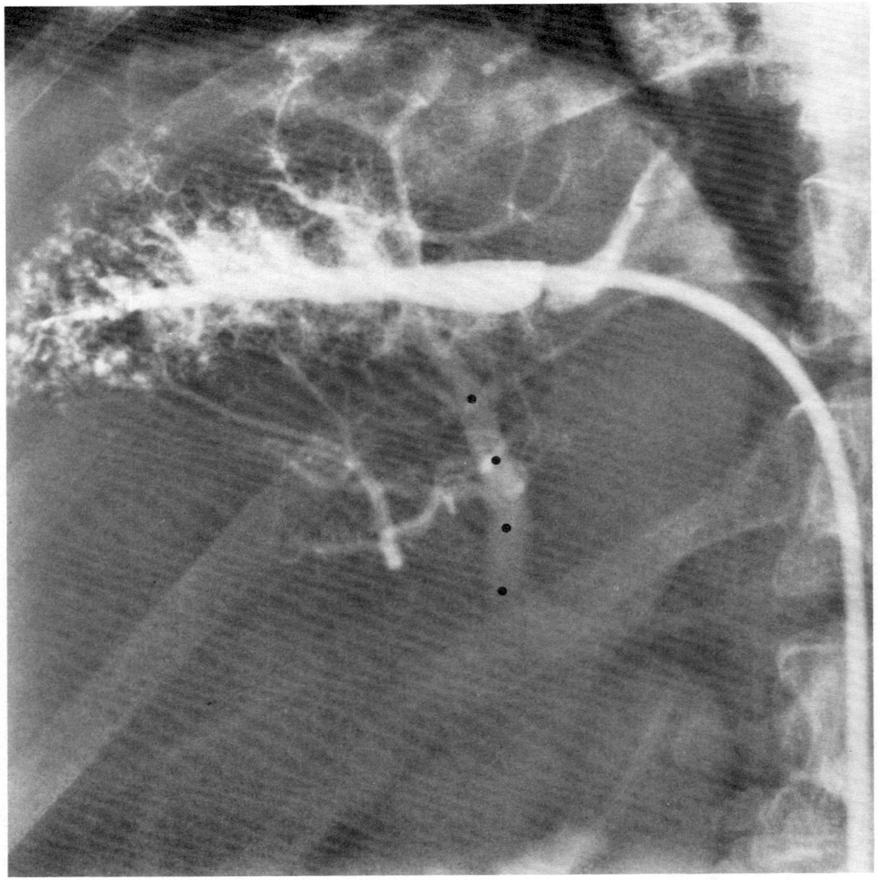

(G)

Figure 10 (continued)

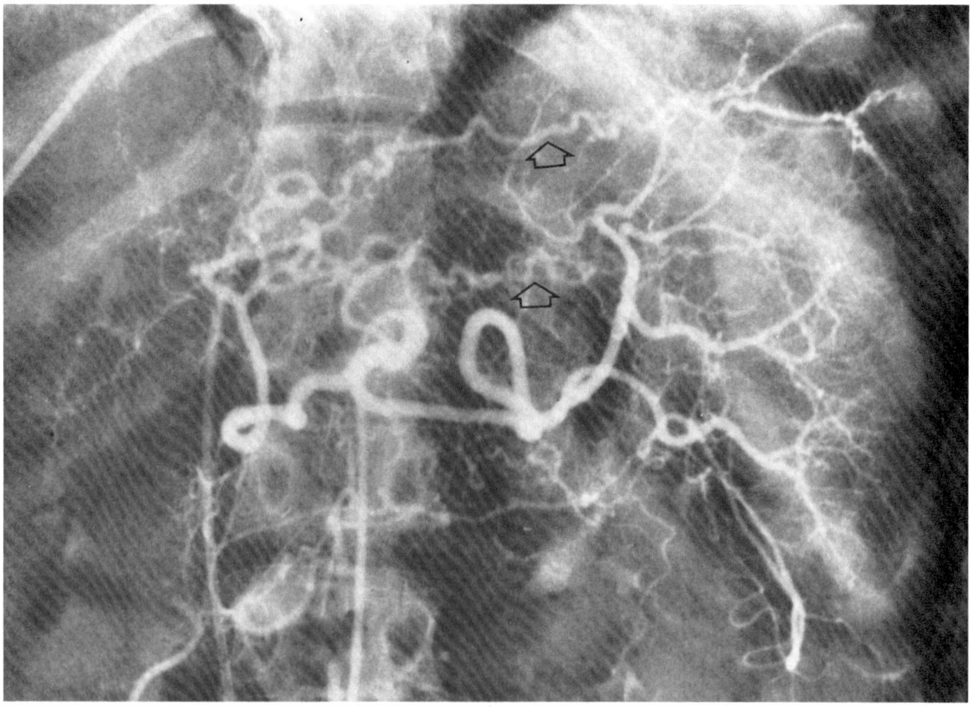

(A)

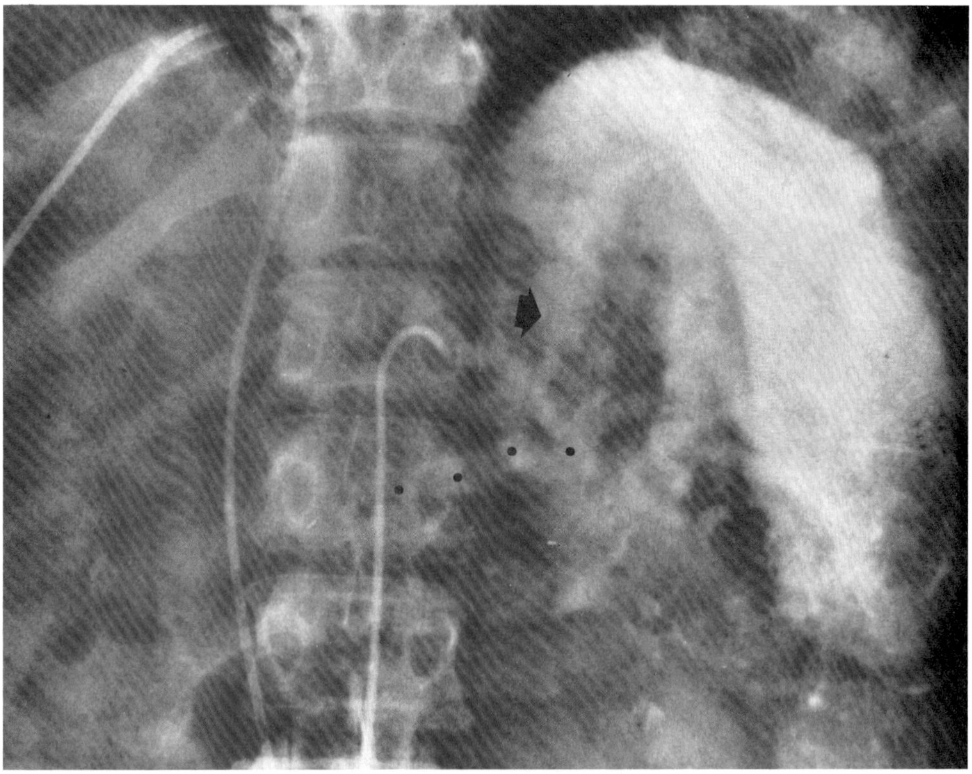

(B)

Figure 11

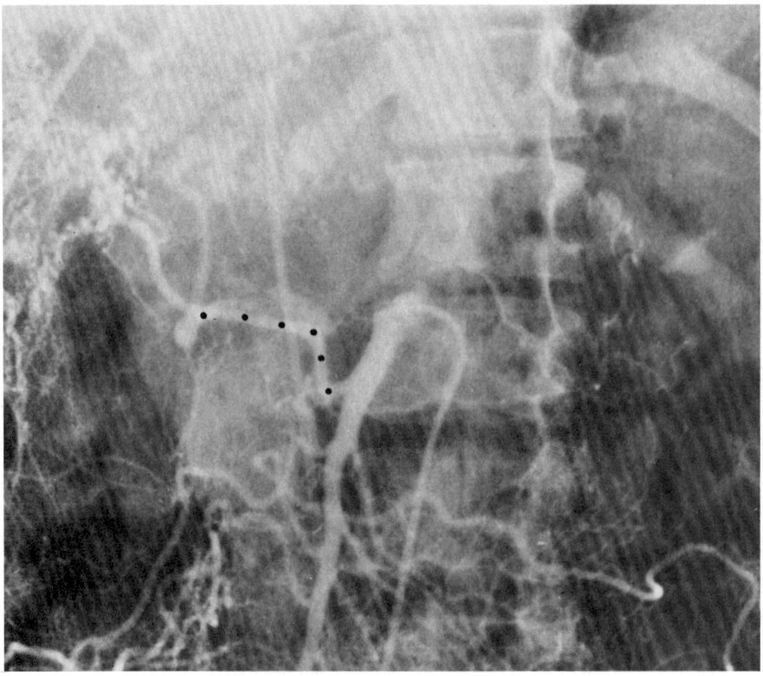

(C)

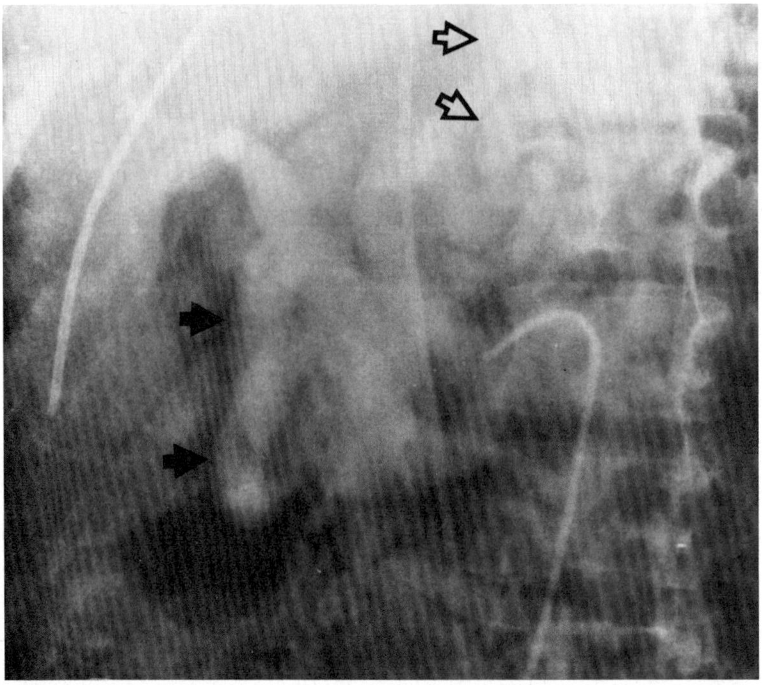

(D)

Figure 11 (continued)

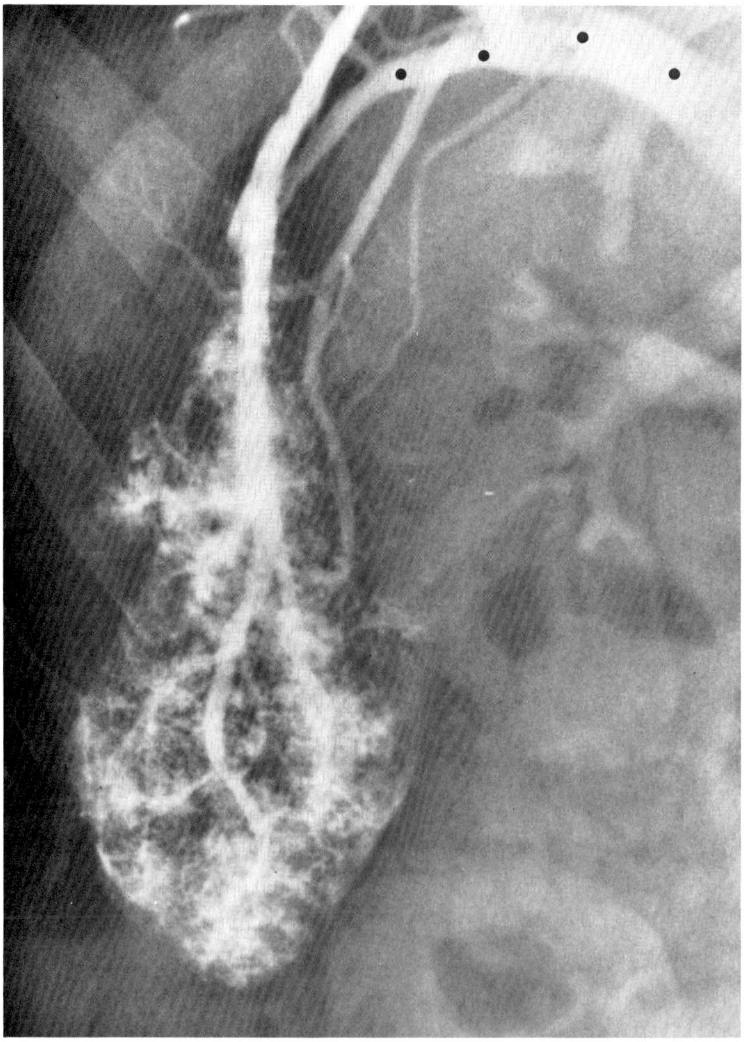

(E)

Figure 11 Stage IIB cirrhosis. (A) Celiac arteriogram, arterial phase. The left hepatic arterial branches are tortuous and irregular (arrows). (B) Celiac arteriogram, venous phase. Faint opacification of splenic vein (dots). Varices around the spenic hilus and the fundus of stomach are noted (arrow). (C) Superior mesenteric arteriogram, arterial phase. A replaced right hepatic artery (dots) supplies the right lobe, and its branches are very tortuous and irregular. (D) Superior mesenteric arteriogram, venous phase. The portal vein is patent; the umbilical vein (closed arrows) is enlarged and esophageal varices (open arrows) are present. (E) Wedged hepatic venography. Marked distortion of sinusoidogram and opacification of the portal vein (dots) up to the porta hepatis. The corrected sinusoidal pressure was 22 mmHg.

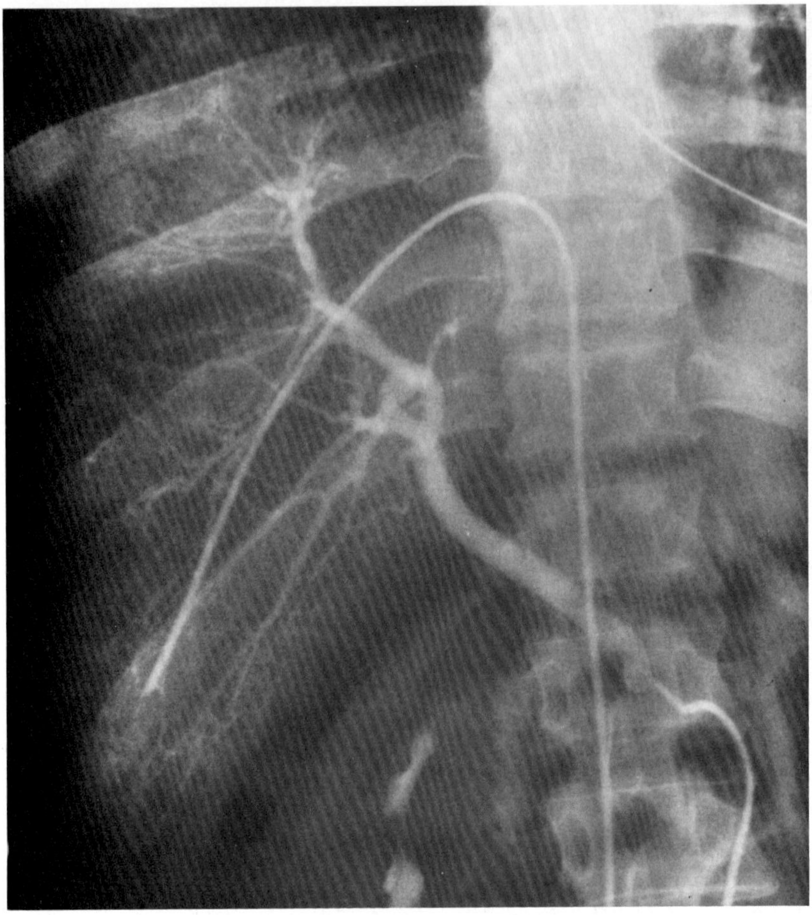

Figure 12A Stage III cirrhosis. Right hepatic arteriogram, arterial phase. The liver is hypervascular. Ascites.

by one of the following methods: (1) wedged hepatic venography, (2) percutaneous hepatography (see Chap. 17), and (3) hepatic venography with a balloon catheter. The wedged hepatic venogram is the method used most frequently and is usually part of the routine liver panangiography. Wedged hepatic venographic findings in cirrhosis are classified as follows (2,4):

Stage I: Hepatopetal portal flow: portal vein not opacified, or opacification lasting at most 2 sec (Fig. 9D).

Stage II: Bidirectional portal flow: opacification of both hepatic and portal veins. Because the majority of cirrhotic patients (70–80%) belong to this stage, it is further subdivided into:

IIA. Mild form: opacification of the portal vein for 2–4 sec (Fig. 10G).

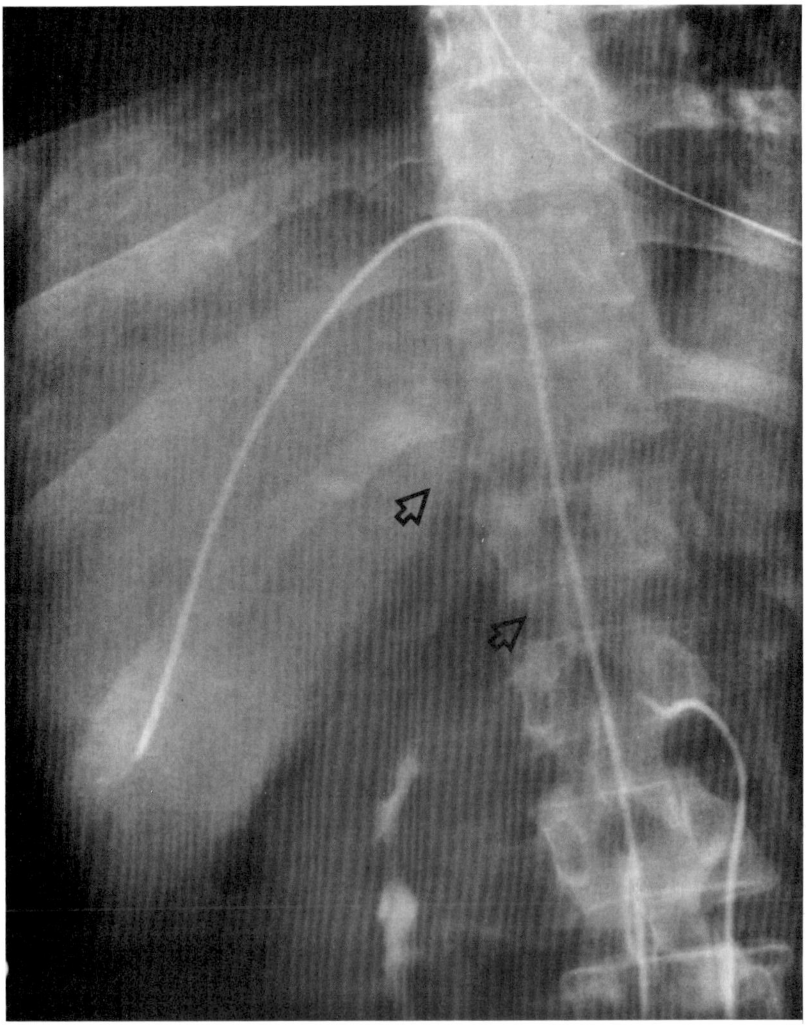

Figure 12B Right hepatic arteriogram, venous phase. Faint opacification of the portal vein (arrows), indicative of hepatofugal portal flow.

IIB. Severe form: opacification of the portal vein for longer than 4 sec, contrast medium stagnant in the intrahepatic portal vein (Fig. 11E)

Stage III: Hepatofugal flow: retrograde opacification of the entire portal system (i.e., both intrahepatic and extrahepatic) (Fig. 12C).

Hepatic venography has been considered to be more accurate than arterioportography in the evaluation of portal flow direction because (1) wedged hepatic venography directly opacifies the sinusoids, and (2) the use of vasodilator drugs to assist

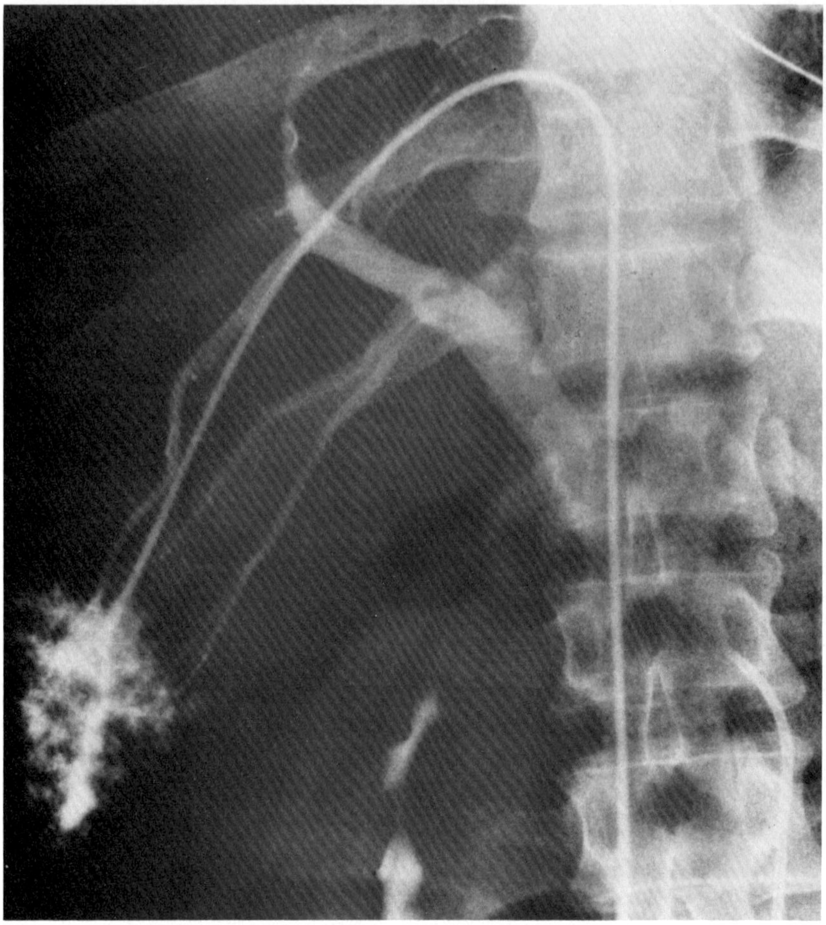

Figure 12C Wedged hepatic venography. Preferential hepatofugal portal flow is shown. The sinusoids are severely distorted. The corrected sinusoidal pressure was 19 mmHg.

portal vein opacification in arterioportography may transiently increase the portal flow and alter the hemodynamics.

If venographic staging of cirrhosis is to be meaningful, overinjection must be avoided. The ideal injection rate through a wedged hepatic vein catheter is 1 ml/sec for 4 sec, with a filming sequence of one film per second for 10–12 sec. Using an injection rate of 2 ml/sec for 4 sec, as has been employed in several departments of radiology, transient regurgitation of the contrast medium into the portal vein may occur in stage I cirrhosis. The manometric measurements in the wedged hepatic vein position and at other sites are important in the differentiation of intrahepatic and extrahepatic portal hypertension (see Table 1).

The panangiographic staging of cirrhosis is summarized in Table 4.

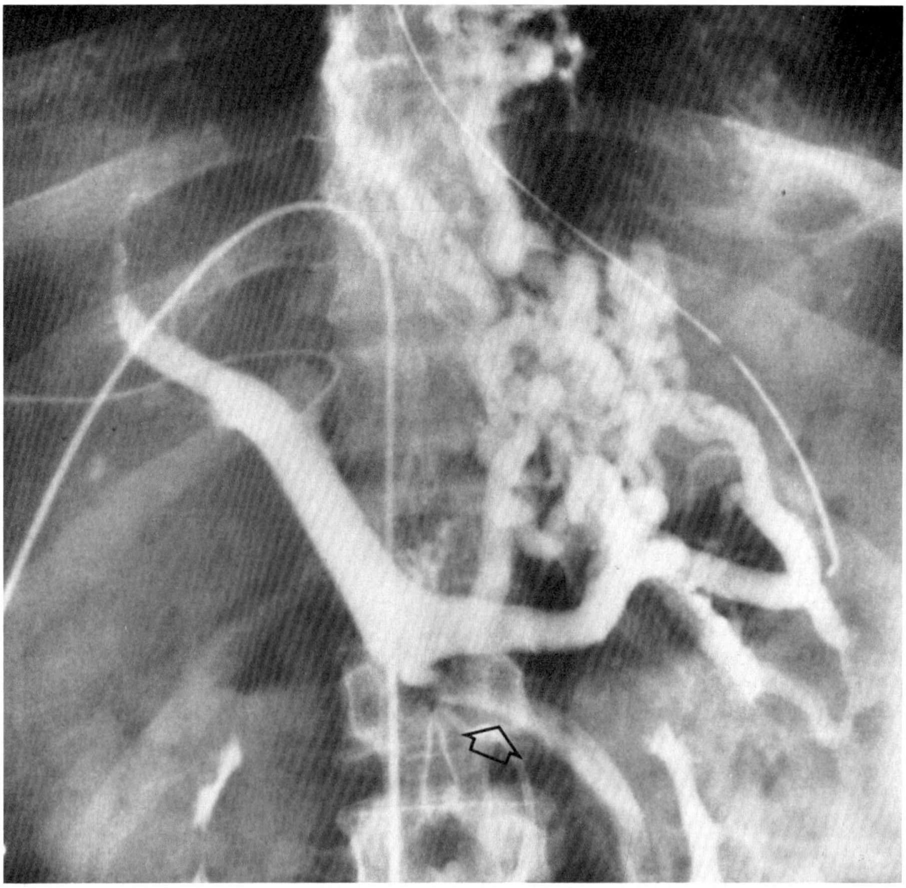

Figure 12D Percutaneous transhepatic portal venography. Well-opacified portal, splenic, and variceal veins. Note the preferential flow toward the esophageal varices instead of the inferior mesenteric vein (arrow).

Hepatic Vein Obstruction (Postsinusoidal)

Hepatic venous outflow obstruction, known as the *Budd-Chiari syndrome*, can be due to intrahepatic obstruction of major hepatic veins or their radicles or may relate to post-hepatic obstruction. The causes of hepatic vein obstruction can be classified as: (1) hyper-coagulation state (e.g., polycythemia vera, sickle cell disease, use of oral contraceptives, and nocturnal paroxysmal hemoglobinuria) (18) (Fig. 14); (2) occlusion by a tumor mass [e.g., hepatoma (Fig. 15), metastatic hepatic neoplasms, and inferior vena cava extension of renal carcinoma]; (3) veno-occlusive disease from certain plant poisons (*Crotalaria* or *Senecio*); and (4) idiopathic.

The clinical manifestations of the syndrome may be acute or subacute and the degree of hepatic vein obstruction may be complete or partial. Acute, complete occlusion

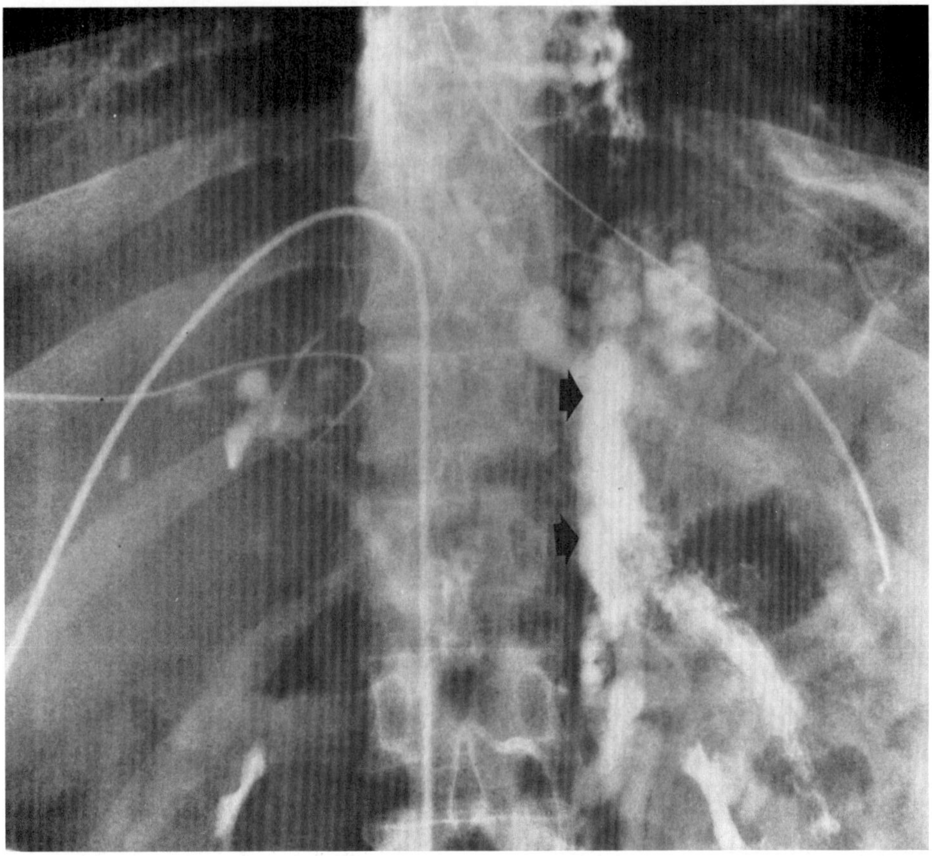

Figure 12E Late phase of percutaneous portal venography. Extravasation of contrast medium from the gastric varices into the stomach (arrows), demonstrating active variceal bleeding.

Table 3 Arteriographic Features in Cirrhosis

1.	Hypervascularity and a nonhomogeneous hepatogram
2.	Increased tortuosity of hepatic artery branches (corkscrew appearance)
3.	In the fatty liver, hepatomegaly with stretched arteries
4.	Apparent duplication of hepatic artery branches
5.	Splenomegaly
6.	A small and contracted liver
7.	Evidence of ascites
8.	Regenerating macronodules
9.	Hepatoma
10.	Arterioportal shunting

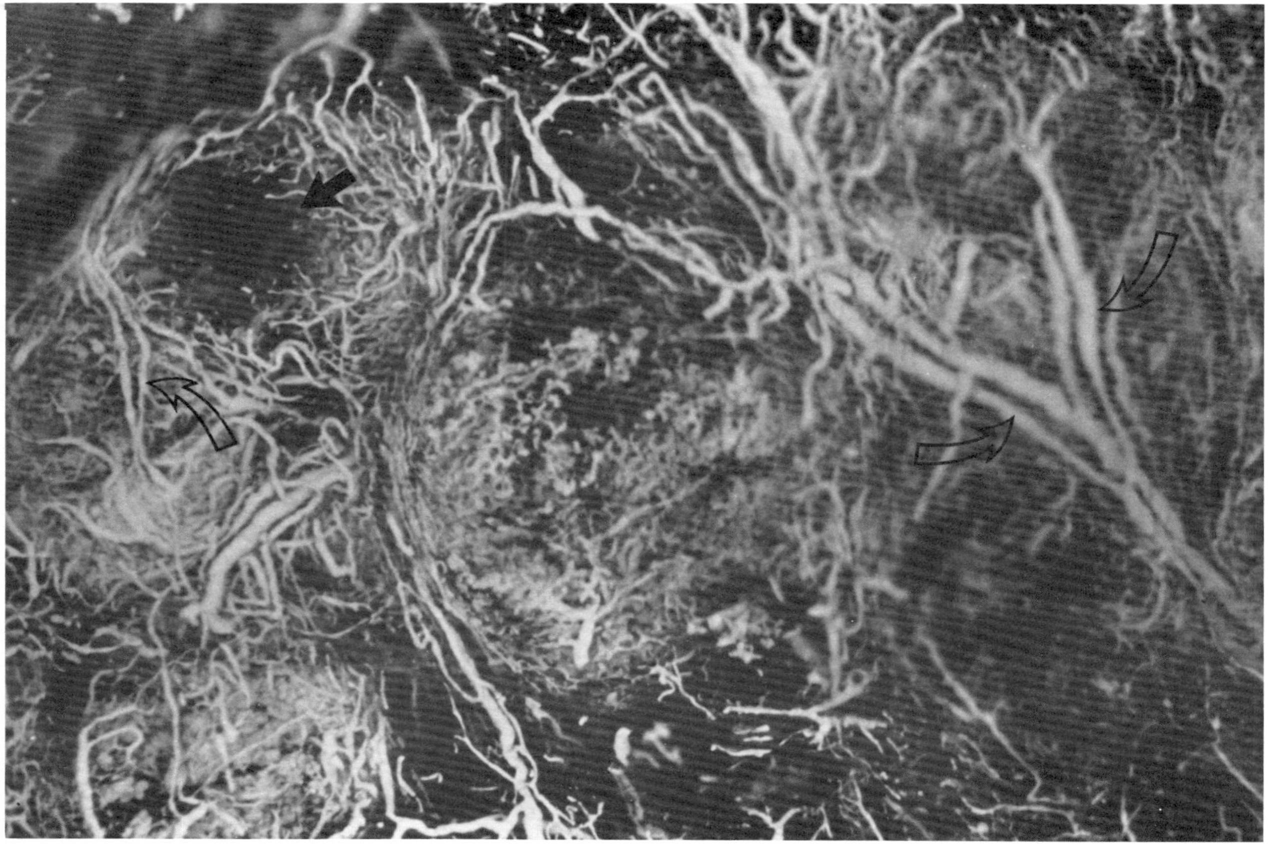

Figure 13 Microfil-injected cirrhotic liver, cleared specimen. ''Duplication'' of several hepatic artery branches (open arrows). Also, empty space due to nonfilling of sinusoids (arrow).

Table 4 Panangiography Staging of Cirrhosis

Stage I
- a. Normal or slightly increased vascularity of the liver
- b. Hepatopetal portal flow (normal splenic, superior mesenteric, and portal veins)
- c. No varices
- d. Wedged hepatic venography—drainage via hepatic veins
- e. Normal to mildly elevated corrected sinusoidal pressure (CSP)

Stage II
- a. Mild hypervascularity of the liver
- b. Opacification of both portal vein and *varices* (bidirectional portal flow)
- c. Wedged hepatic venography—opacification of portal vein for 2–4 sec but with eventual drainage into the hepatic vein in stage IIA. In stage IIB, opacification of the segmental or main portal vein for more than 4 sec (almost standstill)
- d. Moderately elevated CSP
- e. Ascites may be present

Stage III
- a. Liver usually small and contracted
- b. Markedly hypervascular liver
- c. Demonstration of varices with nonvisualization of the portal vein at arterioportography
- d. Wedged hepatic venography with drainage into the portal vein
- e. Ascites often present

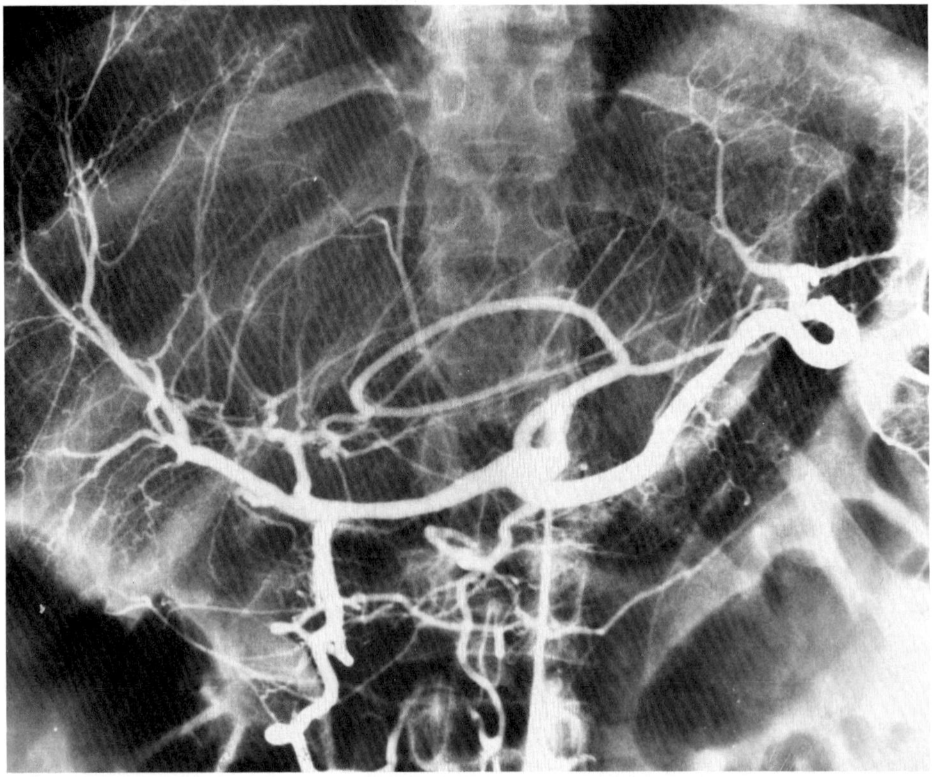

(A)

Figure 14

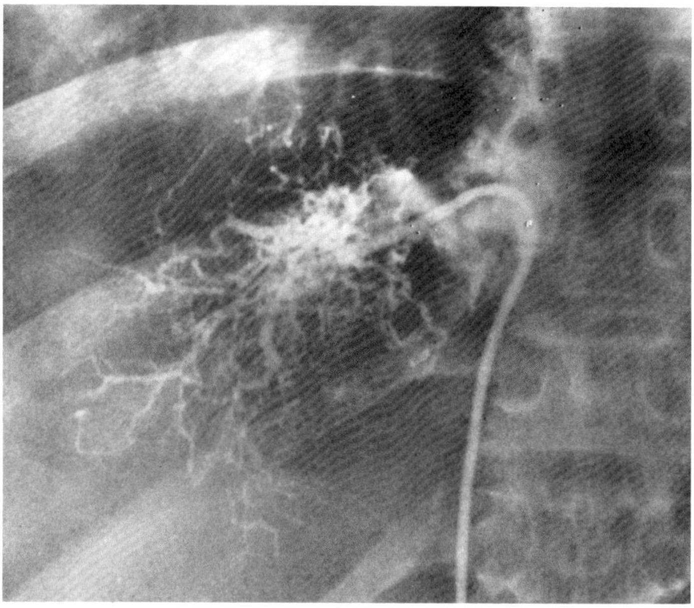

(B)

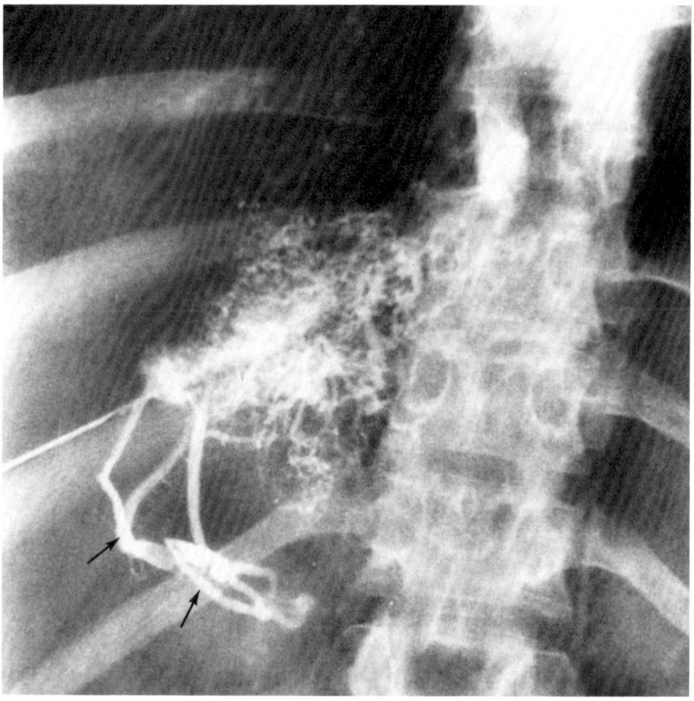

(C)

Figure 14 Patient with paroxysmal nocturnal hemoglobinuria. (A) Celiac angiography. Enlarged liver with stretched hepatic arteries. (B) Retrograde hepatic venography showing hepatic vein thrombosis and a spider's web pattern typical of the Budd-Chiari syndrome. (C) Transhepatic parenchymal injection of contrast medium shows occlusion of the main right hepatic vein with collaterals and a small patent hepatic vein (arrows) draining into the inferior vena cava.

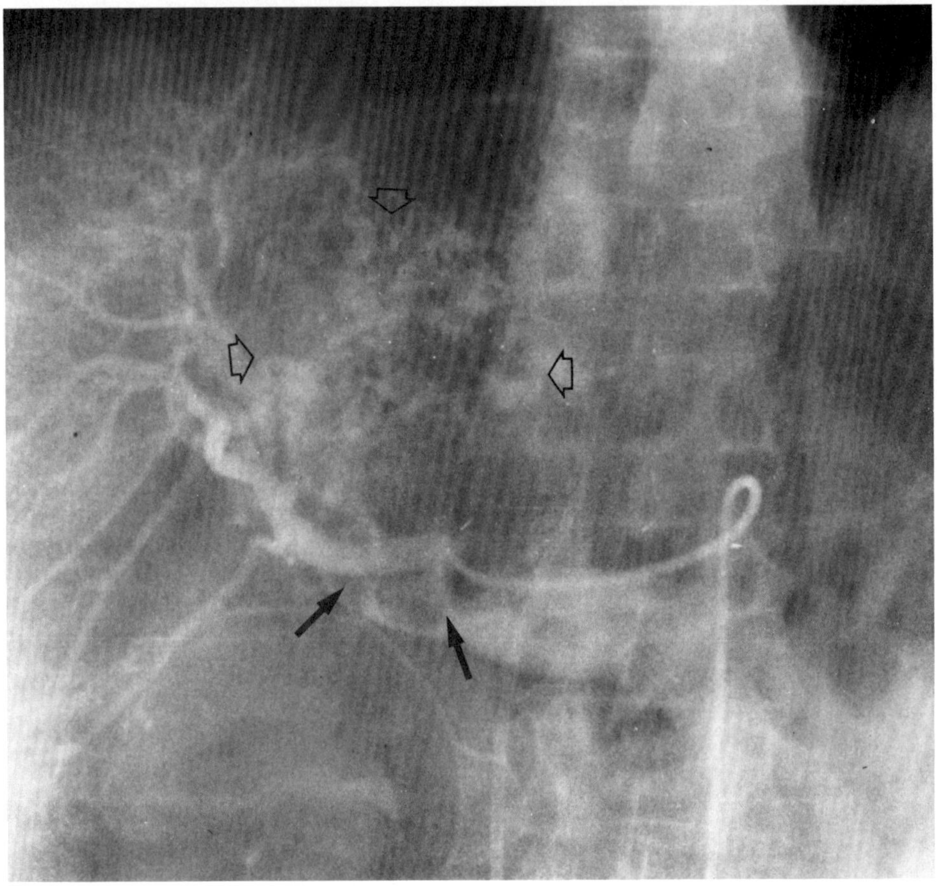

Figure 15A Hepatoma with portal vein, hepatic vein, and inferior vena cava extension. Proper hepatic arteriogram. A hypervascular mass with extensive tumor stain is seen in the medial segment of the left lobe (arrows). The poor arterial opacification of the liver itself results from the markedly increased arterial flow to the hypervascular tumor. Early opacification of the portal vein (closed arrows) is due to arterioportal shunting.

presents with liver failure and shock. In less acute cases, intractable ascites is the major manifestation. Retrograde thrombosis may extend to the portal system and may result in intestinal infarction.

The diagnosis is difficult clinically and many cases are discovered only at autopsy. This applies particularly to the diagnosis of the unilobar form of Budd-Chiari syndrome (19). The *angiographic features* include stretching of the hepatic artery branches, intense hepatic capillary blush, a mottled and prolonged hepatogram, and an enlarged, edematous liver (Fig. 14A), most of these nonspecific findings. Occasionally, the angiographic features are difficult to differentiate from those of metastases (20). Inferior vena cavograms sometimes demonstrate occlusion of the cava by thrombus or tumor.

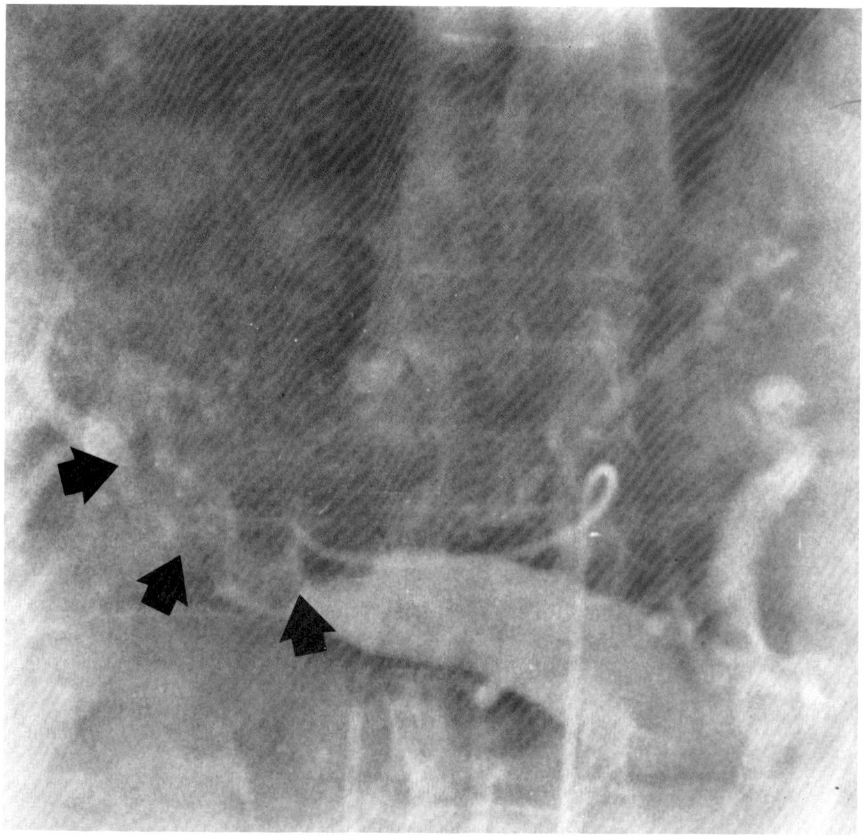

Figure 15B Hepatogram phase. The tumor stain has cleared very early, typical of a hepatoma. The tumor extension to the portal vein (arrows) and the arterioportal shunt are well demonstrated.

Despite the occlusion of the hepatic vein, a *hepatic venogram* can usually be performed and the hepatic venographic findings are more specific. Because of the hepatic vein obstruction, contrast medium injected into the hepatic parenchyma is diverted into multiple irregular collateral channels, giving a typical "spider's web" appearance (19,21) (Fig. 14B).

Posthepatic

Posthepatic portal hypertension results from diseases in the hepatic segment of the inferior vena cava and the heart. The cardiac causes are right heart failure, constrictive pericarditis, and rheumatic heart disease, which can lead to cardiac liver cirrhosis, a consequence of passive congestion. Obstruction of the inferior vena cava by a congenital web (see Fig. 31 in Chap. 2) or a tumor, either a hepatoma extending through the hepatic vein (Fig. 15) or a renal carcinoma extending through the renal vein, may result in portal

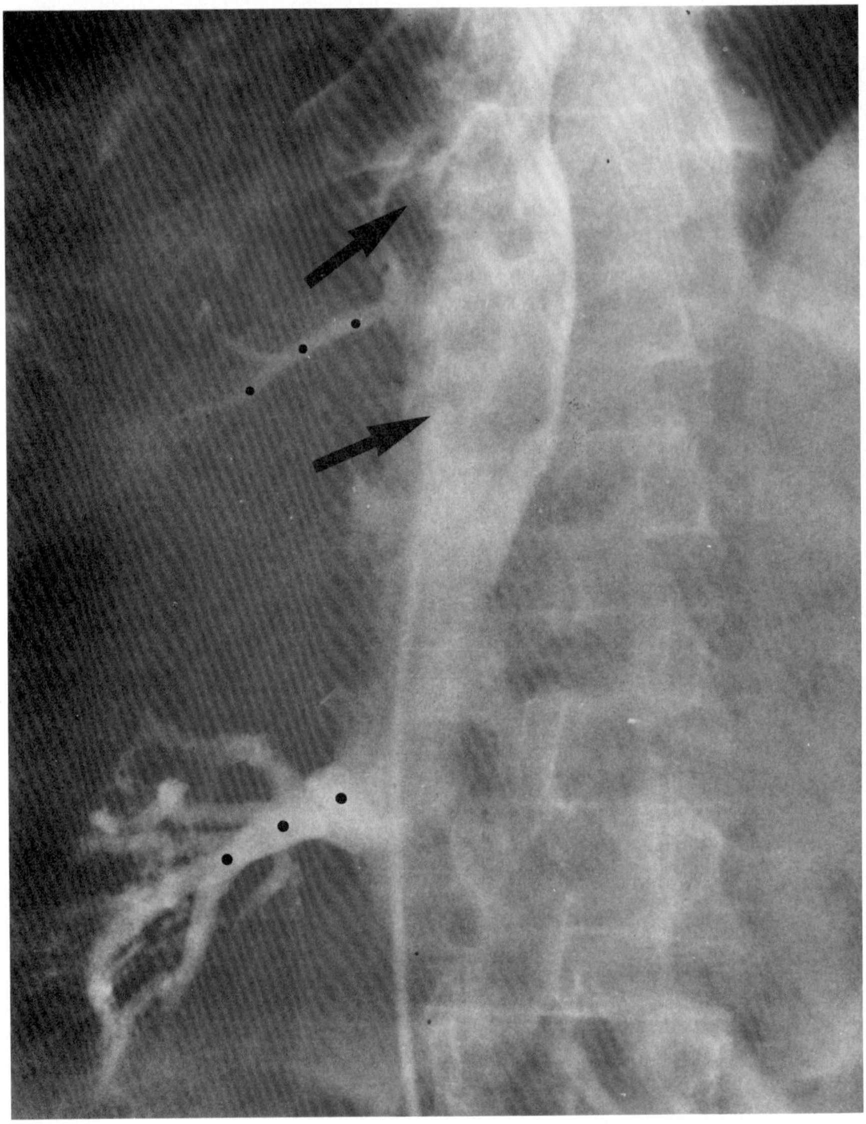

Figure 15C Inferior vena cavogram. Extension of the hepatoma from the hepatic vein into the inferior vena cava (arrows). Note that only a small branch of hepatic vein is still patent (dots).

hypertension of posthepatic type. The clinical manifestations may be indistinguishable from the Budd-Chiari syndrome.

The following case illustrates the value of liver panangiography in the evaluation of liver disease of unknown etiology. A known drug addict was hospitalized for intractable ascites. An arteriogram was requested to exclude Budd-Chiari syndrome. The liver was

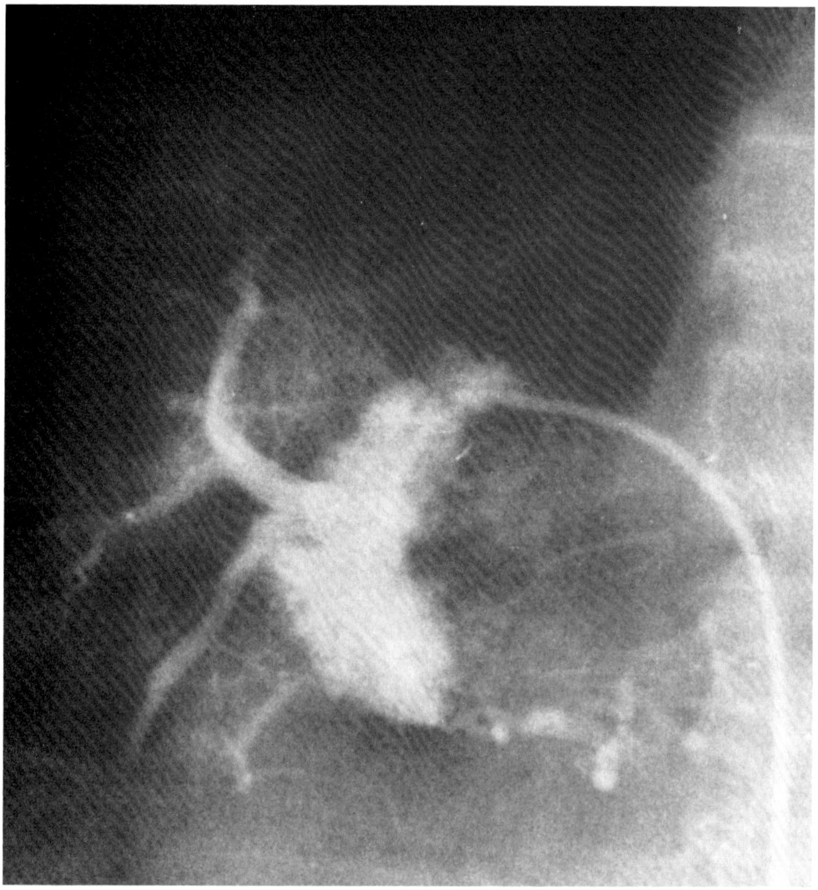

Figure 15D Hepatic venogram. The catheter was passed through a nonoccluded hepatic vein into a wedged position. The study reveals the major portion of the hepatic vein to be occluded by the tumor. A patent segmental hepatic vein and area of normal sinusoids are seen lateral to the mass.

normal except for slowed arterial flow. Hepatic venography showed normal hepatic sinusoids and patent hepatic veins, which ruled out the Budd-Chiari syndrome (Fig. 16). The manometric recordings were of diagnostic value, the WHVP was notably elevated at 23.5 mmHg, and the pressures in the right atrium, free hepatic vein, and high and low inferior vena cava were biphasic (systole and diastole) and elevated, similar to the pressure in the right ventricle. The findings were consistent with tricuspid insufficiency, subsequently confirmed by cardiac catheterization. The inferior vena cavogram showed right atrial flow to be directed to the inferior vena cava and hepatic veins in systole (cardiofugal) and directed to the heart in diastole (cardiopetal). The tricuspid insufficiency was secondary to drug-induced endocarditis.

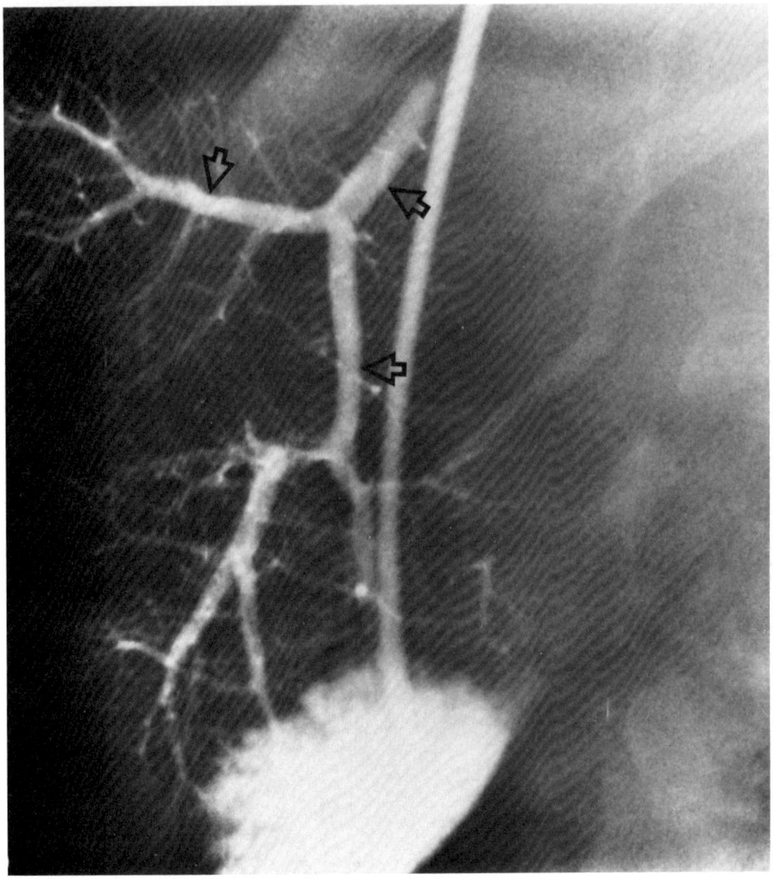

Figure 16A Tricuspid insufficiency in a drug addict with intractable ascites. Wedged hepatic venogram, early phase. Normal homogeneous hepatic sinusoidogram. Regurgitation of contrast medium into portal vein branches (open arrows) partly due to injection pressure and partly due to passive congestion of the hepatic vein.

Venous Collaterals

When the hepatic venous outflow can no longer cope with the entire hepatic arterial inflow, the direction of the portal flow will reverse to become hepatofugal. This change in direction is preceded by a segmental hepatofugal flow within the liver, usually in the dorsocaudal segment of the right lobe (Fig. 17). The hepatofugal portal flow can be reversed to hepatopetal if the arterial inflow is transiently reduced by administering a vasoconstrictor (22). Occasionally, the flow in the main stem of the portal vein is

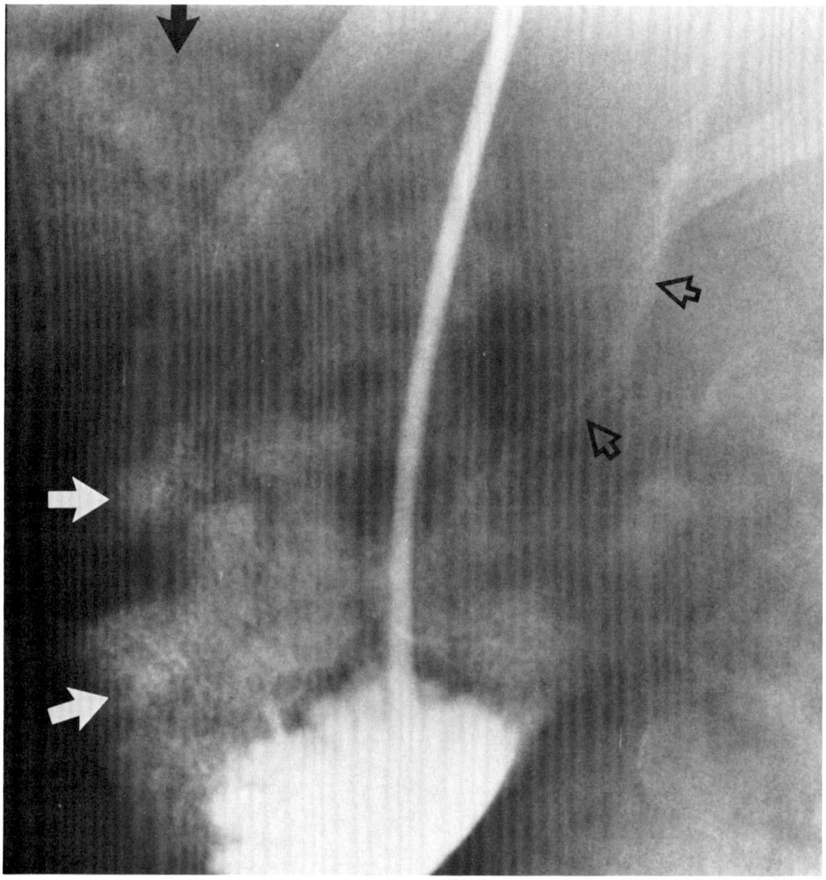

Figure 16B Contrast medium in the portal vein flows in the hepatopetal direction (toward hepatic sinusoids) and results in a lighter secondary sinusoidogram (closed arrows). The contrast medium in the primary sinusoidogram drains to a hepatic vein (open arrows). The patent hepatic vein and normal sinusoidogram ruled out Budd-Chiari syndrome.

hepatopetal in spite of total hepatofugal flow within the liver itself. This may occur when the umbilical vein is capable of draining not only the arterial inflow but also part of the venous return from the spleen and the gastrointestinal tract (Fig. 18).

The *major collateral channels* in portal hypertension are (23):

1. The coronary, or left gastric vein (Fig. 19) and the short gastric veins, leading to esophageal varices and the azygos or hemiazygos
2. The paraumbilical vein (Figs. 20, 21)

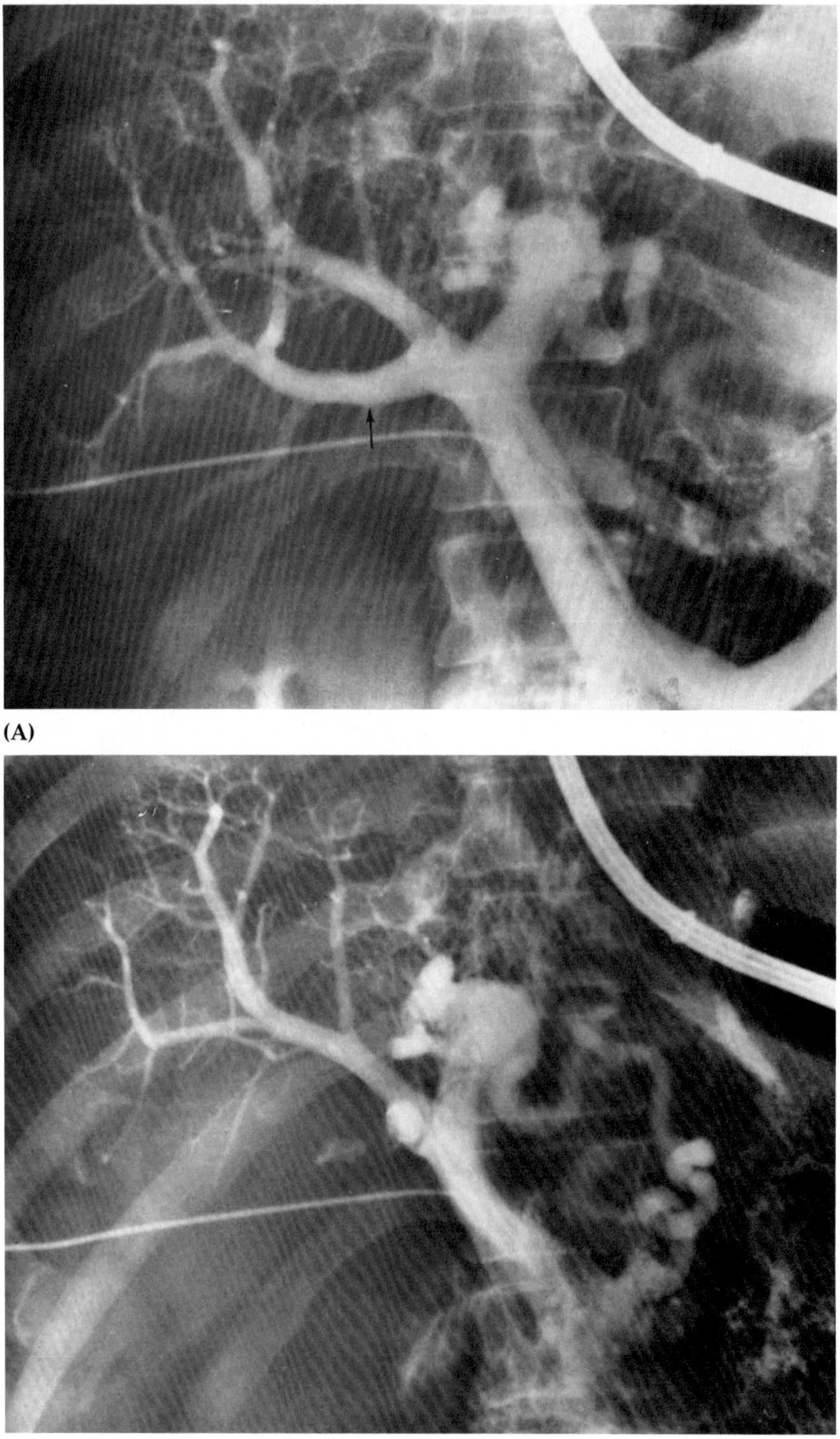

(A)

(B)

Figure 17

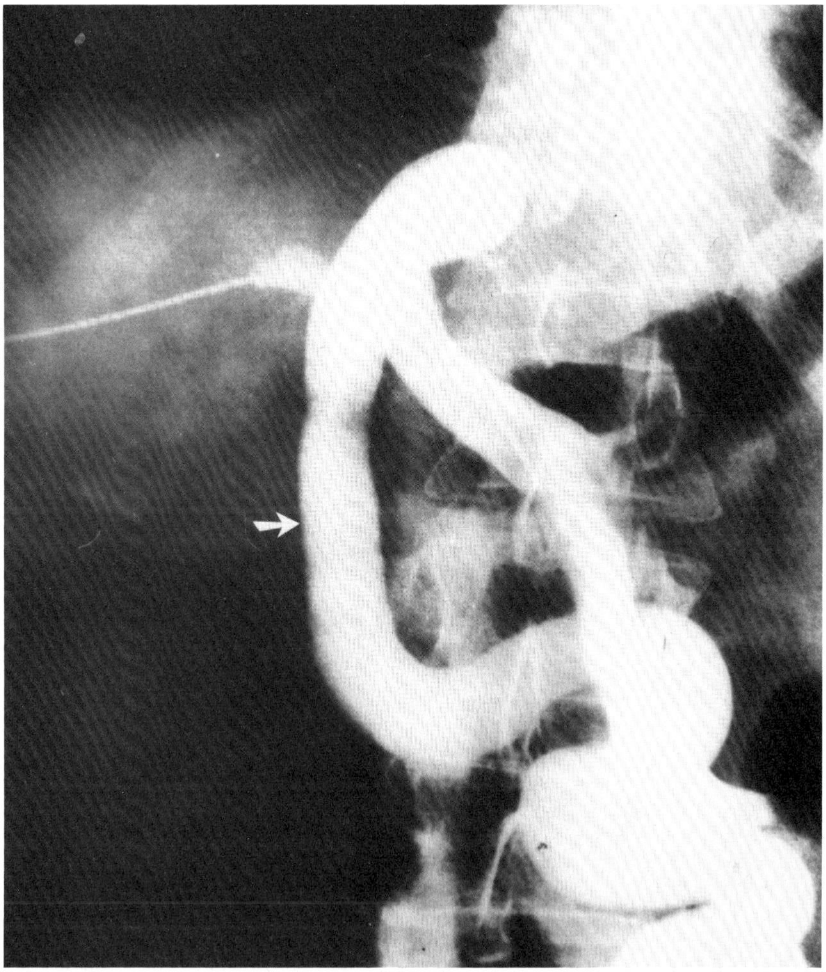

Figure 18 Transhepatic portography in a patient with portal hypertension. Total hepatofugal flow within the liver in spite of hepatopetal flow in the main stem of the portal vein, due to substantial fugal flow in a wide paraumbilical vein (arrow).

Figure 17 Transhepatic portography in a patient with portal hypertension. (A) The slight increase in pressure caused by the injection of contrast medium produces transient hepatopetal flow in a portal vein branch to the dorsocaudal segment of the right lobe (arrow). (B) A few seconds later, with the pressure reduced at the end of injection, hepatofugal flow has cleared contrast from this segmental branch.

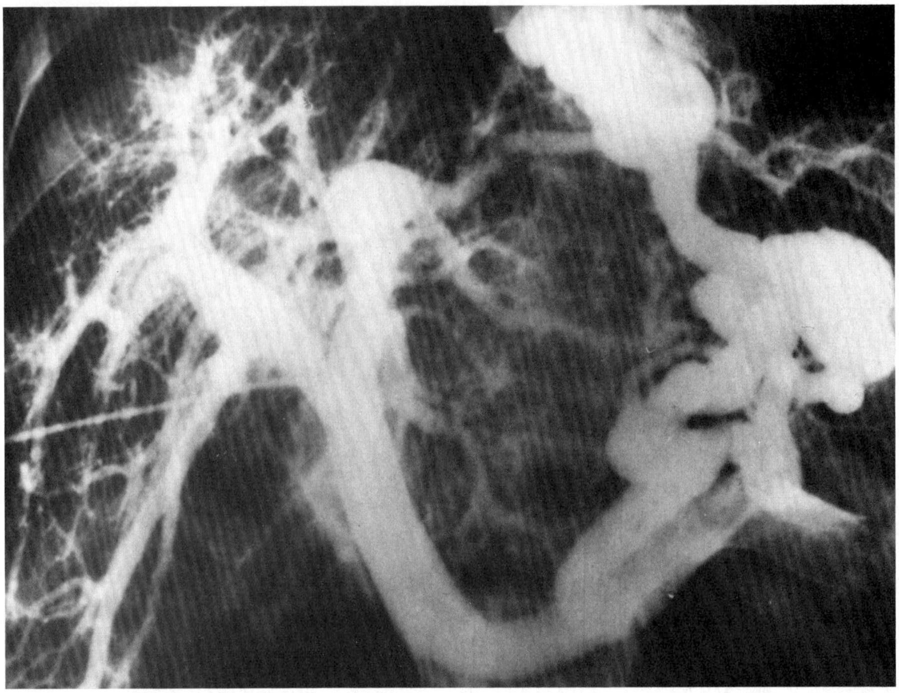

Figure 19 Patient with portal hypertension and esophageal varices. Transhepatic portography. Retrograde flow in a wide left gastric vein, tortuous collaterals in the fundus of the stomach, and wide esophageal varices.

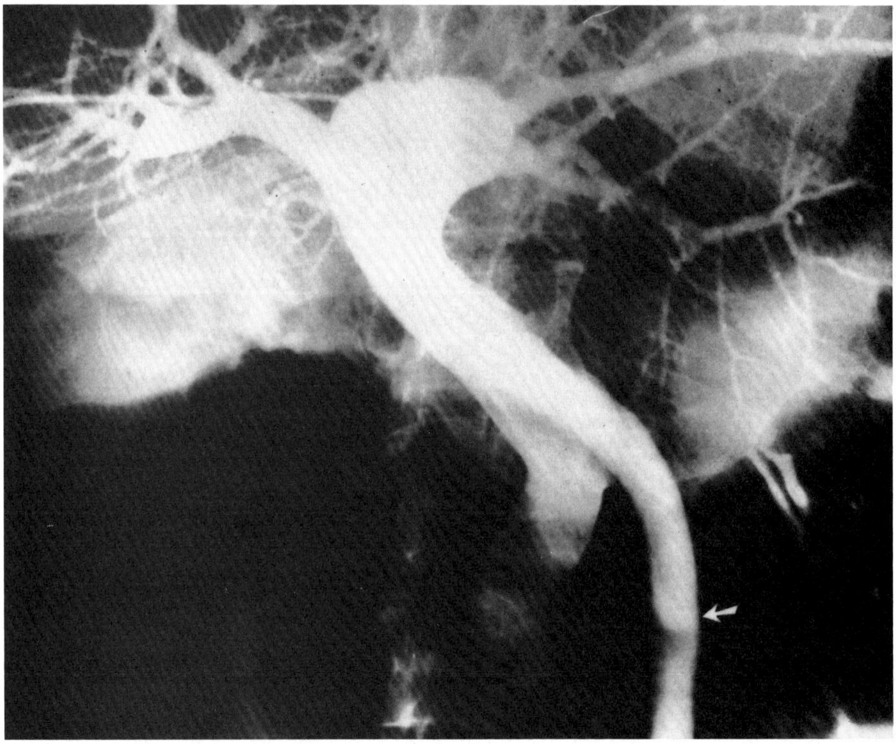

Figure 20A Transhepatic portography in a patient with portal hypertension. Retrograde flow into the upper portion of a paraumbilical vein (arrow).

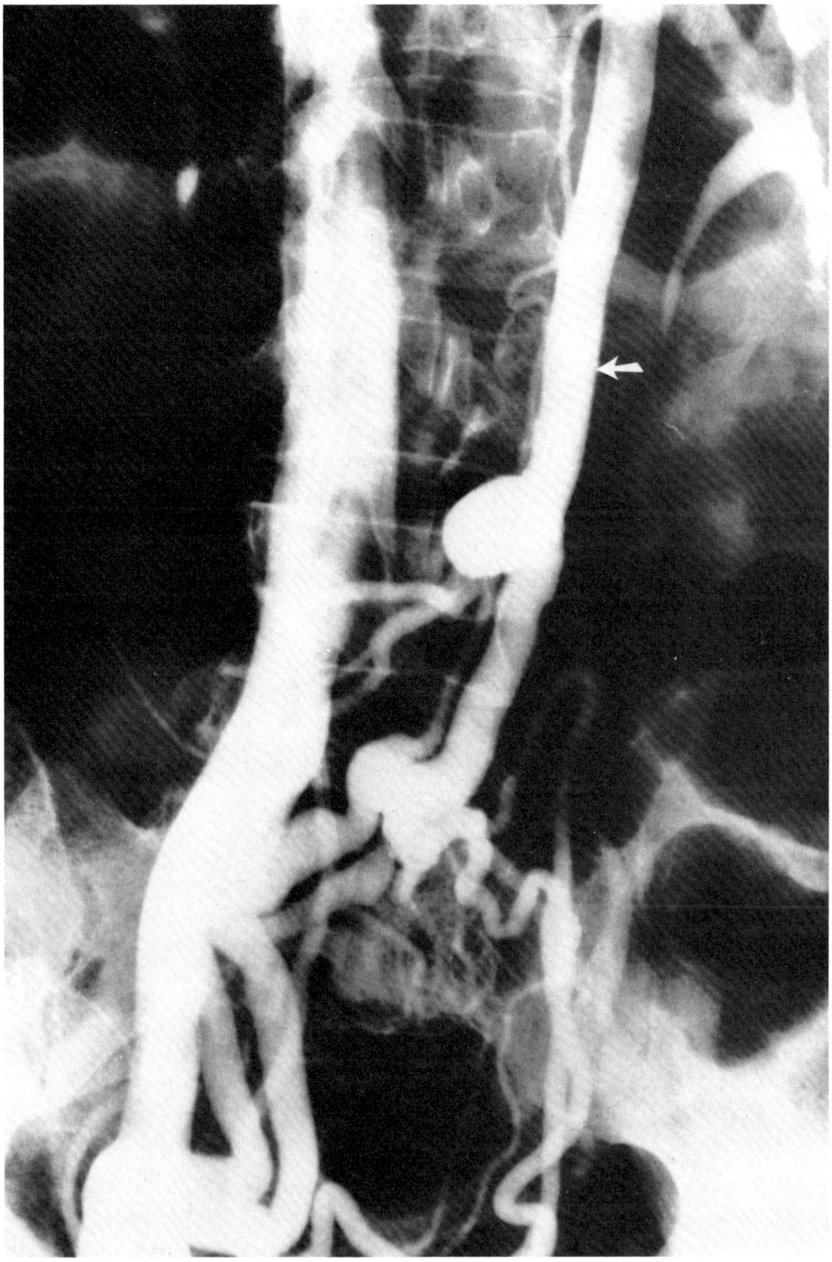

Figure 20B Retrograde flow through the lower portion of the paraumbilical vein (arrow) with wide connections to the inferior vena cava.

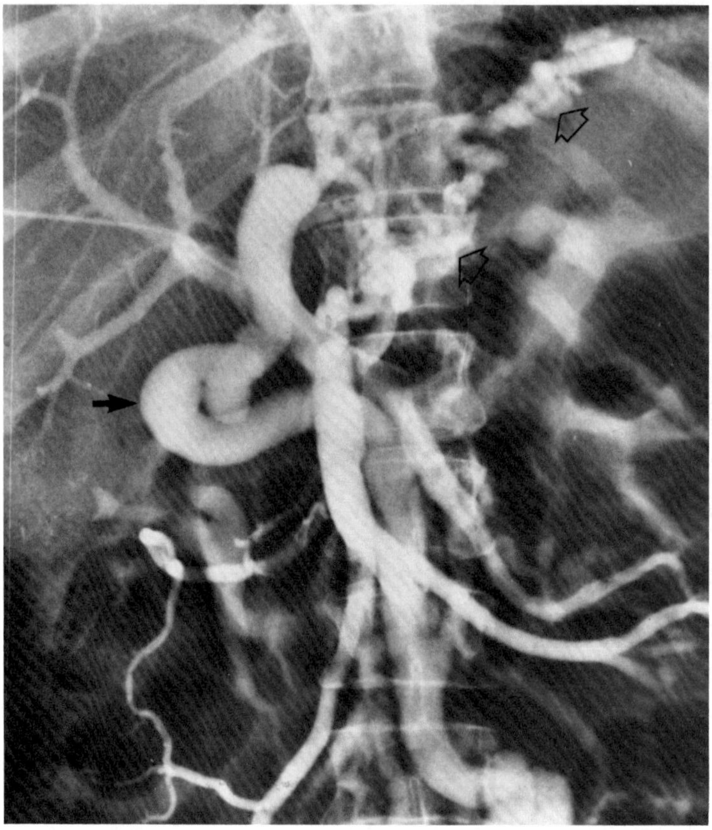

Figure 21 Patient with portal hypertension, portal venous pressure 31 cm H_2O. Transhepatic portography. Retrograde flow through a wide paraumbilical vein (arrow). Flow rate 1.350 ml/min (measured with Lipiodol droplets). Coronary vein opacified (open arrows).

3. The inferior mesenteric vein (Fig. 22)
4. The superior mesenteric vein (Fig. 23)
5. Retroperitoneal veins, which include several groups:
   a. The vein of Sappy (from liver to diaphragm)
   b. The veins in the splenorenal ligament to adrenal and left renal veins (Fig. 24)
   c. The lumbar veins or veins of Retzius (6,24)

Many other unnamed collaterals are often present. CT and ultrasound (24) are capable of demonstrating major hepatofugal venous collaterals with increasing confidence.

Of all the portosystemic collaterals, the left gastric and short gastric veins are the most frequently encountered and the most important because they drain to the esophageal varices. They comprise the shortest route to the lower-pressure systemic veins. The clinical importance of the esophageal varices is due to their potential for gastrointestinal hemorrhage and exsanguination.

Downhill esophageal varices are a rare abnormality. Portal hypertension-related varices reach only as far as the midthoracic level of the esophagus, where they communicate with the azygos and hemiazygos system. Downhill varices are formed to bypass superior vena cava obstruction and to communicate with the azygos system, when they occupy the upper half of the esophagus, or with the inferior vena cava through the portal system, when they extend through the entire length of the esophagus (25). Caval obstruction is usually due to malignant disease, more rarely to a mediastinal goiter or sclerosing mediastinitis (Fig. 25).

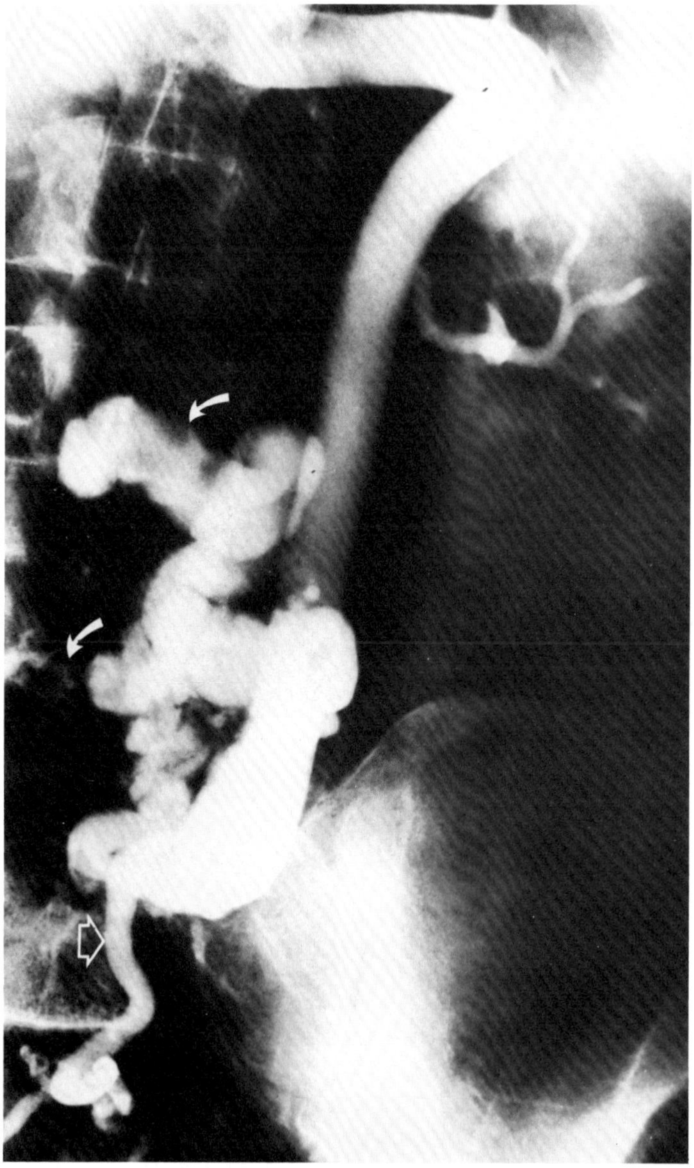

Figure 22 Transhepatic portography in a patient with portal hypertension and hepatofugal flow in the portal vein. Retrograde flow in a large inferior mesenteric vein. Wide collaterals to the inferior vena cava (arrows) and superior hemorrhoidal vein (open arrow).

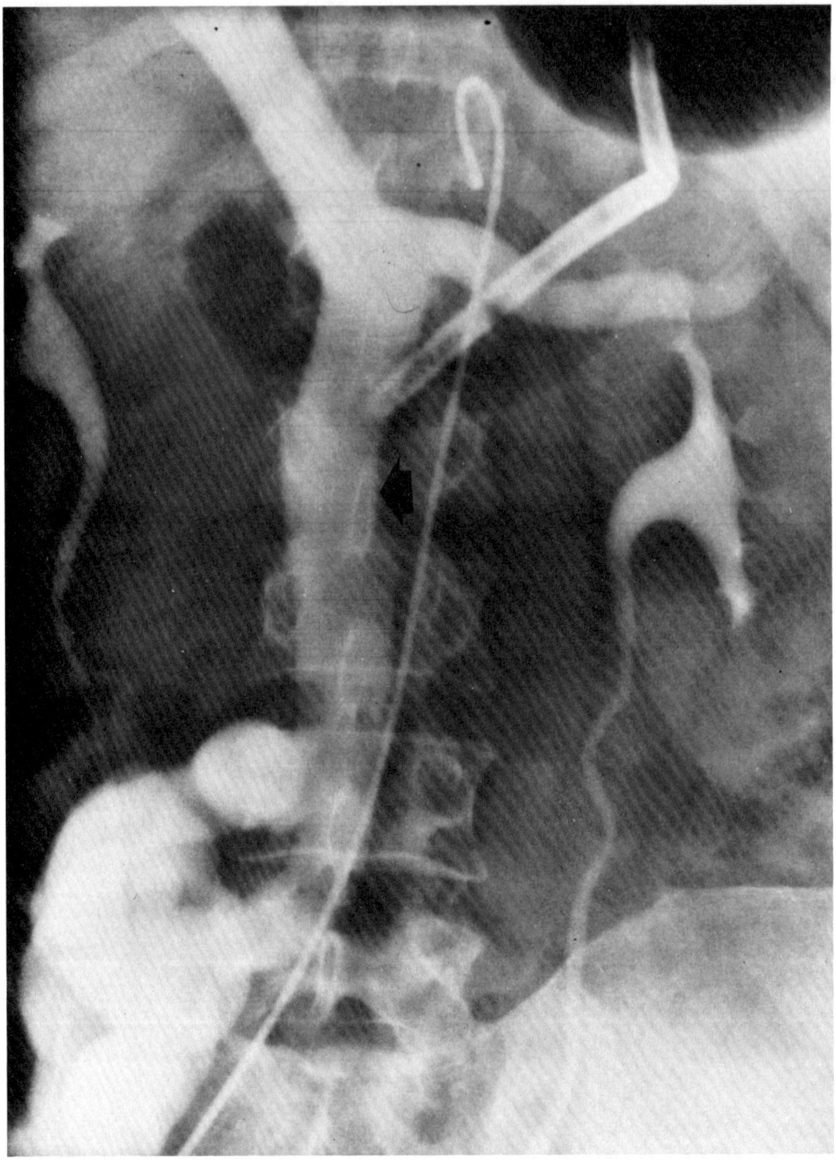

Figure 23A Spontaneous portosystemic shunt through the superior mesenteric vein. Percutaneous transhepatic portal venography with injection into the portal vein. Retrograde flow into the superior mesenteric vein (arrow) and ileocolic vein.

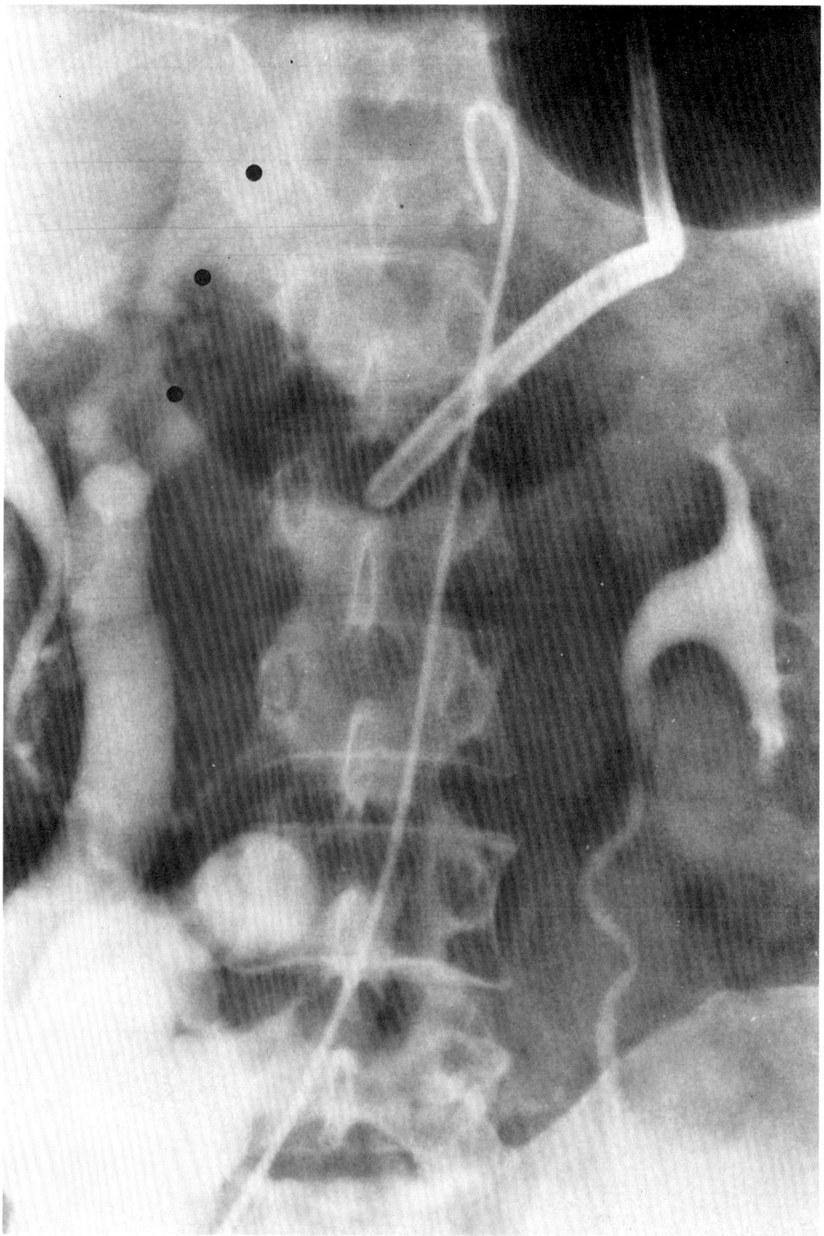

Figure 23B A large varicose venous channel leads to a retroperitoneal (or ovarian) vein, then communicates with the inferior vena cava (dots).

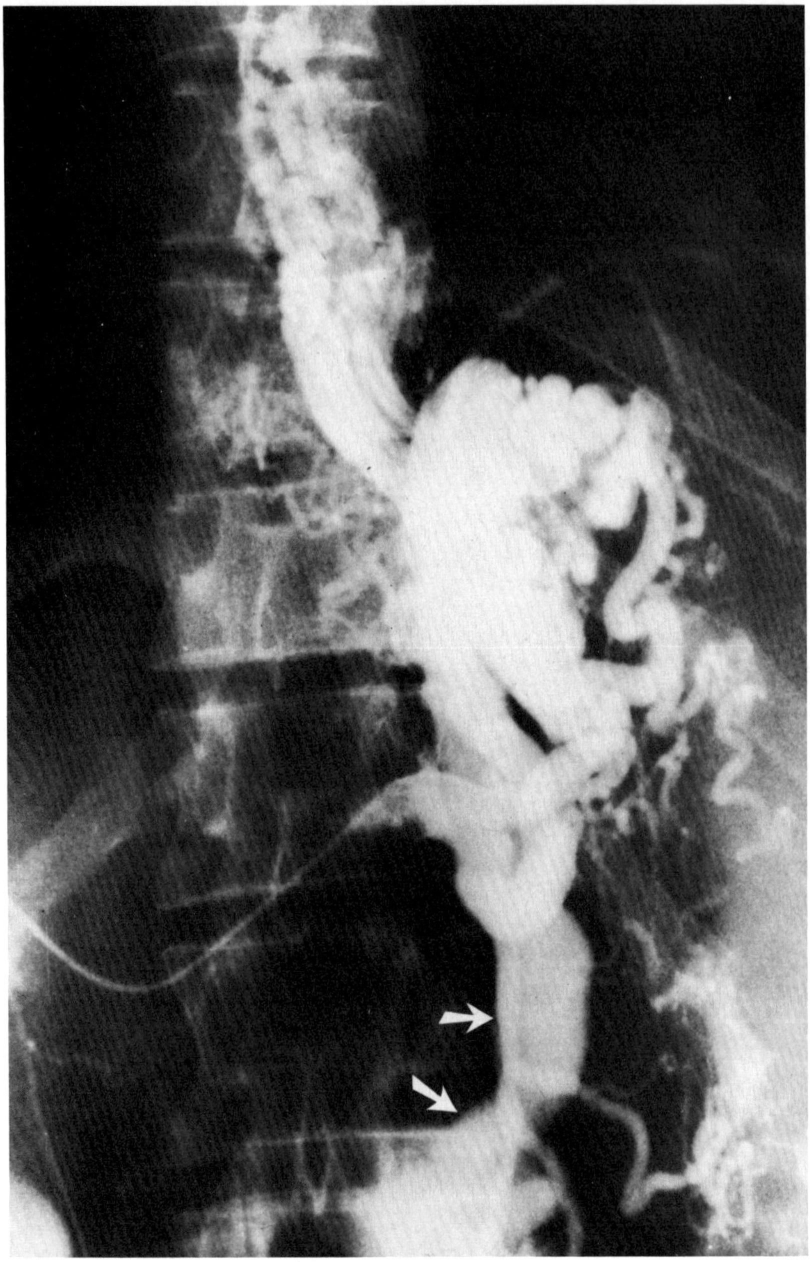

Figure 24 Transhepatic portography in a patient with portal hypertension. The injection of contrast into the left gastric vein shows collaterals in the fundus of the stomach, esophageal varices, and a wide spontaneous anastomosis to the left renal vein (arrows).

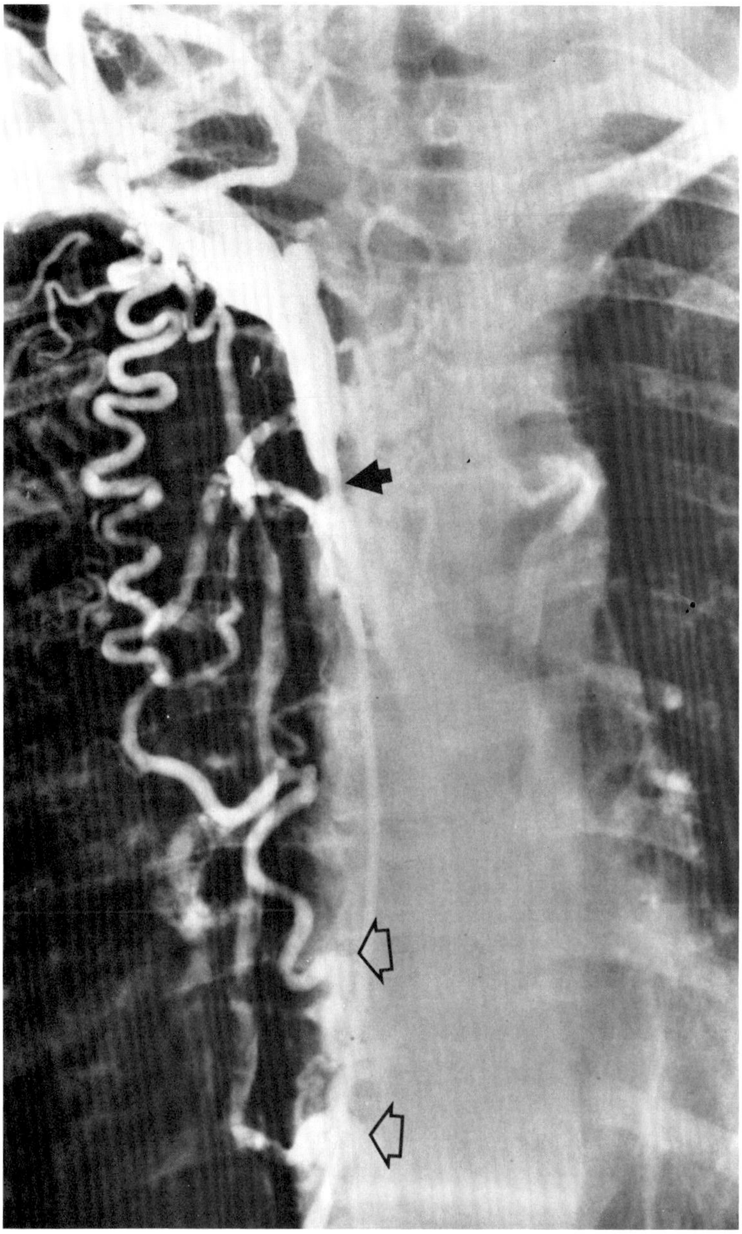

Figure 25 Downhill varices. Superior vena cava stenosis (arrow). Multiple collateral veins are shown in the mediastinum and the esophagus (open arrows).

Upper Gastrointestinal Hemorrhage

The upper gastrointestinal barium series is employed only rarely in the diagnosis of acute gastrointestinal bleeding. Although it is possible, provided that an excessive amount of blood is not present, to demonstrate evidence of active or recent bleeding by the double-contrast barium technique and to identify the causative lesion in this way (26), endoscopy is generally regarded the superior and more appropriate method of diagnosis in these circumstances. The barium used would frequently be retained in the gastrointestinal (GI) tract for several days, making subsequent use of angiography impossible. In contrast, angiography can be utilized not only to demonstrate an arterial bleeding site or the presence of varices, but also to control GI bleeding by arterial infusion or embolization. Thus in the workup of a patient with portal hypertension and active upper gastrointestinal hemorrhage, endoscopic examination is usually the first step, followed by angiography. If the patient bleeds massively and transcatheter control is desired, endoscopy can be bypassed.

The demonstration of esophageal varices by endoscopy and/or angiography does not always mean that the varices have been the cause of the bleeding. McCray et al. (27) have shown that approximately 20% of patients with massive gastrointestinal hemorrhage and known cirrhosis and portal hypertension bled from sources other than the varices–erosive gastritis, ulcers, or the Mallory-Weiss syndrome. The increased use of angiography in recent years has indicated that the actual figure approaches 50%. The incidence of nonvariceal bleeding in individual patients has been shown to relate to the severity of hepatic failure, being about 68% in the advanced stage and 36% if liver function is only mildly impaired (28).

Differentiation of arterial bleeding (erosions, ulcers, Mallory-Weiss tear) from variceal bleeding is of clinical management importance. Although endoscopy can be difficult in the actively bleeding patient, the experienced endoscopist can, in the majority of circumstances, localize the bleeding site and identify the lesion. If bleeding has stopped, the endoscopist may be able to find signs of recent hemorrhage related to a varix or a source of arterial bleeding.

In active arterial bleeding, the extravasation of contrast medium during arteriography provides an accurate method of diagnosis (Fig. 26). Moreover, bleeding from erosive gastritis is best treated by vasopressin or Pitressin infusion, which has given a response rate of 84% (29). Because of the marked dilution of contrast medium in the venous phase of an arteriogram, extravasation of contrast medium from bleeding varices has never been demonstrated by arteriography. With the angiographic demonstration of esophageal varices in a patient bleeding actively from the upper gastrointestinal tract, the varices become the presumptive source of the hemorrhage after arterial bleeding has been excluded.

Active extravasation of contrast medium from varices has been shown only by percutaneous transhepatic portography (Fig. 12E) and by splenoportography. A dual isotope technique has been developed to differentiate arterial from venous bleeding. A mixture of ^{99m}Tc sulfur colloid and ^{85}Sr microspheres is injected into the celiac artery during active esophagogastric bleeding. Blood samples are aspirated through an NG tube. With arterial bleeding the ratio of microspheres to sulfur colloid approaches that of the isotopes in the injectate; in venous hemorrhage this ratio is significantly reduced (30).

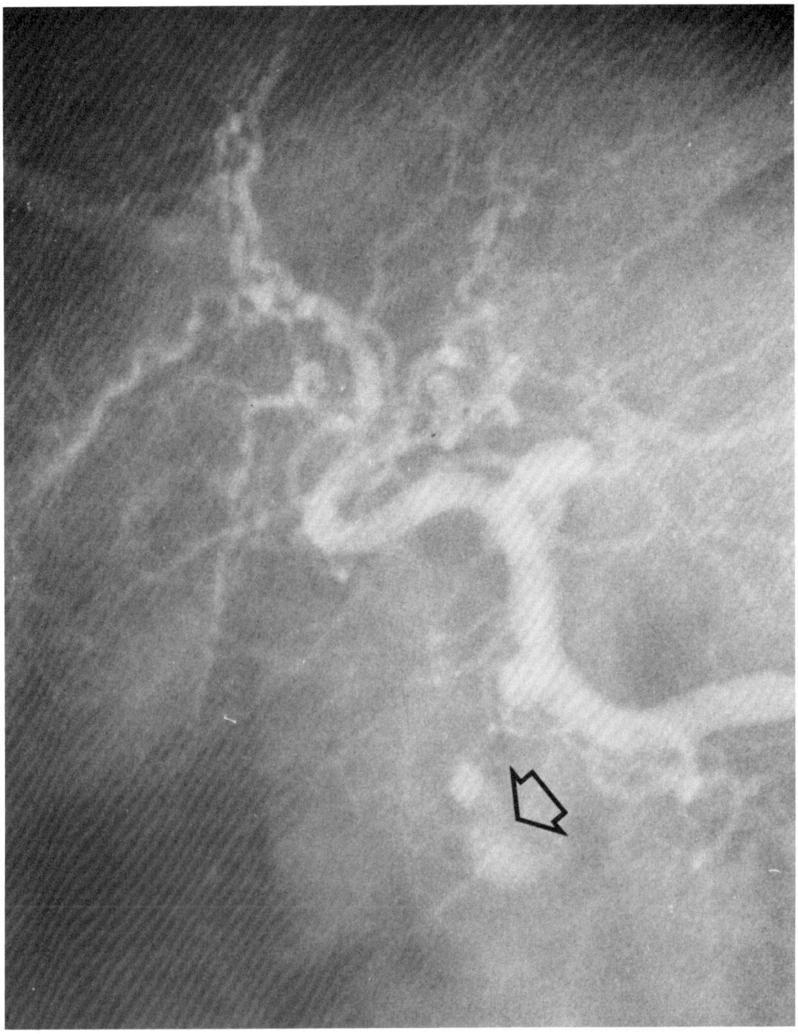

Figure 26A Active upper gastrointestinal bleeding in a patient with portal hypertension. Common hepatic artery injection shows corkscrew deformity of hepatic artery branches and extravasation of contrast medium in the duodenal bulb area (arrow).

Vasopressin infusion of the superior mesenteric artery at 0.2 unit/min (range = 0.1–0.4 unit/min) has controlled variceal bleeding in 71% of patients (31). It is postulated that vasopressin causes vasoconstriction of mesenteric arteries, with subsequent decrease of the volume of portal flow and reduction of the portal pressure. In 10 patients with cirrhosis and demonstrable esophageal varices, the superior mesenteric artery was infused with vasopressin at a dose of 0.2 unit/min for 20–30 min and the wedged hepatic vein pressure (WHVP) was monitored. The WHVP decreased by 2–3 mmHg in the majority of

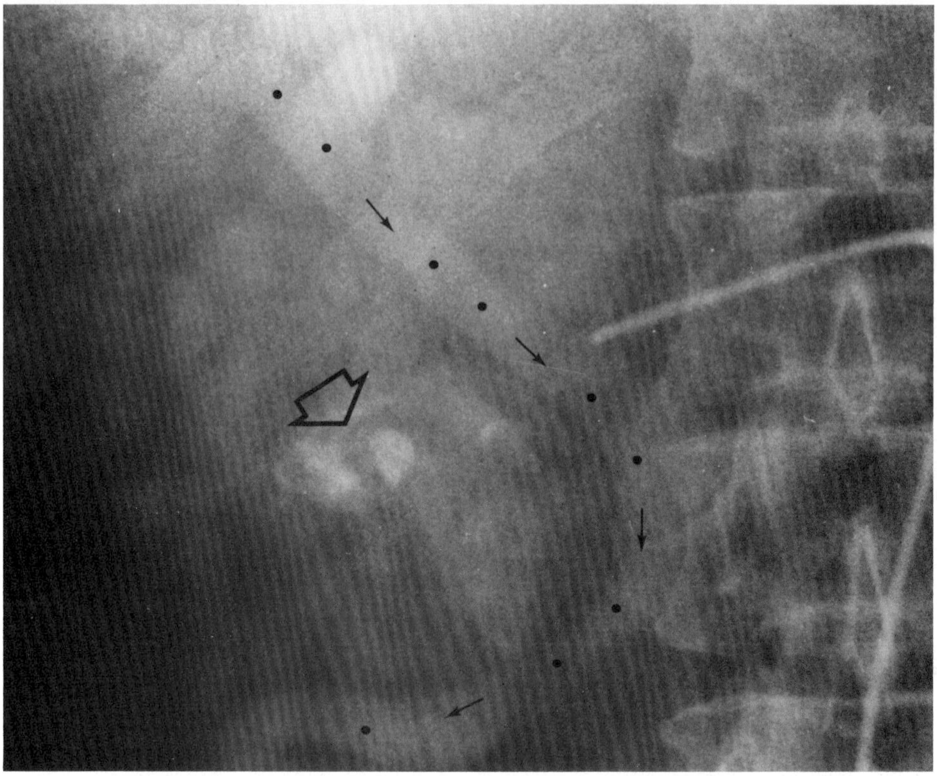

Figure 26B Extravasated contrast (arrow) seen at the same time as hepatofugal portal vein outflow (dots and arrows). Stage III cirrhosis. (Courtesy of Dr. Stanley Baum.)

the patients; some showed no change of pressure and none had more than 4 mmHg decrease. Repeat superior mesenteric arteriography, however, revealed excellent vasoconstriction together with decreased opacification of the varices (32) (Fig. 10E,F). The study suggests that decrease of portal flow is a constant finding following vasopressin infusion, but decrease of portal pressure is minimal and inconsistent. The portal flow decrease seems to be one of the factors that cause varices to cease bleeding following vasopressin infusion therapy.

Another vasopressin effect is the alteration of muscle tone in the lower esophagus. Both increased and decreased muscle tone of the lower esophageal sphincter have been reported with vasopressin infusion (22,33–35). Pentagastrin is known to increase the lower esophageal sphincter tonus; its use in a single case showed blockage of variceal flow at the lower esophageal sphincter level (22) (Fig. 27).

Comparison of intravenous with intra-arterial infusion of vasopressin in experimental animals has shown no difference in the degree of portal blood flow reduction (36,37). Successful control of variceal bleeding in patients has been reported with intravenous vasopressin infusion (38). Thus intravenous vasopressin can be used on all patients suspected of variceal bleeding. As arterial bleeding can also respond to intravenous vasopressin, arteriography may now be reserved for patients with possible arterial bleeding who do not respond to the intravenous infusion.

Catheter Management

Angiography and/or transcatheter treatment of bleeding related to portal hypertension has a restricted management application;

1. The diagnosis of the site and cause of bleeding should be made by endoscopy whenever possible. Intravenous vasopressin, a Sengstaken-Blakemore balloon, and blood and coagulation factor replacement should be the first line of treatment.
2. If bleeding fails to arrest, arterioportography may have to follow as emergency procedure, either to control an arterial bleed by embolization or to precede

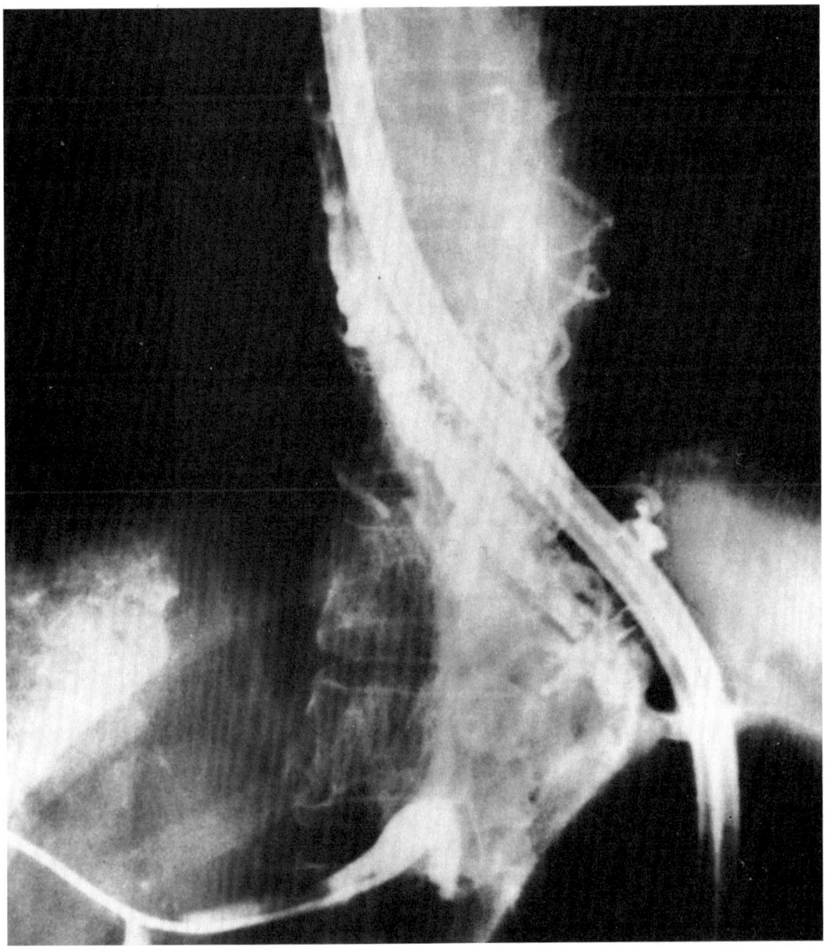

Figure 27A Transhepatic catheterization of a left gastric vein in a patient with portal hypertension and esophageal varices. Sengstaken-Blakemore tube positioned. Injection of contrast into the left gastric vein demonstrates esophageal varices.

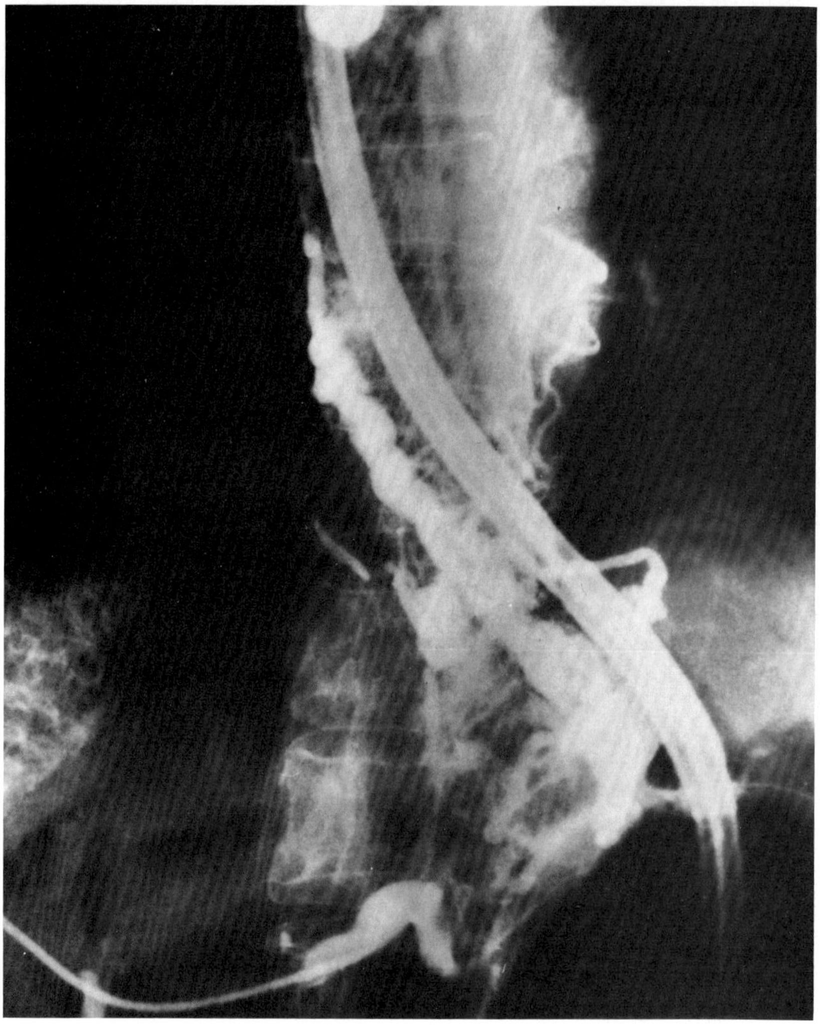

Figure 27B Contrast injection into the left gastric vein after infusion of 0.25 unit of vasopressin intravenously. No reduction of flow.

transhepatic portal catheterization and establish portal vein patency and exclude hepatic tumor presence.

3. Transhepatic variceal occlusion carries a significant complication rate (see Chap. 15). However, it must be preferred to emergency shunt surgery, with its excessively high mortality (39), and is, together with endoscopic sclerotherapy, the emergency treatment of choice in unremitting variceal bleeding.
4. Transhepatic variceal occlusion can be only a temporizing measure, and rebleeding is likely to occur unless elective surgery follows in suitable patients. Of 85 patients followed up after successful transhepatic variceal obliteration, rebleeding occurred in 55 (65%) after a mean interval of 4.6 months (40). However, it has recently been claimed that the continued oral administration of propranolol can produce a sustained reduction of portal pressure and a significant decrease in the incidence of rebleeding from varices or erosions (41).

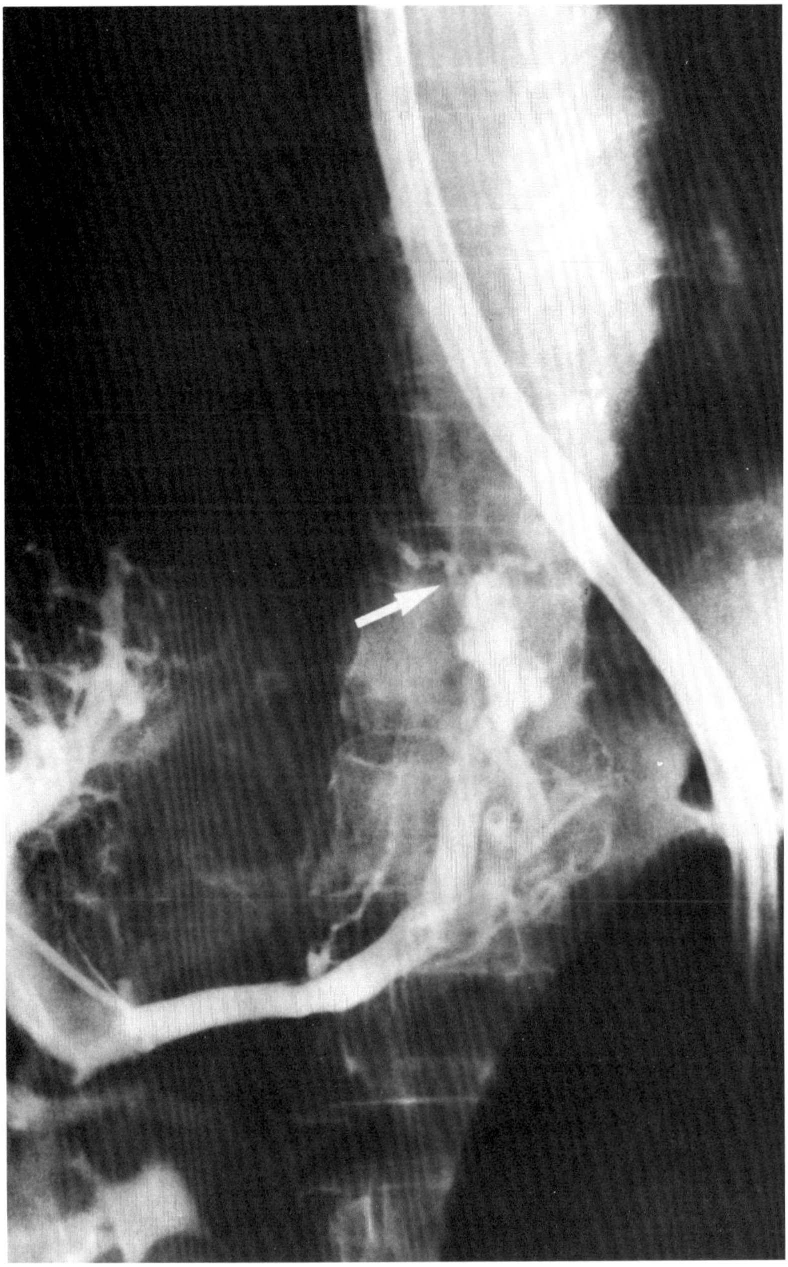

Figure 27C Injection into the left gastric vein after intravenous injection of 0.25 μg of pentagastrin. Blood flow to esophageal varices is totally blocked at the lower esophageal sphincter level (arrow).

Selection of Patients for Portal Decompression

It is generally agreed that the degree of residual normally functioning parenchyma determines the chances of survival of a patient with a portocaval shunt. Marked hepatic parenchymal dysfunction from cirrhosis usually manifests as hyperbilirubinemia, hypoalbuminemia, hypoprothrombinemia, hepatic encephalopathy, and malnutrition. Child (42) has introduced a classification for the evaluation of the hepatic function reserve in patients with liver cirrhosis:

	Group A	Group B	Group C
Serum bilirubin (mg%)	<2.0	2.0–3.0	>3.0
Serum albumin (mg%)	>3.5	3.0–3.5	<3.0
Ascites	None	Easily controlled	Poorly controlled
Neurologic disorder	None	Minimal	Advanced, "coma"
Nutrition	Excellent	Good	Poor, "wasting"

For years, Child's classification was considered the best criterion to predict the likely success of a shunt procedure. In a series of 128 patients who underwent elective end-to-side portal decompression, the mortality was 0% in class A, 9% in class B, and 53% in class C (43).

However, Child's classification is difficult to use because in the majority of cirrhotic patients, each of the five criteria tend to fall into a different class. For example, a patient might have a bilirubin 1.7% (A); serum albumin 2.8 mg%2 (C); ascites, easily controlled (B); neurological disorder, none (A); and nutrition state, good (B).

A simplified point system has been advocated to predict the outcome of emergency surgery in patients with cirrhosis and nonvariceal bleeding. Each of the following results scores one point:

Serum bilirubin >2 mg%

Serum albumin <3 mg%

Prothrombin time >16 sec

Presence of encephalopathy

Presence or history of varices

A score of one point is associated with a 43% mortality rate, 3 points with 85% mortality, and 4 points with 100% mortality (44).

Angiographic evaluation of the portal flow rate and direction has not proved as valuable as clinical signs and liver function tests in predicting the optimal shunt procedure and the chance of encephalopathy following shunt surgery (45). However, liver panangiography has contributed greatly to the understanding of portal hypertension and continues to be the best modality in giving a panoramic view of the entity. It is also helpful in determining individual patient suitability for certain types of shunt surgery (see Chap. 14).

Evaluation of Portosystemic Shunts

Surgical methods for the long-term prevention of variceal bleeding are generally of two types:

1. Those aimed at obliterating or interrupting the hepatofugal pathways through the varices. Esophageal transection, gastroesophageal resection, and most successfully, the Sugiura procedure of paraesophagogastric devascularization, esophageal transection, and splenectomy (46,47). A presurgery angiographic workup is not required, provided that the diagnosis of variceal bleeding has been established by other means.
2. Portosystemic shunting procedures, which can be divided into two categories:
   a. Standard shunts to decompress the portal system and prevent subsequent variceal bleeding, this at the cost of decreased blood flow to the liver and a high incidence of encephalopathy.
   b. Selective decompression shunts such as the distal splenorenal shunt (48,49), which aims to decompress gastrointestinal varices while maintaining the elevated mesenteric and portal venous pressure required for liver perfusion.

The various portosystemic shunting procedures have been described in Chapter 22. Each procedure has its advantages and disadvantages. The selection of a shunt procedure and the interrelationship of surgery to radiology are based on the patient's individual problems and the surgeon's clinical experience and preference. It has been suggested (50) that patients whose bleeding has stopped spontaneously should undergo elective surgical decompression to prevent its recurrence; such surgery should be a distal splenorenal shunt unless arterioportographically contraindicated. Patients who continue to bleed slowly and do not respond to vasopressin infusion may require urgent shunt surgery or endoscopic sclerotherapy (51). The long term administration of propranolol may yet prove to be a possible alternative to shunt surgery (41). Patients whose more profuse blood loss fails to be arrested by tamponade with a Sengstaken-Blakemore tube can be given an emergency mesocaval interposition shunt or, if at high surgical risk, should be referred to transhepatic or endoscopic sclerotherapy (52).

When occlusion of a portosystemic shunt is suspected, angiography remains the best method for confirming the diagnosis. The angiography can be done through the arterial side or the venous side. From the arterial side, it is preferable that arterioportography be augmented by a vasodilator (e.g., tolazoline). The patency (Fig. 28) or thrombosis (Fig. 29) of the portal system can be demonstrated easily. From the venous caval side, a catheter can be advanced into the portal system through the patent shunt; a narrowed or occluded shunt can also be passed with the catheter and dilated with a balloon (53) (Fig. 30). Transhepatic portal vein catheterization offers another route for portocaval shunt evaluation (Fig. 31).

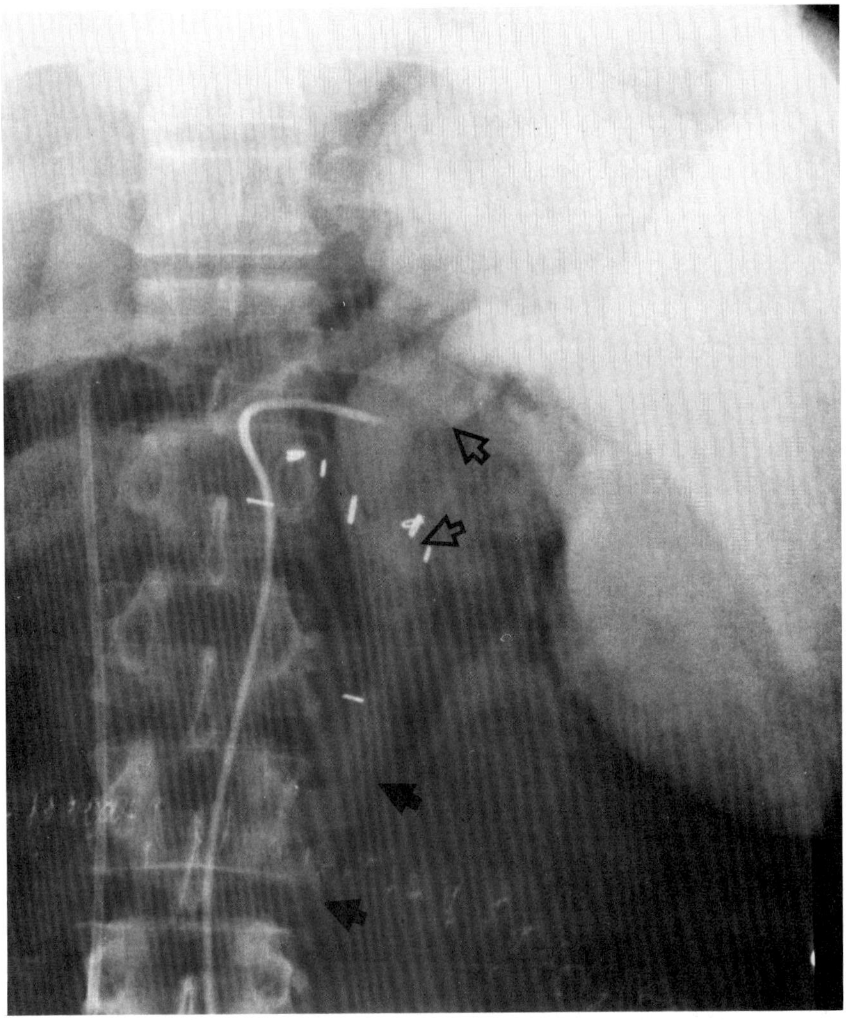

Figure 28A Distal splenorenal shunt (Warren shunt). Venous phase of a splenic arteriogram. The distal splenic vein (open arrows) is anatomosed to the proximal left renal vein (closed arrows) in an end-to-side fashion. The left renal vein (a retroaortic left renal vein) drains inferiorly and medially to join the inferior vena cava.

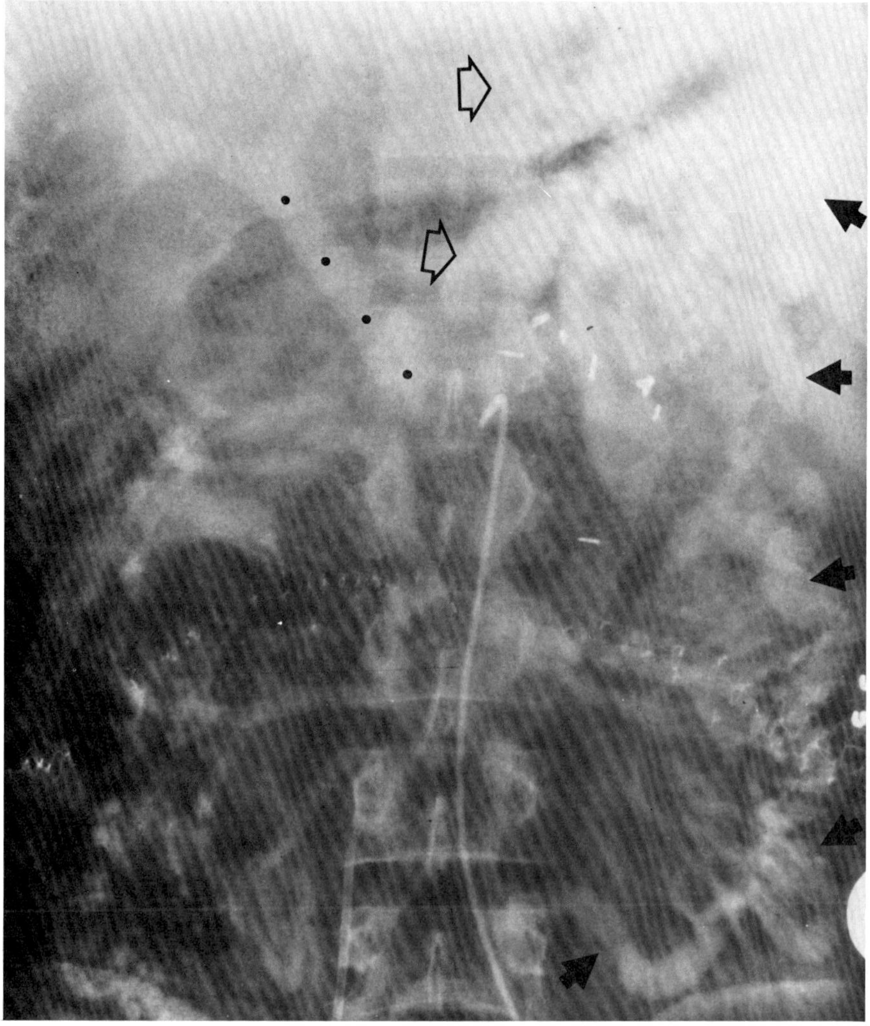

Figure 28B Venous phase of the superior mesenteric arteriogram. Both superior mesenteric vein and portal vein (dots) are patent. However, the portal vein diameter is decreased and an enlarged marginal vein (arrows) drains to the superior hemorrhoidal vein. Collateral channels (open arrows) are also seen, leading toward esophageal varices.

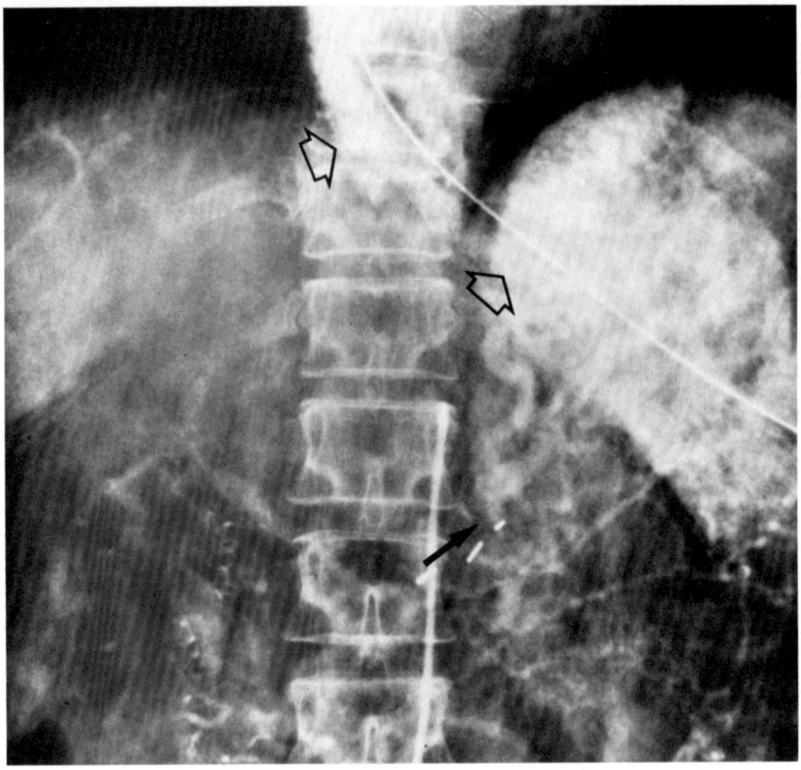

(A)

Figure 29

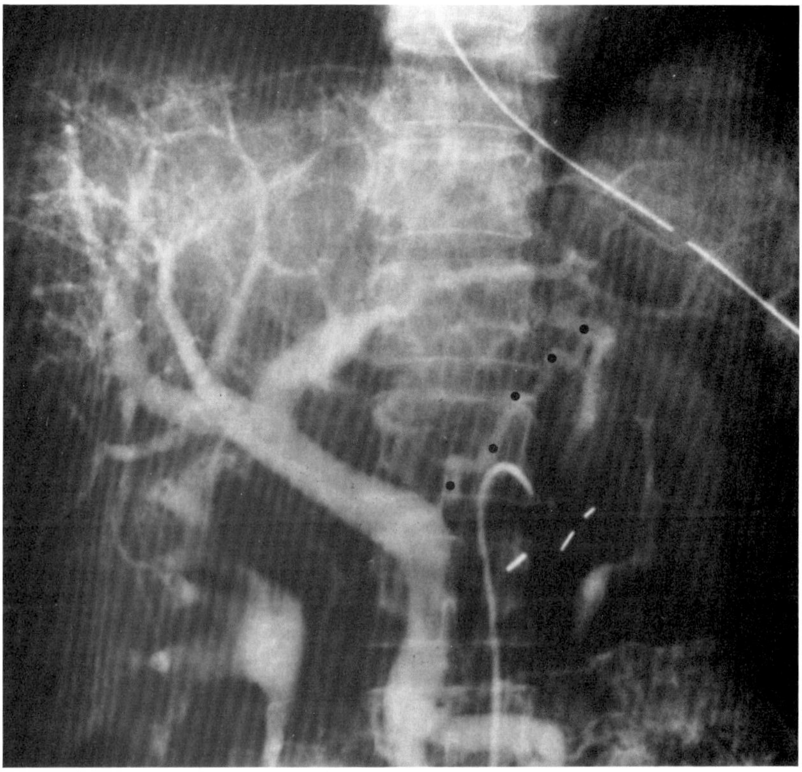

(B)

Figure 29 Thrombosed distal splenorenal shunt. (A) Celiac arteriogram, venous phase. The shunt (at the site of metal clips, arrow) is thrombosed. Esophagogastric varices are prominent (open arrows). (B) Superior mesenteric arteriogram, venous phase. Patent superior mesenteric and portal veins. A small recurrent collateral vein (dots) connects the portal vein to left gastric vein.

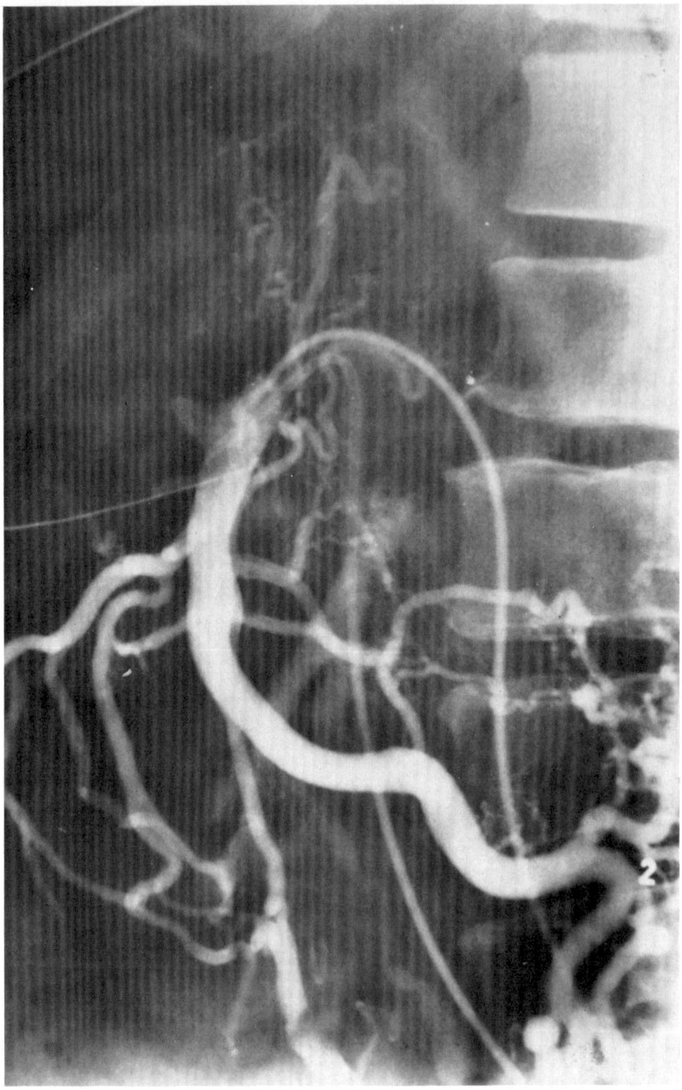

Figure 30A Patient with portal hypertension and an occluded mesocaval shunt. Transcaval catheter could be passed through the occluded mesocaval shunt into the superior mesenteric vein. Injection of contrast medium shows retrograde flow without any contrast entering the inferior vena cava.

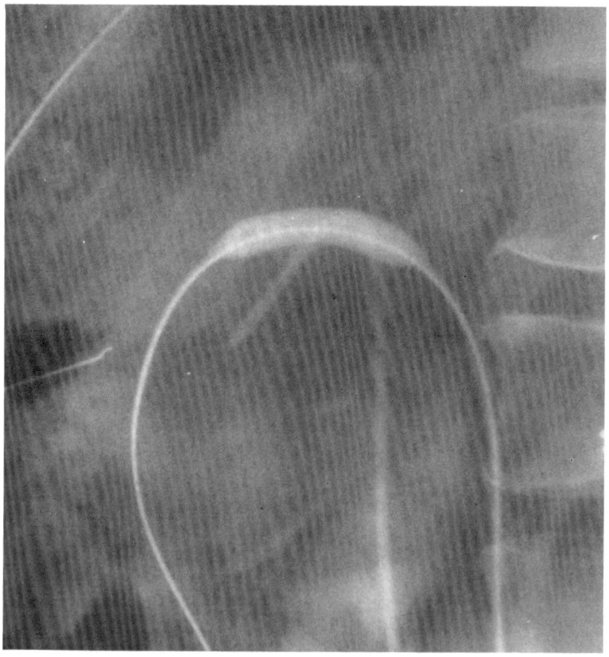

Figure 30B Balloon dilatation of the mesocaval shunt.

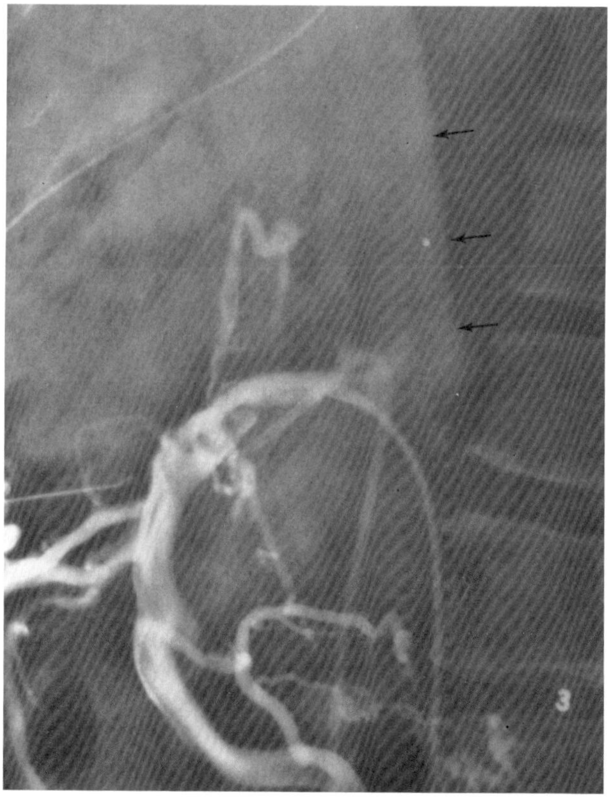

Figure 30C After balloon dilatation, injection into the superior mesenteric vein shows flow of contrast medium into the inferior vena cava (arrows). Balloon dilatation will have to repeated at intervals.

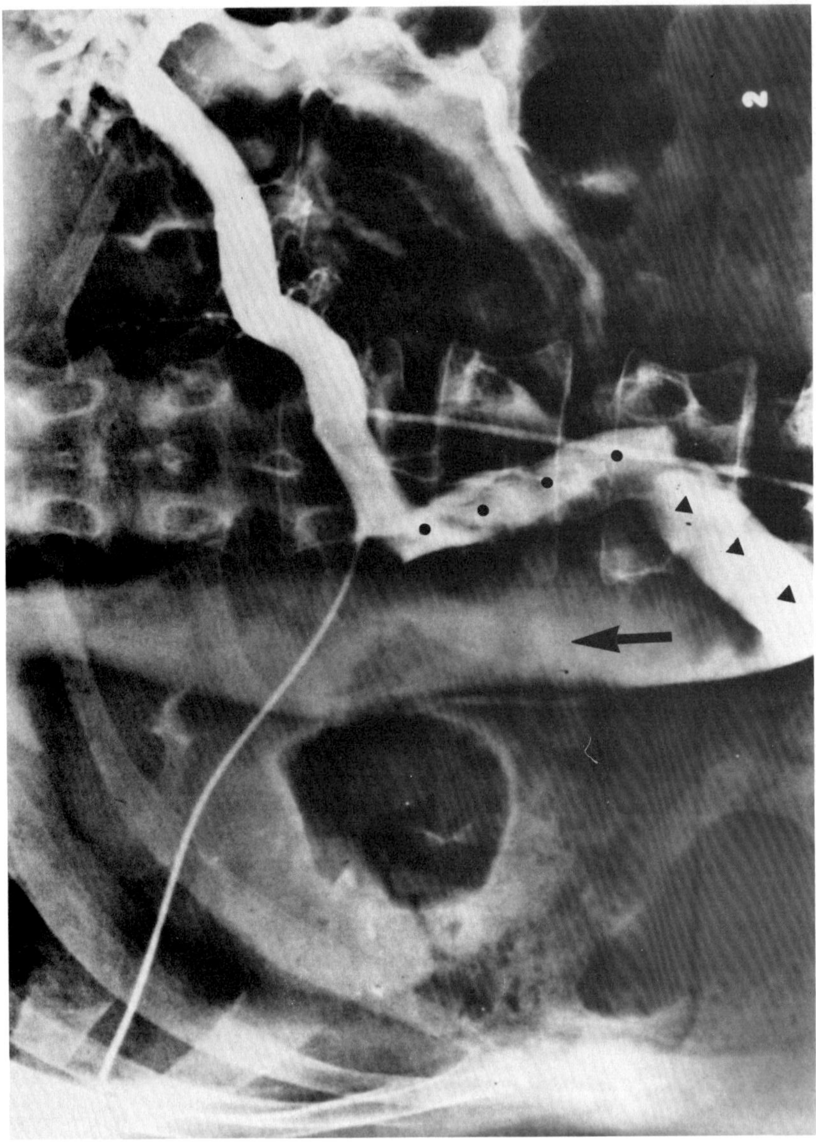

Figure 31 A patent mesocaval shunt (H-type interposition shunt). Transhepatic catheterization of the portal and splenic veins. The portal flow is from the superior mesenteric vein (dots) through the H graft (arrowheads) into the inferior vena cava (arrow).

References

1. Reynolds TB: Portal hypertension: In *Diseases of the Liver*, 4th ed, Schiff L (Ed). J. B. Lippincott, Philadelphia, 1975.
2. Reuter SR and Redman HC: Cirrhosis and portal hypertension. In *Gastrointestinal Angiography* W. B. Saunders, Philadelphia, 1977.
3. Lunderquist, A, Koolpe H, Mendez G, Russell E: Wedged pressure recording and injection of contrast in the hepatic veins. A study performed on cadaver livers to explain clinical finding. *Radiology 136*:619, 1980.
4. Viamonte M Jr, Warren WD, Fomon JJ: Liver panangiography in the assessment of portal hypertension in liver cirrhosis. *Radiol Clin North AM 8*:147, 1970.
5. Viamonte M Jr, Warren WD, Fomon JJ, Martinez LO: Angiographic investigations in portal hypertension. *Surg Gynecol Obstet 130*:37, 1970.
6. Viamonte M Jr, LePage JR, Russell E, Roen SA, Pereiras R, Zeppa R, Viamonte M: the hemodynamics of diffuse liver disease. *Semin Roentgenol 10*:187, 1975.
7. Cavaluzzi JA, Sheff R, Harrington DP, Kaufman SL, Barth K, Maddrey WC, White R Jr: Hepatic venography and wedge hepatic vein pressure measurements in diffuse liver disease. *Am J Roentgenol 129*:441, 1977.
8. Chuang VP, Mena CF, Hoskins PE: Congenital anomalies of left renal vein. Angiographic considerations. *Br J Radiol 47*:214, 1974.
9. Maddrey WC, Sen Gupta KP, Basu Mallik KC, Iber FL, Basu AK: Extrahepatic obstruction of the portal venous system. *Surg Gynecol Obstet*:989, 1968.
10. Chuang VP, Pulmano CM, Walter JF, Cho KJ: Angiography of pancreatic arteriovenous malformation. *Am J Roentgenol 129*:1015, 1977.
11. Stone HH: Portal arteriovenous fistulas: review and case report. *Am J Surg 109*:191, 1965.
12. Van Way CW, Crane JM, Riddell DH, Foster JH: Arteriovenous fistula in the portal circulation. *Surgery 70*:876, 1971.
13. Reuter S and Redman H: Vascular disease. In *Gastrointestinal Angiography*. W. B. Saunders, Philadelphia, 1977, p 84.
14. Viamonte M Jr, Danner P, Warren WD, Fomon J: A new technique for the assessment of hyperkinetic portal hypertension. *Radiology 96*:539, 1970.
15. Anthony PP, Ishak KJ, Nayak NC, Poulsen HE, Scheuer PJ, Sobin LH: The morphology of cirrhosis. *J Clin Pathol 31*:395, 1978.
16. Reuter SR and Chuang VP: The location of increased resistance to portal blood flow in obstructive jaundice. *Invest Radiol 11*:54, 1976.
17. Hales MR, Allan JS, Hall EM: Injection—corrosion studies on normal and cirrhotic livers. *Am J Pathol 35*:909, 1959.
18. Staab EV, Hartman RC, Parrott JA: Liver imaging in the diagnosis of hepatic venous thrombosis in nocturnal hemoglobinuria. *Radiology 117*:341, 1975.
19. Galloway S, Caserella WJ, Price JB: Unilobar veno-occlusive disease of the liver. *Am J Roentgenol 119*:89, 1973.
20. Hungerford GD, Hamlyn AN, Lunzer MR, Dick R, Sherlock S: Pseudometastases in the liver: a presentation of the Budd-Chiari syndrome. *Radiology 120*:627, 1976.
21. Kreel L, Freston JW, Alain D: Vascular radiology in the Budd-Chiari syndrome. *Br J Radiol 40*:755, 1967.
22. Lunderquist A: Portal vein flow pattern in portal hypertension. *Clin Radiol 31*:395, 1980.
23. Hoevels J, Lunderquist A, Tylen U, Simmet G: Porto-systemic collaterals in cirrhosis of the liver. Selective percutaneous transhepatic catheterization of the portal venous system in portal hypertension. *Acta Radiol (Diagn) 20*:865, 1979.
24. Dach JL, Hill MC, Pelaez JC, LePage JR, Russell E: Sonography of hypertensive portal venous system: correlation with arterial portography. *Am J Roentgenol 137*:511, 1981.

25. Johnson LS, Kinnear DG, Brown RA, Mulder DS: Downhill esophageal varices. *Arch Surg 113*:1463, 1978.
26. Fraser GM: The double contrast barium meal in patients with acute upper gastrointestinal bleeding. *Clin Radiol 29*:625, 1978.
27. McCray RS, Martin F, Amir-Ahmadi H, Sheahan DG, Zamcheck N: Erroneous diagnosis of hemorrhage from esophageal varices. *Am J Dig Dis 14*:755, 1969.
28. Franco D, Durandy Y, Deporte A, Bismuth H: Upper gastrointestinal hemorrhage in hepatic cirrhosis, causes and relationship to hepatic failure and stress. *Lancet 1*:218, 1977.
29. Athanasoulis CA, Baum S, Waltman AC, Ring EJ, Imbembo A, Van der Salm TJ: Control of acute gastric mucosal hemorrhage: intra-arterial infusion of posterior pituitary extract. *N Engl J Med 290*:597, 1974.
30. Alavi, A, Goldstein HA, Baum R, Baum S: Differentiation of arterial and venous bleeding using dual radioisotopes. Presented at the 66th Scientific Assembly and Annual Meeting of the Radiological Society of North America, Dallas, November 18, 1980.
31. Conn HO, Ramsby GR, Storer EH, Mutchnick MG, Joshi PH, Phillips MM, Cohen GA, Fields GN, Petroski D: Intraarterial vasopressin in the treatment of upper gastrointestinal hemorrhage: a prospective, controlled clinical trial. *Gastroenterology 68*:211, 1975.
32. Chuang VP: Personal data, 1980.
33. Aronsen KF and Nylander G: The mechanism of vasopressin hemostasis in bleeding esophageal varices. An angiographic study in the dog. *Acta Chir Scand 131*:443, 1966.
34. Cincotti JJ: Reduction of portal hypertension by nonshunting methods in patients with cirrhosis. *Surg Forum 11*:276, 1960.
35. Cho KJ and McGinnis B: Effect of superior mesenteric arterial and intravenous vasopressin infusions on esophageal motor function: a study on hemostatic mechanism of vasopressin in bleeding esophageal varices. Presented at the 65th Scientific Assembly and Annual Meeting of the Radiological Society of North America, Las Vegas, 1979.
36. Barr, JW, Larkin RC, Rosch J: Similarity of arterial and intravenous vasopressin on portal and systemic hemodynamics. *Gastroenterology 69*:13, 1975.
37. Davis GB, Bookstein JJ, Hagen PL: The relative effects of selective intra-arterial and intravenous vasopressin infusion. *Radiology 12*:537, 1976.
38. Athanasoulis CA, Waltman AC, Novelline RA, Krudy AG, Sniderman KW: Angiography: its contribution to the emergency management of gastrointestinal hemorrhage. *Radiol Clin North Am 14*:265, 1976.
39. Bengmark S, Barjesson B, Hoevels J, Joelsson B, Lunderquist A, Owman T: Obliteration of esophageal varices by PTP—a follow up of 43 patients. *Ann Surg 190*:549, 1979.
40. Smith-Laing G, Scott J, Long RG, Dick R, Sherlock S: Role of percutaneous transhepatic obliteration of varices in the management of hemorrhage from gastroesophageal varices. *Gastroenterology 80*:1031, 1981.
41. Lebrec D, Poynard T, Hillon P, Benhamou J-P: Propranolol for prevention of recurrent gastrointestinal bleeding in patients with cirrhosis. *New Engl J Med 305*:1371, 1981.
42. Child CG III: *Portal Hypertension as Seen by Seventeen Authorities*. W. B. Saunders, Philadelphia, 1974.
43. Campbell DP, Parker DE, Anagnostopoulos CE: Surgical prediction in portacaval shunts: a computerized statistical analysis. *Am J Surg 126*:748, 1973.
44. Wirthlin LS, Urk HV, Malt RB, Malt RA: Predictor of surgical mortality in patients with cirrhosis and nonvariceal gastroduodenal bleeding. *Surg Gynecol Obstet 139*:65, 1974.
45. Smith GW: Use of hemodynamic selection criteria in the management of cirrhotic patients with portal hypertension. *Ann Surg 179*:782, 1974.
46. Sugiura M and Futagawa S: A new technique for treating esophageal varices. *J Thorac Cardiovasc Surg 66*:677, 1973.

47. Koyama K, Takagi Y, Ouchi K, Sato T: Results of esophageal transection for esophageal varices. Experience with 100 cases. *Am J Surg 139*:204, 1980.
48. Warren WD, Zeppa R, Fomon JJ: Selective transhepatic decompression of gastroesophageal varices by distal splenorenal shunt. *Ann Surg 166*:437, 1967.
49. Warren WD, Salam AA, Smith RB III: The mesospleno-renal shunt procedures: a comprehensive approach to portosystemic decompression. *Ann Surg 179*:791, 1974.
50. Hanna SS, Warren DD, Galambos JT, Millikan WJ Jr: Bleeding varices: elective management. *Can Med Assoc J 124*:42, 1981.
51. Terblance J, Northover JM, Bornman P, Kahn D, Barbezat GO, Sellars SL, Saunders SJ: A prospective evaluation of injection sclerotherapy in the treatment of acute bleeding from esophageal varices. *Surgery 85*:239, 1979.
52. Hanna SS, Warren WD, Galambos JT, Millikan WJ Jr: Bleeding varices: emergency management. *Can Med Assoc J 124*:29, 1981.
53. Cope C: Balloon dilatation of closed mesocaval shunts. *Am J Roentgenol 135*:989, 1980.

26

Liver Tumors: Diagnosis and Management

Sidney Wallace and Vincent P. Chuang
M.D. Anderson Hospital and Tumor Institute
Houston, Texas

Introduction

Radiological methods for the diagnosis of the presence, nature, and location of an hepatic mass have been presented in the preceding chapters. The diagnostic armamentarium includes conventional radiography, scintigraphy (NM), sonography (US), computed tomography (CT), angiography, and percutaneous biopsy. Extending these diagnostic capabilities, the radiologist has become increasingly involved in the therapeutic management of patients with an hepatic mass by employing interventional techniques of percutaneous drainage, intra-arterial infusion of chemotherapeutic agents, embolization, and occlusion of the hepatic arterial supply. This chapter reiterates the contributions of the diagnostic radiologist to the diagnosis of an hepatic tumor by a correlation of available modalities and the utilization of this information in the management of the patient by

Table 1 Diagnostic Approach to a Hepatic Mass

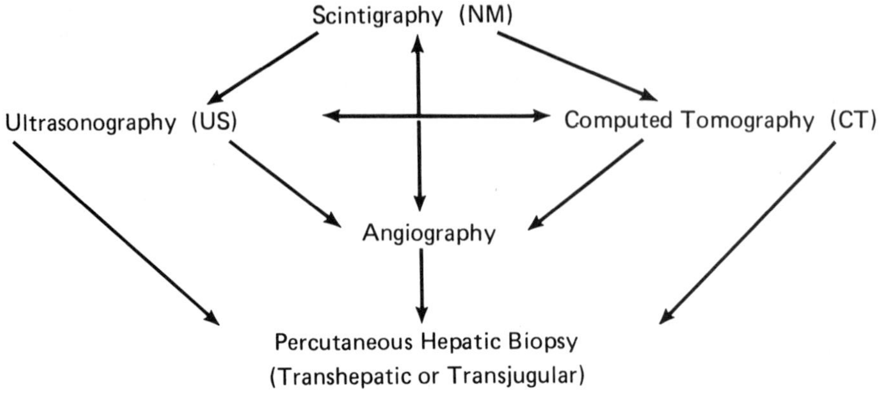

interventional techniques. Additional experience in hepatic embolization is presented in Chapter 27.

The recommended diagnostic approach to an hepatic mass is outlined in Table 1. The sequence of studies is dictated by the available facilities, the personnel, its technical and professional expertise, the patient's clinical status and habitus, as well as the financial burden. Undoubtedly, the diagnosis must be established with the minimum of discomfort and expense to the patient. The rewards must warrant the risk and cost.

Radiologic Screening Techniques

Computed Tomography (CT)

CT is superior in sensitivity, specificity, and accuracy in diagnosis (1,2). CT results in the lowest rate of false positive and false negative diagnoses. CT is also the procedure of choice to define and differentiate intra- from extrahepatic masses. Inherent limitations are a paucity of abdominal fat and artifacts due to motion and metallic clips. False negative evaluation is related to the size and location of the lesions and their relationship to the dome of the diaphragm. An extrahepatic neoplasm originating in the right kidney or adrenal may project into the liver, presenting on CT as an intrahepatic tumor (Fig. 1). This diagnostic difficulty can be minimized by the rapid scanners with dynamic capabilities, by reconstruction in multiple planes, and by the use of newer contrast agents (e.g., emulsified Ethiodol) (3) (Fig. 2).

Sonography (US) (4–6)

US is less sensitive and less specific than CT and presents difficulty in interpreting the inhomogeneous sonographic architecture (Fig. 3). The major problem with US is interference by abdominal gas, which is present in 15–30% of patients. Real-time sonography reduces the difficulties created by intestinal gas and peristalsis. In large retroperitoneal masses, especially on the right, ultrasound has the advantage of displaying the information in multiple projections, better defining the plane of cleavage between the liver and the adjacent mass (see Fig. 1B). Post data processing (PDP) may increase the

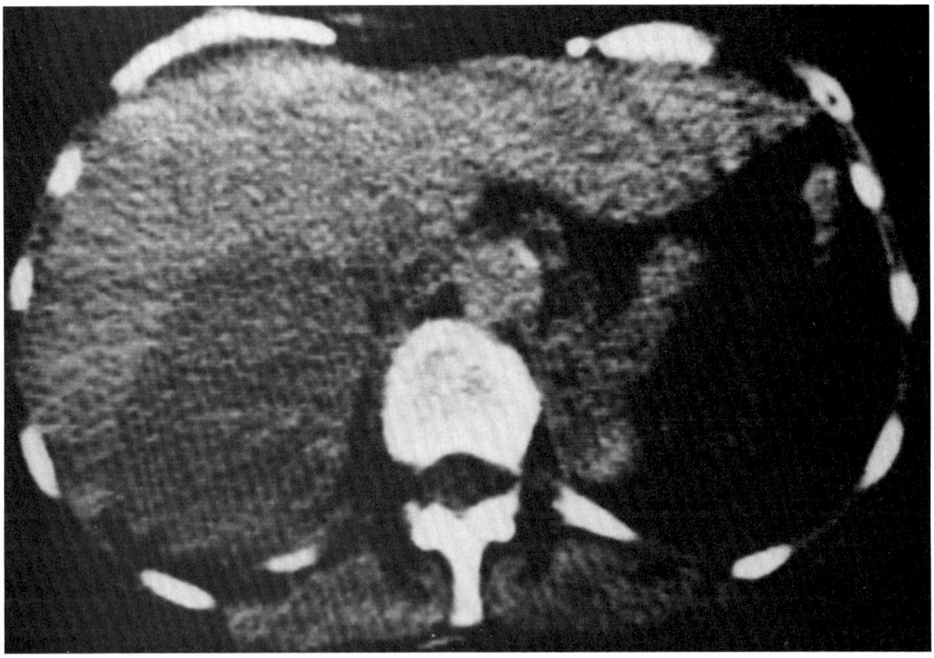

(A)

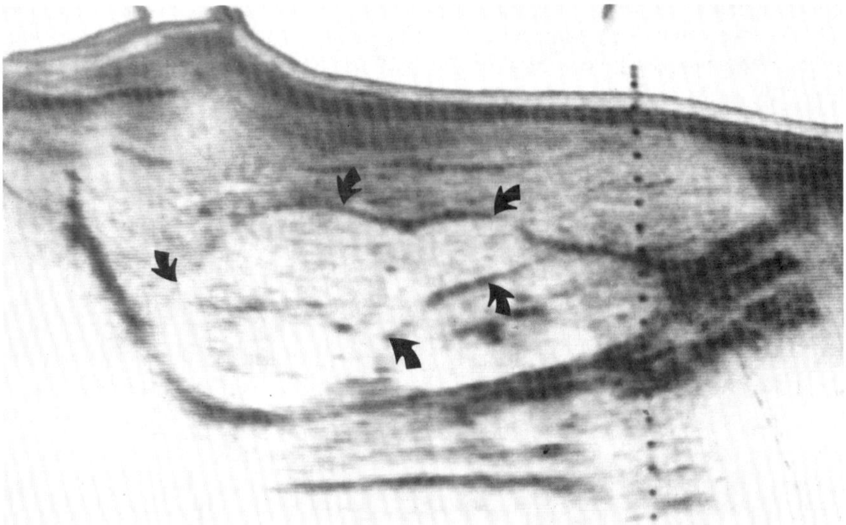

(B)

Figure 1 Diagnostic approach. Carcinoma right adrenal. (A) The CT suggests a mass within the parenchyma of the liver. (B) The longitudinal projection of the US clearly defines the plane of cleavage between the right adrenal neoplasm and the kidney as well as that between the neoplasm and the liver (arrows). The ability of US to depict the lesion in multiple planes is a decided advantage. Reconstruction of the CT image will assist in correcting this difficulty.

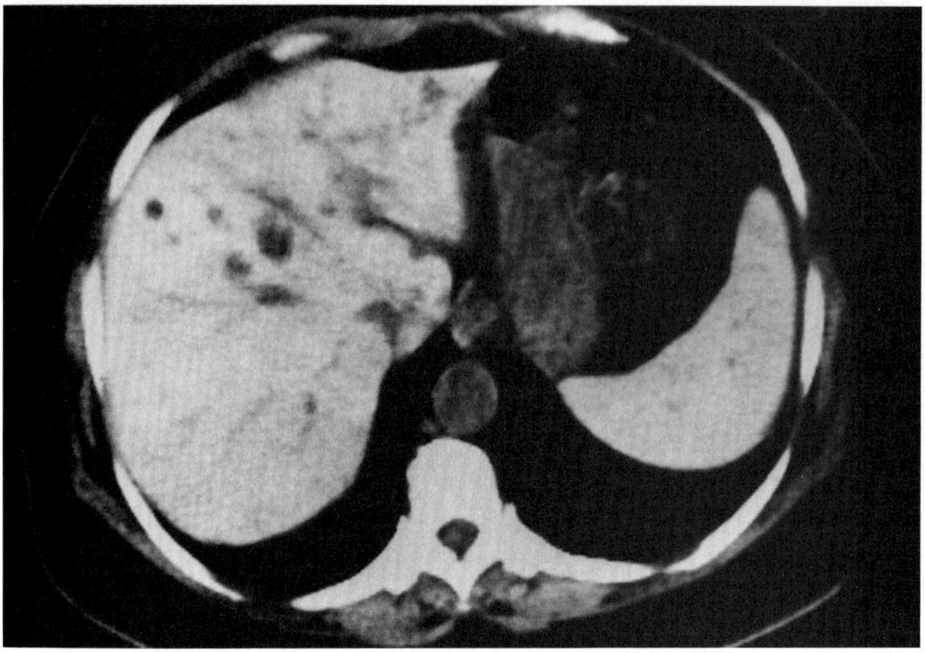

Figure 2 Diagnostic approach. Cysts of the liver: the sensitivity of CT can be enhanced by the use of newer contrast agents. An emulsion of Ethiodol (EOE 13), formulated by Vermess et al. (3), concentrates in the liver and spleen allowing detection of lesions as small as 5 mm in diameter. EOE 13 is an investigational contrast agent not yet commercially available.

accuracy of sonography by better defining the lesions. This is akin to varying the window levels and width on CT for optimal definition (7).

Scintigraphy (NM) (8–12)

NM is very sensitive, but relatively nonspecific, due to limitations in differentiating diffuse parenchymal abnormalities, anatomic variants, and extrinsic masses from hepatic tumors. Technetium sulfur colloid (^{99m}Tc-SC) scan is used to detect hepatic masses (Fig. 3A). Flow studies may demonstrate increased radionuclide activity in highly vascular lesions. Gallium citrate (^{67}Ga-citrate) scans may be of value in defining certain hepatic neoplasms especially in the differentiation of a hepatoma in a cirrhotic liver.

Comparison of Screening Techniques

Despite their high sensitivity, each of these techniques has difficulty in differentiating diffuse from unilobar disease. The significance of this information in those cases in whom

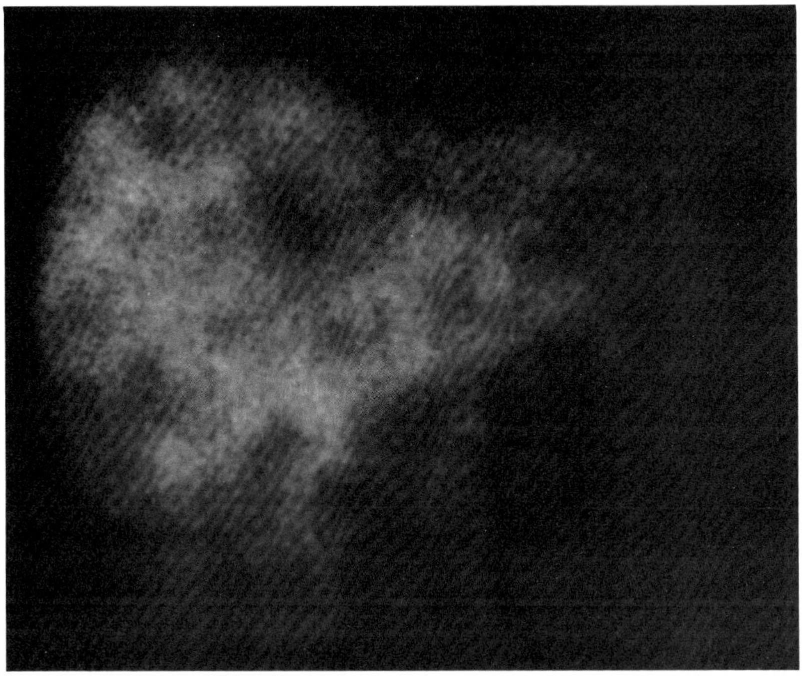

(A)

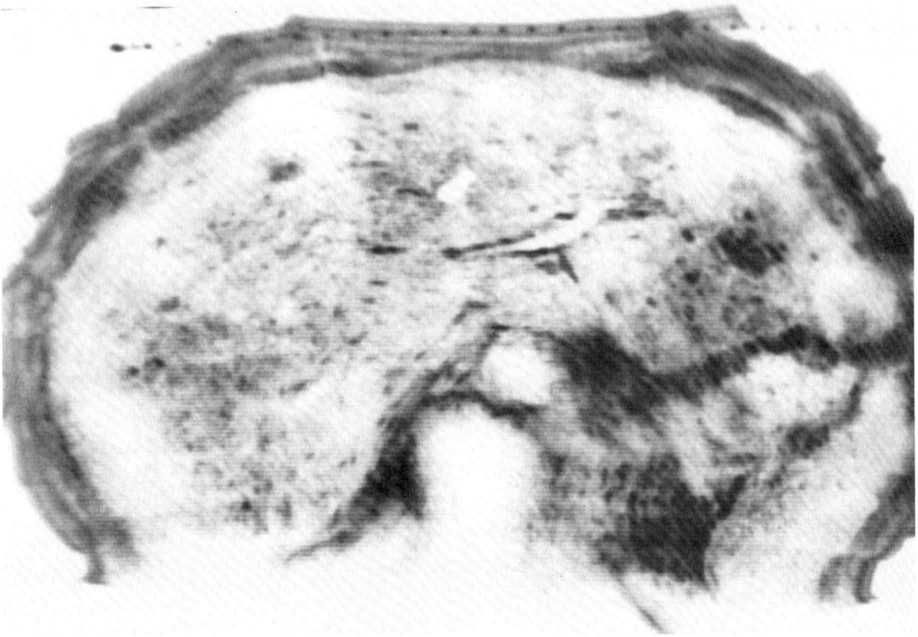

(B)

Figure 3 Diagnostic approach: hepatocellular carcinoma. (A) Scintigram: the multiple discrete nodules are obvious. Although nonspecific, the radionuclide scan is extremely sensitive for intrahepatic masses. (B) Sonogram: the complex pattern seen in this same patient with a hepatocellular carcinoma is difficult to interpret although definitely abnormal. In a categorical institution such as the M. D. Anderson Hospital and Tumor Institute, the most likely diagnosis of the US image is neoplasm. However, in a general hospital, this scan might justifiably be considered a diffuse infiltrative disease like cirrhosis.

Table 2 Comparison of Screening Methods

	Examinations/results (%)		
Performance standards	CT	US	NM
Sensitivity	96	75	94
False positive interpretations	12	17	26
Accuracy of abnormal interpretations	91	85	82
Specificity	86	50	67
False negative interpretations	4	10	6

Source: Ref. 1.

hepatic lobectomy is contemplated emphasizes the necessity for angiography. The nonspecificity of the screening methods, even in combination, is demonstrated by their inability to differentiate some benign lesions (hepatic adenoma, focal nodular hyperplasia, cirrhosis, cavernous hemangioma, abscess, etc.) from malignancy. This may be resolved by angiography, but at times only by histologic evaluation after biopsy or aspiration.

Comparison of the three screening techniques demonstrates that CT is the best single examination to determine the presence and extent of an hepatic mass (Table 2).

When all things are considered, a practical and accurate screening plan would consist of scintigraphy, followed as clinically indicated, by computed tomography. The large volume of cases at an institution such as the M. D. Anderson Hospital and Tumor Institute, as well as the cost considerations, have dictated the sequence of diagnostic procedures. Scintigraphy is performed as the initial examination and is also often used to follow the course of disease because it is very sensitive and can cope with the largest number of patients per single scanning unit. Sonography often follows to confirm the isotopic findings and to resolve problems whenever possible. Because of its greater expense and limited patient capacity, CT is used in those situations in which conflicts occur between scintigraphy and sonography. Angiography is reserved as the last resort to solve a problem of diagnosis or in preparation for management (Figs. 4–6).

Conventional Radiography

Radiographic findings depend on the location and extent of the intrahepatic process (13). As the liver enlarges locally, there is an alteration in its contour, with the edge becoming more rounded or undulated. (See also Chapter 7.)

Signs of right lobe enlargement:

1. Shadow of a mass in the right upper abdomen
2. Displacement of the stomach and duodenal bulb to the left
3. Downward displacement of the right kidney and the transverse colon
4. Downward and posterior displacement of the hepatic flexure of the colon
5. No displacement of the second part of the duodenum
6. Normal position of the duodenojejunal flexure

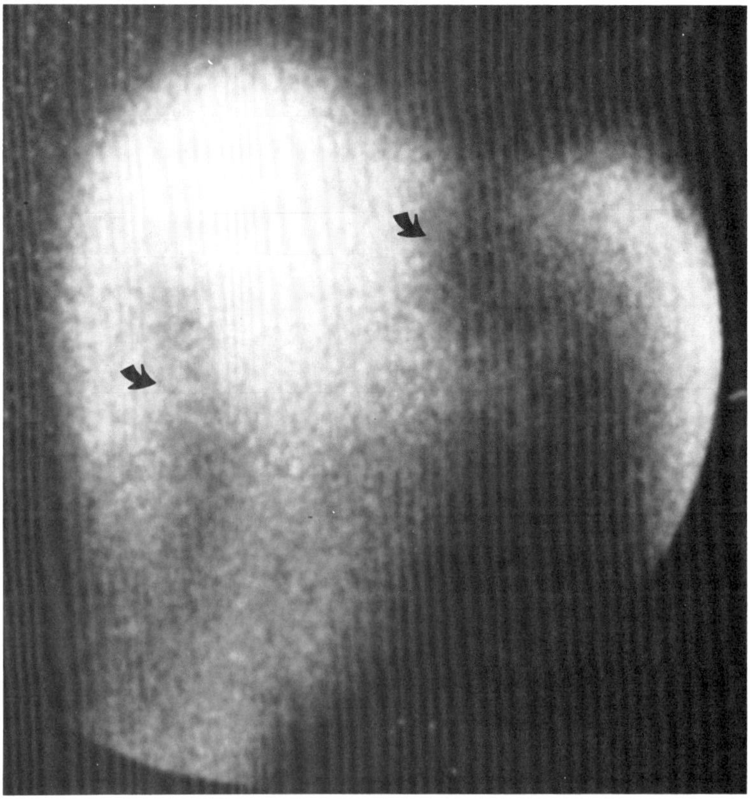

(A)

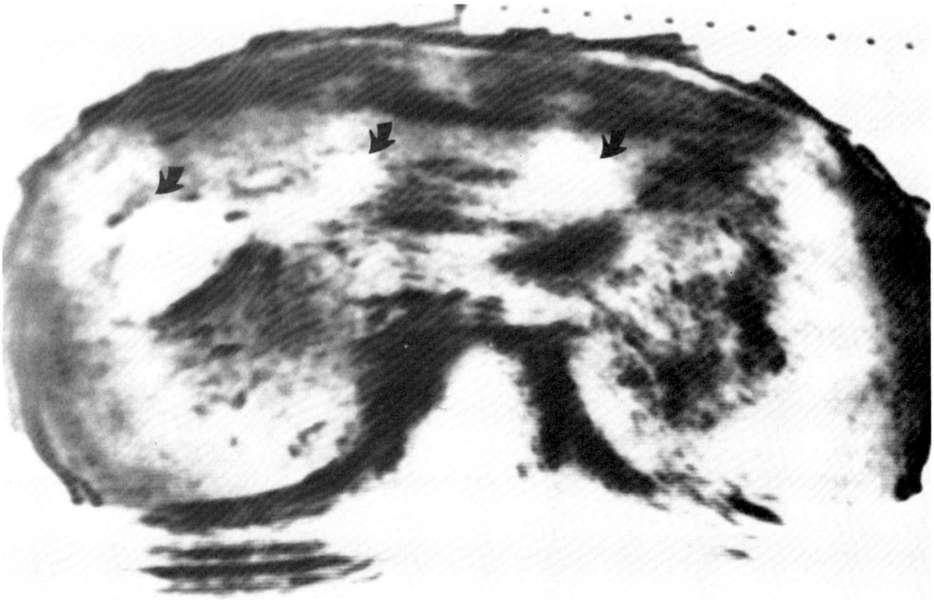

(B)

Figure 4

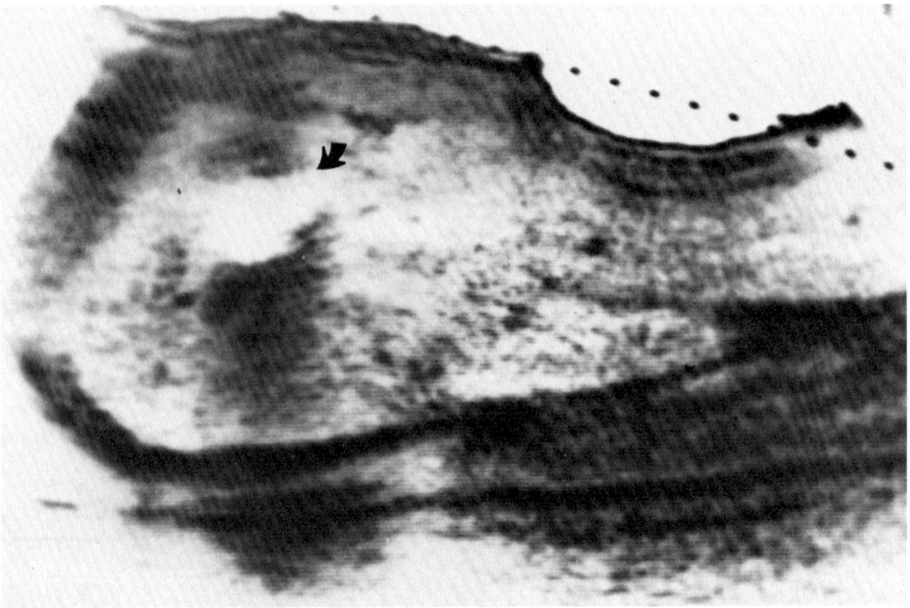

(C)

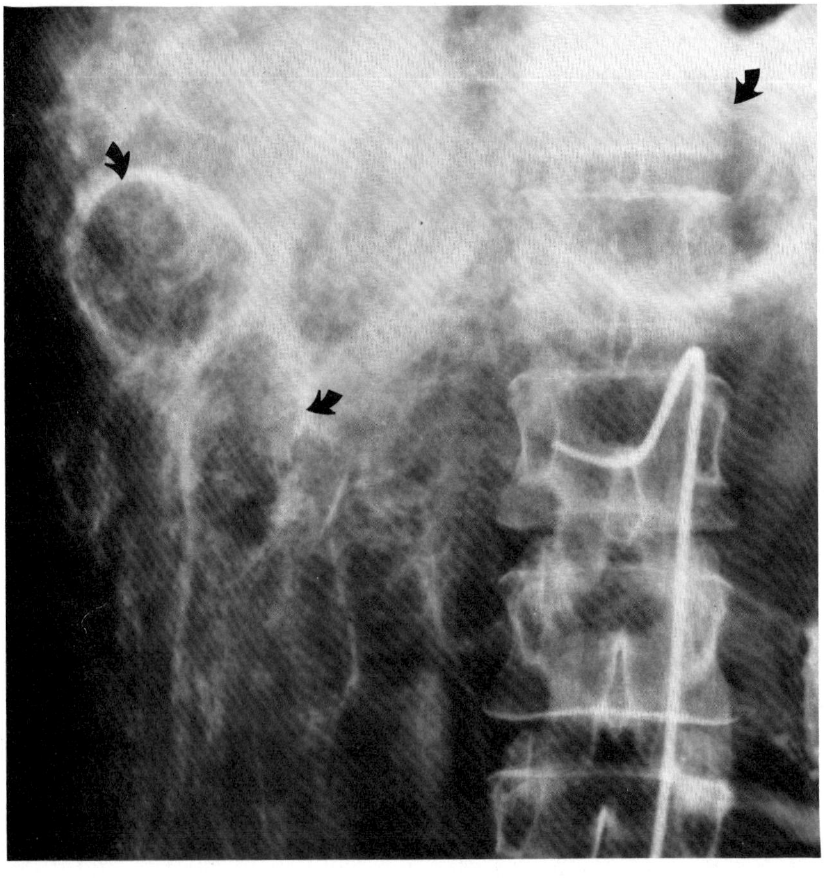

(D)

Figure 4 (continued)

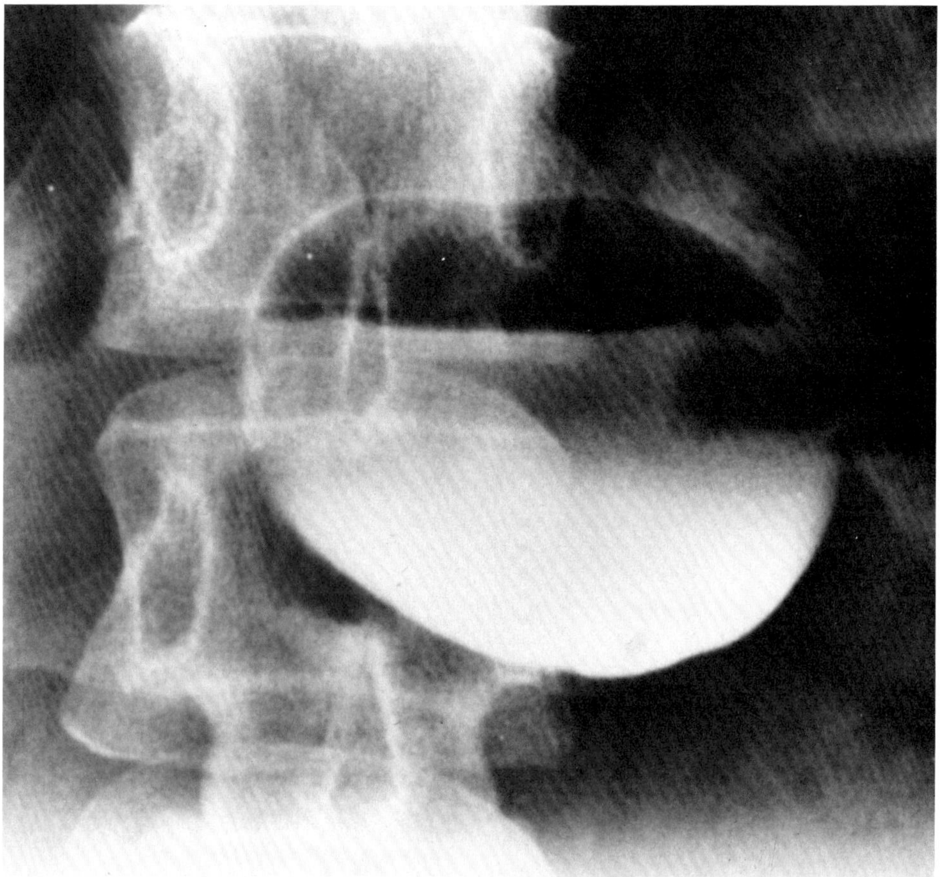

(E)

Figure 4 Diagnostic approach. This 47-year-old female was seen at MDAH because of an adenocarcinoma of the breast, which was 2 cm in diameter and freely movable. (A) As part of the diagnostic evaluation, the scintiscan of the liver revealed multiple lesions (arrows). Multiple metastases to the liver would be most unusual as an initial finding in a patient with a small carcinoma of the breast. (B,C) Sonography, transverse and longitudinal, revealed multiple lesions which were sonolucent with a slightly irregular posterior margin and through transmission (arrows). These were most consistent with hepatic cysts. The slight irregularity of the margins and the possibility of necrotic metastases required further investigation. Once again, metastases, especially necrotic metastases, are most unusual in the presence of a small carcinoma of the breast. (D) Angiography: selective hepatic arteriography demonstrated multiple thin-walled lesions in each lobe of the liver (arrows). No neovascularity was noted. The wall of each lesion had some irregularity. The most likely diagnosis was multiple benign hepatic cysts. (E) Transhepatic puncture and aspiration of the contents with injection of water-based contrast material and air definitely established the diagnosis of hepatic cysts. The aspirated material was yellowish brown and contained no bile or tumor cells. When there is a discrepancy between the clinical picture and the radiographic evaluation, a further pursuit of the diagnosis must be undertaken. Once there is reasonable agreement, the pursuit is curtailed. There is no necessity to do all the examinations on every patient. This is too costly, too time consuming, and unnecessary.

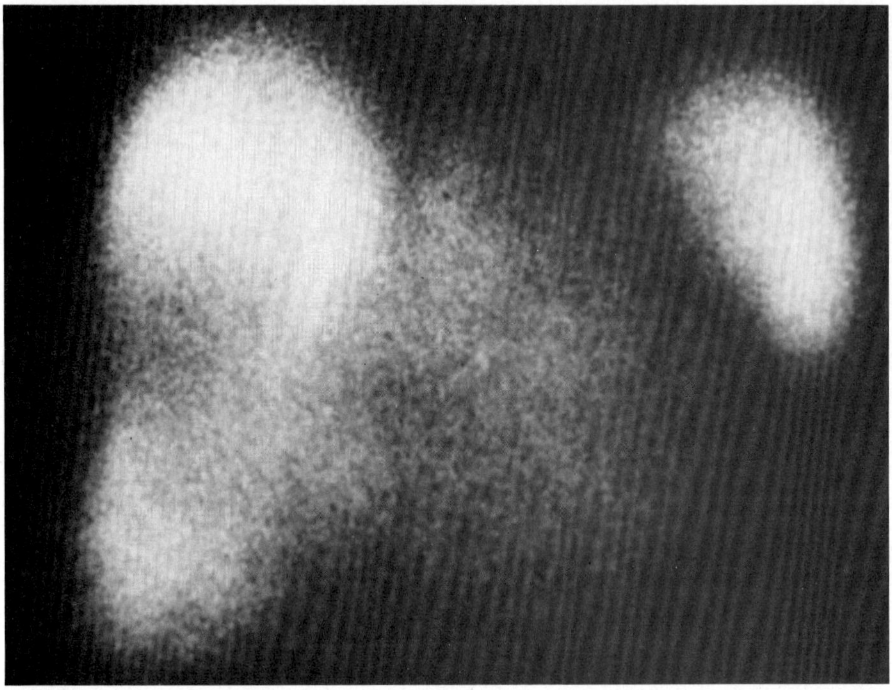

(A)

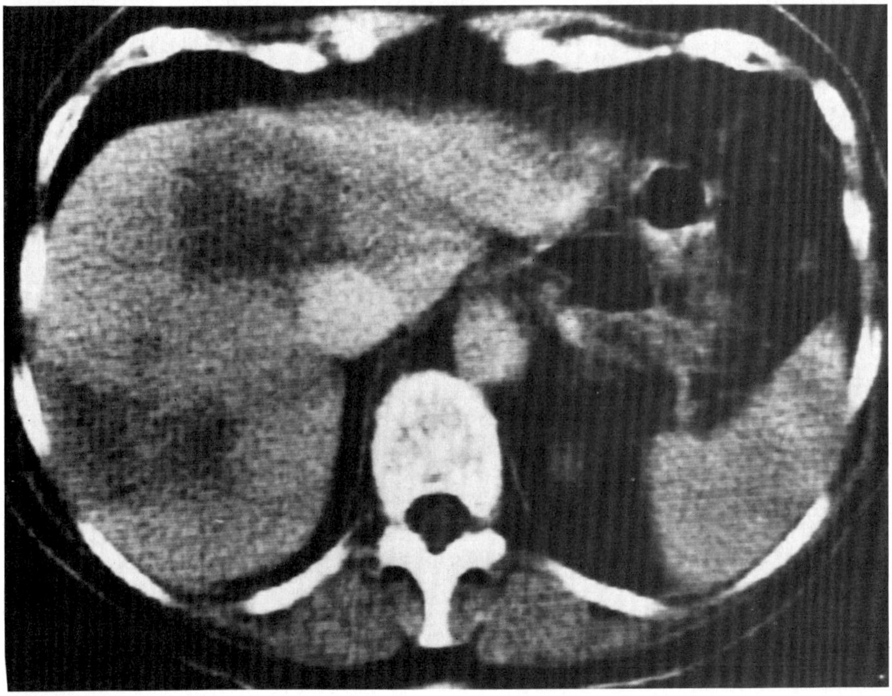

(B)

Figure 5

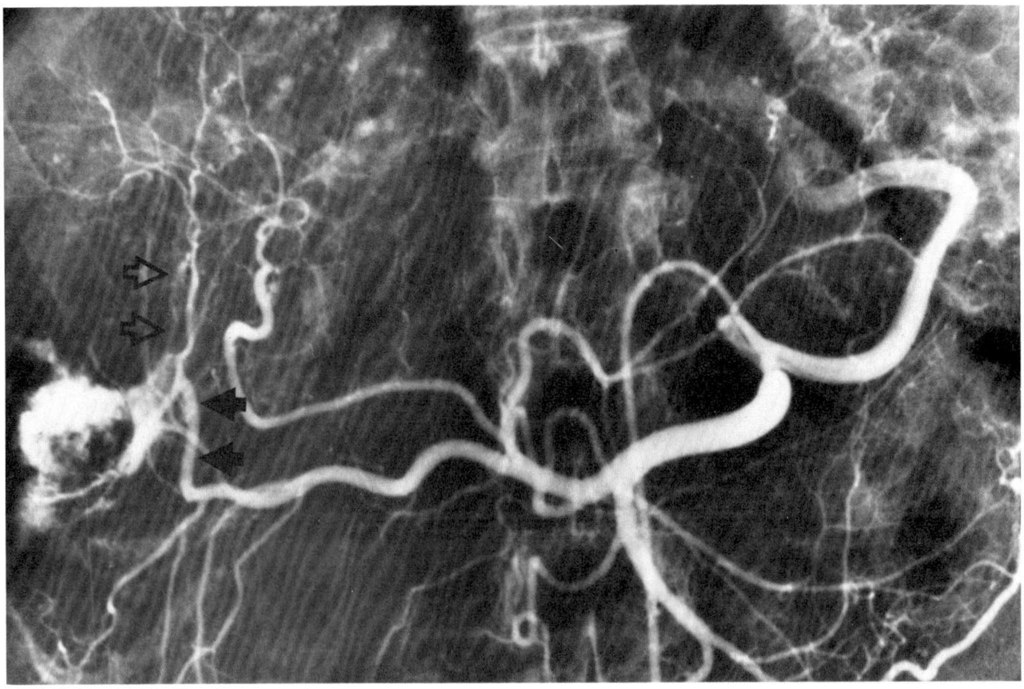

(C)

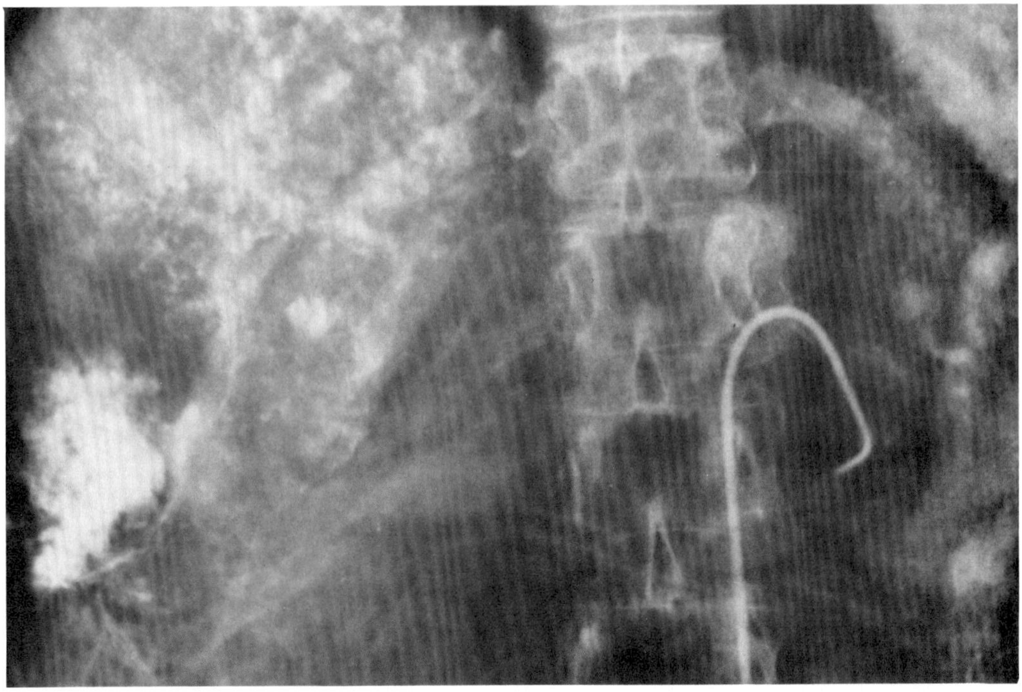

(D)

Figure 5 (continued)

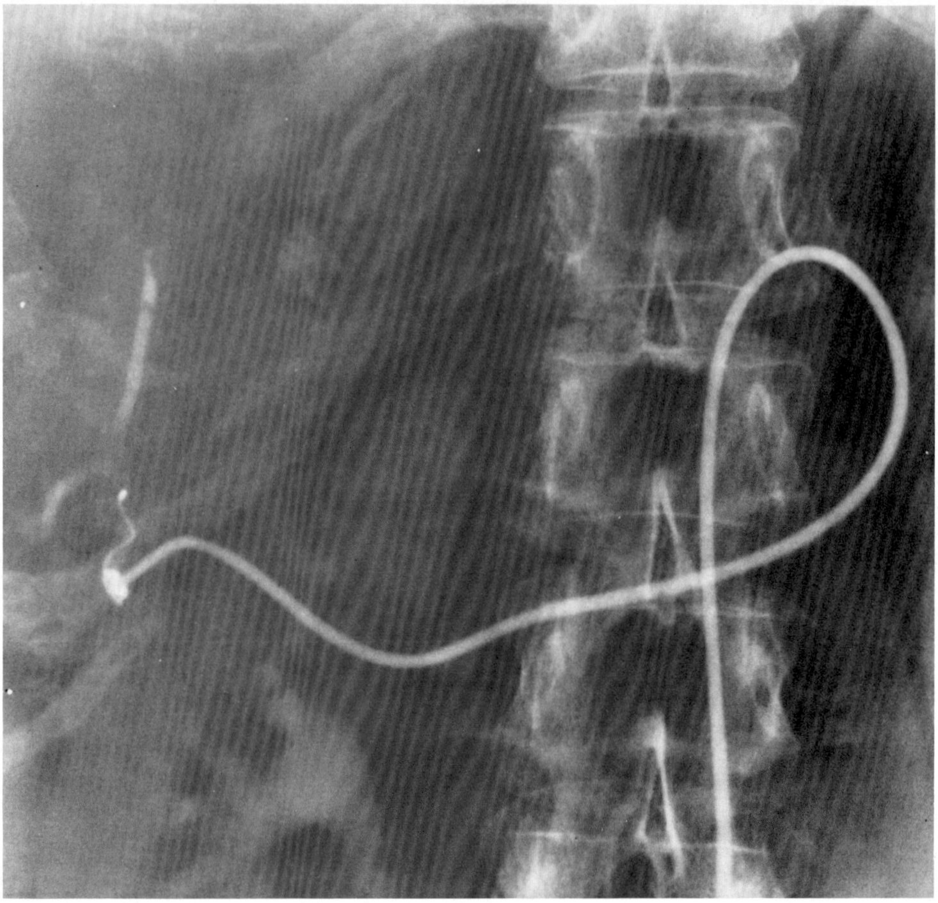

(E)

Figure 5 Diagnostic approach. This female patient also had a small carcinoma of the breast. An exploration of the extent of disease revealed on: (A) Scintigraphy: multiple lesions of the liver. (B) CT confirmed the existence of these multiple lesions. The combination of NM and CT is the most accurate in our hands. However, they still lack specificity. The gastroenterologist performed a percutaneous Menghini needle biopsy which disclosed no evidence of tumor. (C,D) Angiography: because of the discrepancy in clinical and radiographic information, the hepatic arteriogram was performed. This demonstrated hemangiomas of the liver. A hematoma and an arteriovenous fistula were opacified (artery: closed arrow; vein: open arrow). (E) Interventional radiologic management: the catheter was advanced along the right hepatic artery and the fistula was occluded using a 3-mm steel coil.

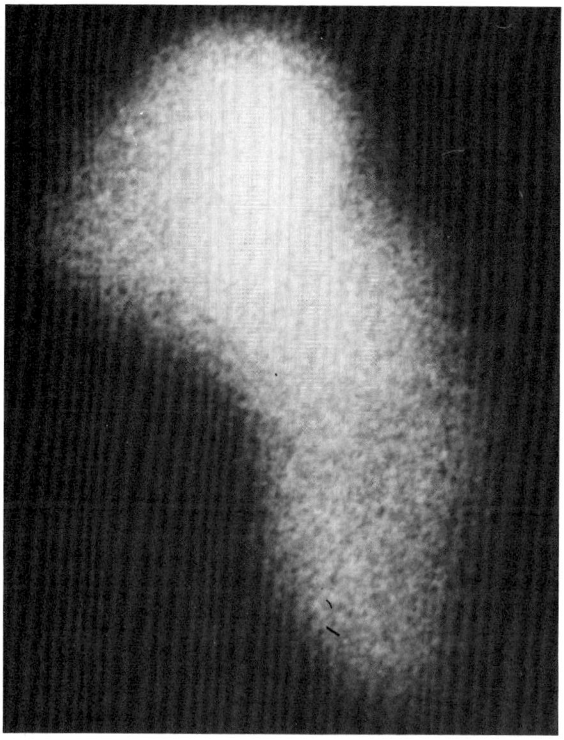

Figure 6A Diagnostic approach. This patient with an insulin-producing islet cell carcinoma of the pancreas, previously treated by hemipancreatectomy, experienced renewed episodes of hypoglycemia. Scintiscan of the liver was considered normal, which did not solve the clinical problem.

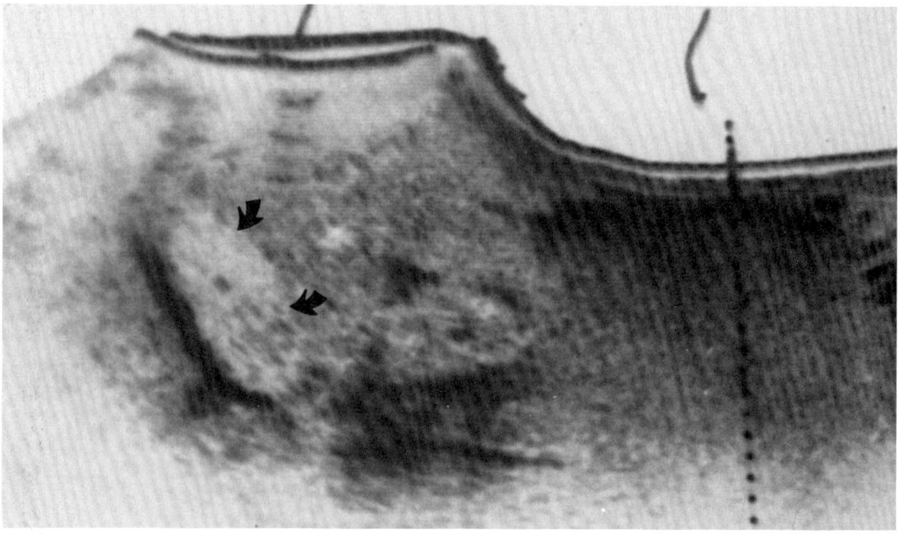

Figure 6B Sonography demonstrated an area of decreased echogenicity in the right lobe of the liver at the dome (arrows).

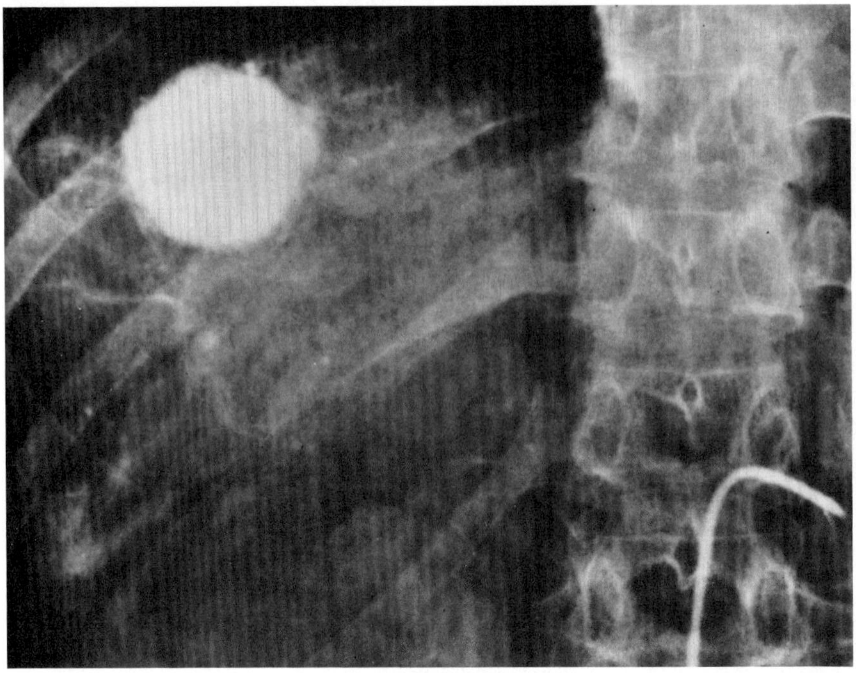

Figure 6C Angiography documented the existence of a single hypervascular metastasis in the dome of the right lobe.

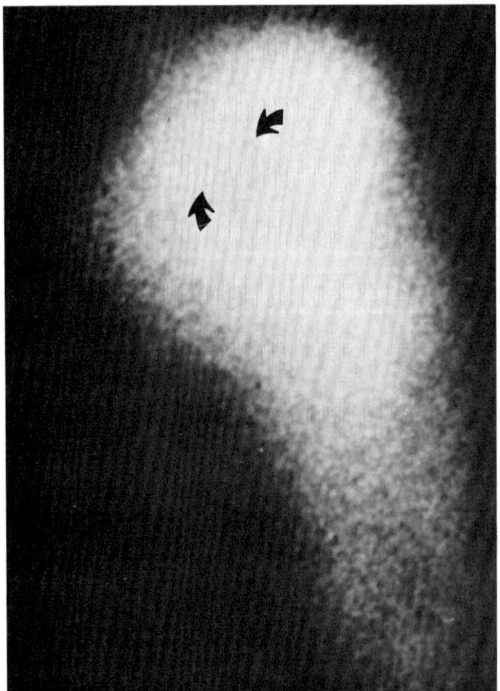

Figure 6D Follow-up scintiscan 6 months later demonstrated the metastatic focus (arrows). In a view of the hypervascularity of islet cell tumors, confirmation was best accomplished by angiography. In the process, the pancreas was reevaluated for residual or recurrent disease.

Signs of left lobe enlargement:

1. Central upper abdominal mass extending toward the left lateral abdominal wall, inseparable from the liver outline
2. Downward displacement of the splenic flexure of the colon
3. Anterior displacement of the transverse colon, which may be pushed upward or downward around the mass
4. Marked displacement of the entire stomach to the left
5. No displacement of the second part of the duodenum
6. Downward displacement of the duodenojejunal flexure
7. Downward and posterior displacement of the left kidney

A diffusely enlarged liver produces a combination of the organ displacements described. Pedunculated masses arising from the undersurface of the liver will impinge on the adjacent viscera. Projection into the retrogastric space will displace the stomach anteriorly and to the left. The pedunculated tissue may be normal liver or a variety of benign or malignant neoplasms, including hamartoma (Fig. 7), hemangioma, adenoma, focal nodular hyperplasia, and hepatoma.

Calcification

The presence and configuration of calcification within an hepatic mass may be helpful in determining the cause. Calcification in the upper abdomen in a child is more common with neuroblastoma or Wilm's tumor. In adults, calcifications in the right upper quadrant are more frequently associated with calculi, biliary or renal. Calcifications within the liver may be related to abscesses, hydatid cysts, granulomas, metastases, hepatocellular neoplasms, hemangiomas, infantile hemangioendotheliomas, simple cysts, and teratoma (Fig. 8A).

Calcifications occur in approximately 25% of children and 10% of adults with malignant hepatocellular neoplasms and may be multiple, irregular, nodular, or discrete (14). In children, the osteoid component of a hepatocellular neoplasm is frequently responsible for the calcium deposition (Fig. 8B), whereas in adults, calcification is usually a manifestation of tumor necrosis. Hemangiomas may contain linear, stellate, speckled, or rounded calcifications which may rarely have the appearance of phleboliths. Benign hepatic cysts (Fig. 8C), and hydatid cysts may have curvilinear calcifications in the wall. Calcification in a teratoma has been described as irregular and faint (15). In infants and children, metastases to the liver containing calcifications are more frequently from a neuroblastoma. Metastases showing calcification in adults usually originate from the colon, ovary, pancreas, APUD (amine precursor uptake dehydrogenase) tumors, and thyroid.

Osteoporosis

Osteoporosis has been described in children with primary malignant hepatic tumors, glycogen storage disease, and hepatic cirrhosis (16,17). This is probably related to loss of functioning liver tissue and associated with disturbed lipid metabolism, hyperlipidemia, and hypercholesterolemia (16). In hepatic neoplasms, osteoporosis need not be associated with extensive tumor invasion (17).

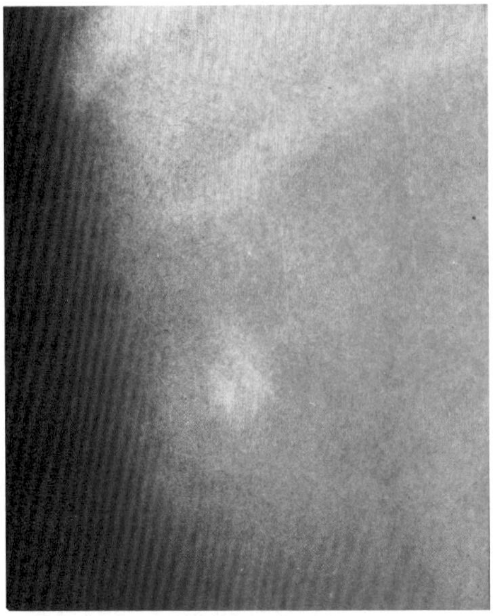

(A)

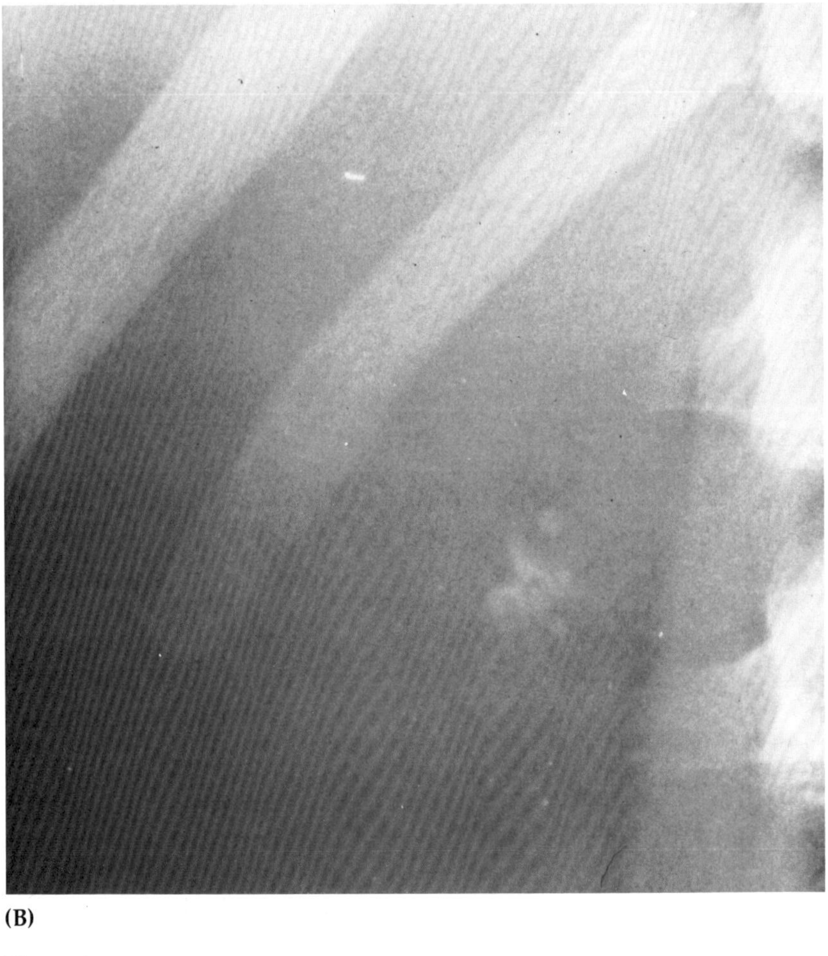

(B)

Figure 8

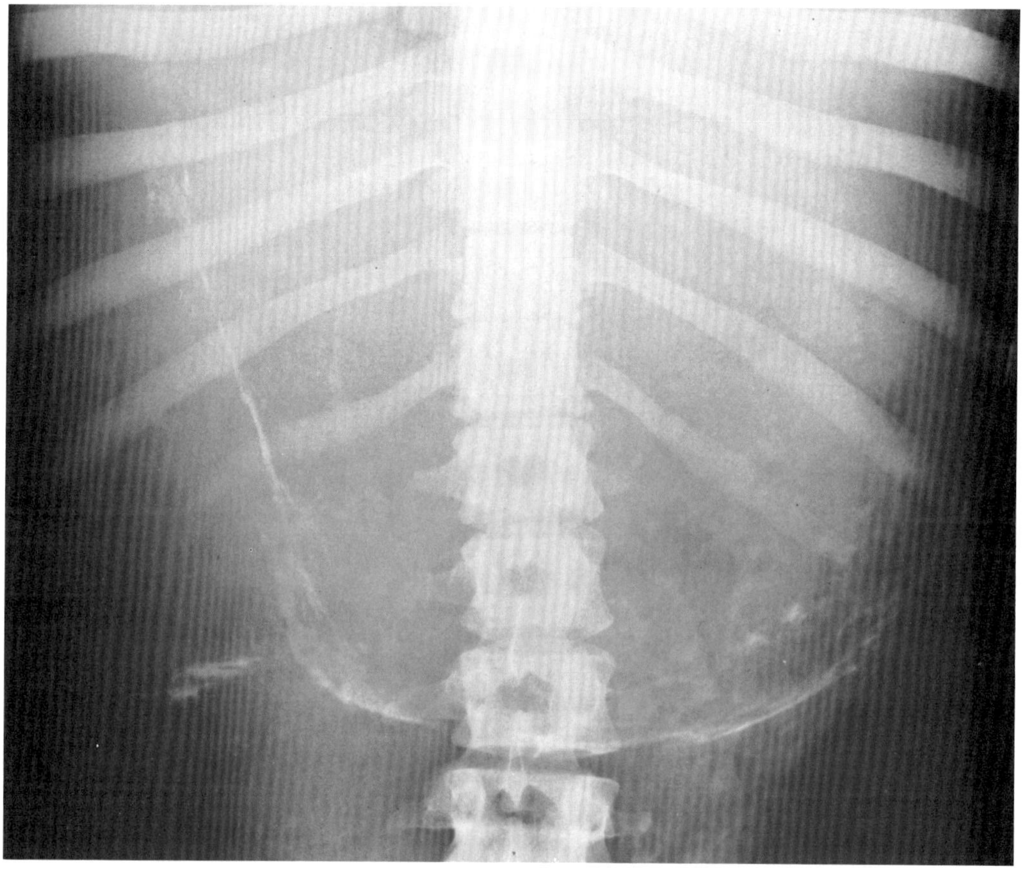

(C)

Figure 8 Hepatic calcifications. (A) Cystic hamartoma. (B) Hepatocellular carcinoma. (C) Multiple benign cysts.

Specific Techniques

Total Body Opacification

The intravenous injection of water-soluble radiopaque contrast material, 60% methylglucamine diatrizoate (1 ml per pound of body weight by drip infusion or bolus injection), will increase the radiodensity of the liver as it does of other solid viscera. Tomography can enhance the visualization of both normal and abnormal densities in the liver. Radiographs exposed during the injection are useful for a better appreciation of the nature of the mass. During the hepatogram phase, the line of demarcation between the mass and surrounding liver may be better discerned (Fig. 9). This technique is particularly applicable to newborns and infants, especially in the diagnosis of cysts or abscesses which are avascular, and of hemangiomatous or hepatocellular neoplasms, which are frequently hypervascular (18).

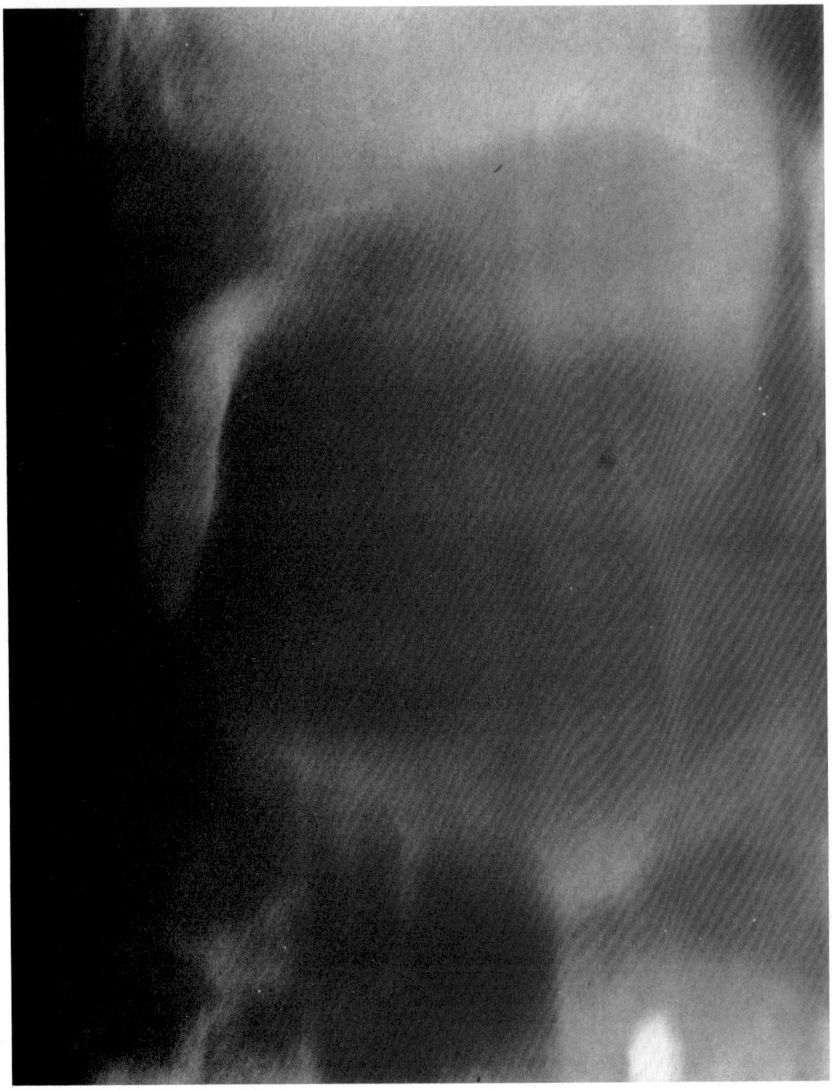

(A)

Figure 9

Angiography

Hepatic angiography is now reserved for problem solving or in preparation for therapeutic management. It is the most invasive of the diagnostic methods, requires hospitalization, and is, therefore, expensive. More sophisticated techniques in angiography include superselective catheterization, magnification, infusion, and pharmacoangiography (see Chap. 12). Still, there are limitations.

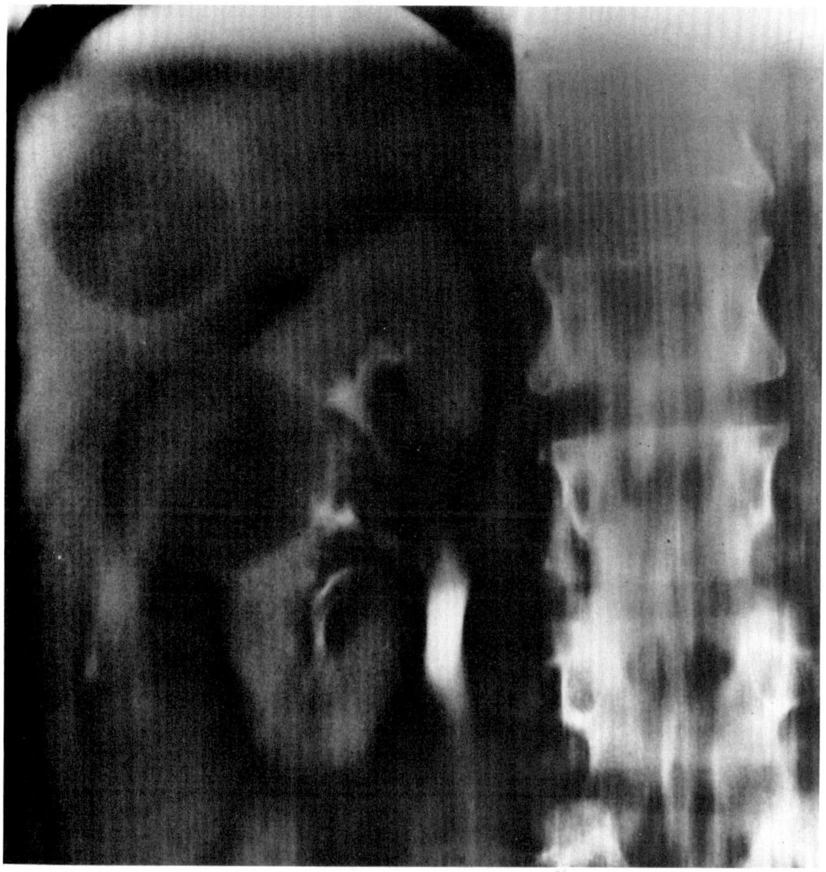

(B)

Figure 9 Total body opacification. (A) Simple hepatic cyst in the left lobe of the liver. The line from the gallbladder bed to the inferior vena cava delineates the right from the left lobe of the liver. The position of the gallbladder defines the localization of the cyst. (B) Simple cysts of the liver and kidney in another patient.

Value of Supraselective Catheterization

Most neoplasms have some degree of neovascularity which at times can be demonstrated only by more selective catheterization. Superselective catheterization of the hepatic arteries can be accomplished in 95% of patients. Angiography remains the most specific of all diagnostic radiologic procedures (Fig. 10). Hypervascular neoplasms, as small as 5 mm, can be defined, whereas hypovascular lesions still require a diameter minimum of 2 cm for detection. The angiographic evaluation of the left lateral segment of the liver remains difficult. It is small, comprising 10–15% of the liver substance, is horizontal in position, and is supplied by the superior and inferior subsegmental branches. These are approximately parallel and frequently superimposed on the spine, gastric fundus, or the spleen. Selective catheterization of the left hepatic artery or the artery to the left lateral

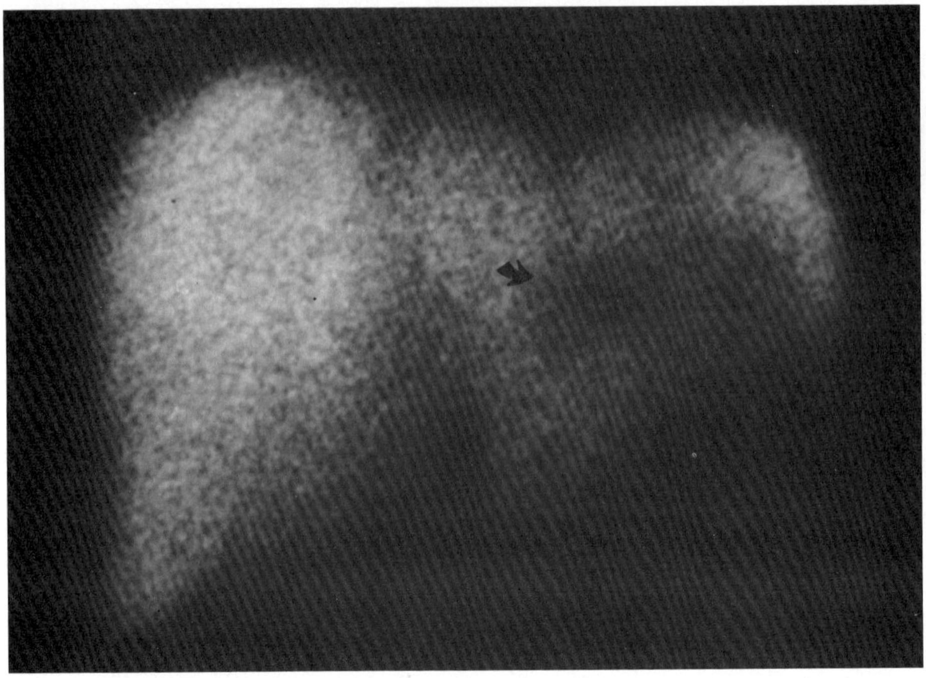

(A)

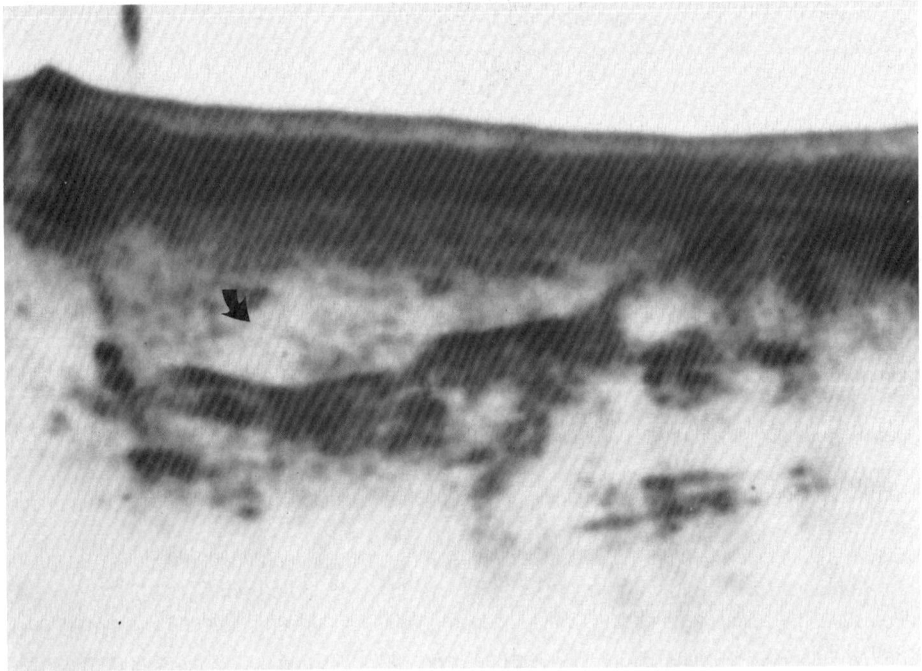

(B)

Figure 10 Diagnostic approach. Workup of a patient with colon carcinoma and metastases to the left lobe of the liver (arrows) as seen by: (A) Scintigraphy. (B) Sonography (longitudinal scan). (C) CT. These modalities confirm the presence of metastases in the left lateral segment. (D) Angiography not only demonstrates the large lesion in the left lobe but also multiple small metastases in the right lobe. This finding will clearly influence management.

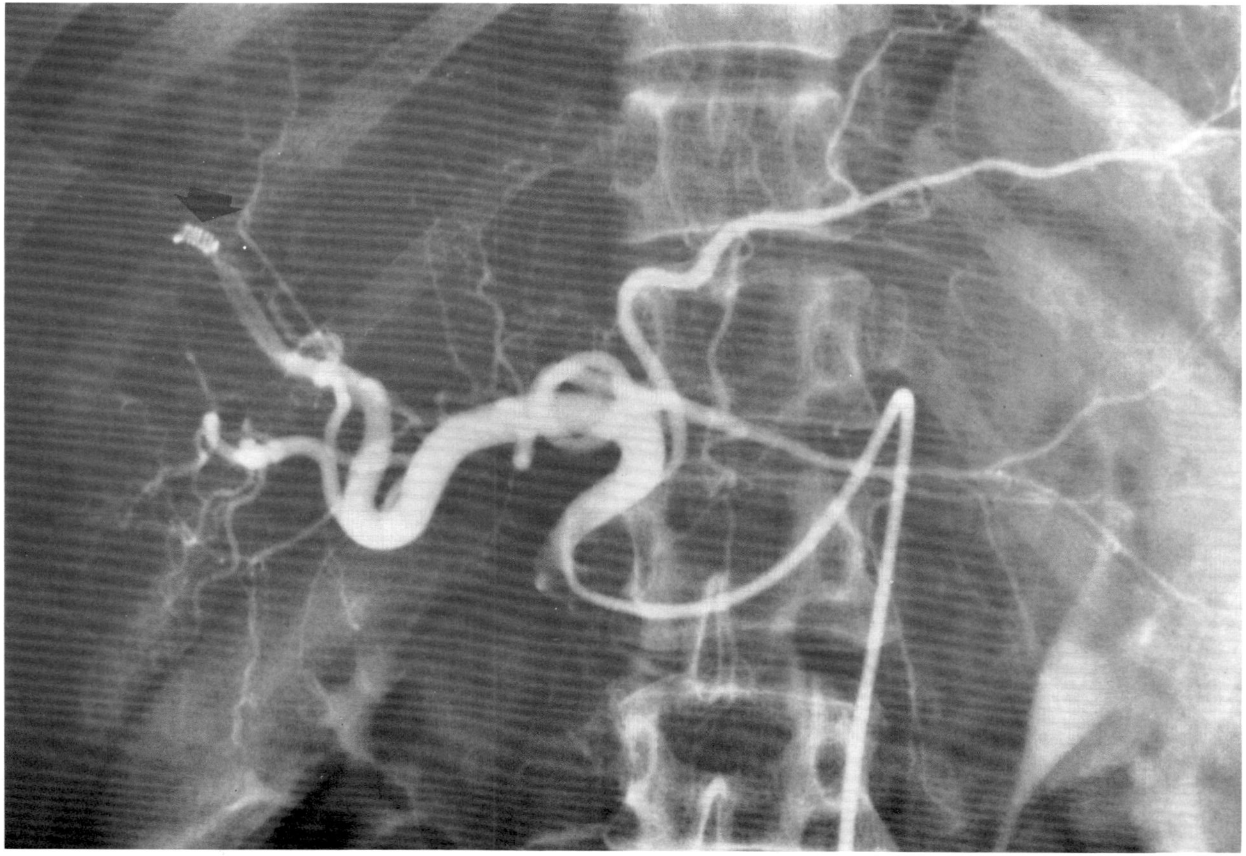

Figure 13D Postocclusion arteriogram no longer opacifies the fistula. The arrow indicates the coil which occludes the right hepatic artery.

Comparison of Biopsy Methods

Conventional liver biopsy techniques remain the procedure of choice with diffuse parenchymal disease. However, accuracy decreases in the presence of focal malignant disease (40,43), due primarily to a reluctance to change from the usual puncture site and the relatively short length of the needles. Fine needle aspiration biopsy employs longer needles, smaller gauge, and can be assisted by such methods of localization as CT, US, NM, and angiography. Johansen and Svendsen (40) reported a correct diagnosis of malignancy in 94% with material obtained by fine needle aspiration of the liver guided by radionuclide scan. The combined method of biopsy using ultrasound has also been found to be helpful. Our results of 83% accuracy compared favorably; the cases were usually selected when Menghini biopsy attempts were inconclusive or the lesions were located in areas difficult to approach by the more conventional procedures. Aspiration biopsy allows the puncture of lesions of the left lobe of the liver as well as biopsy in jaundiced patients; it is easier to perform because the lesions can be accurately localized and the approach is more direct.

Hepatic Tumors

Primary tumors of the liver, although rare, are the third most frequent solid abdominal neoplasms in children, following Wilm's tumor and neuroblastoma. The incidence of hepatic malignancies has been reported as 0.06–0.16 per 1000 admissions to children's hospitals (44,45). In adults, primary carcinoma of the liver displays a remarkable geographic distribution. Its relative frequency among all cancers has been 1.4–2.5% in America, 1.2% in Europe, 16.9% in Singapore, and 50.9% in the Bantu in Africa (46). Benign tumors are reported approximately one-tenth as frequently (47). On the other hand, the liver is the most common site of metastatic disease. Among all patients who die of cancer, about 50–75% have liver metastases (48–51).

Classification

In view of the rarity of benign hepatic tumors, some confusion exists over their histological classification. Table 3 lists benign masses in the liver by combining the classifications of Edmondson (52) and Ishak and Rabin (53). A classification of the malignant hepatic tumors is given in Table 4.

Benign Hepatic Tumors

Incidence and Presentation

Benign tumors of the liver may be found at any age, but the majority are detected in adults of middle age. In children, benign tumors are discovered mainly under 2 years of age. The most frequent tumors of the newborn period are the hemangioendotheliomas, solitary cysts, and cavernous hemangiomas. In adults, benign tumors are more common in females than in males, approximately 5:1, while the malignancies are more frequent in males (54). In their clinical presentation, benign tumors are relatively asymptomatic, except for acute catastrophic hemorrhages seen in hepatic adenomas and hemangiomas, while malignant neoplasms are more generally symptomatic. Benign tumors are often

Table 3 Benign Masses of the Liver

I. Nonparasitic cysts, cystic dystrophies
  A. Solitary cysts
  B. Polycystic disease
  C. Congenital dilatation of intrahepatic biliary ducts (Caroli)
  D. Congenital hepatic fibrosis

II. Tumors of hepatocellular origin
  A. Focal nodular hyperplasia
  B. Hepatocellular adenoma

III. Tumors of cholangiocellular origin
  A. Bile duct adenoma
  B. Bile duct cystadenoma

IV. Tumors of fibrous tissue
  A. Fibroma

V. Tumors of adipose tissue
  A. Lipoma

VI. Tumors of muscle tissue
  A. Leiomyoma

VII. Tumors of blood vessels
  A. Hemangioma
  B. Infantile hemangioendothelioma

VIII. Tumors and tumorlike lesions of lymph vessels
  A. Lymphangioma

IX. Tumors of mesothelial tissues
  A. Benign mesothelioma

X. Miscellaneous tumors and tumorlike lesions
  A. Heterotopias—adrenal cell rests
  B. Benign teratomas
  C. Mesenchymal hamartoma
    Cystic
    Solid
  D. Myxoma

Table 4 Malignant Tumors of the Liver Primary

I. Hepatocellular neoplasms
  A. Hepatoblastoma
  B. Hepatocarcinoma (hepatoma)
  C. Hepatic mixed tumors

II. Cholangiocellular neoplasms
  A. Cholangiocarcinoma

III. Mesenchymal neoplasms
  A. Malignant mesenchymal tumors
    1. Embryonal rhabdomyosarcoma
    2. Malignant counterparts of benign tumors (e.g., leiomyosarcoma, fibrosarcoma, etc.)
  B. Hemangiosarcoma (angiosarcoma)

discovered incidentally by the patient, the parents, or during the physician's examination for unrelated complaints. The normal growth of the child and the general health of the patient are usually not disturbed. Physical examination reveals a well-delineated epigastric mass without splenomegaly. In spite of the enlarged liver, the liver function studies are usually normal.

Benign vascular tumors are almost always incidental findings, at times associated with cutaneous hemangiomas. The average age of the female patient with a symptomatic hemangioma is 45 years. Symptoms are created by the size of the mass or an acute hemorrhage. On the other hand, when symptomatic, infantile hemangioendotheliomas and cavernous hemangiomas are diagnosed before 6 months of age. These children may present with high output congestive failure, thrombocytopenia, and acute intra-abdominal hemorrhage due to rupture (see Chap. 30).

Cystlike Masses

Solitary Unilocular Cysts

Solitary cysts of the liver are most commonly discovered in adult females and most frequently in the right lobe. They tend to be silent and innocuous. When symptomatic, abdominal pain is the most outstanding complaint. Acute severe pain may result from intracystic hemorrhage or rarely from the twisting of the pedicle of a pedunculated cyst. The pain may be episodic and simulate biliary colic. Abdominal fullness, nausea, and vomiting may also be experienced. Examination of the abdomen reveals a palpable mass. Jaundice occurs only if there is bile duct obstruction, which is not unusual. Curvilinear calcifications in the wall of the cyst may occasionally be discerned radiologically (Fig. 8C).

Radiologic appearance Radionuclide scanning usually reveals a round area of decreased uptake of isotope. Ultrasound will define a rounded sonolucent mass with through transmission with echoes building up beyond the smooth distal wall (Fig. 4). A hepatic cyst as seen by computed tomography is a rounded area of decreased attenuation measuring 0–10 HU, the density of water. Total body opacification studies demonstrate the relative lucency of the cyst and a smooth sharp demarcation at the margin as seen in a renal cyst (Fig. 9). Tomography might enhance the demonstration of the cyst. Hepatic angiography reveals a curvilinear displacement of intrahepatic vessels. Portal venography and hepatic venography will demonstrate the smooth distortion of these vessels by the cyst, a mass of relative lucency with a sharp delineation from the surrounding parenchyma.

Diagnosis Puncture of the hepatic cyst can be accomplished with aspiration of its contents, which are usually yellow to brown in color with little, if any, bile. The injection of carbon dioxide or air and water-soluble contrast material allows evaluation of the cyst wall (Fig. 14). The contents should be examined for neoplastic cells and bile. Attempts at sclerosing the cyst may be made with the injection of an oil-based material such as Pantopaque (Fig. 14D,E). However, surgical treatment may become necessary because of the large size of a cyst.

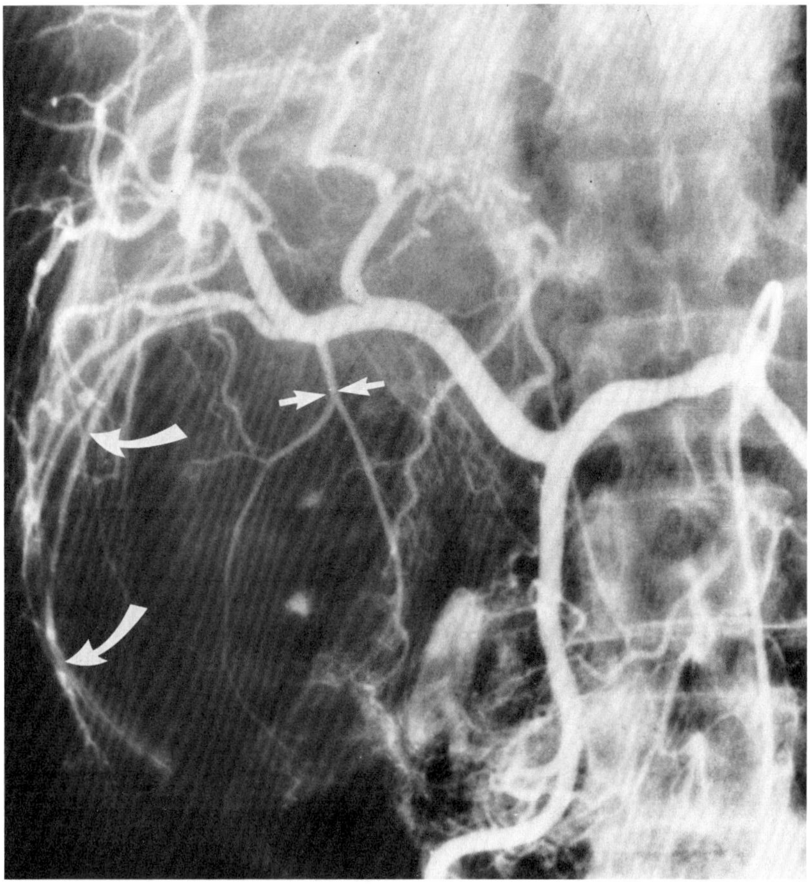

Figure 14A Hepatic cyst puncture. The arterial phase demonstrates displacement of the anterior inferior branch (curved arrows) of the right hepatic artery and, to a lesser degree, of the posterior inferior branch. The cystic artery (arrows) overlies the mass. Therefore, the cyst lies in both the right and left lobes of the liver.

Polycystic Disease

Polycystic disease is the most common nonparasitic cyst formation of the liver. It is also relatively asymptomatic, depending on the extent of involvement; even when extensive, liver function studies are seldom impaired. Polycystic disease in childhood can be classified according to the age of presentation into perinatal, neonatal, infantile, and juvenile (55,56). There is a frequent association with polycystic disease of the kidneys (adult type), where the prognosis is determined by the renal disease. Of patients with polycystic kidneys, 19–33% have polycystic kidneys (55). Cysts may also be found in the

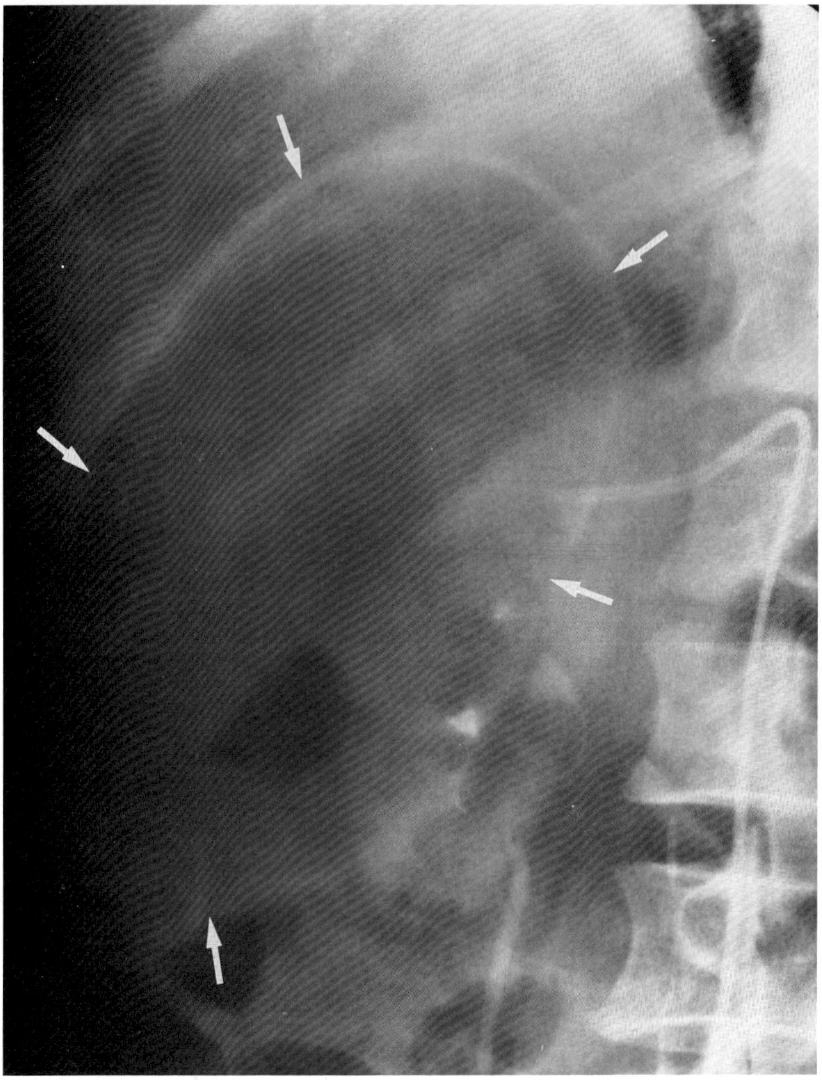

Figure 14B The hepatogram phase defines the fine line of the cyst wall (arrows).

pancreas and lung. On rare occasions, polycystic disease of the liver can be associated with congenital hepatic fibrosis and portal hypertension (57).

Radiologic Diagnosis The diagnosis of polycystic disease of the liver can be established by scintigraphy, ultrasonography, or computed tomography; angiography is not often required. The incidence of cystic disease has been found to be greater than previously considered because of the identification by these screening techniques. Scintigraphy merely defines rounded areas of decreased uptake indistinguishable as to

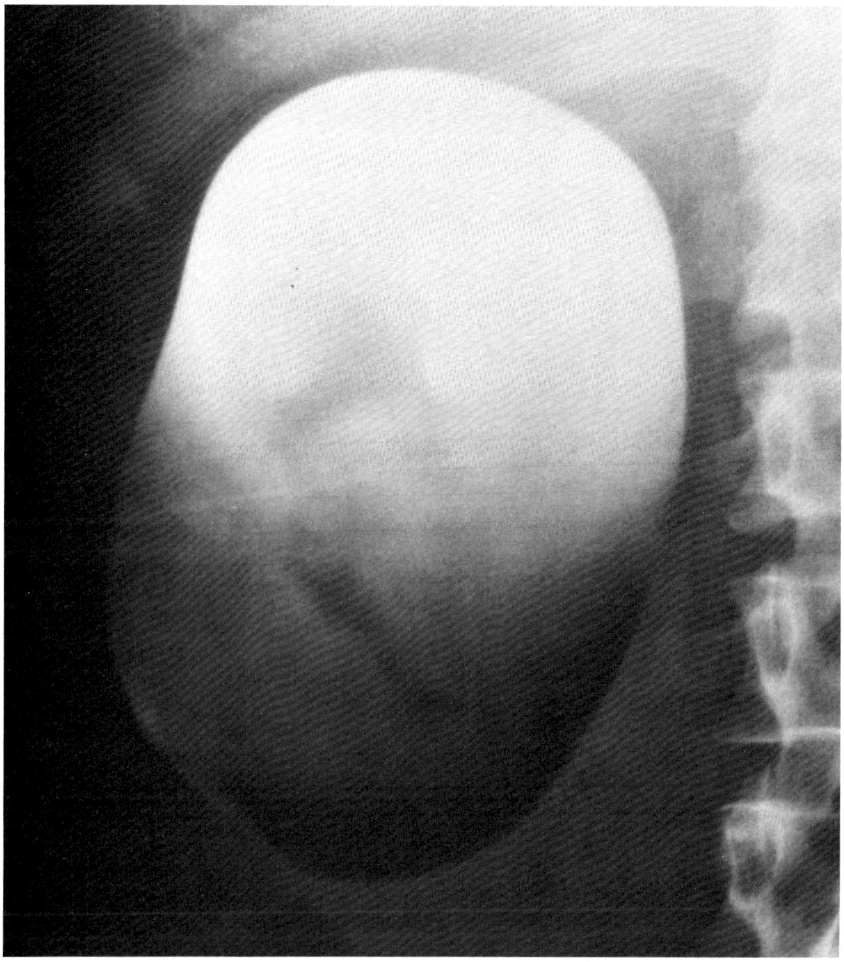

Figure 14C The cyst was punctured, aspirated, and contrast material and air injected, demonstrating a smooth wall.

etiology. Ultrasound establishes the cystic nature of the lesions as smooth, rounded, sonolucent masses with through-transmission. Computed tomography confirms the nature, and when large enough (i.e., greater than 2 cm), the attenuation coefficient is 0, that of water. However, when smaller or located deep within the liver parenchyma, the volume averaging will yield a higher coefficient.

Differential diagnosis Differentiation must be made from multiple abscesses and multiple necrotic neoplasm (57) (Fig. 15); this may require biopsy, guided by US or CT. Angiography may become necessary should confusion persist. Curvilinear displacement and stretching of the hepatic arteries and portal veins with multiple sharply circumscribed

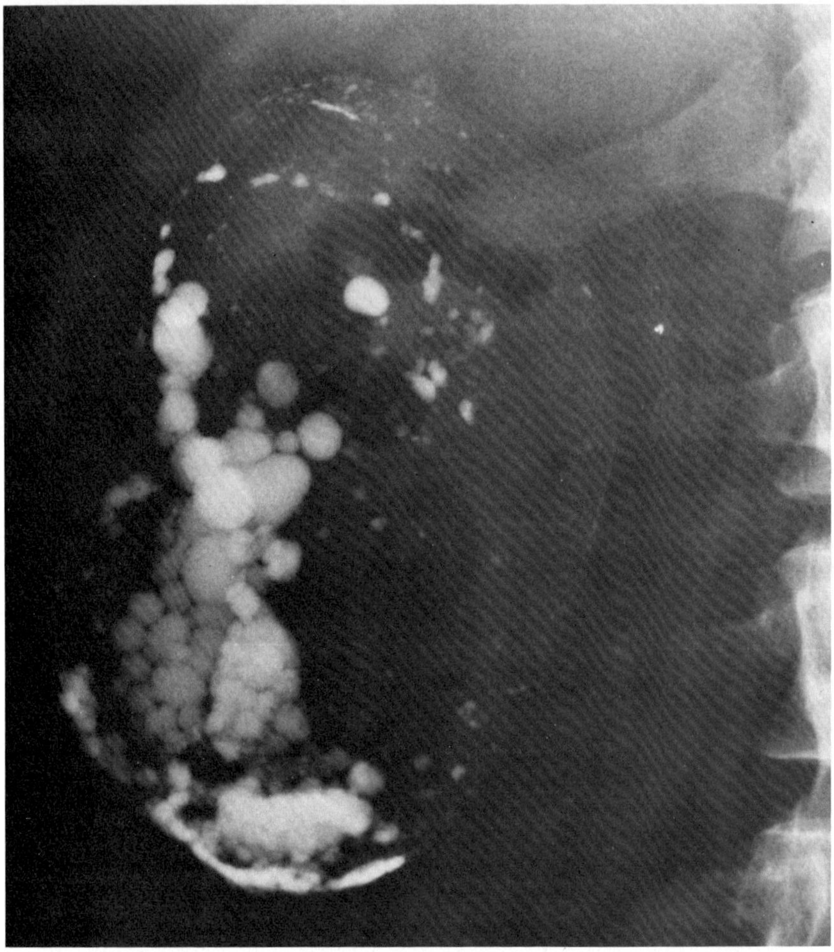

Figure 14D Pantopaque was injected in an attempt to sclerose the wall and decrease the size of the cyst to alleviate the patient's complaint of pain.

lucencies are seen in the hepatogram phase. The cysts may be surrounded by a hypervascular rim, representing the cyst wall or compressed parenchyma.

Congenital Dilatation of Intrahepatic Ducts (Caroli's Disease)

This disease is familial, probably due to an inherited Mendelian recessive trait (58,59). The congenital nature is suggested by its occurrence in newborns and its frequent association with cystic disease of the kidneys and pancreas and congenital hepatic fibrosis (59,60). In the absence of hepatic fibrosis, afflicted children live to be adults, but are predisposed to biliary calculi, cholangitis, and liver abscess.

Cystic dilatation of the intrahepatic ducts has been shown to follow peripheral embolization of the livers of monkeys with silicone (61). The radiographic picture was indistinguishable from Caroli's disease, providing a possible etiological basis.

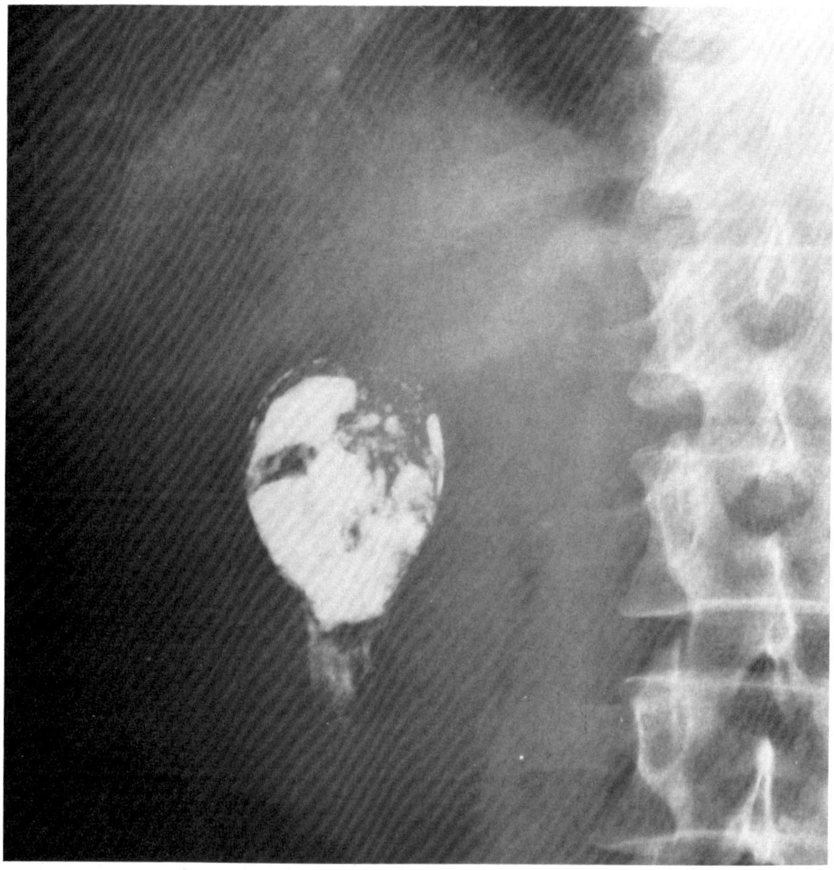

Figure 14E Six months later, there was marked reduction in the size of the cyst and relief of pain.

On US, CT, NM, and angiography, dilated bile may simulate polycystic liver disease. However, "cyst" puncture yields bile because of the continuity with the biliary tract. Transhepatic cholangiography provides the definitive diagnosis (Fig. 16).

Liver Abscess

Hepatic abscesses are usually bacterial in origin (gram-negative *Aerobacter* and *Escherichia coli*), while the infestations may be amebic or hydatid, and are most frequently found in the dome of the right lobe. Diagnosis by screening techniques (Figs. 17, 18) is nonspecific and it is frequently impossible to differentiate from benign cysts, benign cystic tumors, or necrotic neoplasms (6,62). Depending on the maturation of the abscess wall and the consistency of the contents, the CT attenuation coefficient will vary. Early in the course of the disease, angiography will merely show displacement of the hepatic arteries and portal veins. As the abscess matures, a definite wall may be portrayed angiographically as a hypervascular ring surrounding a relatively avascular center. The angiographic appearance is at times difficult to differentiate from that of a cystic mass from any other cause, but the febrile clinical course is usually the deciding factor (63).

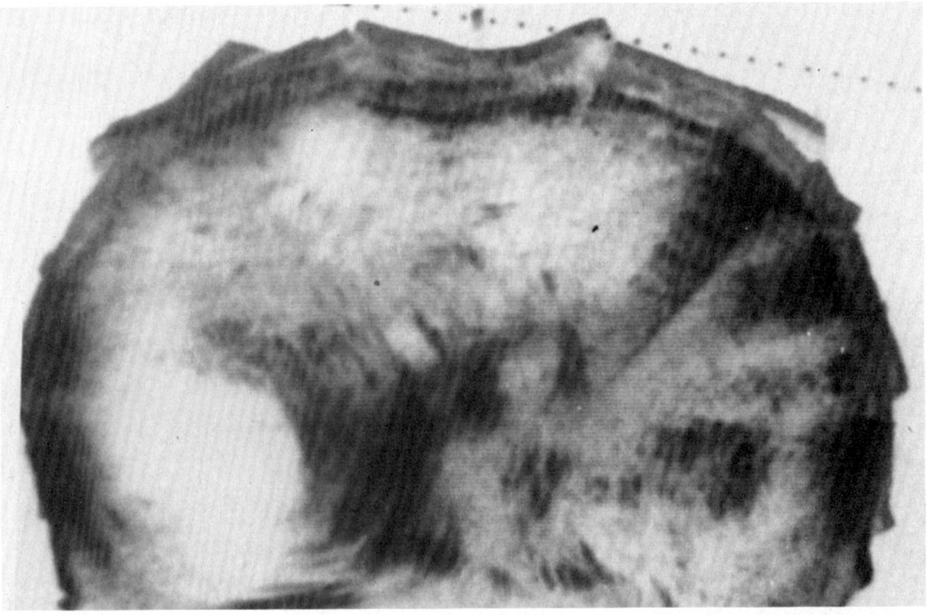

(A)

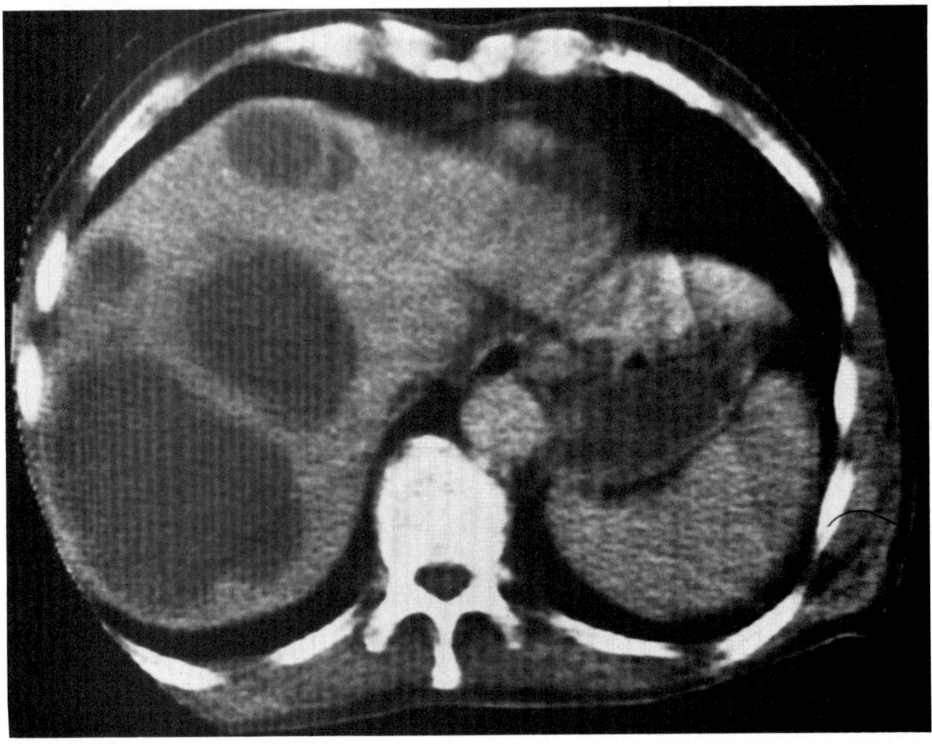

(B)

Figure 15

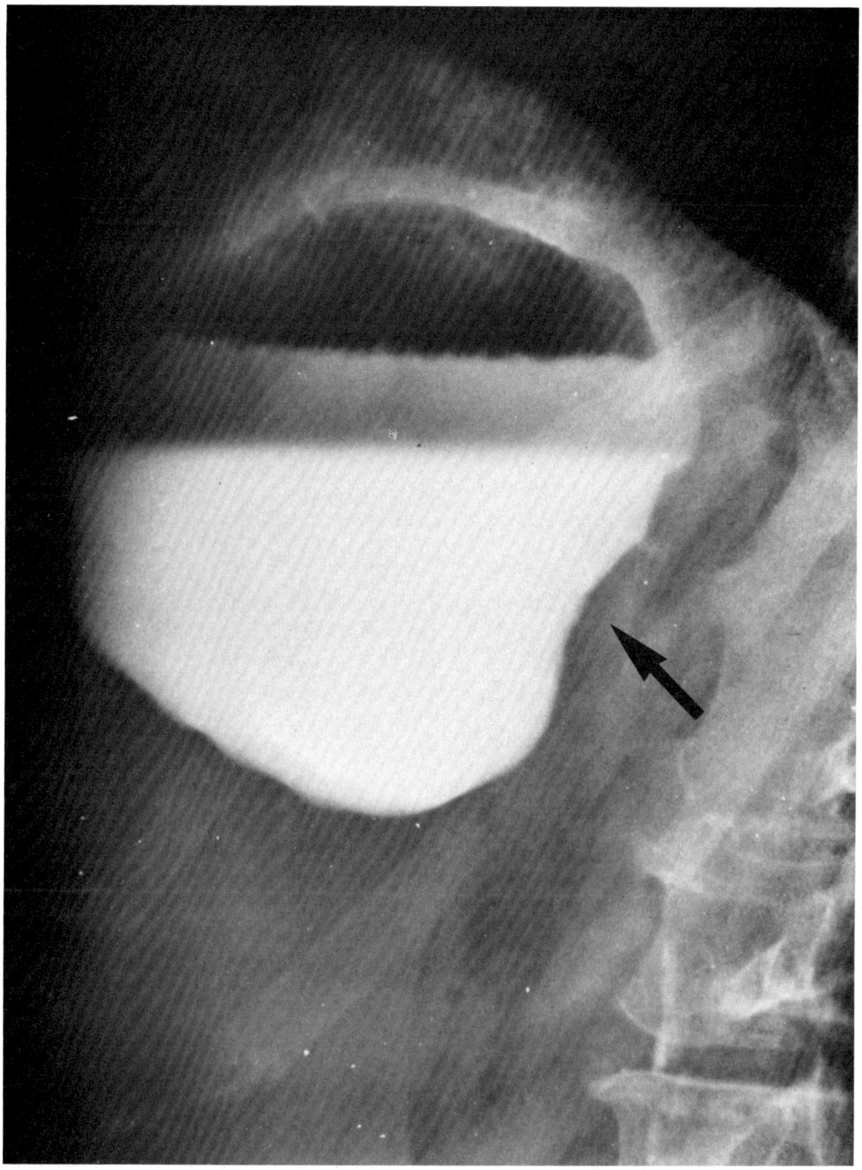

(C)

Figure 15 Cavitating metastatic leiomyosarcoma in a patient with a known leiomyosarcoma of the stomach who experienced right upper quadrant discomfort. (A) US, Sonolucent masses in the liver with some through transmission. (B) CT, Multiple low-attenuation lesion (0–10 EMI units) with relatively smooth margins. The differential diagnosis of benign hepatic cysts from necrotic metastases was not established. (C) Transhepatic puncture, aspiration, and injection of water-based contrast material and air demonstrated slight irregularity of the wall (arrow). The aspirate revealed tumor cells.

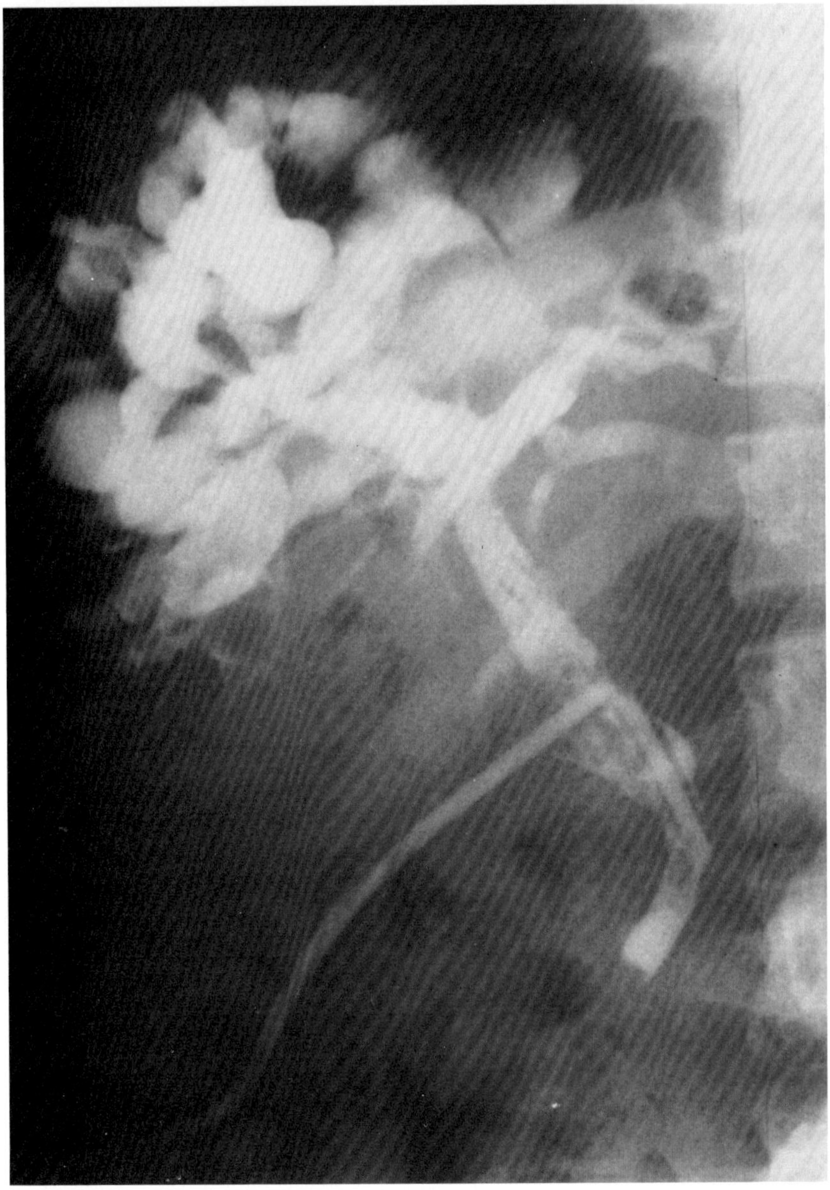

Figure 16 Caroli's disease. The operative cholangiography best defines the saccular dilatation of the intrahepatic bile ducts. (Courtesy of Dr. McIntyre, Houston, Texas.)

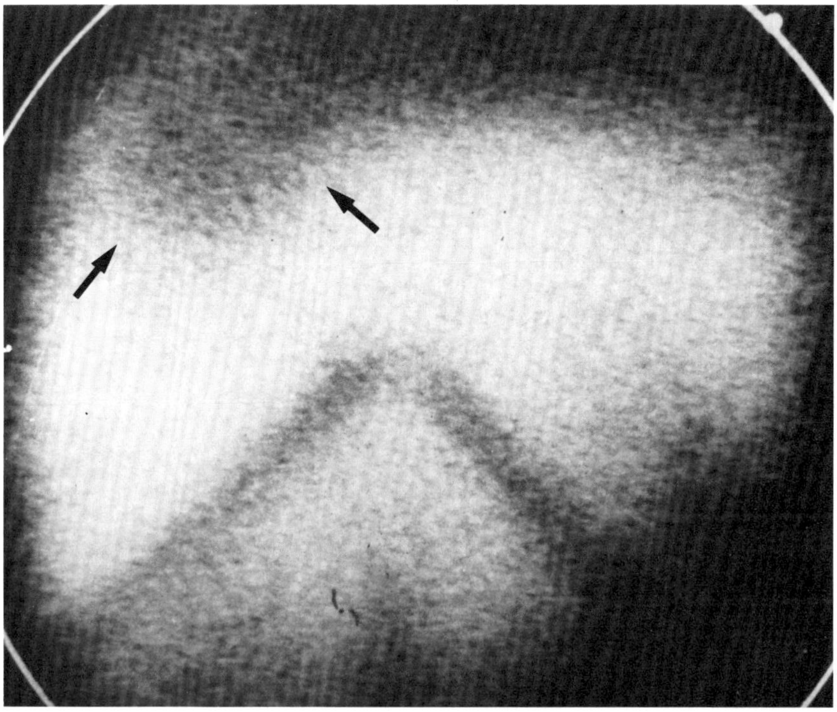

Figure 17A Hepatic abscess (bacterial). A 48-year-old black female who had an ovarian neoplasm removed 6 years earlier, developed generalized weakness, chills, and fever. Anemia and a purulent right pleural effusion were discovered and a subhepatic purulent collection was drained. Chills and fever continued. A liver scan with ^{99m}Tc sulfur colloid revealed a "cold" area in the right lobe (arrows). An upper gastrointestinal examination disclosed an ulcerated submucosal mass in the descending limb of the duodenum.

Diagnosis Percutaneous needle puncture and aspiration of contents will establish the nature of the lesion. At times, injection of water-based contrast and air or CO_2 will delineate the irregular nodular wall seen in both an abscess and a necrotic neoplasm. Bacteriologic and cytologic evaluation may then aid in differentiation and lead to the correct diagnosis.

Percutaneous drainage of an abscess Drainage of an abscess can then proceed (Fig. 19). The Seldinger approach can be adapted with the use of a guide wire and polyethylene catheters (63–67). Utilizing the liver scan and angiogram for localization, drainage is undertaken under fluoroscopic guidance. Under local anesthesia, a small

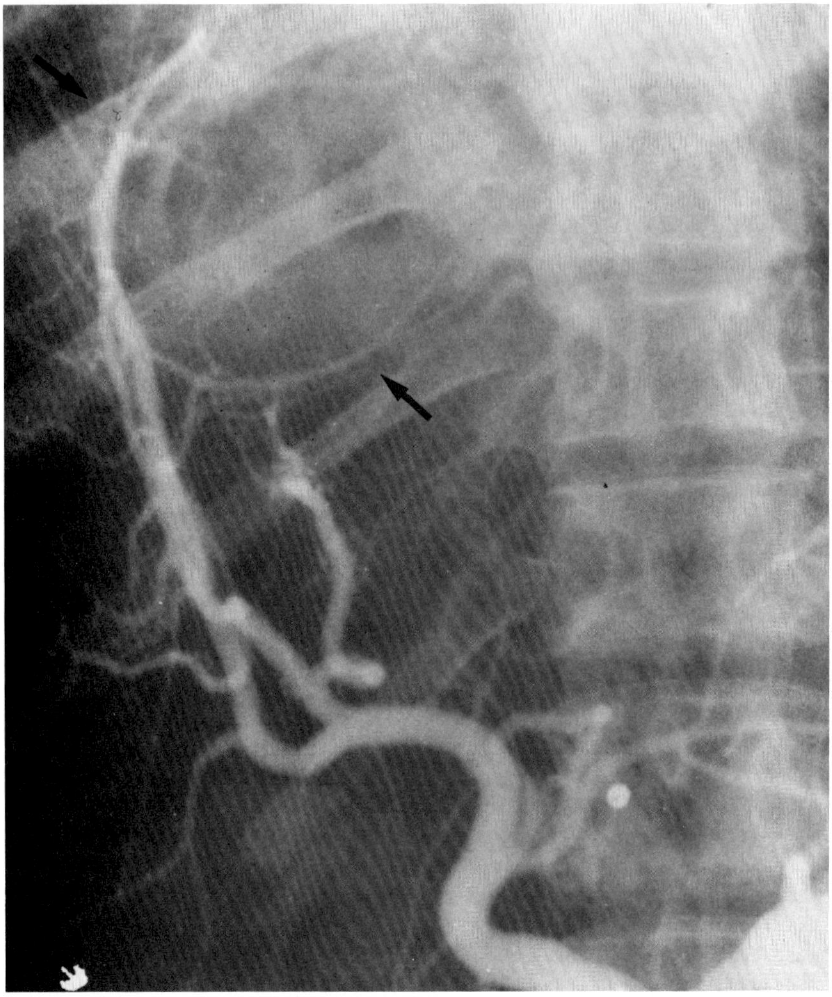

Figure 17B Celiac and superior mesenteric arteriography demonstrated curvilinear displacement of the superior portions of the anterior and posterior segmental branches of the right hepatic artery by an avascular mass (arrows). In addition, a well-defined hypervascular lobulated neoplasm was opacified to the right of the gastroduodenal artery, coinciding with the upper gastrointestinal examination. Exploratory laparotomy confirmed the presence of a hepatic abscess from which *Enterobacter* and anaerobic streptococci were cultured. A perforated leiomyoma of the second portion of the duodenum was resected.

incision is made in the lateral aspect of the abdominal wall at the midpoint of the liver shadow. In suspended respiration a 6-in. polyethylene-sheathed 18-gauge needle is introduced and any purulent material is aspirated and removed for culture and sensitivities. A 0.038-in. guide wire is inserted through the sheath, which is withdrawn and replaced by a 7– 8F radiopaque pigtailed catheter with multiple side holes near the tip. By the same procedure a second catheter is introduced, at a slightly different angle. One of

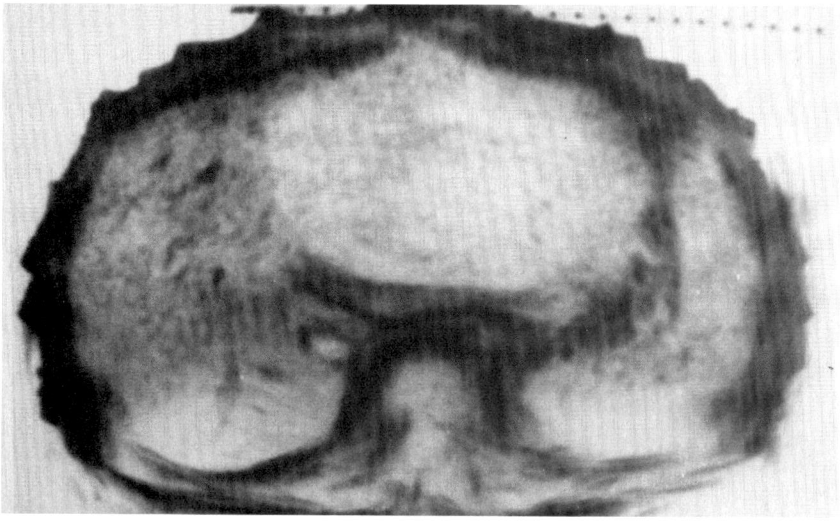

(A)

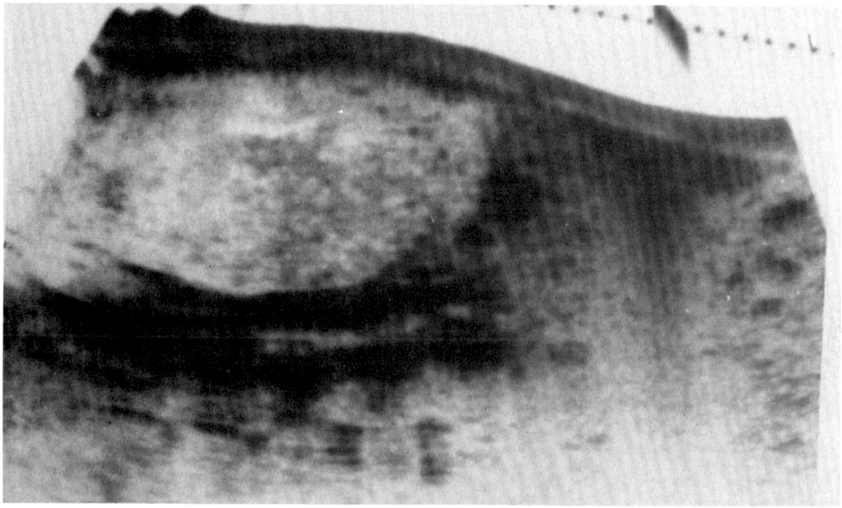

(B)

Figure 18 Amebic abscess in a physician recently returned from South America. Abdominal pain, fever, palpable mass in the midepigastrium. (A,B) US scans, transverse and longitudinal, revealed a mass with a complex echo pattern and minimal through transmission. (C) CT confirmed the presence of a large mass in the left lobe with attenuation of 20 HU.

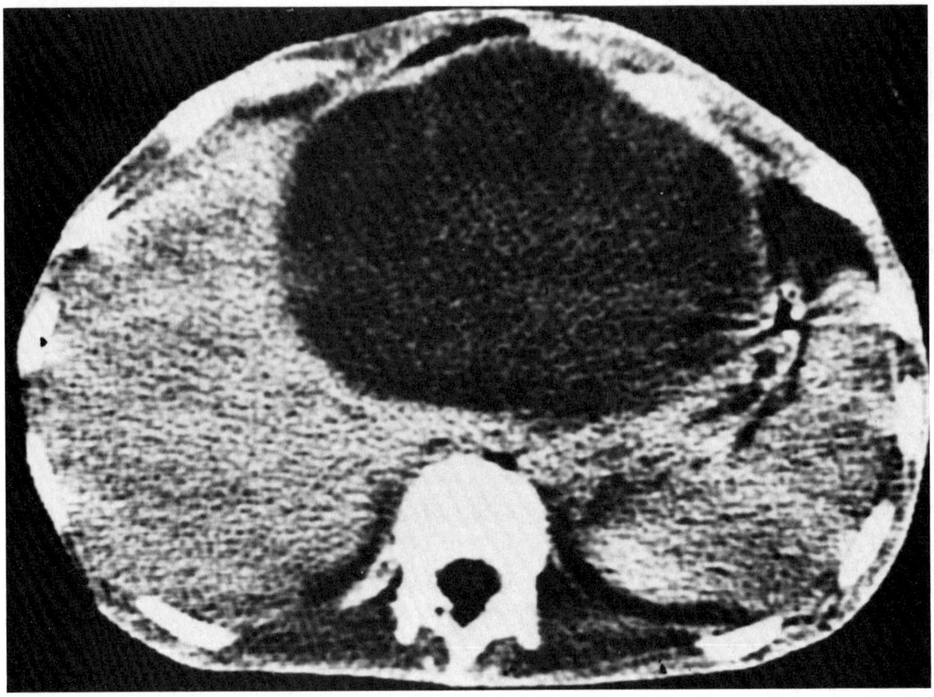

(C)

the two catheters should lead to the most dependent portion of the abscess. This allows for excellent drainage and is used thrice daily for through-irrigation with saline and an appropriate antibiotic.

Multiloculated abscesses must be managed surgically for the interruption of the septa for drainage.

Differential Diagnosis

The differential diagnosis of a cystic mass in the liver should include bacterial abscesses, parasitic infestations, traumatic or hemorrhagic cysts, cystic and necrotic mesenchymal hamartomas, hemorrhage into an hepatic adenoma or focal nodular hyperplasia, teratoid tumors, and cystic alteration in primary and secondary malignancies. Percutaneous needle puncture is indicated in cystlike lesions and is best accomplished by utilizing CT or US for guidance. If the lesion is large enough, fluoroscopic control of the puncture and aspiration procedure is more efficient.

Mesenchymal Tumors

Hamartoma

Cystic Mesenchymal hamartoma This tumor is perhaps lymphangiomatous in origin and is usually discovered before the child is 20 months of age (52,54,68). The relatively symptomless mass in the upper abdomen may rapidly increase in size because of an accumulation of fluid within the lesion. It is usually poorly demarcated from the

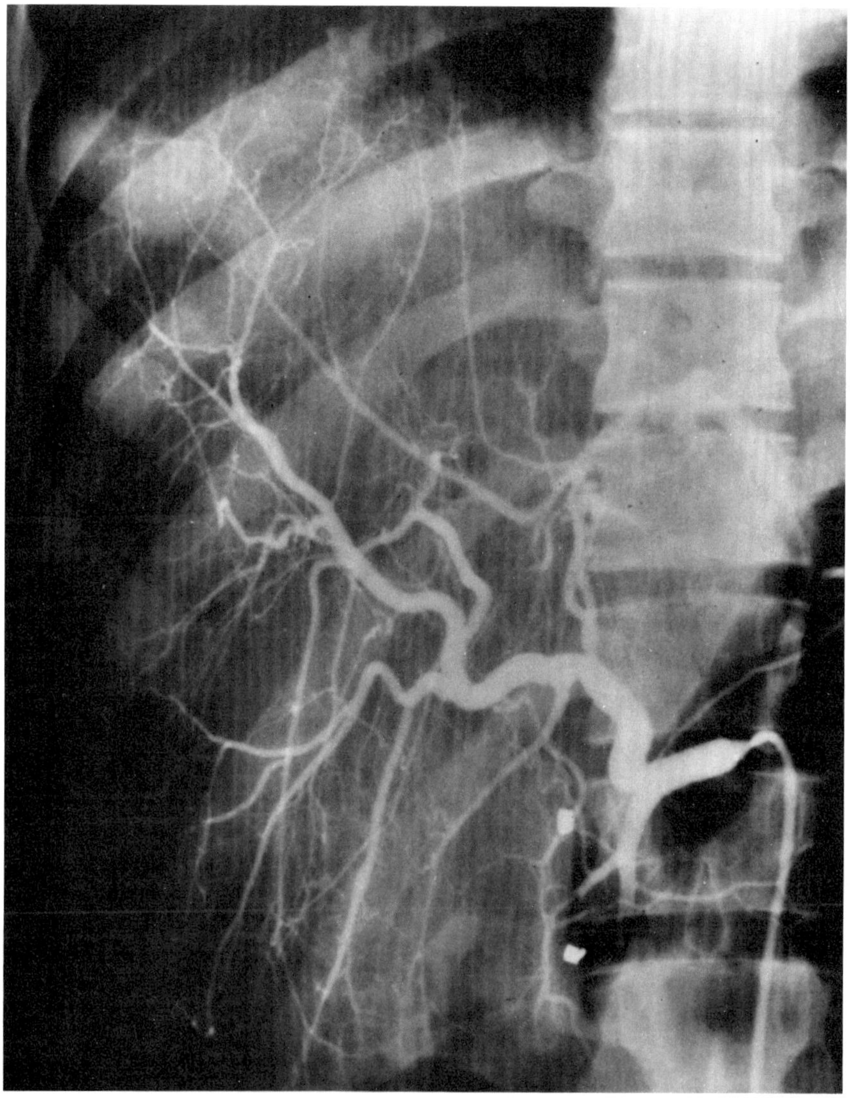

Figure 19A Hepatic abscess drainage (bacterial). A 19-year-old white male was admitted with persistent leukocytosis 4 weeks after an upper respiratory infection. A bone marrow examination revealed acute myelogenous leukemia. Physical examination disclosed lymphadenopathy and hepatopslenomegaly. The patient improved on chemotherapy with COPP, but developed pancytopenia accompanied by a gram-negative sepsis and bilateral pleural effusions which were treated by antibiotics: carbenicillin, Keflin, and kanamycin. Right upper quadrant abdominal pain precipitated an exploratory laparotomy; acute gangrenous cholecystitis and a pericholecystic abscess were found. The abscess was drained and cholecystostomy was done. The patient remained febrile and his condition deteriorated. A ^{99m}Tc sulfur colloid liver scan delineated a "cold" area in the right lobe of the liver. Hepatic arteriography demonstrated curvilinear displacement of the superior branches of the anterior and posterior segments of the right hepatic artery.

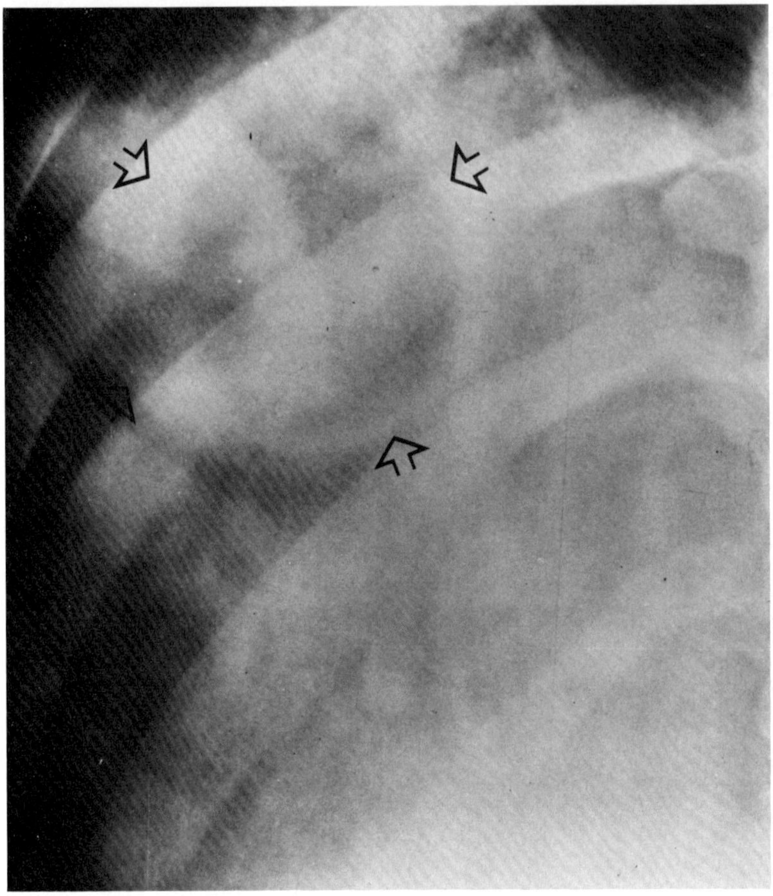

Figure 19B A radiolucent defect surrounded by a relatively thick zone of hypervascularity was visualized (arrows) in the parenchymal phase. These findings, together with his clinical picture, led to the consideration of an hepatic abscess.

surrounding normal liver, but may be pedunculated. The pseudocyst may be loculated and filled with a pale serous fluid. Radiologically, it may be impossible to differentiate cystic mesenchymal hamartoma from a solitary cyst or a polycystic liver (Fig. 20). The hamartoma is less well defined and the margins may be irregular.

Solid hamartoma The tumors have also been designated as cholangiohepatoma or biliary fibroadenoma. These mixed tumors originate from both hepatic cells and bile ducts and show pronounced hyperplasia of the connective tissue elements. Because of progression in size, the remote possibility of malignant transformation, and the danger of hemorrhage or torsion of the pedicle, these hamartomas should be excised (52,54,68). Angiographic findings may reveal a hypervascular tumor mass without obvious neoplastic

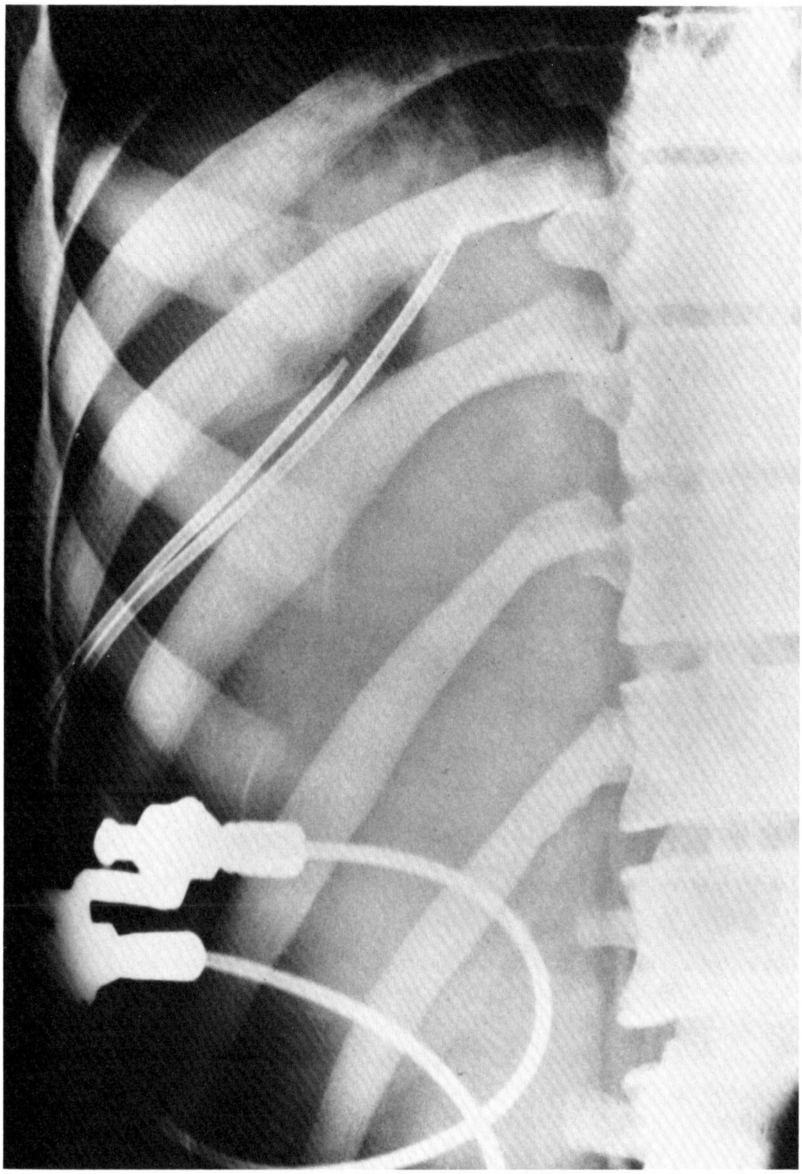

Figure 19C In view of the patient's poor general status, it was felt that he would not tolerate surgical intervention. Utilizing the liver scan and angiogram for localization, percutaneous double catheter drainage under fluoroscopic guidance was undertaken. The catheters were irrigated three times daily with appropriate antibiotics. The first catheter came out spontaneously after 3 days without obvious bleeding. The second catheter remained in the cavity for 10 days and came out uneventfully. The patient responded to this regimen and the chemotherapy was resumed. An elective cholecystectomy was performed 6 weeks later.

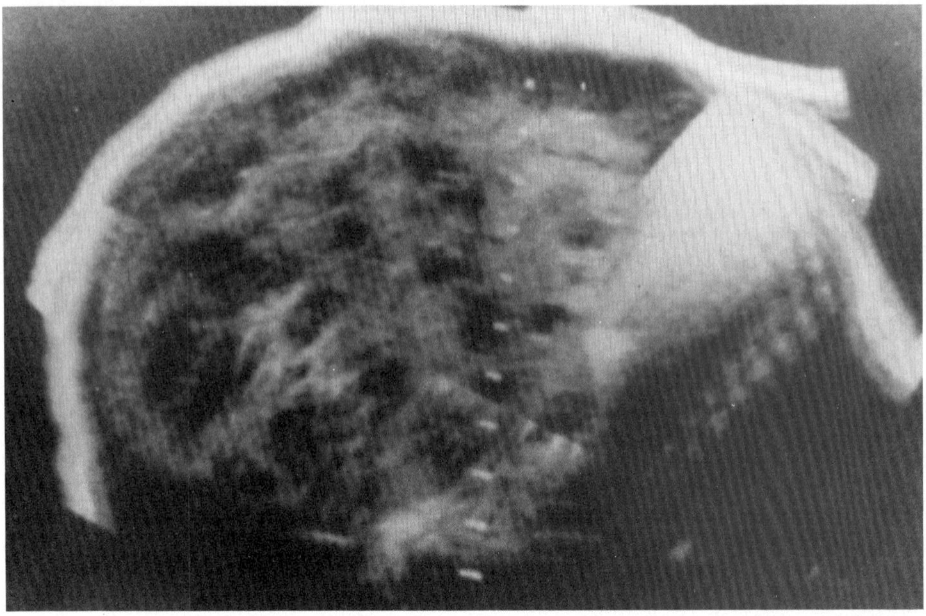

Figure 20 Cystic mesenchymal hamartoma. US scan shows multiple areas of decreased echogenicity. (Courtesy of Dr. Michael Wolverson, St. Louis University, St. Louis, Missouri.)

vessels (Fig. 21). An angiomatous hamartoma attached to the right lobe of the liver by a pedicle is shown in Figure 22.

Cavernous Hemangioma

Vascular tumors comprise approximately 10% of the primary hepatic tumors of childhood; they are usually detected before the child is 6 months of age. This pertains to the more symptomatic giant cavernous hemangiomas or extensive hemangioendotheliomas. Cavernous hemangiomas are more frequently seen in adults, usually females (69–72).

These vascular lesions are more often diagnosed inadvertently in the evaluation of the liver for more serious maladies. They may be found incidentally in children whose deaths are attributed to various congenital anomalies, including renal agenesis, atrial defects, and biliary tract abnormalities (47,52,54). As with cutaneous hemangiomas, cavernous hemangiomas of the liver may progress for a time and then involute (47,52,54). They are most frequently small, but on occasion may be large and multiple, producing an otherwise asymptomatic mass, especially in children. They may rupture, producing intra-abdominal hemorrhage. Thrombocytopenia may be present due to trapping of platelets in the large cavernous spaces.

Radiologic diagnosis Identification of these vascular neoplasms by NM, US, and CT is nonspecific. A defect is seen in the liver by NM. On rare occasions, there may be an increased uptake. An increased echogenicity has been a frequent finding by US, but this varies considerably. Recent reports suggest a more characteristic finding by dynamic CT scanning with a defect in the noncontrast scan and a prolonged increase in uptake with a bolus injection. This, however, is still not specific and can be found in primary and secondary neoplasms. The most reliable and diagnostic study is accomplished by angiography (Figs. 5, 23, 24). The hepatic arterial branches to the cavernous hemangioma are normal in caliber, tapering toward the periphery. In the later arterial phase, small or larger vascular spaces fill and form ringlike clusters. Relatively avascular areas are frequently present and are due to thrombotic or hyalinized portions of the hemangioma. Unlike other hypervascular tumors, these vascular pools remain filled with contrast material throughout the venous phase. Early venous drainage rarely occurs.

Treatment of hemangiomas depends on the extent of involvement and clinical status of the patient. Surgical resection, ligation or banding of the hepatic artery, radiotherapy, hepatic artery embolization, and corticosteroids have been employed (69,70). Surgical

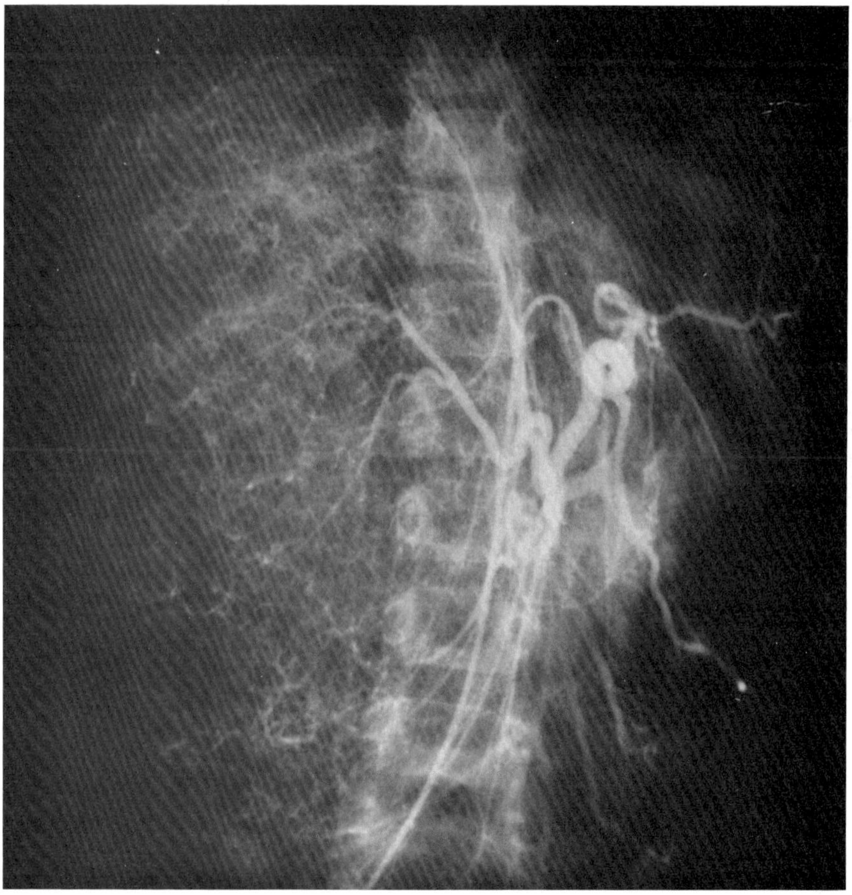

Figure 21 Solid mesenchymal hamartoma. Celiac arteriogram in a 4.5-year-old girl opacified a fairly well defined hypervascular mass in the right lobe of the liver which proved to be a benign solid mesenchymal hamartoma. (Courtesy of Dr. Klaus Bron, University of Pittsburgh, Pittsburgh, Pennsylvania.)

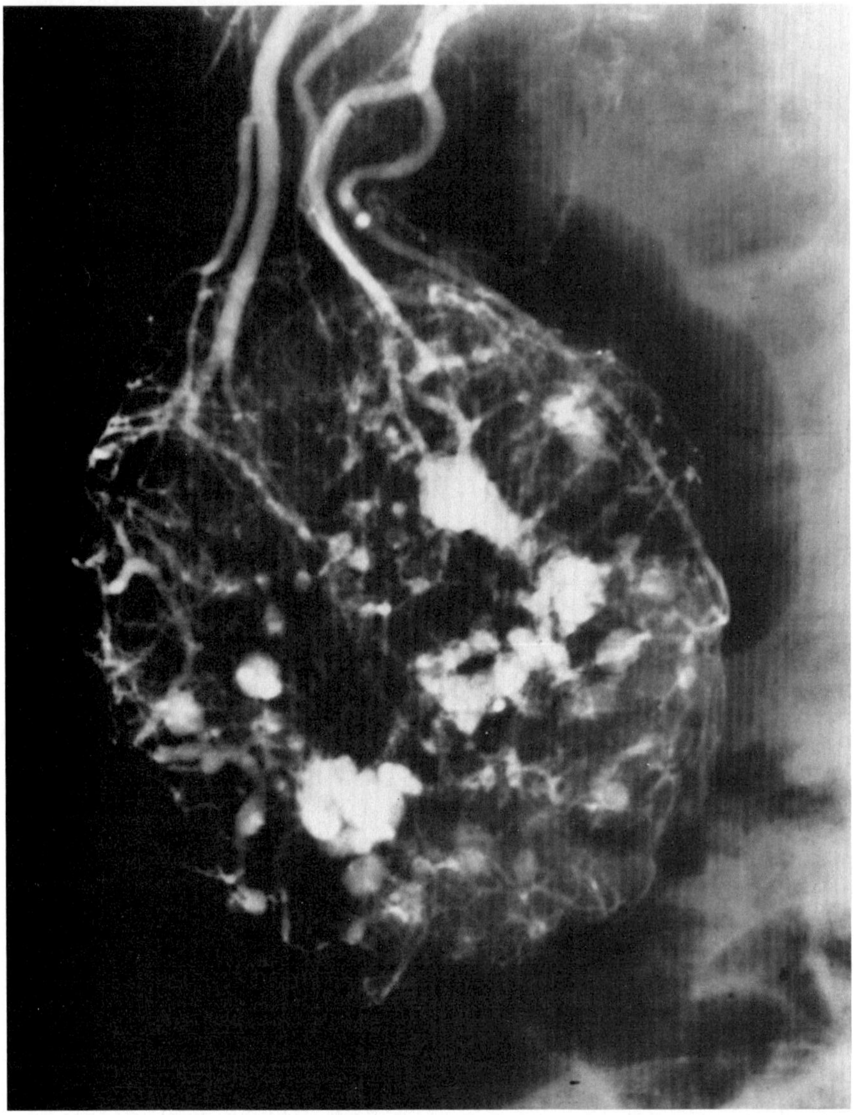

Figure 22 Pedunculated angiomatous hamartoma. This hypervascular neoplasm projected from the under surface of the right lobe of the liver. The hepatic arteriogram best demonstrated the nature and extent of this lesion in preparation for local resection.

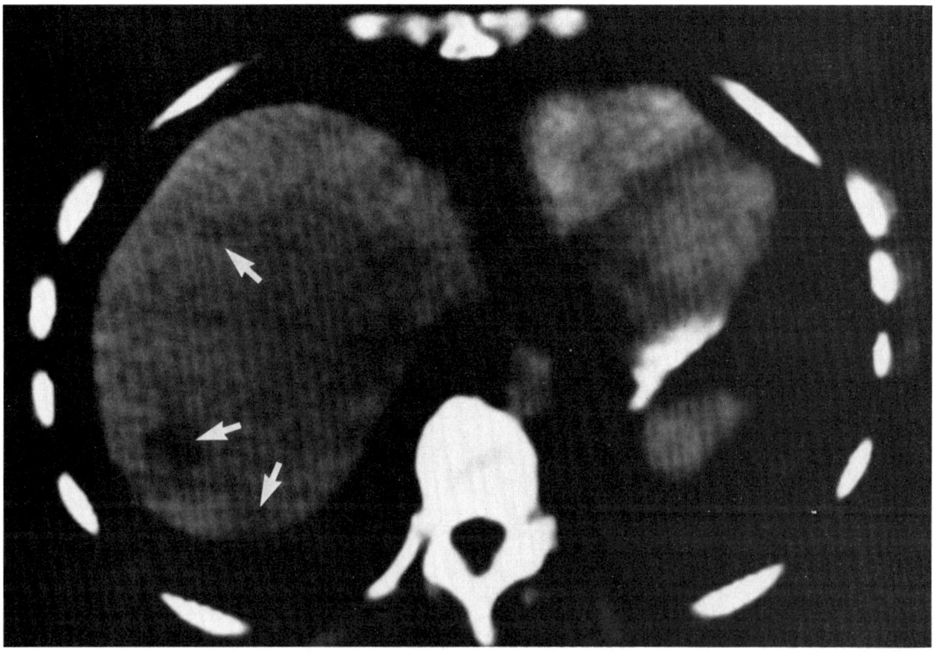

(A)

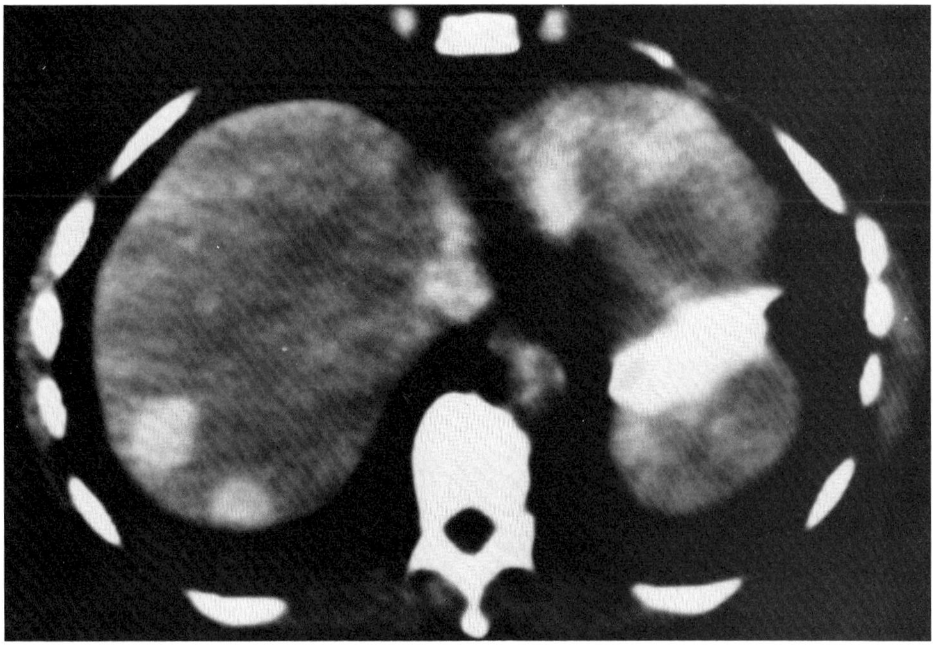

(B)

Figure 23

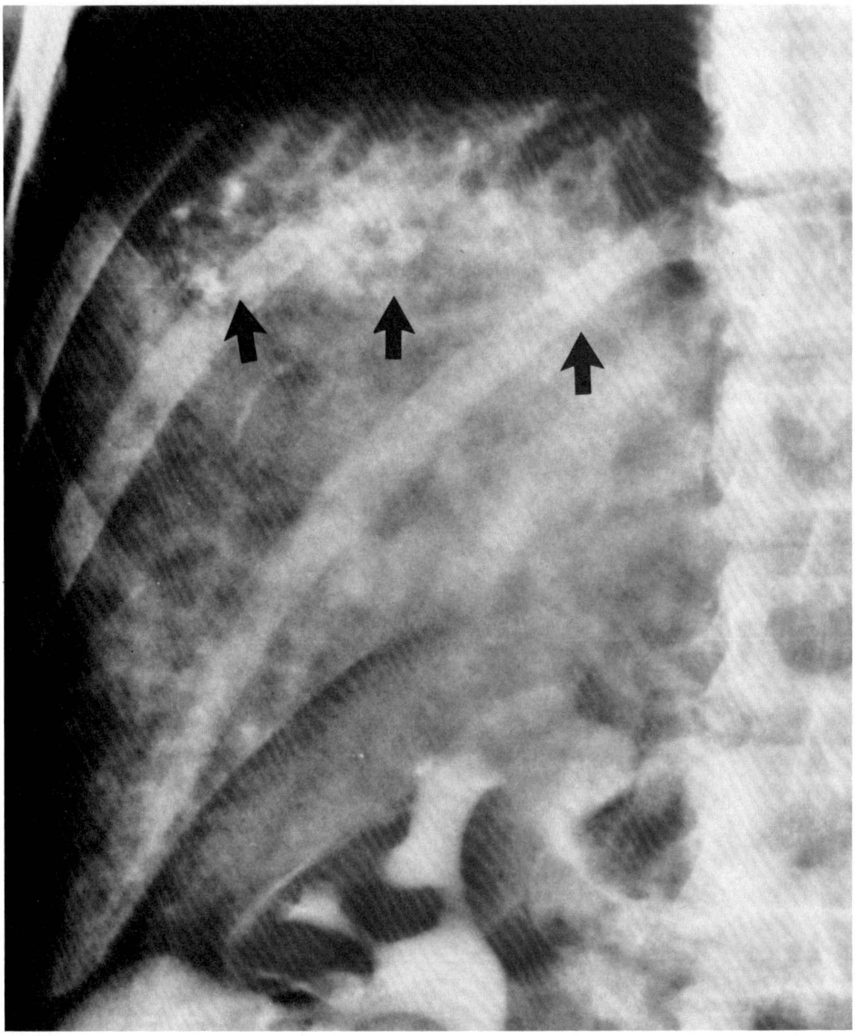

(C)

Figure 23 Cavernous hemangiomas. (A) CT scan without contrast material reveals small areas of decreased attenuation in the dome of the right lobe (arrows). (B) Enhancement of these lesions is noted following infusion of contrast material. (C) Arteriography definitely establishes these lesions to be cavernous hemangiomas. (Courtesy of Dr. M. Granmayeh, Houston, Texas.)

resection of a localized lesion that is symptomatic is the preferred approach. Preoperative embolization may control the symptoms and facilitate the subsequent surgical procedure (Fig. 25).

Infantile Hemangioendothelioma

Infantile hemangioendotheliomas are usually more aggressive, although they too may be incidental findings or appear as an upper abdominal mass. A precordial murmur, cough,

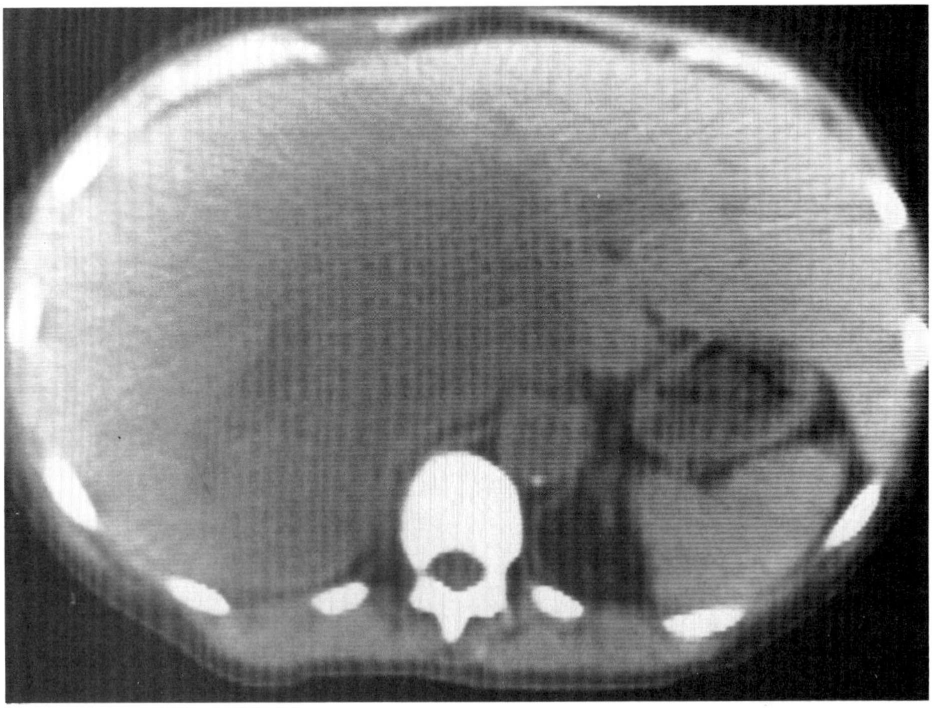

(A)

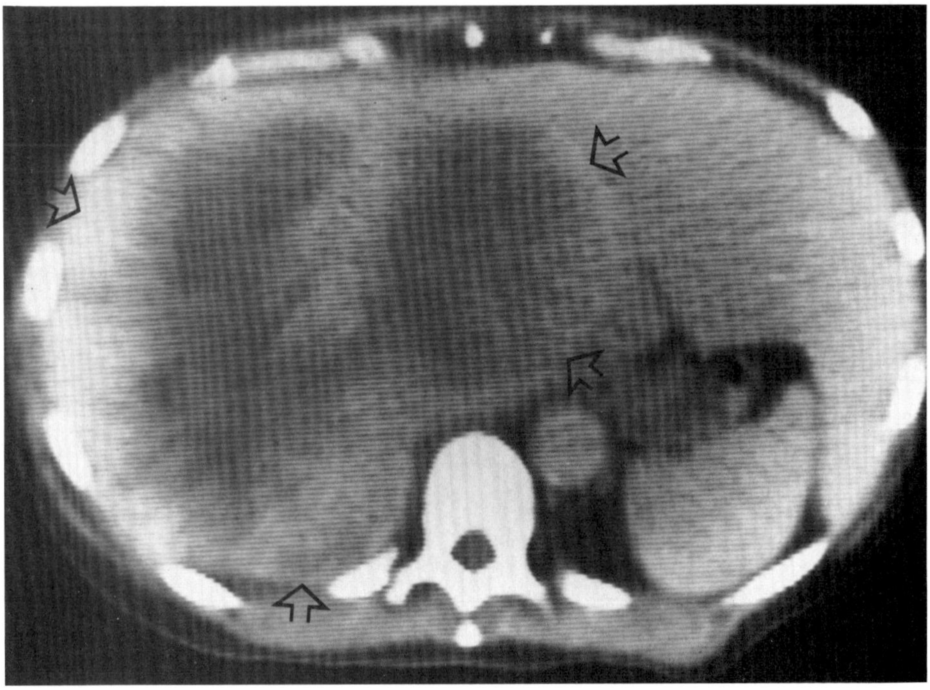

(B)

Figure 24

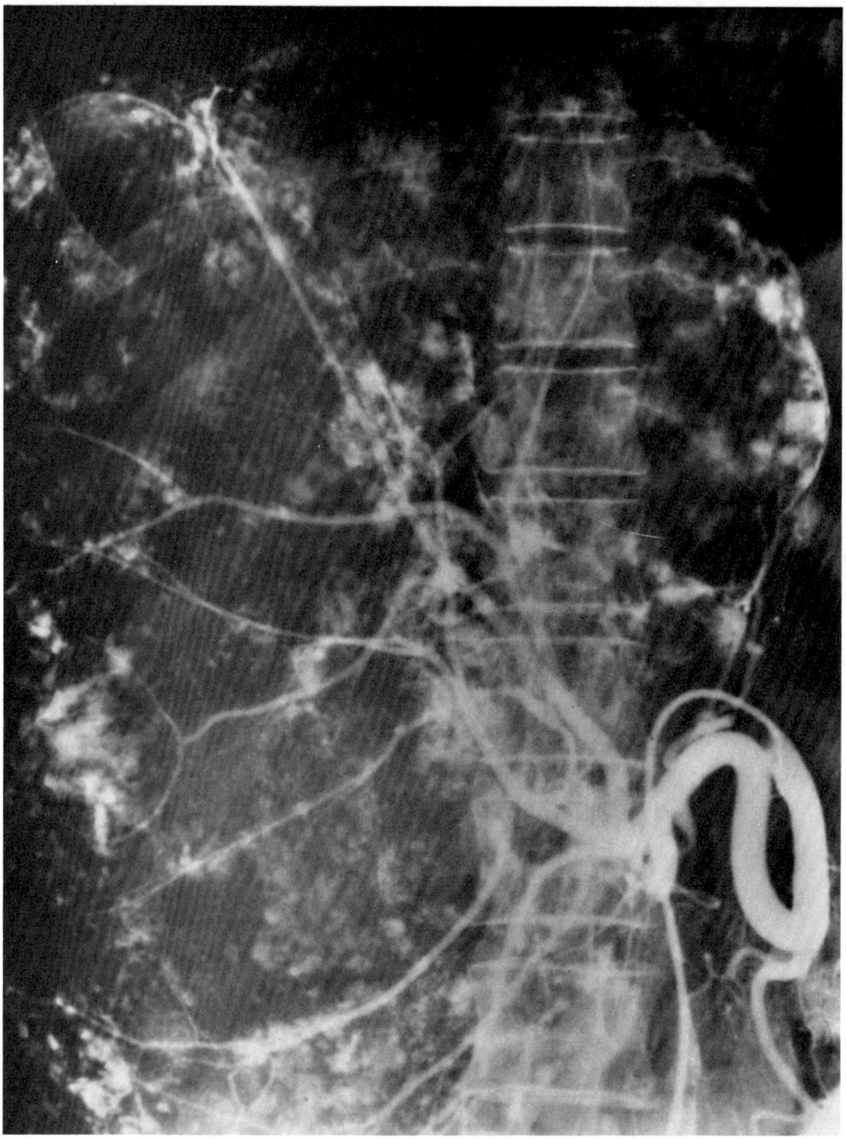

(C)

Figure 24 (continued)

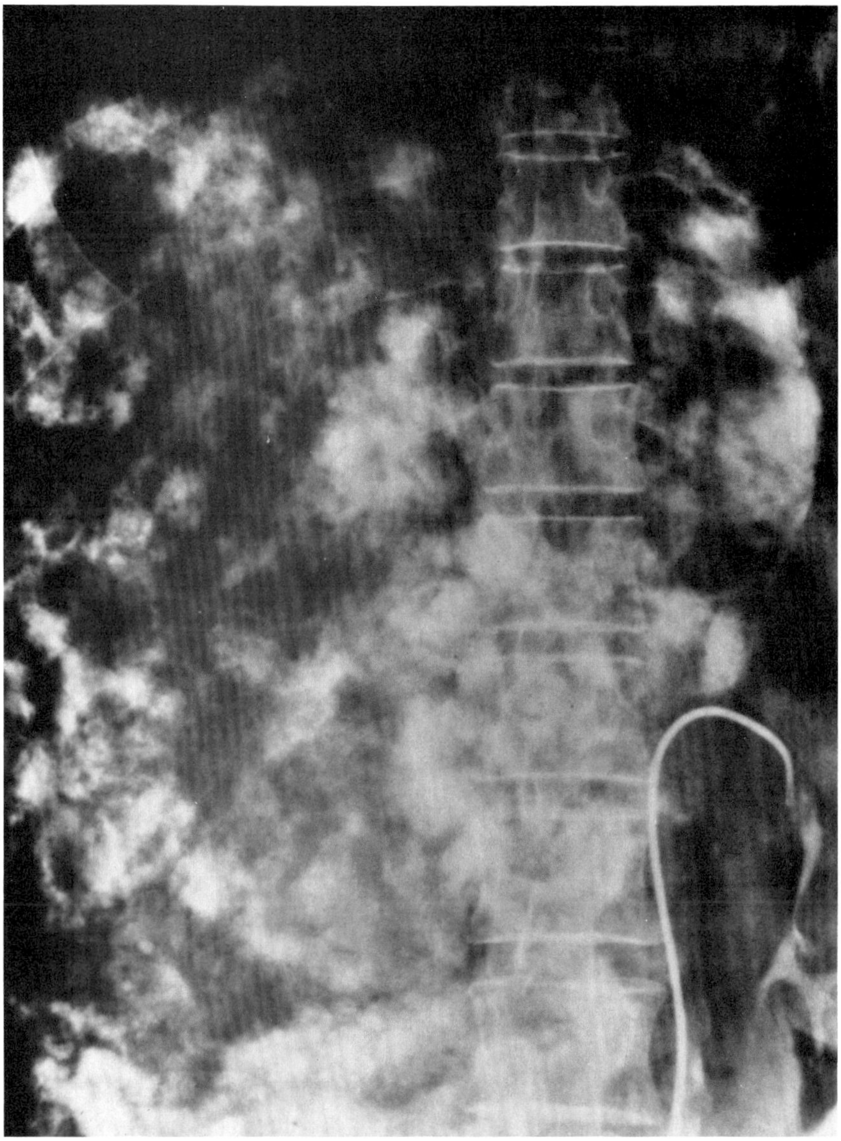

(D)

Figure 24 Cavernous hemangioma. (A) CT prior to contrast material demonstrated a large mass of decreased attenuation replacing most of the liver. (B) CT following contrast enhancement better defines the margins of the lesion (arrows), more in keeping with a hemangioma. (C,D) Selective hepatic arteriography clearly establishes the diagnosis of cavernous hemangioma.

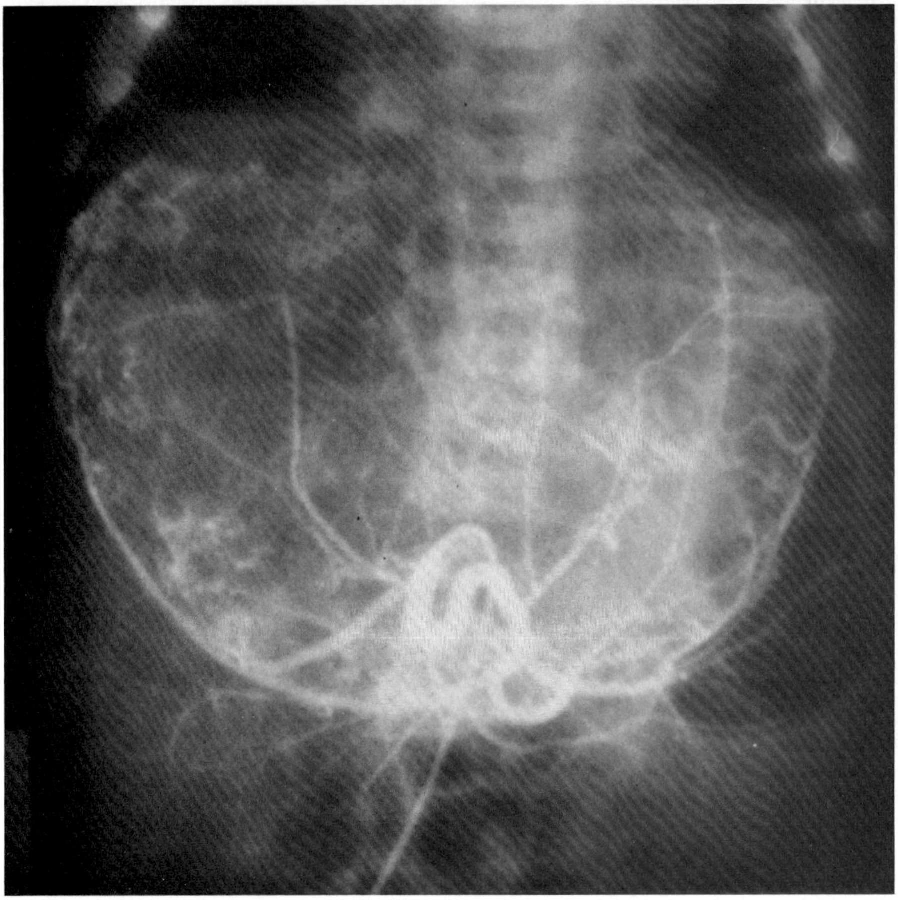

Figure 25A Cavernous hemangioma—preoperative management. This infant had a large hypervascular lesion involving the left lobe of the liver which, on selective left hepatic arteriography, demonstrated normal vessels tapering toward the periphery.

dyspnea, or congestive heart failure are the more typical presentations. Congestive heart failure is presumably due to arteriovenous shunting in the tumor (47,52,54). Gastrointestinal tract symptoms of jaundice, vomiting, and diarrhea may predominate (71). Like cavernous hemangiomas, these vascular neoplasms may rupture with fatal intra-abdominal hemorrhage, or they may manifest thrombocytopenia with anemia.

Angiographic findings are similar to those described for large cavernous hemangiomas. These tumors may be solitary or multiple, with a tendency to form hypervascular nodules containing vascular pools. Rapid arteriovenous shunting, although theoretically the explanation for congestive failure, is demonstrated only occasionally.

Infantile hemangioendotheliomas are not considered entirely benign and may rarely metastasize, especially to lymph nodes and lungs (72). A high mortality rate is associated with this neoplasm.

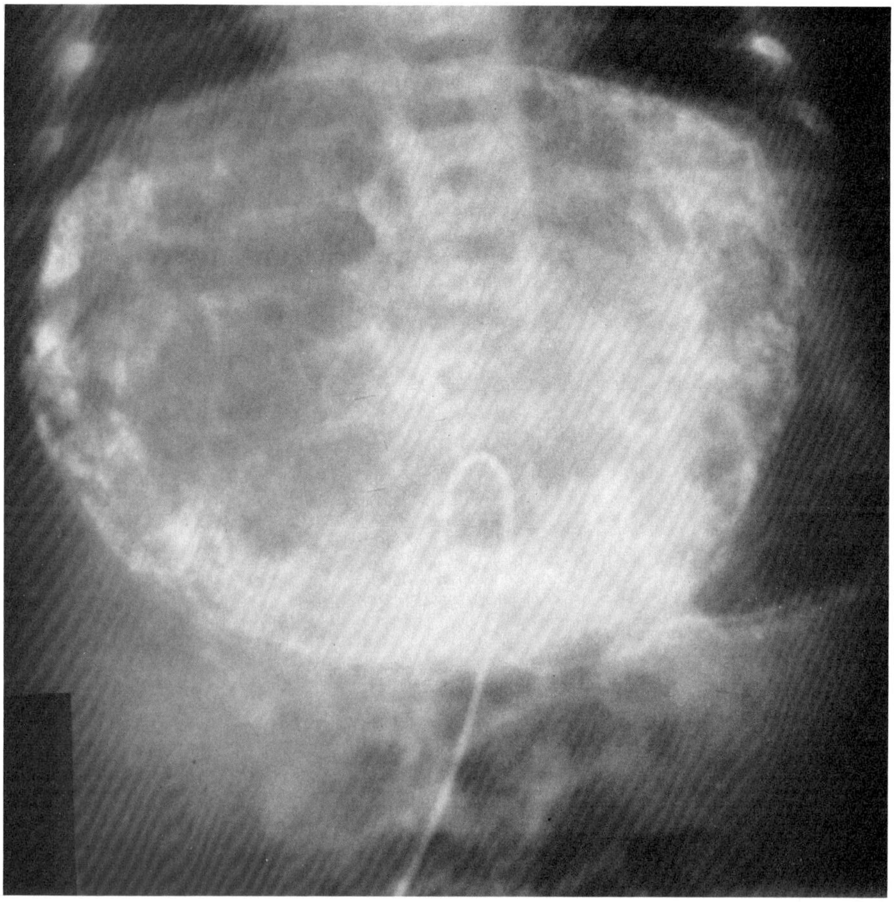

Figure 25B Pools of contrast material opacify primarily at the margin of the cavernous hemangioma.

Differential Diagnosis

Peliosis hepatis, or livid liver, resembles hemangioma angiographically (Fig. 26). There is still considerable dispute as to these findings in that they may also be seen in apparently normal livers. Small rounded collections of contrast material are found in the late arterial and hepatogram phases (73). Peliosis was initially reported in patients with chronic debilitating disease, such as tuberculosis. More recently, it has been associated with hormonal intake (i.e., estrogen and testosterone) (74). Histologically, these vascular pools are enlarged hepatic sinusoids, at times with evidence of necrosis.

Rendu-Osler-Weber disease, hereditary telangiectasia, is difficult to differentiate from hemangiomas. These telangiectatic lesions usually occur in the skin or mucosa and may also be found in the alimentary tract, lungs, liver, pancreas, spleen, brain, arachnoid membranes, and the genitourinary tract. Painless hematemesis and melena are seen in

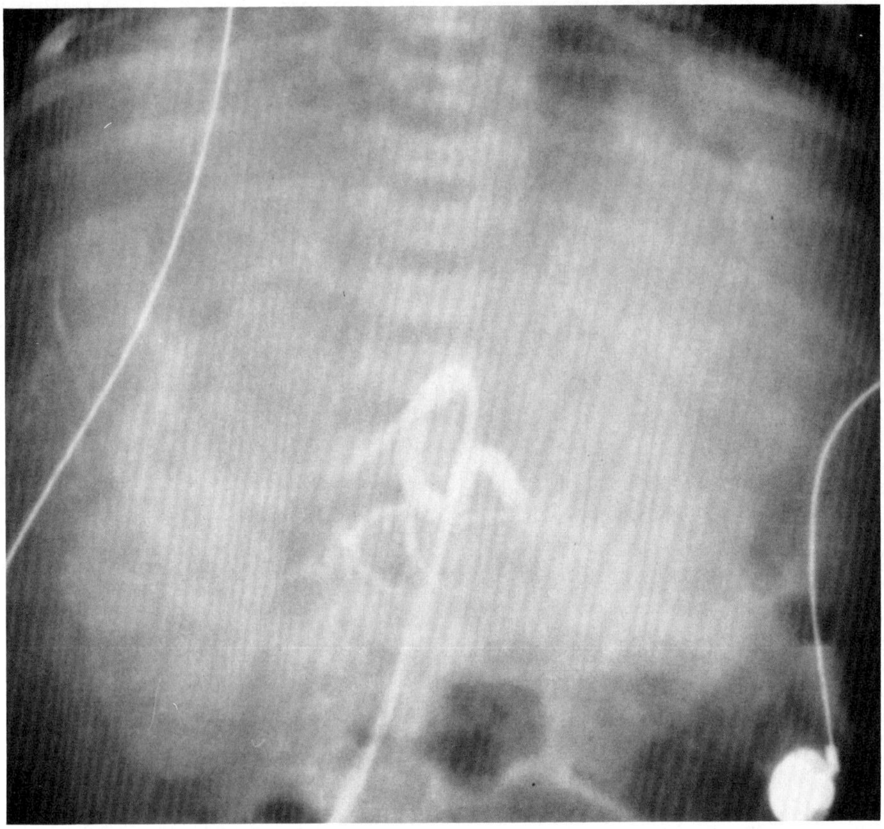

Figure 25C Preoperatively, the neoplasm was embolized with Gelfoam, creating a relatively hypovascular tumor, markedly reducing the expected blood loss. The infant tolerated surgery well. (Courtesy of Mitchell Vinson, Norfolk, Virginia.)

15–30% (75). Involvement of the liver can be complicated by intra-abdominal hemorrhage. The hemodynamic significance of visceral lesions lies in the frequency of associated arteriovenous shunts. Arteriography is usually essential to establish the vascular nature, the extent of the lesions, and their arterial and venous components (Fig. 27 and Fig. 4 of Chap. 29). Control of bleeding from the liver has been accomplished by transcatheter embolization of the hepatic artery (76).

Epithelial Tumors

Although no malignant potential has been established for benign epithelial liver tumors, it is difficult to distinguish these lesions from certain hepatocellular malignancies. Both

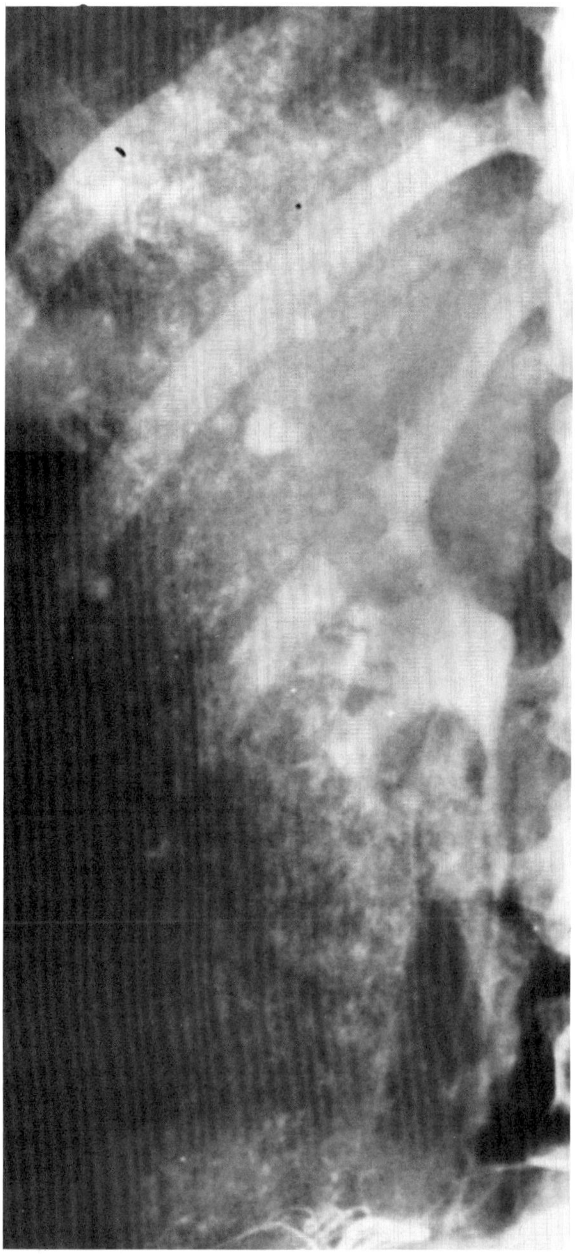

Figure 26 Peliosis hepatis. This young female on oral contraceptives was found to have an enlarged liver. Hepatic arteriography demonstrated multiple rounded collections of contrast material scattered throughout the liver. Operative biopsy was interpreted as peliosis hepatis. (Courtesy of Dr. M. Pliskin, Houston, Texas.)

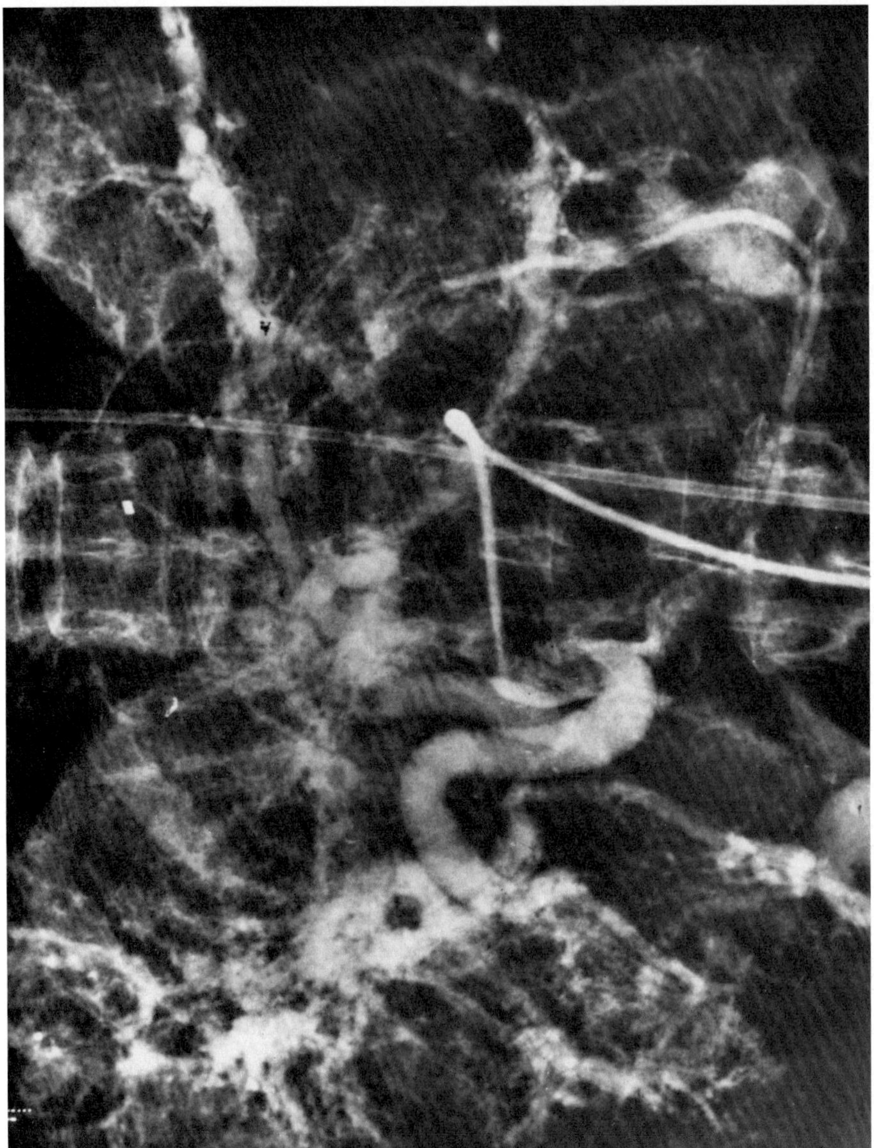

Figure 27A

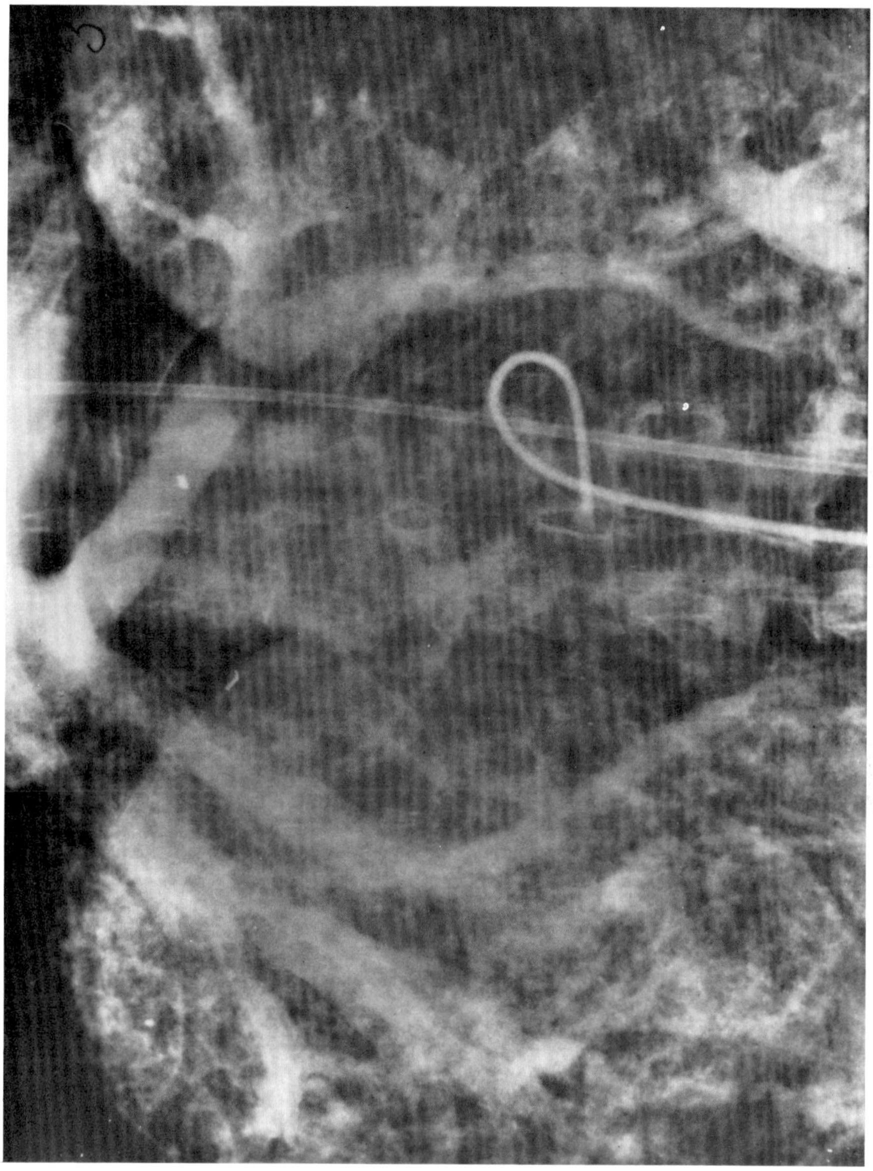

Figure 27B

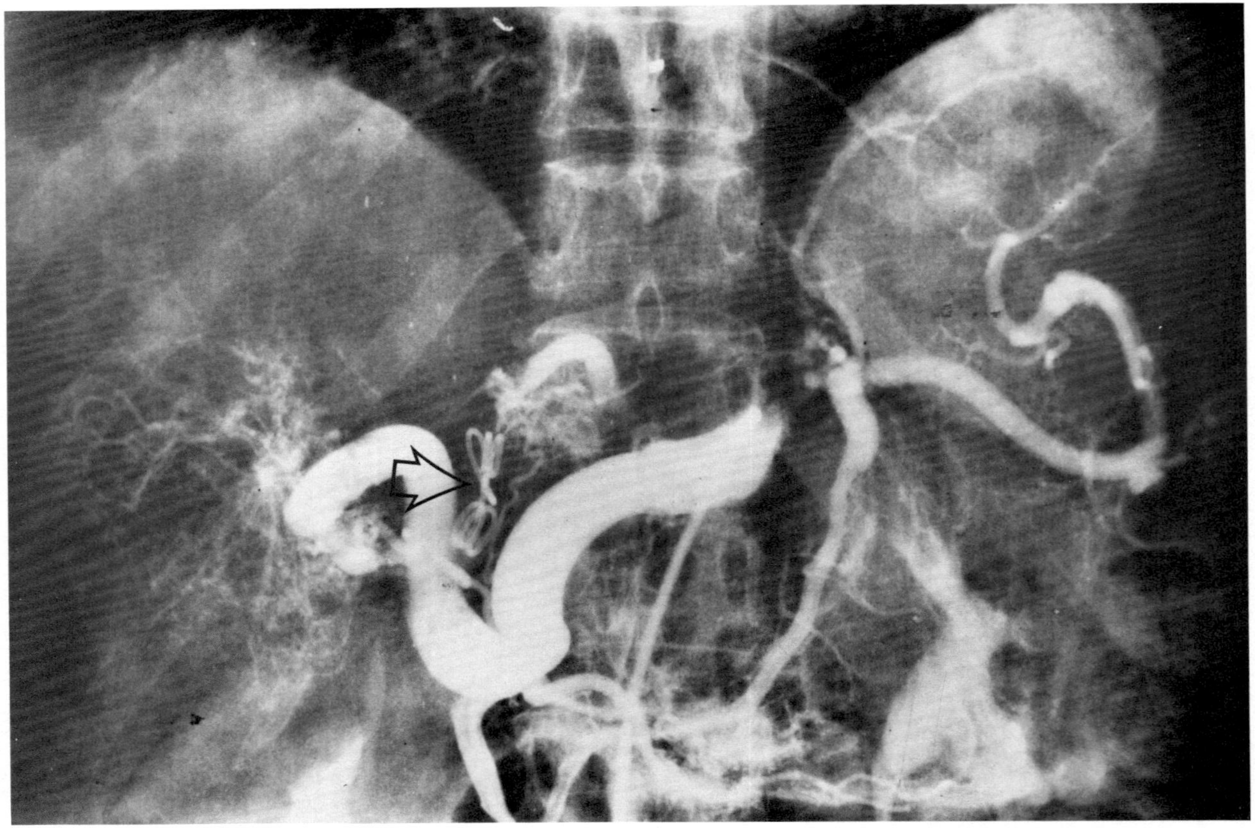

(C)

Figure 27 Rendu-Osler-Weber disease. (A) The hepatic arteriogram was done to define the cause of an intra-abdominal hemorrhage. Extensive vascular changes are seen in the arterial phase. (B) The parenchymal abnormalities and opacification of the hepatic veins were dramatic. (C) The hemorrhage was controlled by embolization of the hepatic artery with Gelfoam and steel coils (arrow). The patient succumbed to another hemorrhage originating from lesions in the small bowel. (Courtesy of Dr. K. Jonsson, Malmö, Sweden.)

hepatic adenoma and focal nodular hyperplasia may grow and undergo hemorrhage and rupture, this more frequently with hepatic adenomas; surgery is, therefore, indicated (52–54,74–84).

Hepatic Adenoma

These epithelial tumors are extremely rare in childhood but more commonly occur in young women of childbearing age (52–54,78–89). A causal relationship with oral contraceptive agents seems very likely (79,81,83–85,89). Patients may have a mass, pain, or an acute catastrophe due to rupture and intra-abdominal bleeding. An hepatic adenoma is usually solitary, sharply marginated, often an encapsulated mass composed of well-differentiated, uniform liver cells, without portal triads or central veins. Well-differentiated hepatocellular malignant neoplasms and focal nodular hyperplasia may create difficulties in differential diagnosis.

Angiographic features Angiography will usually demonstrate that the vascular supply enters from the periphery of the adenoma (Fig. 28). The vessels are not neoplastic in character, but occasionally seem bizarre (Fig. 29). The hypervascularity produces an increased, fairly homogeneous parenchymal stain in a sharply marginated mass. There may be a fine zone of relative radiolucency separating the adenoma from the surrounding normal liver, probably representing the capsule. Frequently, the vasculature to the remainder of the liver is unusual in that the vessels may be more tortuous and there may be small collections of contrast material seen in the hepatogram phase similar to that seen in peliosis hepatis. Angiographic findings in hepatic adenoma may be indistinguishable from those in focal nodular hyperplasia, hemangioma, certain metastases, or well-differentiated hepatocellular malignant neoplasms.

A significant number of hepatic adenomas are avascular or show diminished vascularity at angiography. This is frequently related to hemorrhage (see Fig. 7).

Focal Nodular Hyperplasia

There is a close similarity to hepatic adenoma. Edmondson (52,54) reported focal nodular hyperplasia in eight children, ranging in age from 7 months to 14 years. More recently, these tumors have also been reported in women of childbearing age (79,80,85–89). Focal nodular hyperplasia has been described in von Gierke's disease (79,83), and in association with pheochromocytomas. These tumors are more often solitary but may be multiple in otherwise normal liver. They are well-circumscribed masses without a definite capsule.

Angiographic appearance The vascular supply may come from the periphery of the mass, as in hepatic adenoma, or may be central in position with radial distribution of the vessels within the tumor (Fig. 30). Fairly homogeneous opacification is shown in the capillary phase, with an avascular zone present if there has been bleeding into the mass. With multiple tumors, metastatic disease must be considered in the differential diagnosis (Fig. 31). The pathologic, clinical, and radiologic features of focal nodular hyperplasia and liver cell adenomas have been compared by Casarella et al. (85) and are presented in Tables 5 and 6. Rogers et al. (87) regard the scintigram as the pivotal diagnostic study and reserve angiography for photon-deficient focal lesions.

We are aware of two patients with focal nodular hyperplasia and von Gierke's disease who eventually manifested hepatocellular carcinomas (Fig. 32).

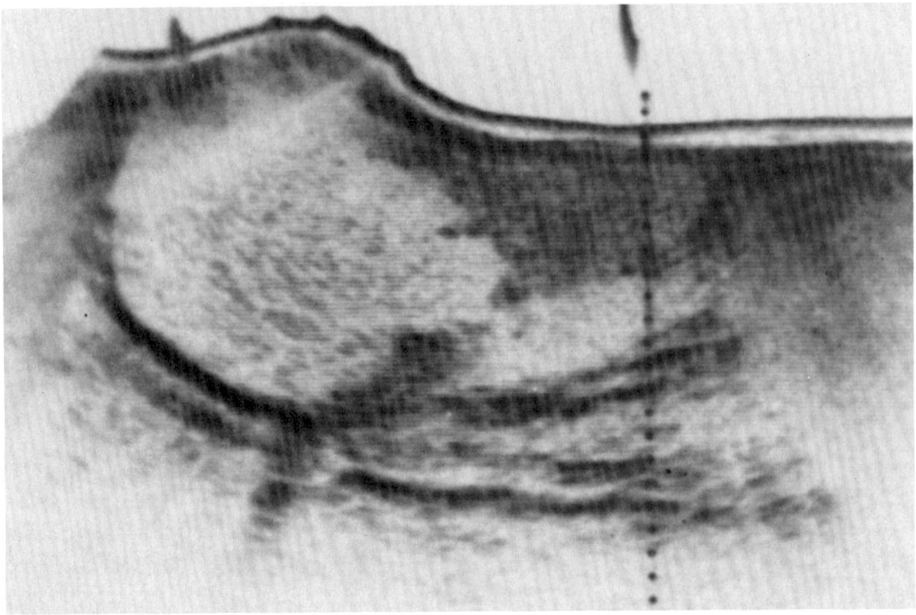

Figure 28A Hepatic adenoma. Forty-year-old female with a history of intake of contraceptive agents was seen because of pain in the right upper quadrant and a "cold" area in the right lobe of the liver on ^{99m}Tc sulfur colloid scan. A large lesion of decreased echogenicity in the right lobe of the liver was demonstrated by sonography (longitudinal scan).

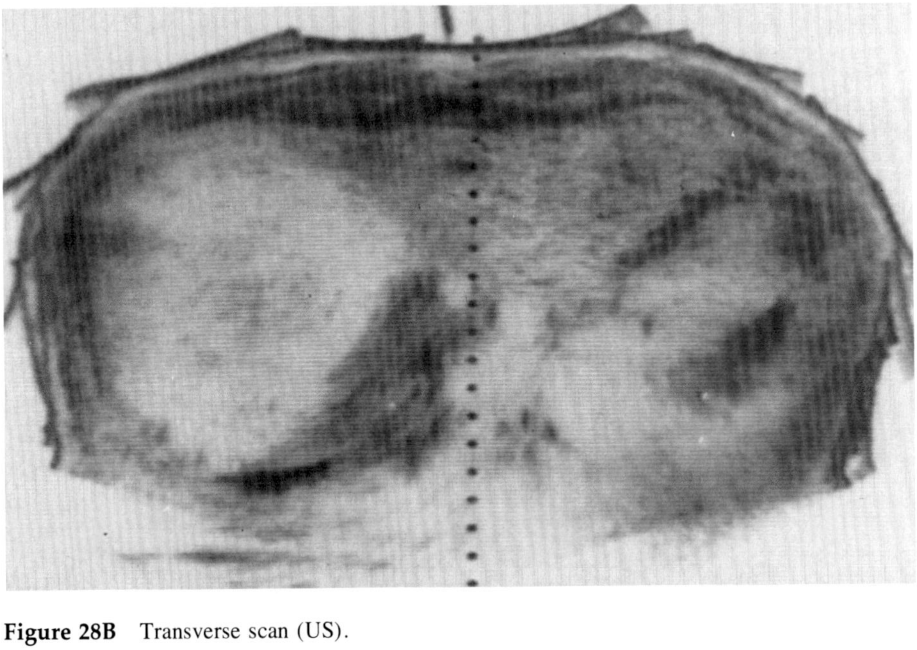

Figure 28B Transverse scan (US).

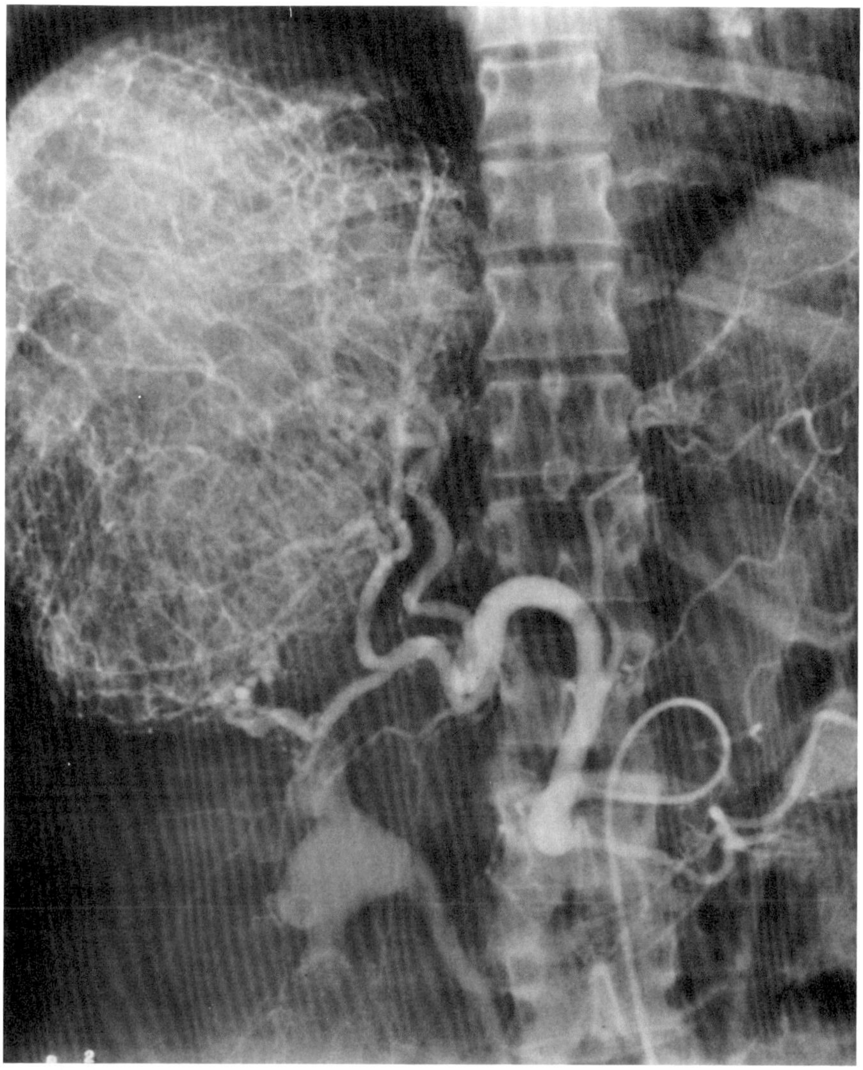

Figure 28C Common hepatic arteriography opacifies a large hypervascular lesion supplied by the superior subsegmental vessels from the anterior and posterior segmental branches of the right hepatic artery.

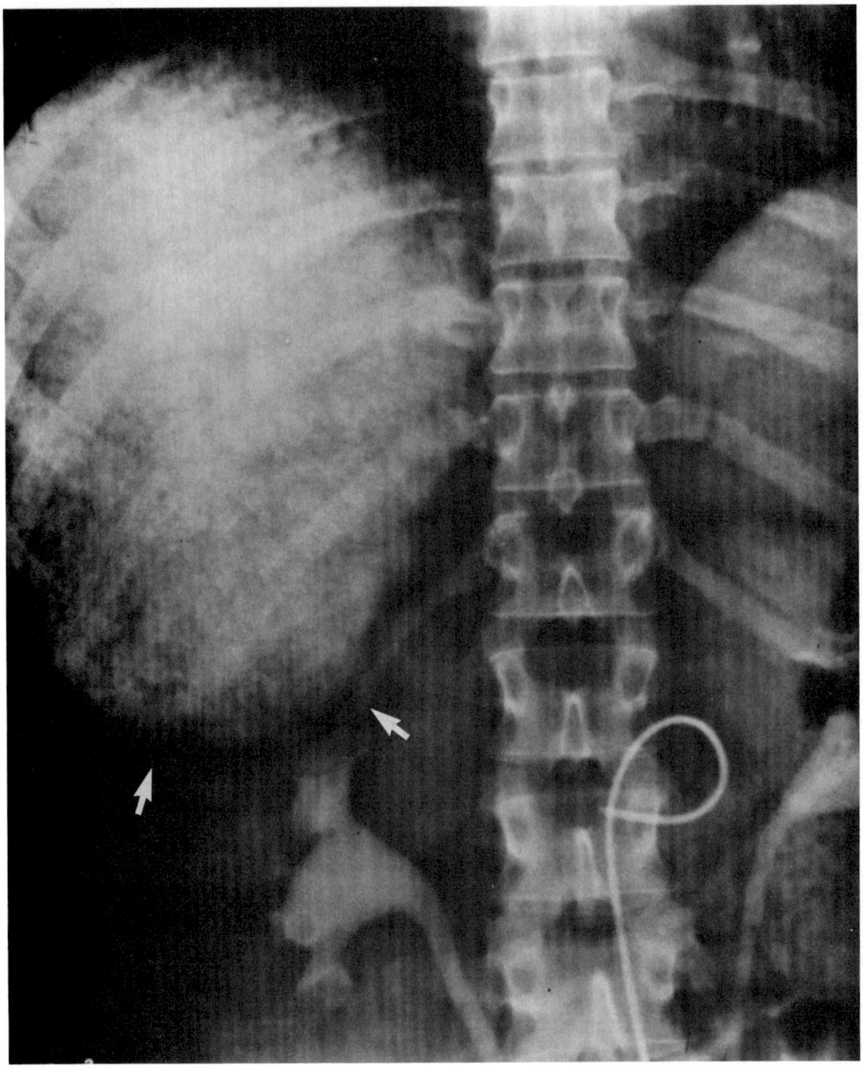

Figure 28D The relatively homogenous tumor stain in a well-circumscribed neoplasm in conjunction with the clinical information suggested the diagnosis of hepatic adenoma. Note the avascular zone around the tumor, most probably depicting the capsule and adjacent compressed normal parenchyma (arrows).

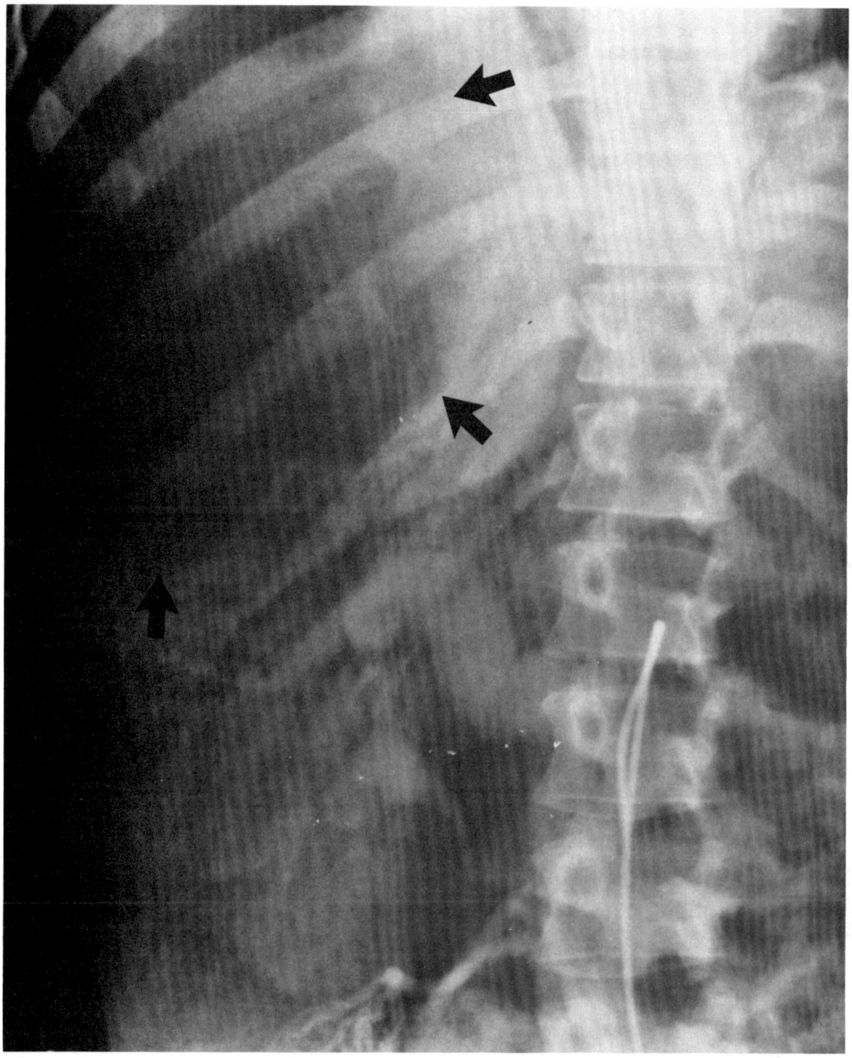

Figure 28E Superior mesenteric artery injection defines the portal vein and the lucency within the liver created by the hepatic artery-supplied hypervascular tumor (arrows).

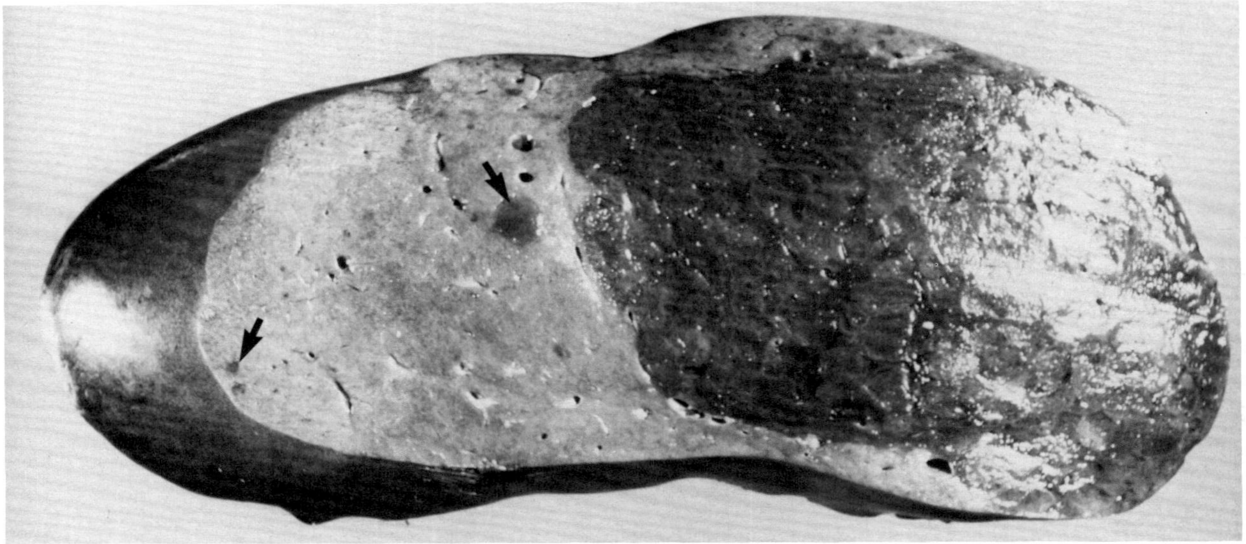

Figure 28F Operative specimen following a right hepatic lobectomy. Note the smaller lesions in the ''normal'' portions of the liver (arrows).

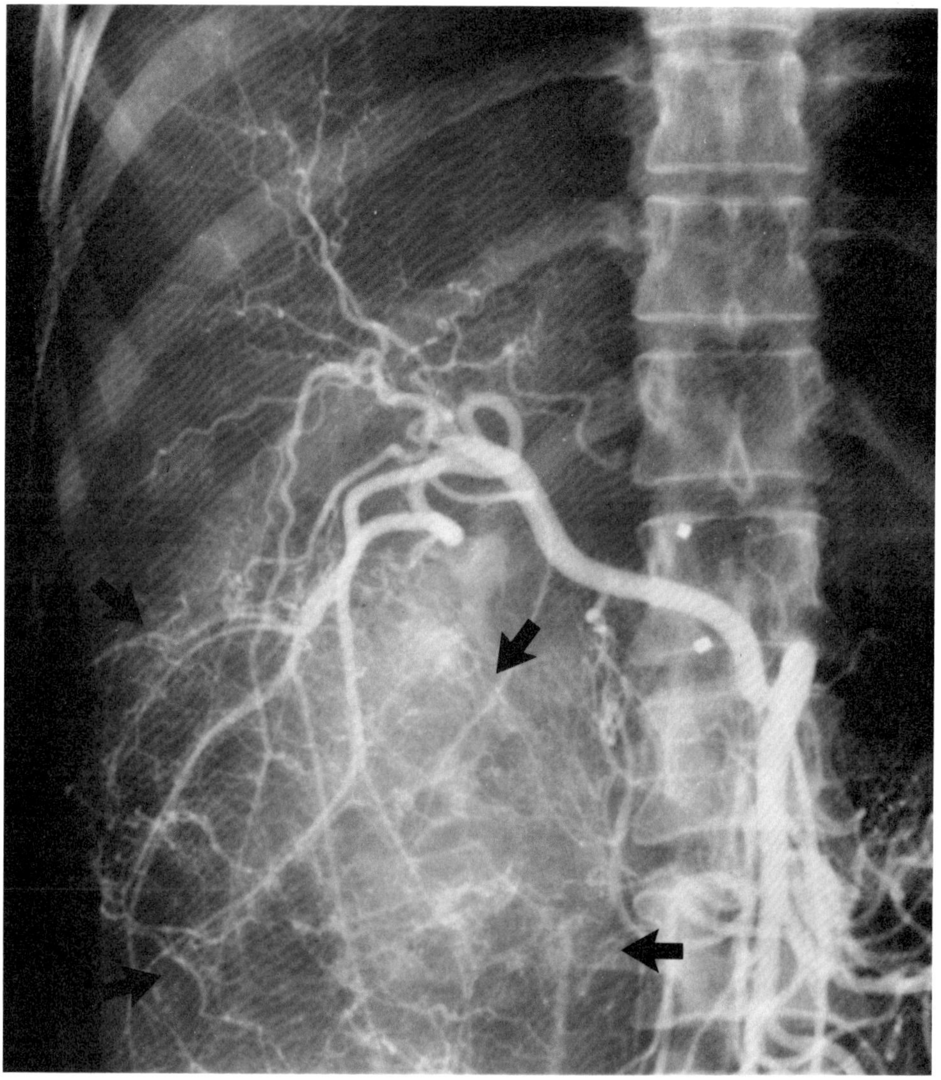

Figure 29A Hepatic adenoma. Arteriography, replaced right hepatic artery. The vascularity of the hepatic adenoma (arrows) is somewhat bizarre. The superior branches are tortuous and irregular, similar to that frequently seen in cirrhosis.

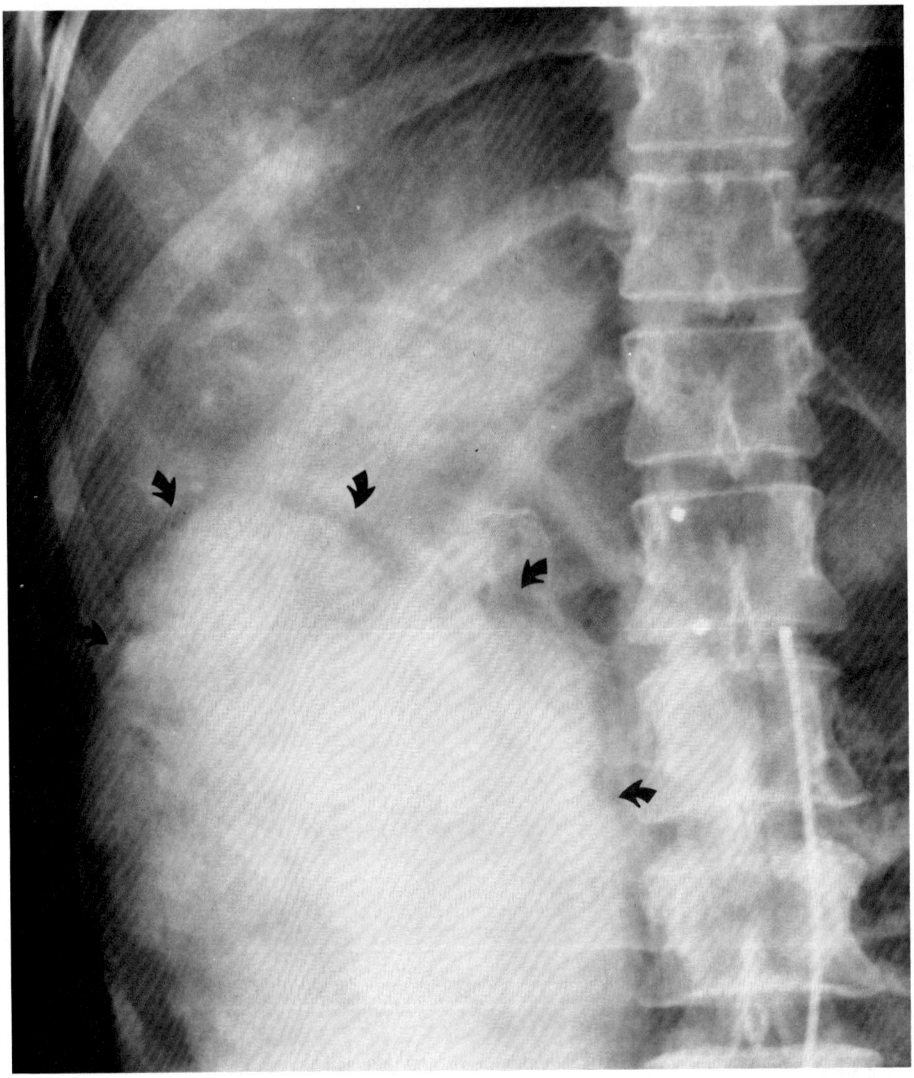

Figure 29B The homogeneous neoplasm in the inferior portion of the right lobe is surrounded by a thin avascular zone (arrows). The superior portion is mottled, suggesting other small adenomas or peliosis hepatis. The tumor was enucleated.

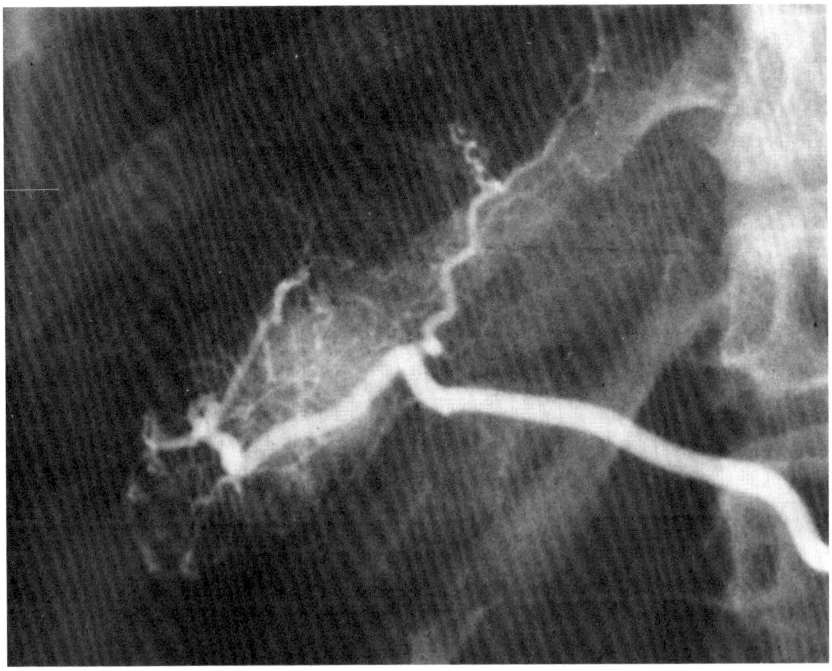

Figure 30A Focal nodular hyperplasia. Opacification of the replaced right hepatic artery from the superior mesenteric artery outlines a hypervascular neoplasm. The arterial pattern is somewhat "radial" in distribution.

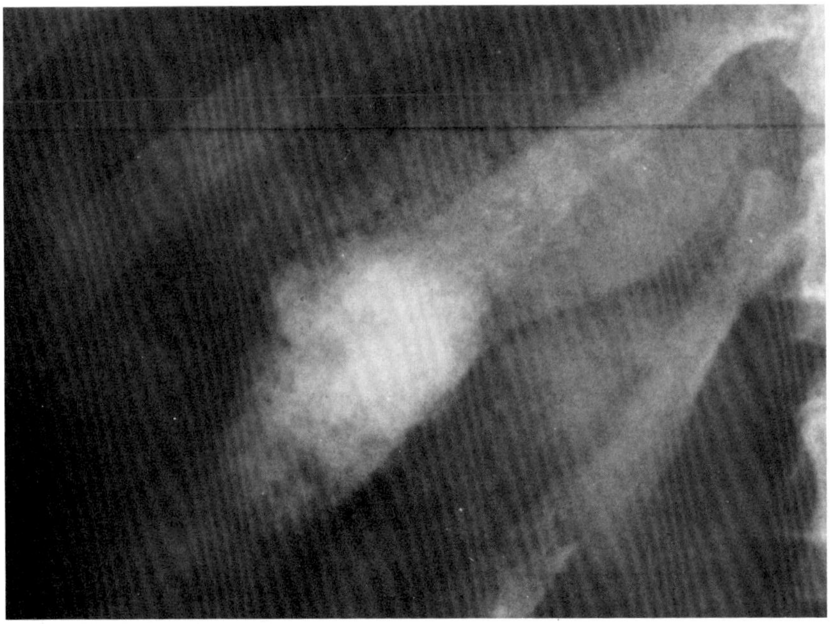

Figure 30B The well-circumscribed mass is fairly homogeneous. The clear zone surrounding the lesion is probably due to compressed hepatic parenchyma, a "pseudocapsule."

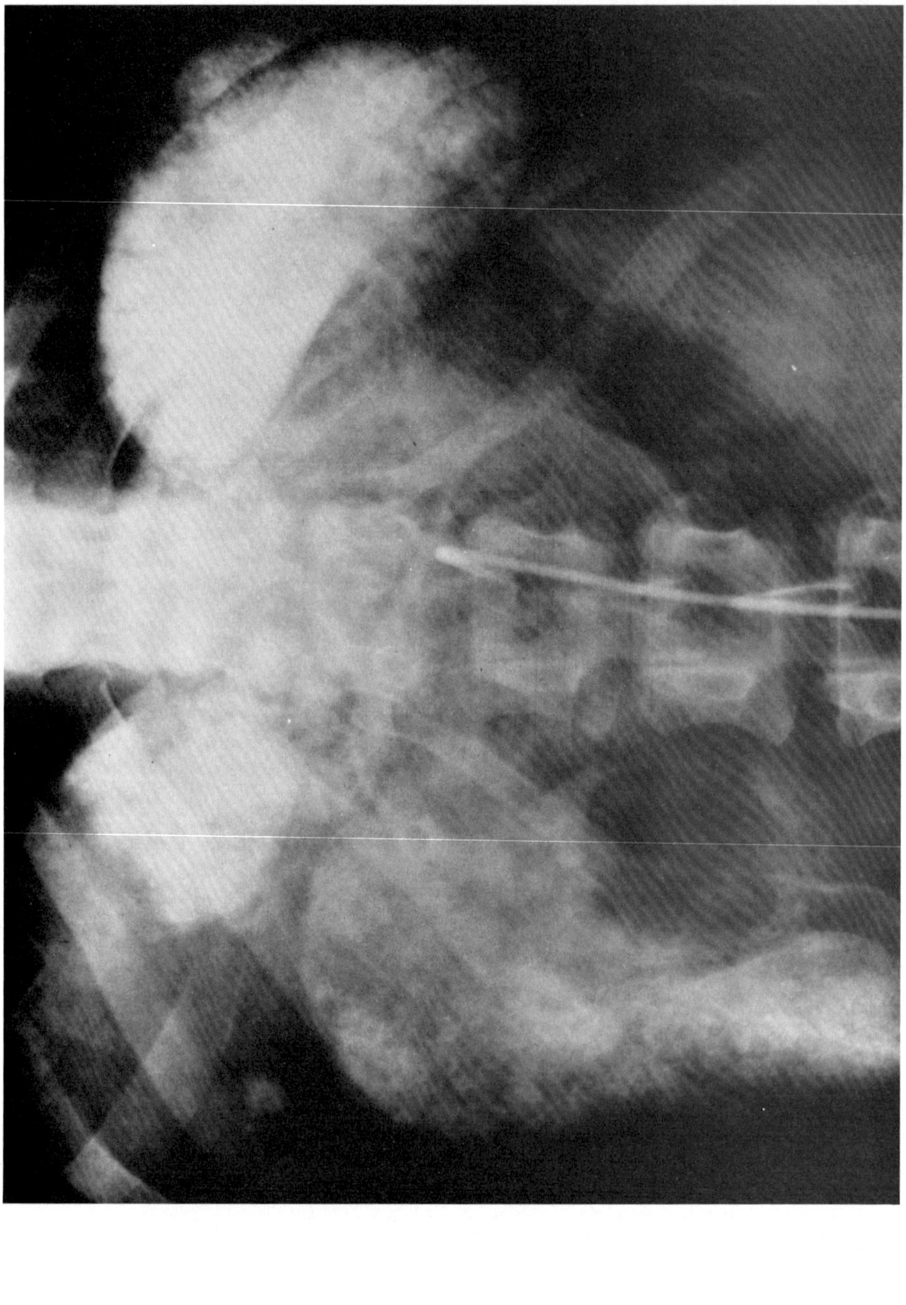

Figure 31

(A)

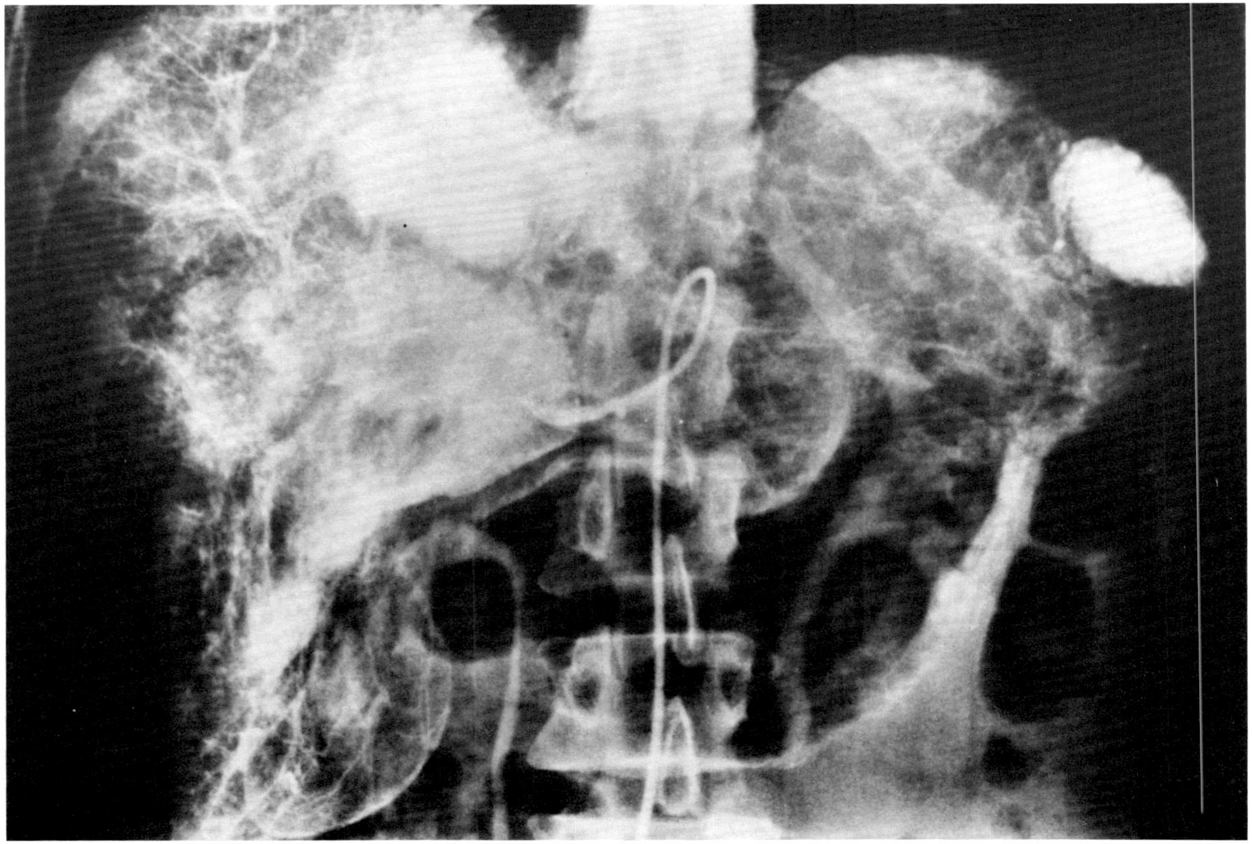

(B)

Figure 31

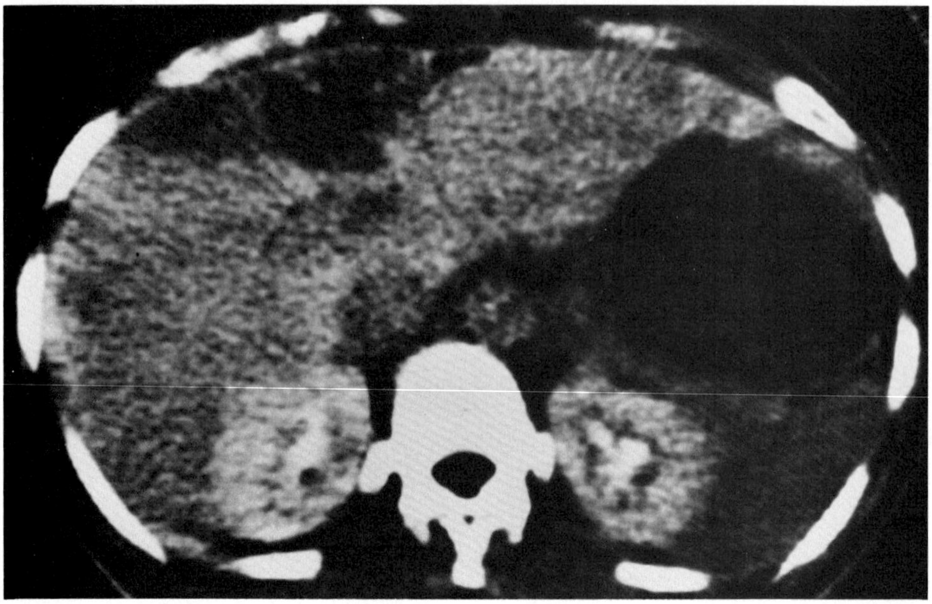

(C)

Figure 31 Focal nodular hyperplasia, multiple lesions. Forty-year-old female, on the contraceptive pill, complained of discomfort, was found to have an enlarged liver. (A) The capillary phase of a celiac arteriogram demonstrates multiple relatively homogeneous masses, probably due to focal nodular hyperplasia. This was impossible to differentiate from hypervascular metastases angiographically. Surgical biopsy confirmed the diagnosis of multiple focal nodular hyperplasia. (B) Hepatic arteriography 2 years later revealed that the multiple lesions were approximately the same in size and distribution. (C) Reexamination by CT after a further 2 years showed multiple lesions of low attenuation, probably unchanged during the last 4 years.

Table 5 Differential Features of Benign Epithelial Tumors

Focal nodular hyperplasia	Liver cell adenoma
Pathology	
Kupffer's cells	Hepatocytes
Fibrous septa	Homogeneous
Bile ducts	Few bile ducts
Often multiple	Rarely multiple
No capsule	Encapsulated
Clinical	
Rarely symptomatic	Hemorrhage
No malignant potential	(?)Malignant potential
Females, 86%	Females, 99%
Birth to 80 years	17–61 years
(?)Hormone-related	Steroid-induced
Radiology	
Always vascular	Frequently vascular
Tortuous neovessels	Hemorrhage, necrosis
Colloid uptake, 40%	No colloid uptake

Source: Ref. 85.

Table 6 Summary of Angiography and Radionuclide Scan Findings in 35 Cases of Focal Nodular Hyperplasia (FNH) and Liver Cell Adenoma (LCA)

	Angiography	
NM scan	Hypervascular	Hypovascular
Uptake of colloid in mass	7 Cases FNH	Nil
Focal defect, no uptake	19 Cases FNH or LCA	9 LCA

Source: Ref. 85.

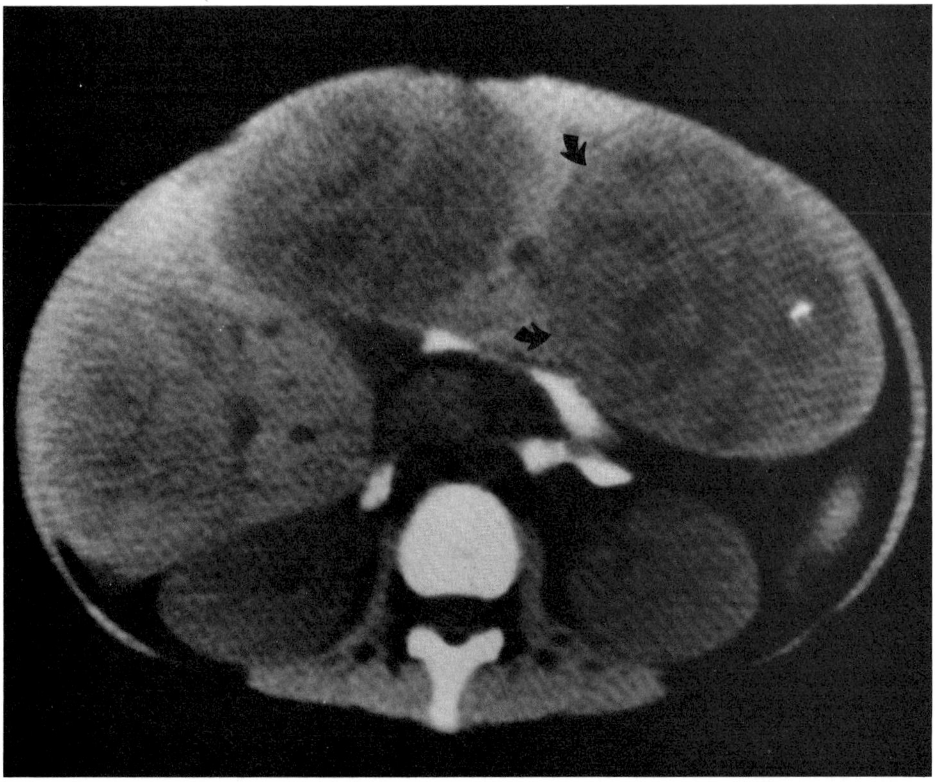

Figure 32A Focal nodular hyperplasia and hepatocellular carcinoma in von Gierke's disease. CT prior to contrast.

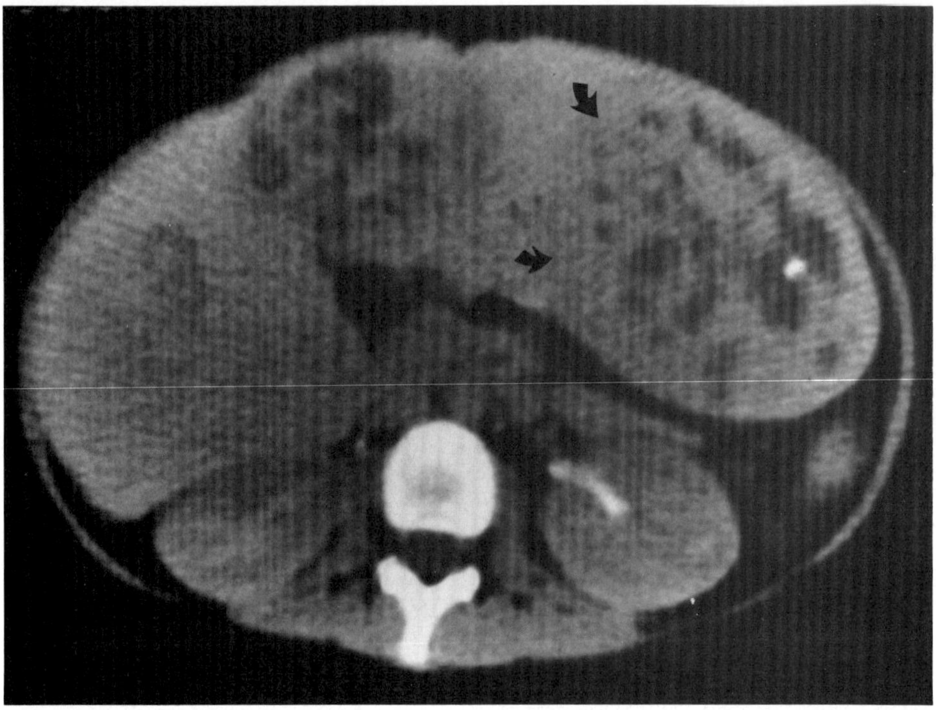

Figure 32B CT following contrast injection (HCC indicated by arrows). FNH is a liver manifestation of von Gierke's disease. It is uncertain whether the HCC is coincidental or is a manifestation of degeneration of the FNH. (Courtesy of Dr. E. Singleton, Houston, Texas.)

Malignant Tumors

Primary Hepatic Neoplasms in Childhood

These neoplasms usually develop in children under 2 years of age and are found more often in males. The children with hepatic malignancy are almost invariably symptomatic, presenting with an abdominal protuberance associated with fever, anorexia, weight loss, and malaise. Spontaneous rupture with hemoperitoneum is not uncommon. Late in the disease or in the presence of cirrhosis, the child may have ascites, jaundice, and hepatic dysfunction. Metastases can occur to the lung, lymph nodes, bones, or peritoneal surface (13,14,16,17,44–46).

Biochemical studies Because of the reserve and regenerative capacity of the liver, extensive involvement is necessary before the abnormality is reflected in the liver function studies. Any elevation of bilirubin is usually due to the intrahepatic process obstructing the biliary tract. Human α-fetoprotein is normally found from 14 to 40 weeks of development and declines until birth. Subsequently, it is absent in healthy children and adults, but does reappear in the serum of patients with hepatocellular carcinoma. Although the frequency of its presence in such patients varies in different parts of the world (46,90,91); in general, it is found in about 50–70% (46). However, an increased fetoprotein may also be found in patients with ovarian or testicular neoplasms and in nonneoplastic disease.

The nonspecificity of these biochemical parameters limits their potential as screening tests.

Hepatoblastoma and Hepatocellular Carcinoma

The differentiation of these two histologic types is, at times, difficult and relates to their degree of cellular maturity (44,45,52). Hepatoblastomas contain relatively small cells resembling embryonal or fetal liver. Hepatocarcinomas are made up of larger pleomorphic, frequently multinucleated cells. The mixed variety of hepatocarcinomas has abundant mitoses, fibrous stroma, and areas of necrosis. Calcification, osteoid tissue, and immature cartilage may be found. Hepatocarcinoma may also be well differentiated. They occur more frequently after 5–6 years of age, whereas hepatoblastomas are usually seen before the age of 2 years.

Radiologic findings Radiologic studies were of greatest assistance in the preoperative evaluation. In a series at the M. D. Anderson Hospital, calcification was seen in 3 of 16 patients. Pulmonary metastases at initial presentation were found in 4 of 16 patients, diffuse osteoporosis in only one.

Hepatic scintigraphy, sonography, and computed tomography were complementary procedures to angiography to establish the presence, number, and distribution of the lesions (92–108). These scans were especially important in hypovascular neoplasms and in those situated in the left lateral segment of the liver. Such studies are more readily accomplished in older children and adults. Scintigraphy and sonography are more rewarding in the infant and smaller child. The lack of body fat and the difficulty in restraining motion places computed tomography at a disadvantage.

Angiographically, hepatocellular neoplasms have a varied pattern with a full range of vascularity. The vast majority are large, solitary, and hypervascular with enlarged feeding arteries, with abundant abnormal vasculature, and increased parenchymal staining (92–102). Although arteriovenous shunting is common in the adult variety, it is not a frequent finding in children. The degree of differentiation may be suggested by the amount of neovascularity and the margination of the mass. The angiographic picture of a hypervascular neoplasm with a well-circumscribed margin may be similar to that of an hepatic adenoma or a focal nodular hyperplexia (see Chap. 30). The differentiation from hemangioendotheliomas, hamartomas, and hypervascular metastases may be difficult. Hemangiomas can usually be differentiated because they typically have normal-appearing arterial vessels that enter into small sinusoidal pools in which contrast material remains late into the venous phase.

Extension into veins Hepatocellular neoplasms in children do extend via the veins (Fig. 33). Inferior venacavography, hepatic venography, and portal venography can offer additional information concerning venous involvement and, therefore, hepatic resectability (92,93,102). Awareness of the projection of the neoplasm into the hepatic veins will alter the surgical procedure to minimize the possibility of tumor embolization. The specific hepatic vein involved should be ligated early in the operation. Extension into the inferior vena cava currently contraindicates surgery. At times, only side-to-side narrowing of the vena cava in its course through the hepatic groove may be seen. It is then often difficult to distinguish between tumor invasion and simple compression, the latter being more usual.

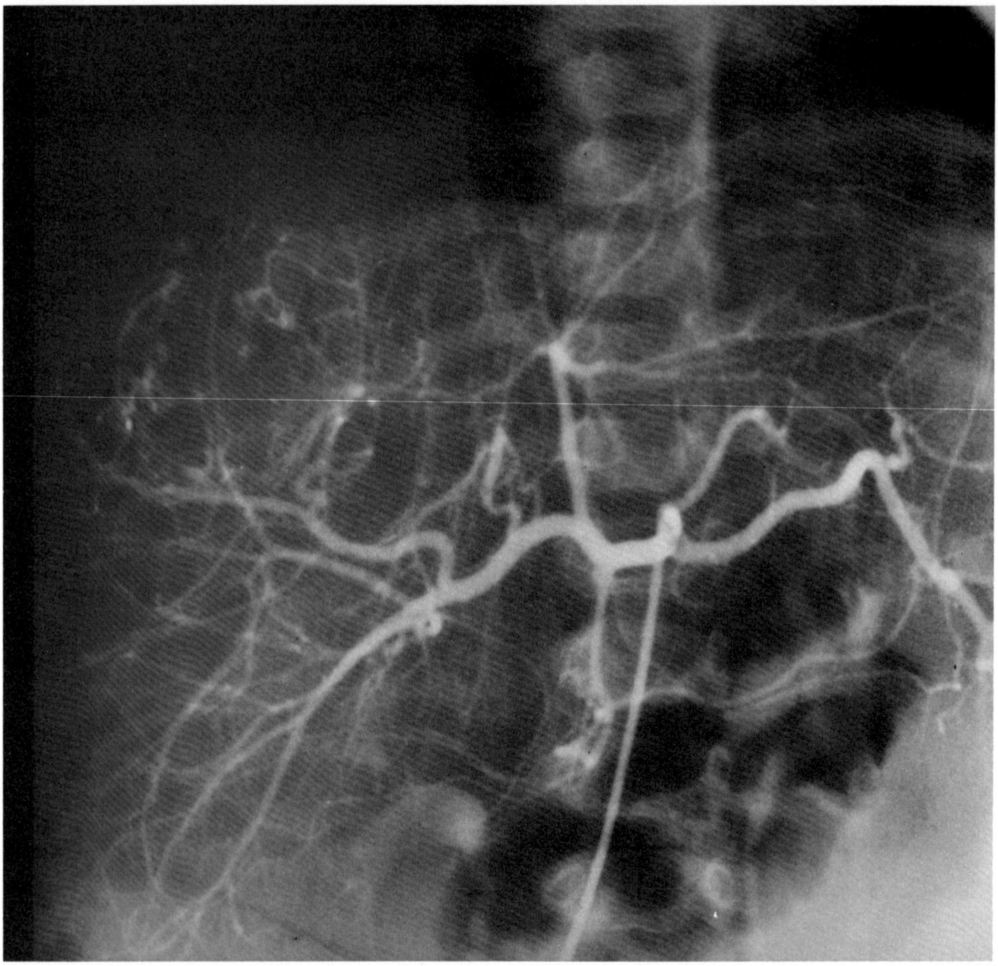

Figure 33A Hepatoblastoma. The hypervascular neoplasm in this 8-month-old boy is supplied by the superior portions of the anterior and posterior branches of the right hepatic artery.

Surgical treatment Once the diagnosis has been made, the treatment of choice in the presence of a localized neoplasm and in the absence of metastases is surgery. The surgeon must be satisfied that the operation is locally curable, that the quantity and quality of liver tissue remaining will support life, and that the general condition of the patient can withstand the surgery. The posterior segment of the right lobe is the only segment that cannot be removed by itself. The hepatic veins draining the superior subsegment of the anterior segment traverses the posterior segment, thus necessitating a right hepatectomy (20). A minimum of 10–15% of normal liver is necessary to sustain life (109,110). The overall operative death rate for extended hepatic resections is approximately 25% (20). The 5-year cure rate for all patients once resection has been accomplished is about 30% (20,110–114). Children tolerate resection better than adults. This is probably because the

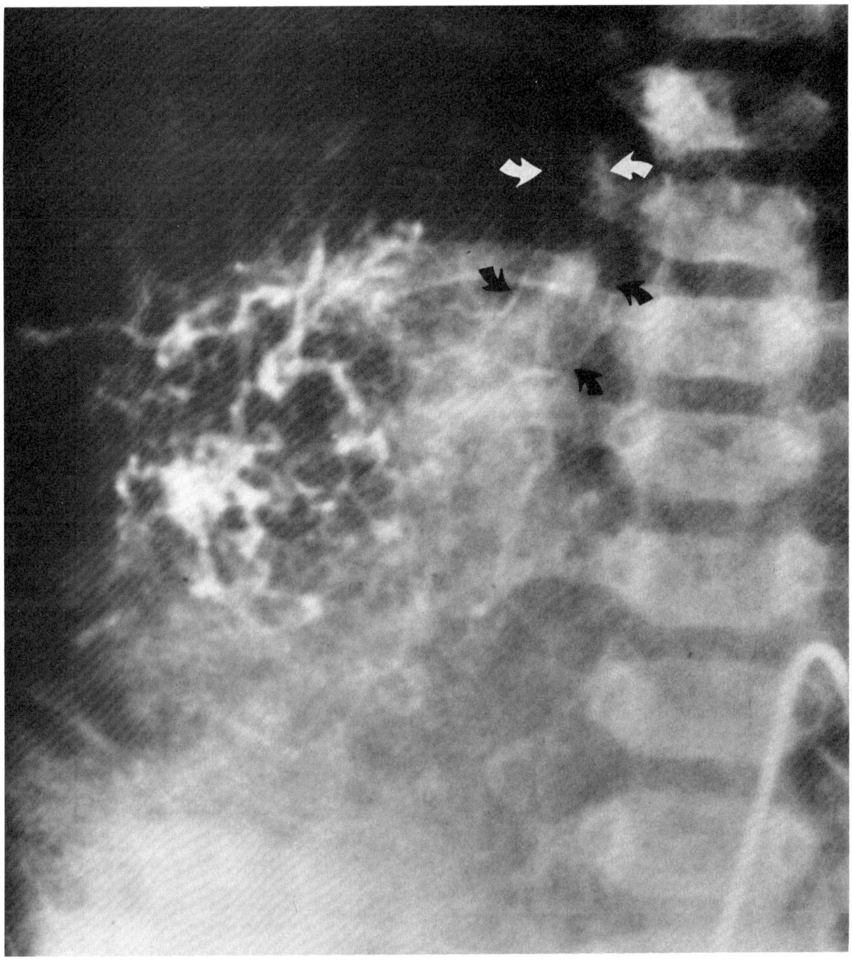

Figure 33B Parallel channels in the distribution of the middle hepatic vein (arrows) suggest intravascular extension of the hepatoblastoma.

residual portion of the child's liver is more likely to be normal and able to regenerate more readily. At the time of resection, the amount of residual normal liver has often been found to be far greater than expected, suggesting hypertrophy and hyperplasia in the presence of the neoplasm. It could be demonstrated that after a 90% resection of the liver in animals, the total mass was regained in 4 months (109,110). Both experimentally and clinically, it has been shown that regeneration begins immediately after surgery. Figure 34 illustrates an 11-year-old child with regeneration occurring within 1 month of hepatectomy. Follow-up examinations are more readily accomplished by means of liver scans. Repeat arteriography is occasionally necessary to determine the presence of recurrent or progressive disease. Metastases usually occur to lungs, lymph nodes, or peritoneum.

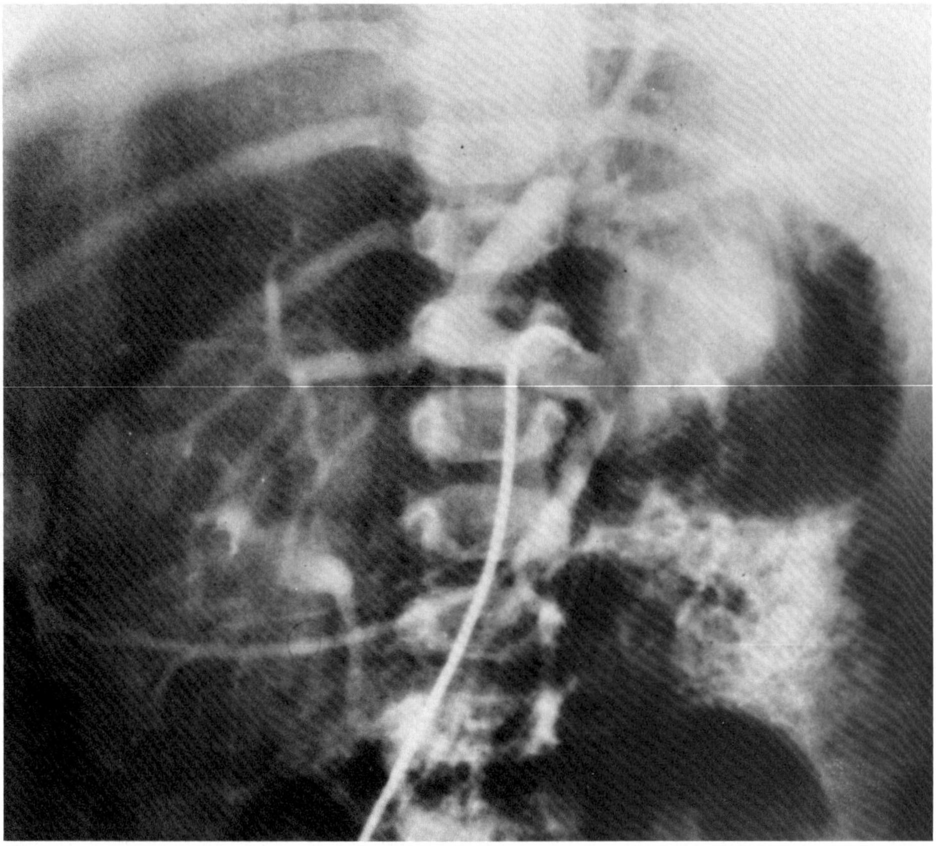

Figure 33C Superior mesenteric arteriogram demonstrates a patent portal vein with displacement of the intrahepatic venous radicles.

Malignant Mesenchymal Tumors

Malignant mesenchymal tumors, such as embryonal rhabdomyosarcoma and malignant mesenchymoma, are rather unusual. The angiographic and pathologic appearance was described by Stanley et al. (1973), in a summary of 12 patients (115). Hepatosplenomegaly, abdominal pain, fever, and weight loss are the usual clinical features.

Angiographically, these tumors are hypovascular, with widely separated minute clusters of neovascularity as well as a lack of prolonged pooling of contrast material. Histologically, there is a combination of epithelium-lined spaces and anaplastic stroma. There are cystic and solid areas with a myxomatous appearance. Bone, cartilage, fat, and smooth and skeletal muscle may be present. There is a high content of acid mucopolysaccharide. Treatment, for the most part, has been surgical, with an overall poor prognosis.

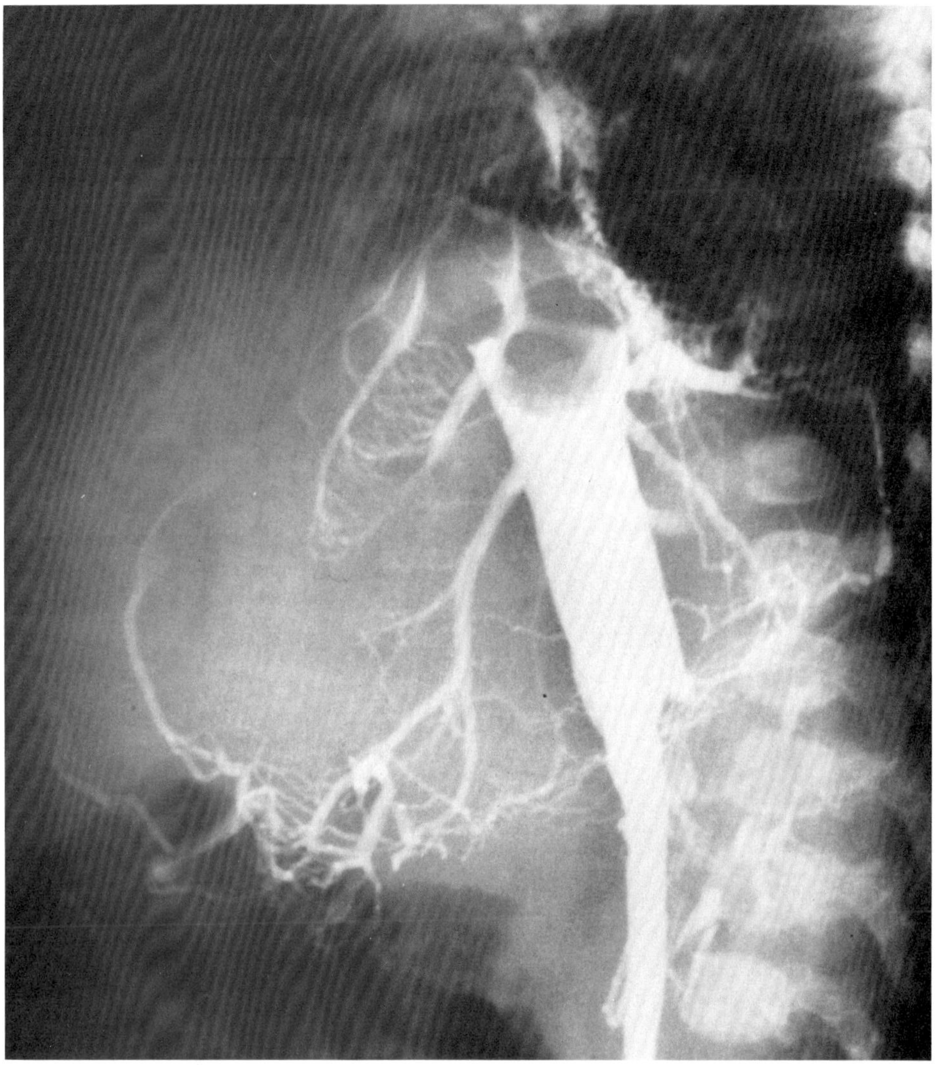

Figure 33D Inferior venacavography reveals an intraluminal mass with opacification of collateral veins. Because of the intravenous extension, the neoplasm was considered nonresectable.

Primary Hepatic Neoplasms in the Adult

Of the primary malignant neoplasms involving the liver, carcinomas (i.e., hepatocellular, cholangiocelluar and mixed) constitute the majority. In the adult, these neoplasms are most common in the sixth decade but may occur at any age and affect men three to seven times as frequently as women (116,117). The patients will usually present with anorexia, weight loss, and abdominal pain associated with hepatomegaly in 75%, splenomegaly in

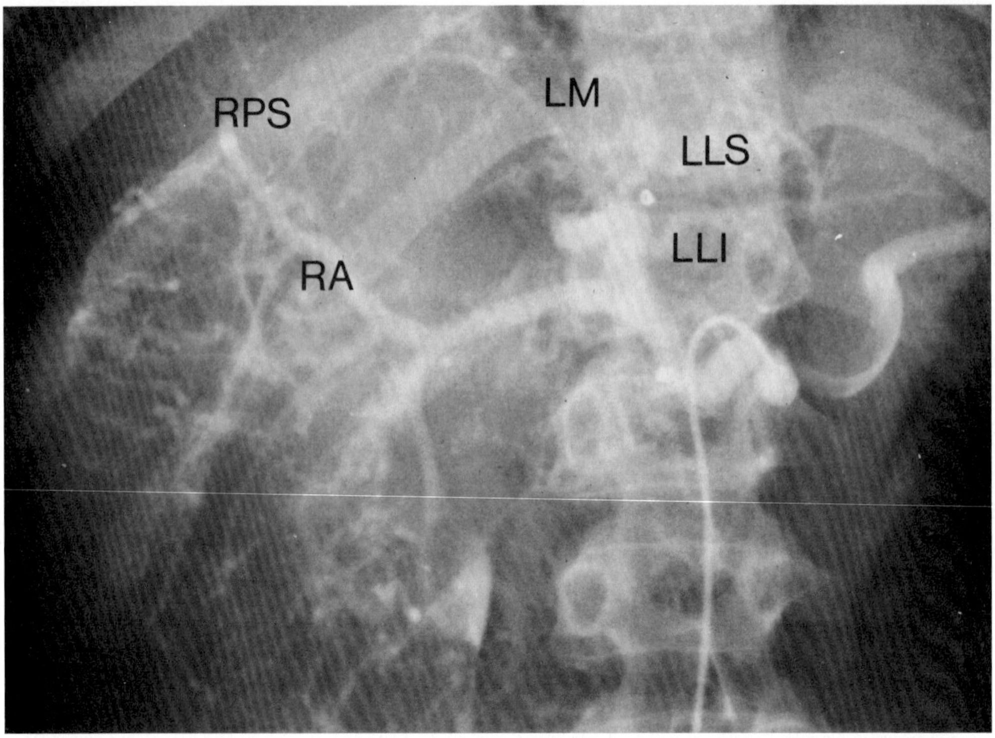

(A)

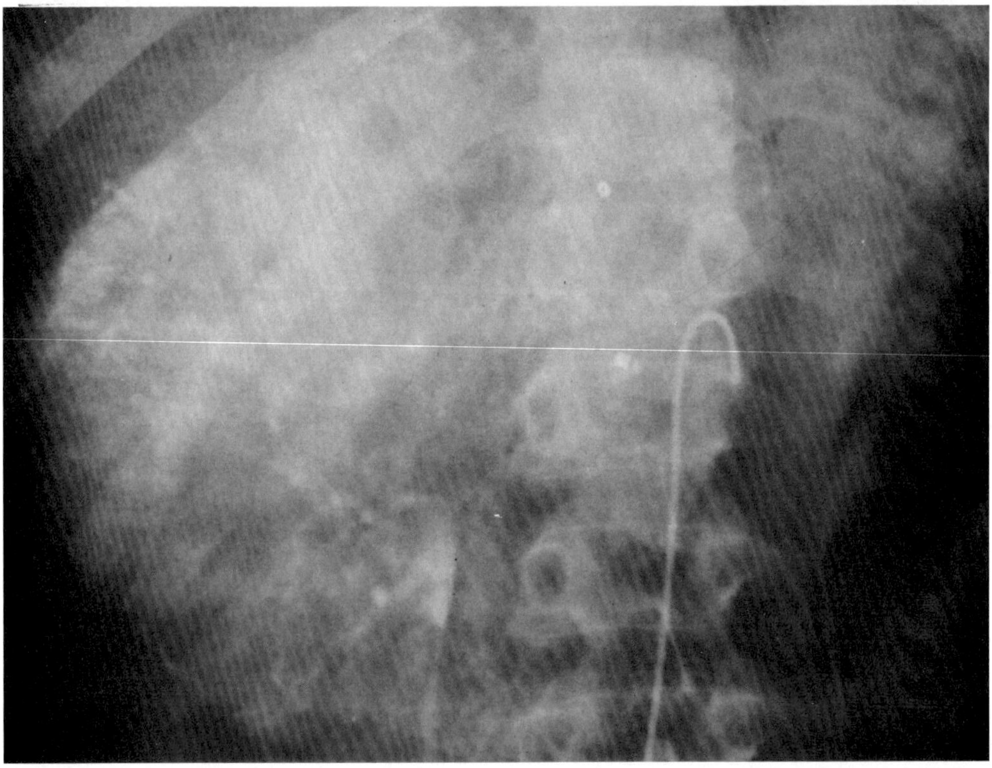

(B)

Figure 34

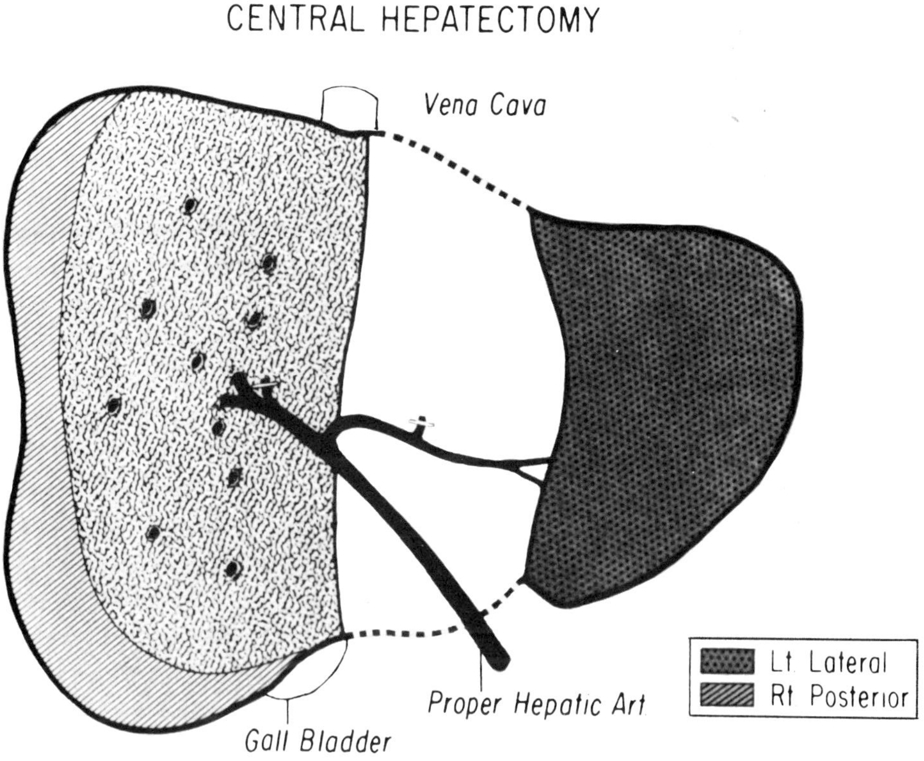

(C)

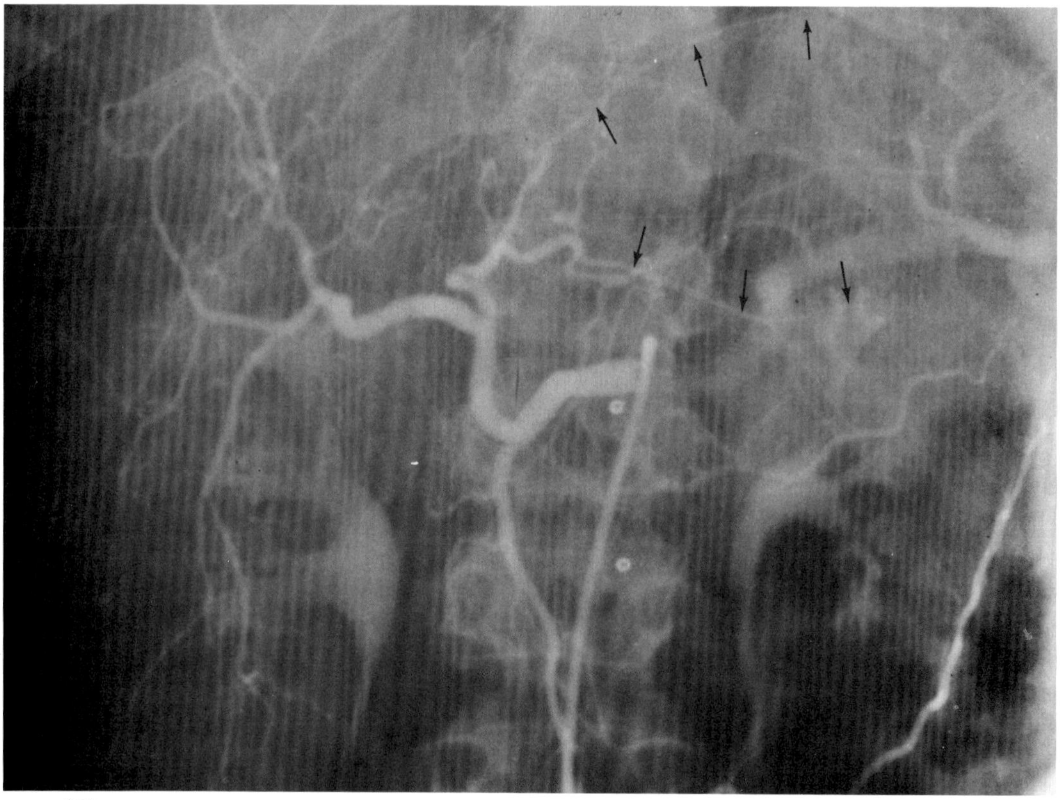

(D)

Figure 34 (continued)

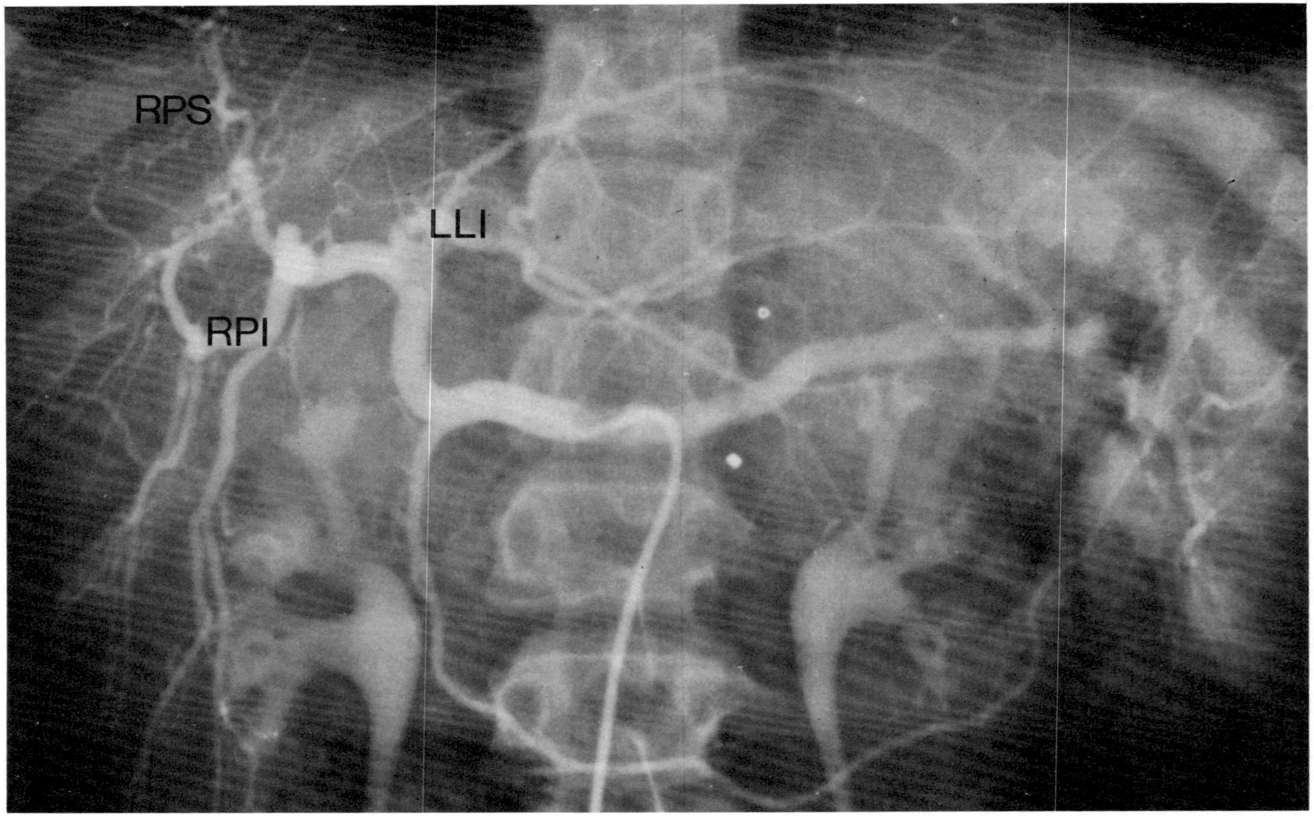

(E)

Figure 34 (continued)

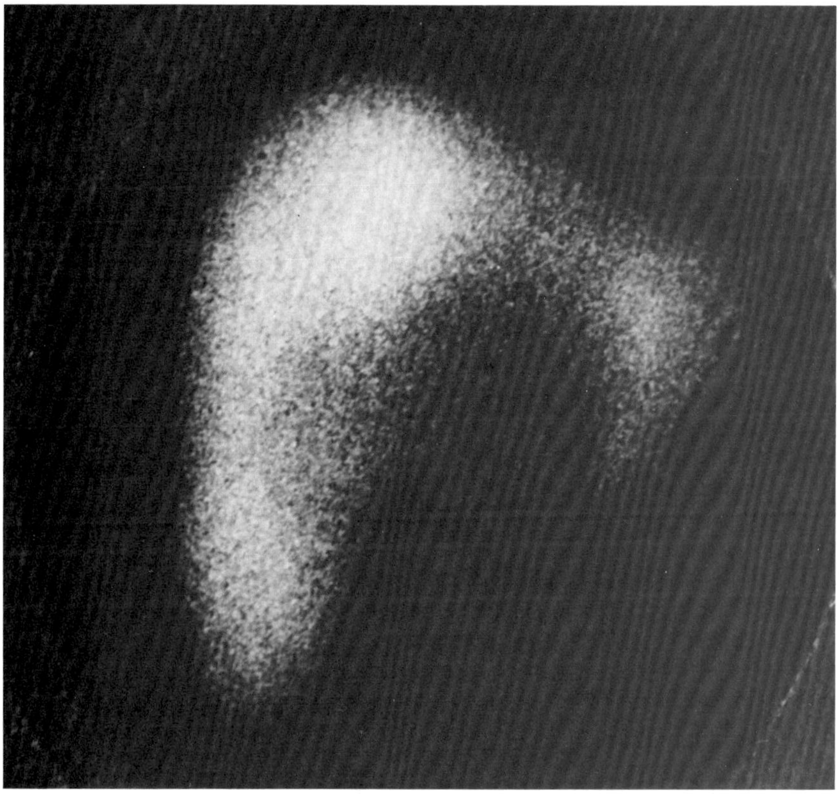

(F)

Figure 34 (continued)

33%, and bloodstained ascites in 50%. Hematemesis and melanoma may be the initial episode and are usually from underlying cirrhosis, which occurs in 50–57%, mostly of the postnecrotic type. The tumors tend to rupture spontaneously with intra-abdominal hemorrhage and shock. Other findings include paraneoplastic syndromes such as hypoglycemia, carcinoid-type syndrome, erythrocytosis, hypercalcemia, hyperlipidemia, and osteoarthropathy (116,117).

Abnormal liver function studies are frequent, especially a raised alkaline phosphatase. A rapid rise in the enzyme in a known cirrhotic should suggest malignant degeneration. An elevated α-fetoprotein (AFP) is found in 30% of patients with hepatocellular carcinoma in the United States, in contrast to up to 70% in the Far East and Africa. Hepatitis virus B has been found in 25–50%. Parasitic infestations, nutritional deficiencies, hemachromatosis, hepatoxic agents, and so on, have been incriminated but not well documented except for clonorchis sinensis, which has been seen in association with cholangiocarcinoma and opisthorchis viverrini with cholangiocarcinoma or mixed hepatocellular cholangiocarcinoma.

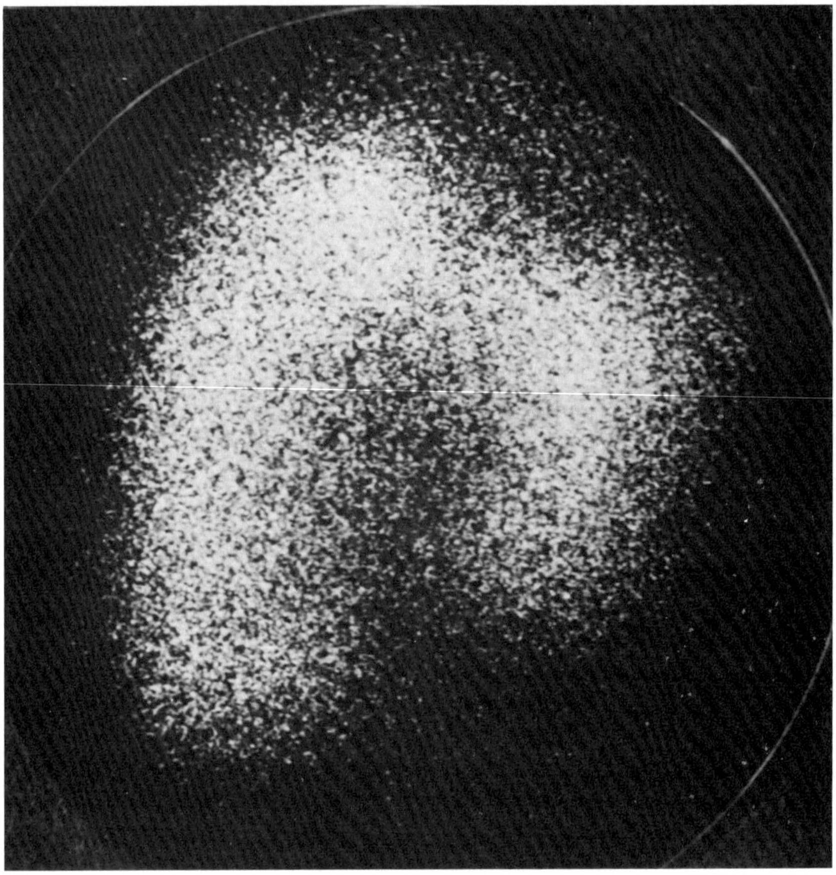

(G)

Figure 34 (continued)

Hepatocellular Carcinoma

These neoplasms mostly present as follows: (1) solitary (usually noncirrhotic), (2) multinodular (more common with cirrhosis), and (3) diffuse without distinct mass. Undoubtedly, the neoplasms most difficult to diagnose are those in patients with diffuse infiltrative disease or in the presence of cirrhosis. They may require the use of all of the scanning procedures (NM, US, and CT) as well as angiography (92–102) (see Chap. 12).

Angiographic appearances As with all other neoplasms, hepatocellular carcinomas run the full gamut of vascularity as demonstrated by angiography, but are predominantly hypervascular with marked neovascularity. Consequently, angiography is most capable of demonstrating smaller lesions (Fig. 35). Infusion angiography is especially applicable in defining the neoplasm arising in a cirrhotic liver. Pharmacoangiography is of assistance at times.

In hepatocellular carcinomas, arteriovenous shunting is relatively common, as is the reversal of flow in the portal vein and intravenous extension of neoplasms. Demonstration

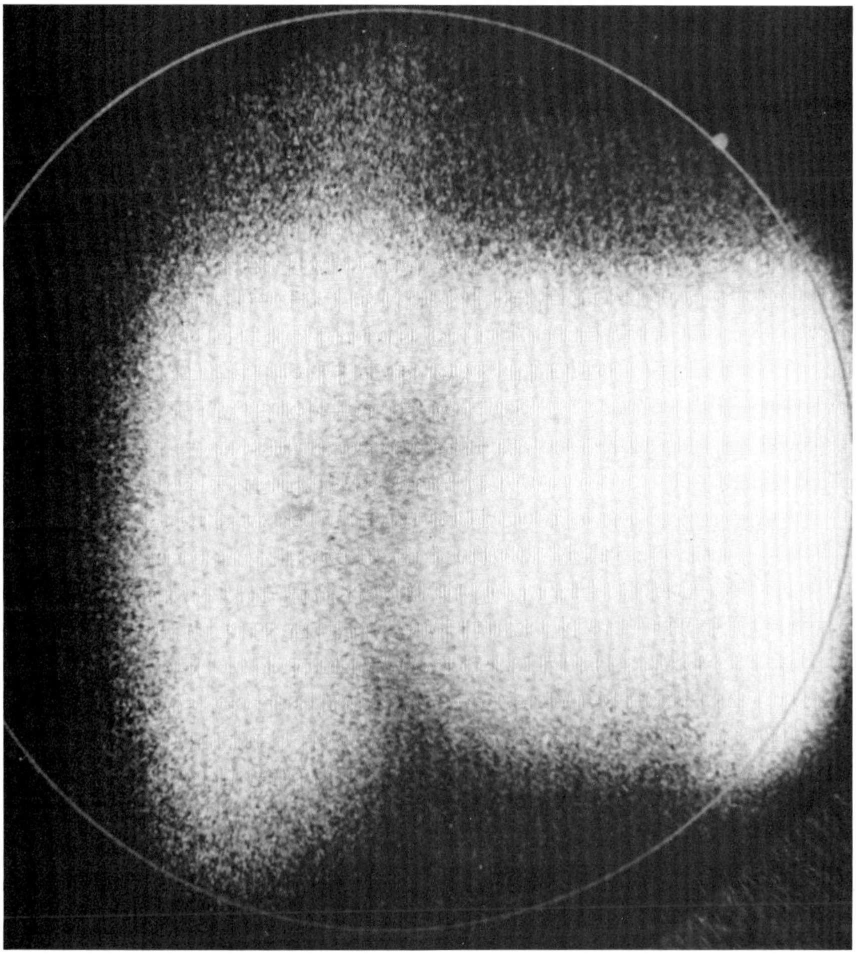

(H)

Figure 34 Hepatocellular carcinoma, pre- and postresection. (A) Hepatic arteriography defines a hypervascular neoplasm supplied by the arterior segmental branch (RA) of the right hepatic artery and the medial segmental branch (LM) of the left hepatic artery. Note the attenuation of the other hepatic arterial branches created by the preferential flow to the neoplasm. (B) The capillary phase reveals a fairly homogeneous vascularity of the neoplasm in the anterior portion of the liver. (C) A central hepatectomy was performed with removal of the anterior segment on the right and the medial segment on the left. Diagrammatic representation. (D) Hepatic arteriogram 1 month postoperatively illustrates regeneration of the left lateral segment and the right posterior segment. Note the wide separation of the normally parallel left lateral subsegmental branches (arrows), a manifestation of the regeneration. (E) Repeat arteriography 1 year following resection reveals further separation of the subsegmental branches (LLS, LLI) of the left lobe due to progressive regeneration. The right posterior superior subsegmental branches (RPS) demonstrate tortuosity, presumably because of contraction of this subsegment. In contrast, there is elongation of the vessels to the inferior subsegment (RPI), also due to regeneration. (F) Preoperative scintigraphy demonstrates a large defect in the central portion of the liver, due to the HCC. (G) Scintigraphy 1 month after resection already documents regeneration. (H) Scintigraphy 1 year after the central hepatectomy illustrates further regeneration of the liver.

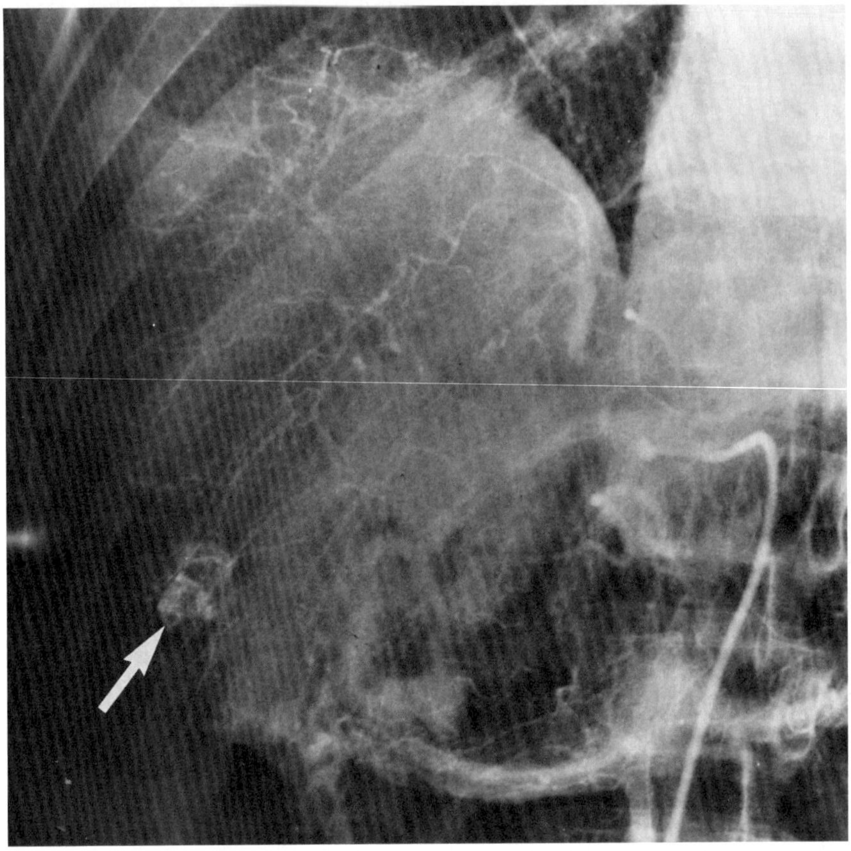

Figure 35 Hepatocellular carcinoma, chance finding. Angiography performed to define a defect shown by screening technique, demonstrated a small hypervascular mass (arrow). The differential diagnosis of the angiographic appearance would include any of the benign or malignant hypervascular neoplasms. However, it does not show the classical features of a cavernous hemangioma. Therefore, surgery was required for a more specific diagnosis, and exploration proved this to be an HCC.

of arteriovenous shunting can be defined by dynamic CT scanning. Intravascular neoplasm projecting into the portal vein, hepatic vein, and inferior vena cava can be demonstrated by US and CT. However, both of these vascular manifestations of tumor extension are most graphically displayed by angiography (Figs. 36, 37). Although most unusual, the same finding can be seen with metastatic disease (Fig. 38).

Metastases from hepatocellular carcinomas are found in the lung in 8.3%, hepatic hilar lymph nodes in 3.4%, central nervous system in 1.5%, and in bones in 0.95% (116).

Cholangiocarcinoma

Most of these neoplasms originate near the hilum of the liver and are manifested by persistent and progressive obstructive jaundice. Anorexia, nausea, fullness, emaciation, and general malaise are the usual signs and symptoms. The abdomen is generally soft and nontender. The liver is frequently, but not always, palpable.

Sonography and computed tomography readily demonstrate biliary duct obstruction and may delineate the primary neoplasm if large enough. Transhepatic cholangiography is, perhaps, most revealing for localization of the biliary obstruction. Differentiation from sclerosing cholangitis is usually established by the focal and hilar location of cholangiocarcinoma. Angiographically, cholangiocarcinoma may cause minor tumor neovascularity, but more often will show invasion or encasement of adjacent vessels (25) (see Fig. 23 in Chap. 12).

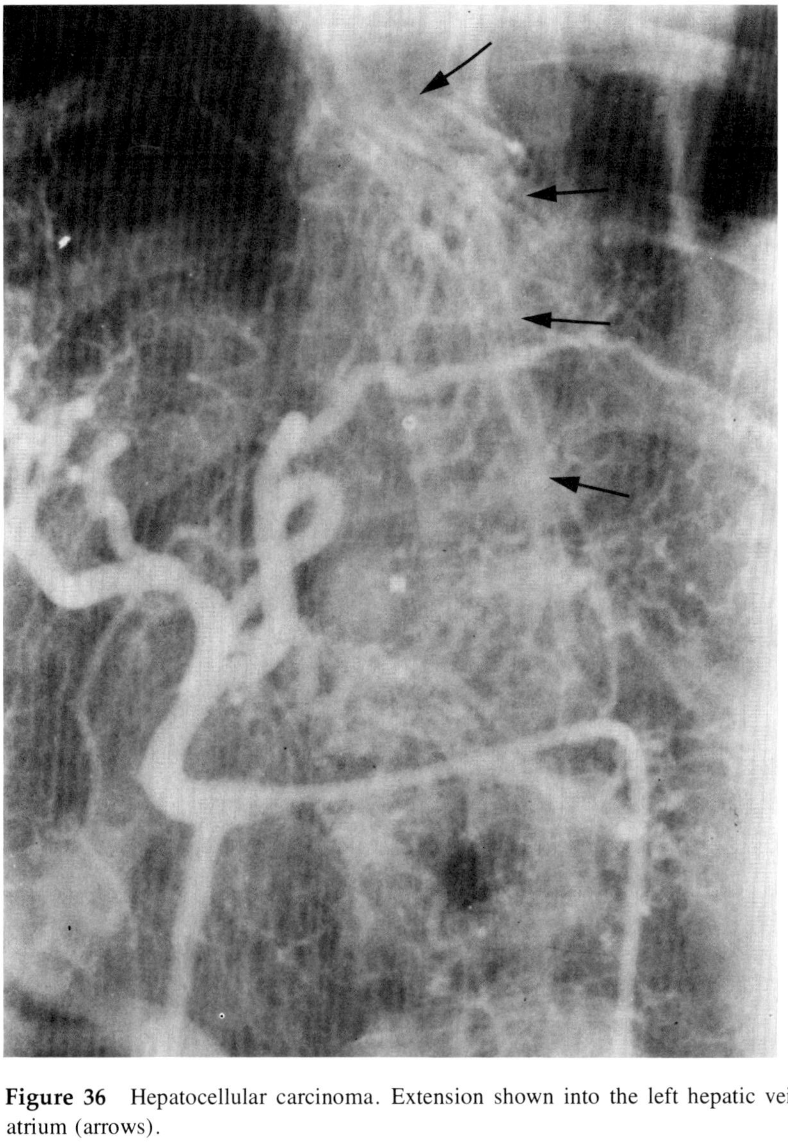

Figure 36 Hepatocellular carcinoma. Extension shown into the left hepatic vein and the right atrium (arrows).

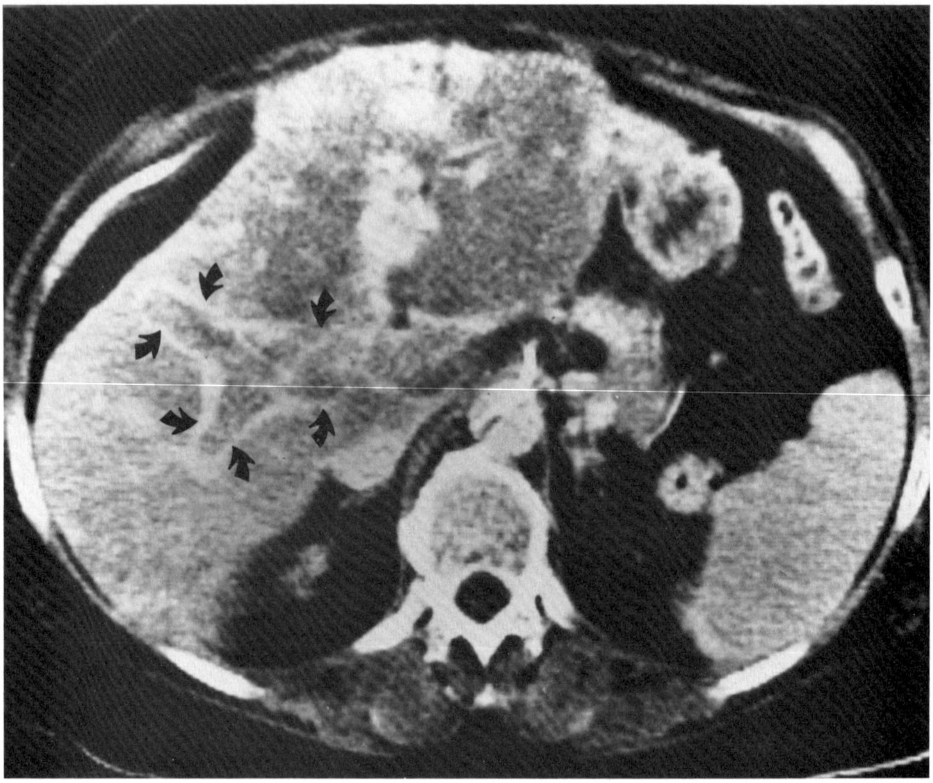

(A)

Figure 37 Hepatocellular carcinoma with tumor extension into the portal vein. (A) Computed angiotomography reveals tumor thrombus in the portal vein (arrows). (B) A hepatic arteriogram confirms the presence of tumor thrombus in the portal vein (arrows). (Courtesy of Dr. Patrick Freeny, Seattle, Washington.)

Sarcomas

Each of the mesenchymal elements of the liver has the potential for malignant proliferation. For example, a leiomyosarcoma may originate from the hepatic capsule or from adjacent structures. In determining the site or origin of the neoplasm, the predominant blood supply is usually a helpful sign. However, parasitization of the hepatic artery supply to neoplasms invading, attached to, or adjacent to the liver at times makes impossible differentiation as to the organ of origin. Ultrasonography, in particular, and computed tomography with reconstruction in multiple planes may better define the line of cleavage between the organs.

Metastases to the Liver

The liver is the major organ most frequently involved by metastatic disease (118–123). Usually, the hepatic metastases and not the primary neoplasm dictate the course of the

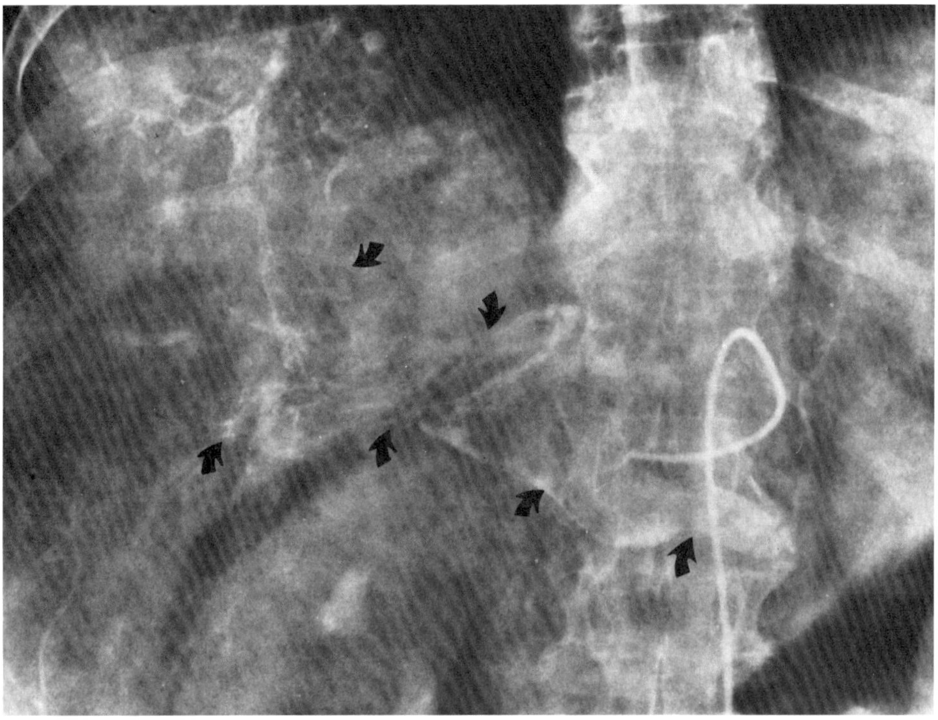

(B)

Figure 37 (continued)

disease and the patient's survival. The median survival for patients with untreated liver metastases from carcinoma of the colon is 150 days; from the stomach, 60 days; and from the pancreas, 50 days (51,118). It has been estimated that in Western countries, metastatic cancer to the liver is 20 times more common than primary hepatic malignancies. From 30–50% of all patients with carcinoma who are examined at necropsy show metastases to the liver (122). The liver involved with metastatic disease is generally enlarged but may be normal in size. The presenting findings in 44% of patients with hepatic metastases are referrable to the liver; nonspecific complaints such as weight loss, anorexia, and fever might also occur. Right upper quadrant abdominal pain is experienced in 36%. Approximately 25% of patients with hepatic metastases have overt jaundice and 33% have ascites. Hematemesis is occasionally found in association with esophageal varices. Intraperitoneal hemorrhage is uncommon (122).

Among the tumor antigens of value in the detection of metastatic disease to the liver is the carcinoembryonic antigen (CEA). CEA is also useful in monitoring therapy for hepatic metastases, especially from cancer of the colon.

Radiologic manifestations Nuclear medicine, US, and CT are sensitive in detecting hepatic metastases; the diagnostic approach is as outlined in Table 1. It must be stressed again that the pursuit of the diagnosis depends on the clinical situation and should be curtailed once a satisfactory correlation has been made. For further specificity and in

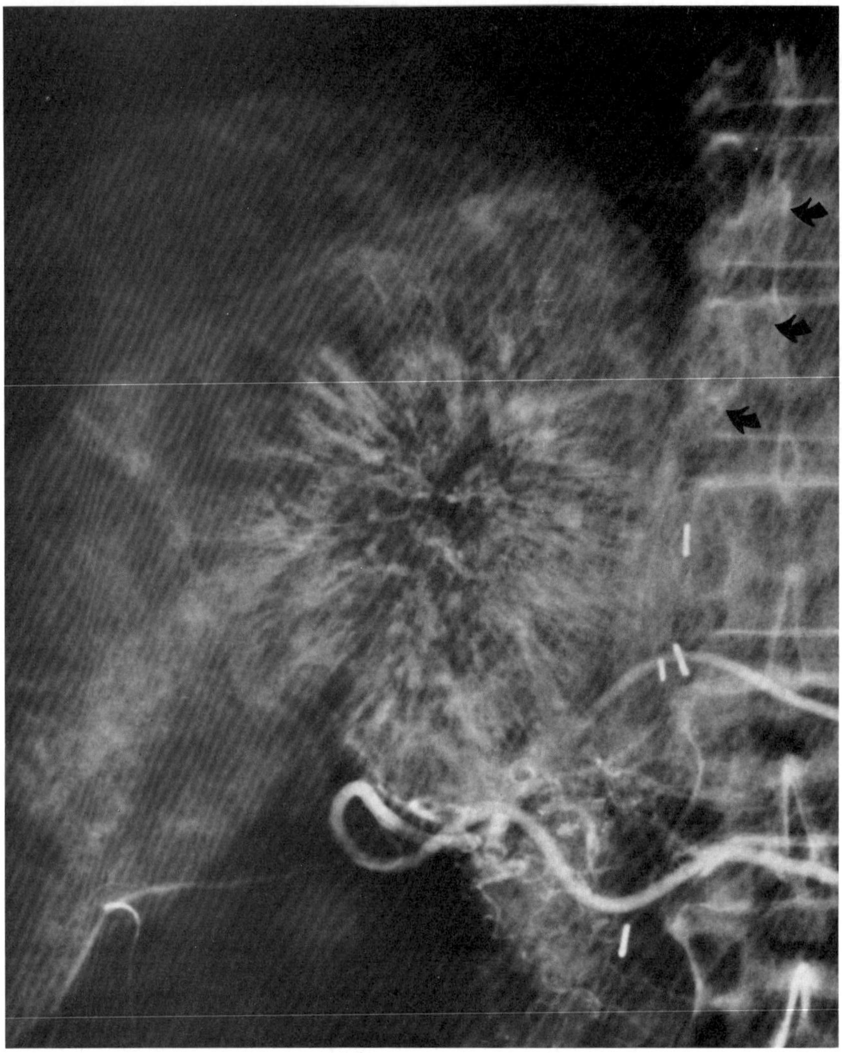

Figure 38 Metastatic renal carcinoma with extension into the hepatic vein (arrows).

the event of a discrepancy between the clinical findings and the scanning procedures, angiography becomes essential (Fig. 34).

The angiography manifestations of metastatic disease have been described (26) in relation to the hepatic parenchyma as (1) hypervascular, (2) isovascular, and (3) hypovascular. The vascularity of the metastases frequently parallels that of the primary. Each primary neoplasm exhibits a range of vascularity, usually with a predominant pattern. This is illustrated by the gamut of vascularity seen in renal neoplasms: 65% hypervascular, 20% isovascular, and 15% hypovascular. Pancreatic adenocarcinomas are most often hypovascular (95%), but occasionally hypervascular. Most metastases to the liver at presentation are multiple (90%) and hypervascular if optimal technique is employed (i.e., selective catheterization, infusion technique, and pharmacoangiography) (Fig. 40).

The left lateral segment creates the most problems in diagnosis by angiography. Selective left hepatic arteriography is frequently necessary for accurate diagnosis. Even with exquisite technique, iso- and hypovascular metastases may be better defined by the scanning procedures (Fig. 12). At times, there is enlargement of the left lateral segment manifested by an increased distance between the superior and inferior subsegmental branches. However, compensatory hypertrophy of this segment may exist when there is replacement by tumor in other areas. Enlargement does, therefore, not necessarily indicate metastases.

Hypervascular Metastases

The majority of metastases can be included in this category. Renal carcinoma (Fig. 39C); thyroid carcinoma; choriocarcinoma (Fig. 5 in Chap. 12); and leiomyosarcoma, especially from the small bowel, frequently demonstrate increased vascularity in their metastases. For the most part, metastases from endocrine-producing tumors, including those of neuroectodermal origin, are hypervascular and best demonstrated by angiography. Epinephrine-enhanced angiography does assist in the opacification of these neoplasms, as illustrated in a patient with metastases from a carcinoid tumor of the small bowel (Fig. 2 in Chap. 12). Hypervascular metastases as small as 2–5 mm (120) are readily demonstrated by angiography.

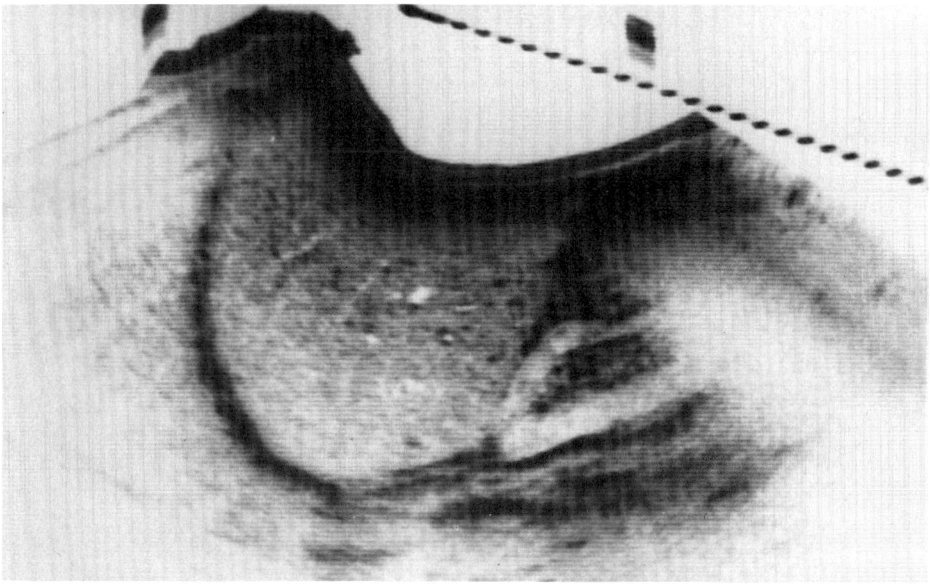

(A)

Figure 39 Metastatic renal cell carcinoma. (A) On US, the liver was considered free of metastatic disease. (B) CT was also considered negative for metastases. The areas of low attenuation appear to branch, in keeping with portal vein structures. (C) Angiography revealed multiple hypervascular metastatic lesions (arrows).

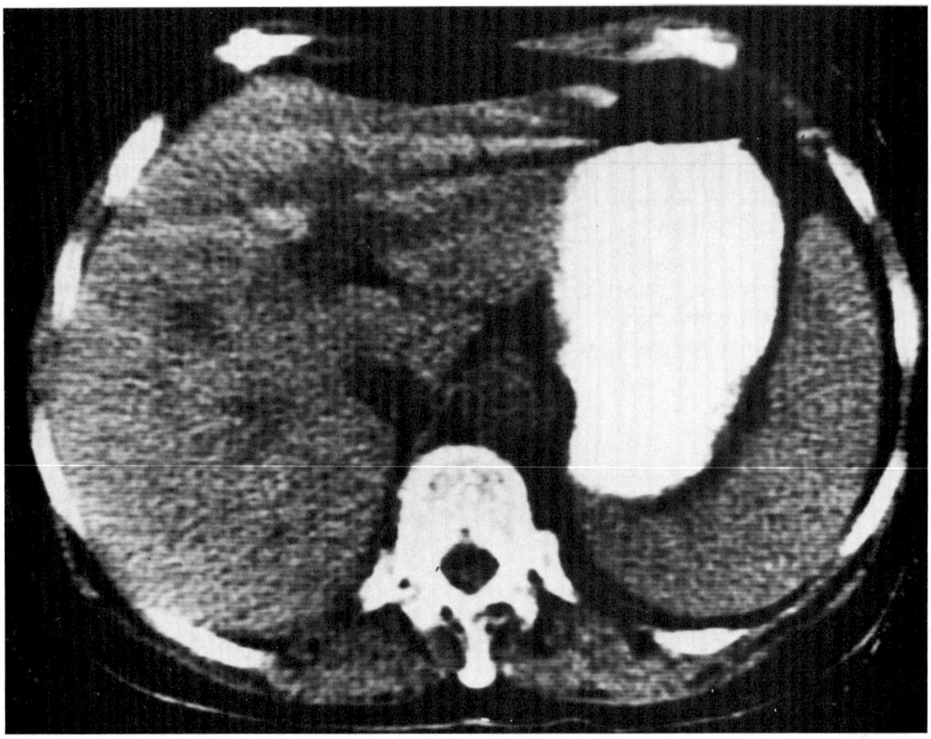

(B)

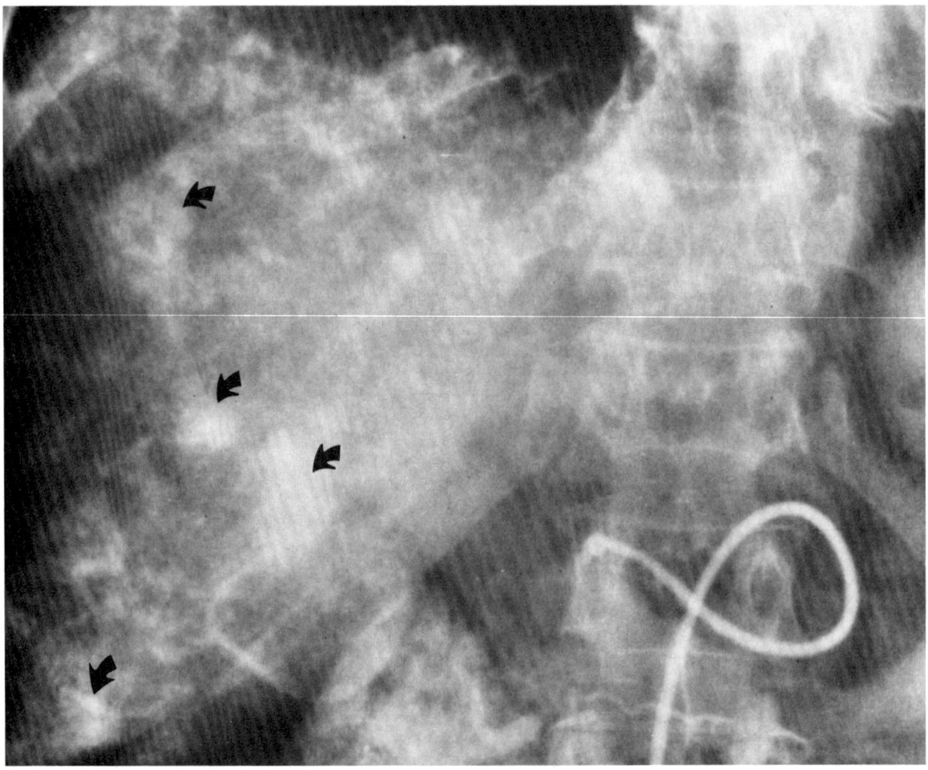

(C)

Figure 39 (continued)

Vein involvement These hypervascular metastases are more likely to be associated with arteriovenous shunting, reversal of flow in the arteries and veins, and tumor extension into the hepatic (Fig. 38) and portal veins as well as into the inferior vena cava. Involvement of the portal vein by obstruction, tumor extension, retrograde opacification, and fistula formation has been described in association with hepatocellular neoplasms, cirrhosis, trauma, congenital malformations (hemangiomas, Rendu-Osler-Weber, etc.), and abscesses. All these angiographic findings of portal vein involvement can occur with hepatic metastases (119).

Metastases from carcinoma of the colon are the most common and usually have a hypervascular rim with a less vascular center (Fig. 40). Intrinsic obstruction of the portal veins is more likely from metastases originating from primary carcinomas drained by the portal system (e.g., colon carcinoma) (123).

The "mottled" liver Hypervascular metastases must be differentiated from the "normal" mottled liver, peliosis hepatis, and nodular hyperplasia as part of the cirrhotic liver, as well as from benign and primary malignant neoplasms of the liver. The mottled

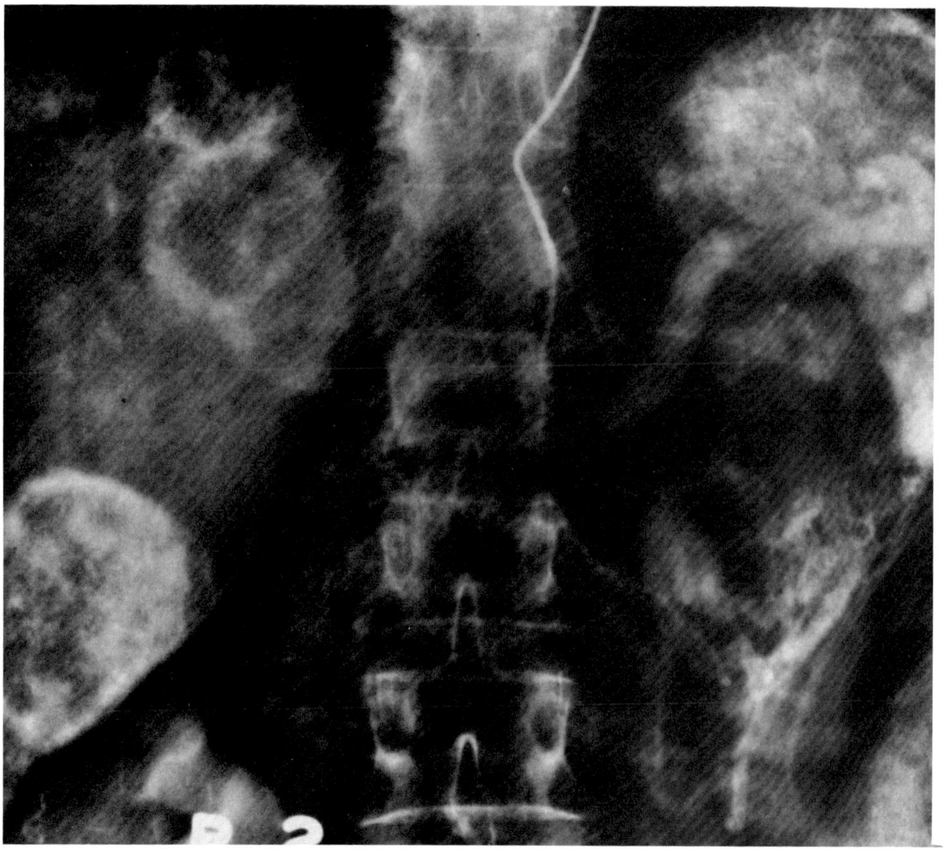

Figure 40A Metastatic colon carcinoma. Effect of hepatic arterial chemotherapy. These lesions represent the usual pattern of colon carcinoma metastases to the liver as demonstrated by the infusion technique (hypervascular rim, hypovascular center).

liver can be seen with selective angiography and following the use of vasodilators. At times, it is difficult to determine whether areas of increased or decreased vascularity are the sites of the metastases. Any discrete rounded lesions are most likely to represent metastases. However, when the diagnosis of metastases is not certain, the patient is given the benefit of the doubt and these mottled areas are considered benign or normal for the purpose of management.

Iso- and Hypovascular Metastases

These lesions must be at least 2–3 cm in diameter to be detected by the usual scanning techniques or by angiography. Angiography depends on the displacement of vessels and distortion, obstruction, invasion, and encasement of normal vessels. In the capillary and hepatogram phases, these tumors create a "Swiss cheese" appearance angiographically (46) (Fig. 41). They are usually caused by infiltrating primary desmoplastic neoplasms, such as carcinoma of the biliary tract, pancreas, and other gastrointestinal carcinomas, scirrhous carcinoma of the breast, and squamous cell carcinoma of the lung.

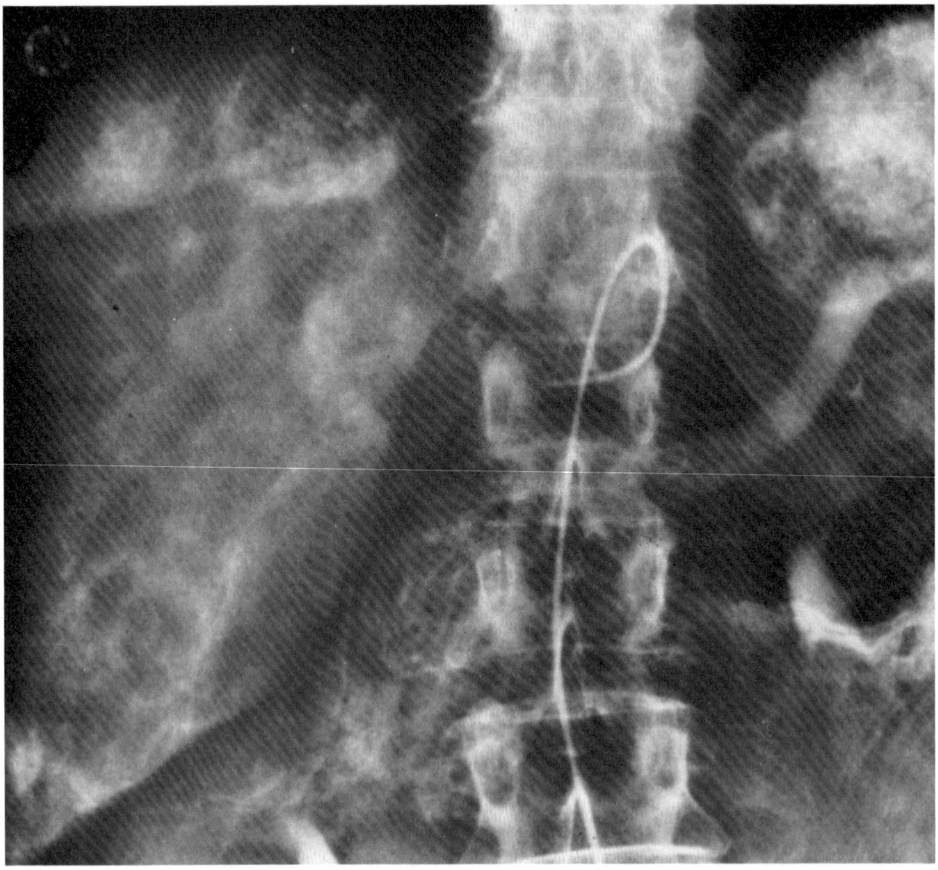

Figure 40B Following intra-arterial chemotherapy, there is a decrease in the size and vascularity of these metastases. The infusion angiographic technique has remained the same.

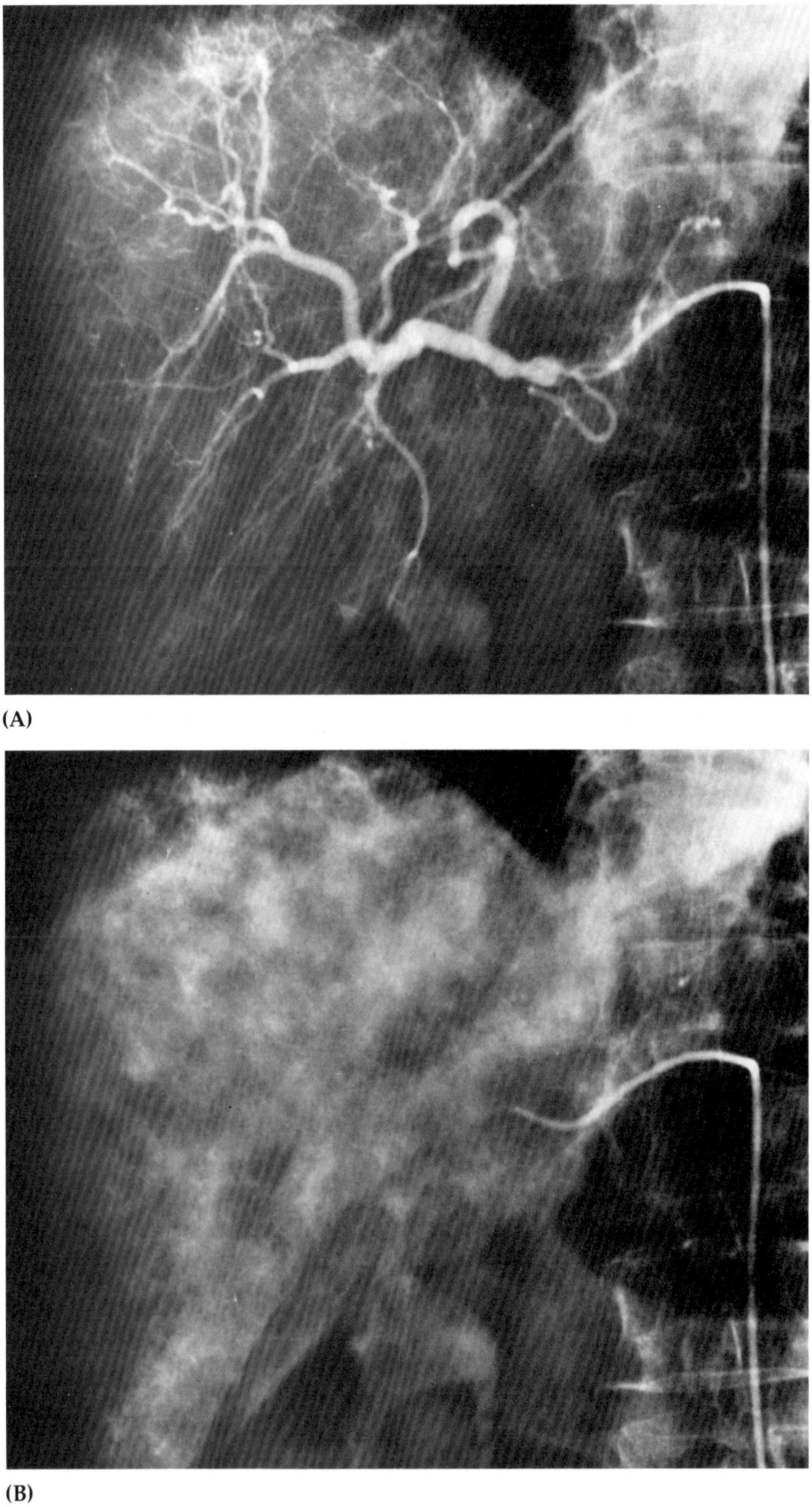

(A)

(B)

Figure 41

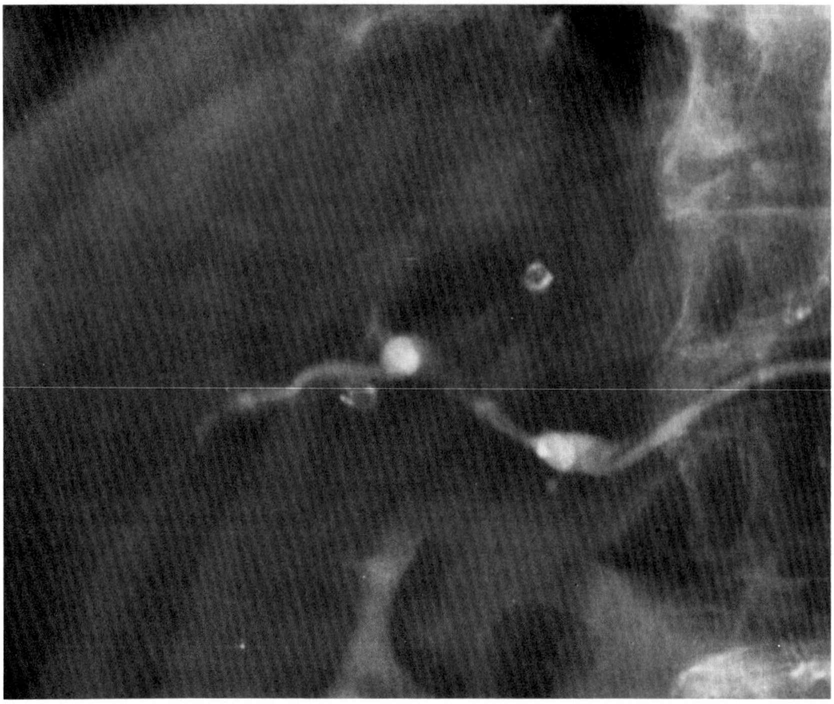

(C)

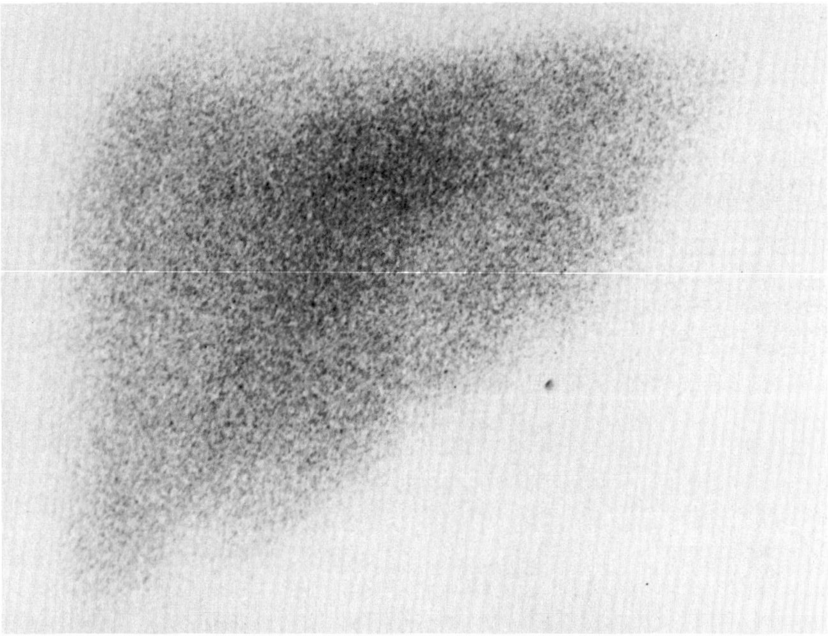

(D)

Figure 41 (continued)

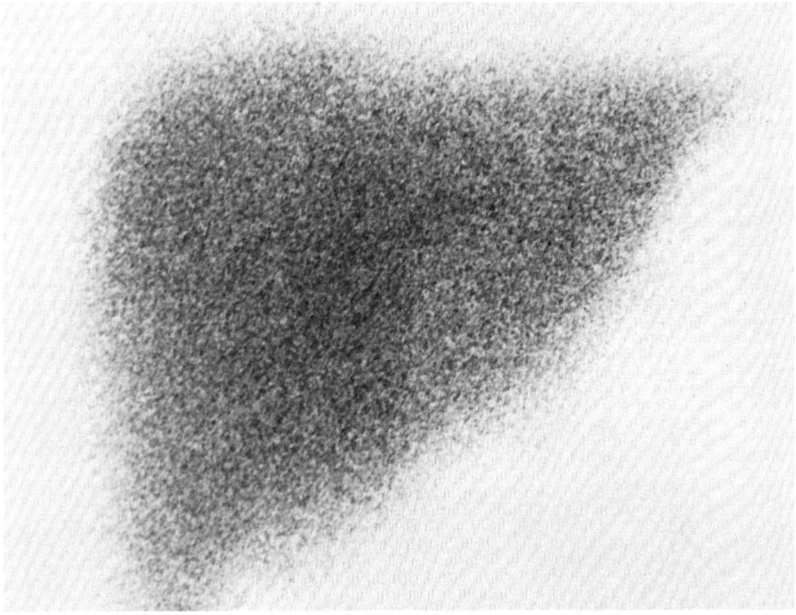

(E)

Figure 41 Metastatic colon carcinoma of the liver. Management by hepatic artery embolization. (A) Selective hepatic arteriogram, arterial phase. (B) Parenchymal phase. A "Swiss cheese" appearance is produced by the multiple hypovascular metastases. (C) Embolization with Gelfoam particles and steel coils. (D) Scintigraphy scan on admission shows uneven uptake consistent with metastatic disease. (E) One year following embolization, there is no evidence of metastatic disease at scintigraphy. The patient had refused chemotherapy.

Leukemia and Lymphoma

Leukemia and lymphoma, when discrete and nodular, will frequently present a feathery pattern which is iso- or hypovascular (Fig. 42). Diffuse infiltration by these neoplasms may not be recognizable in any way other than by hepatomegaly and stretching of the vessels. Similar findings can appear in neuroblastoma, melanoma, and carcinoma of the breast. Such neoplasms may be better defined by the scanning procedures (124,125). Follow-up examinations should be done by the modality that best demonstrates the disease process in the liver.

Transcatheter Management of Hepatic Malignancy

The futility of much of the existing therapy of malignant hepatic tumors stimulated exploration by interventional radiologic techniques. Many interventional procedures were initially performed out of desperation, but soon were incorporated into the primary therapeutic management. At the M. D. Anderson Hospital and Tumor Institute, of five patients referred for angiography each day, four are for interventional procedures. In the majority of these, percutaneous transcatheter intra-arterial infusion of chemotherapeutic agents is employed, while 12–15 arterial embolizations are performed each month. With

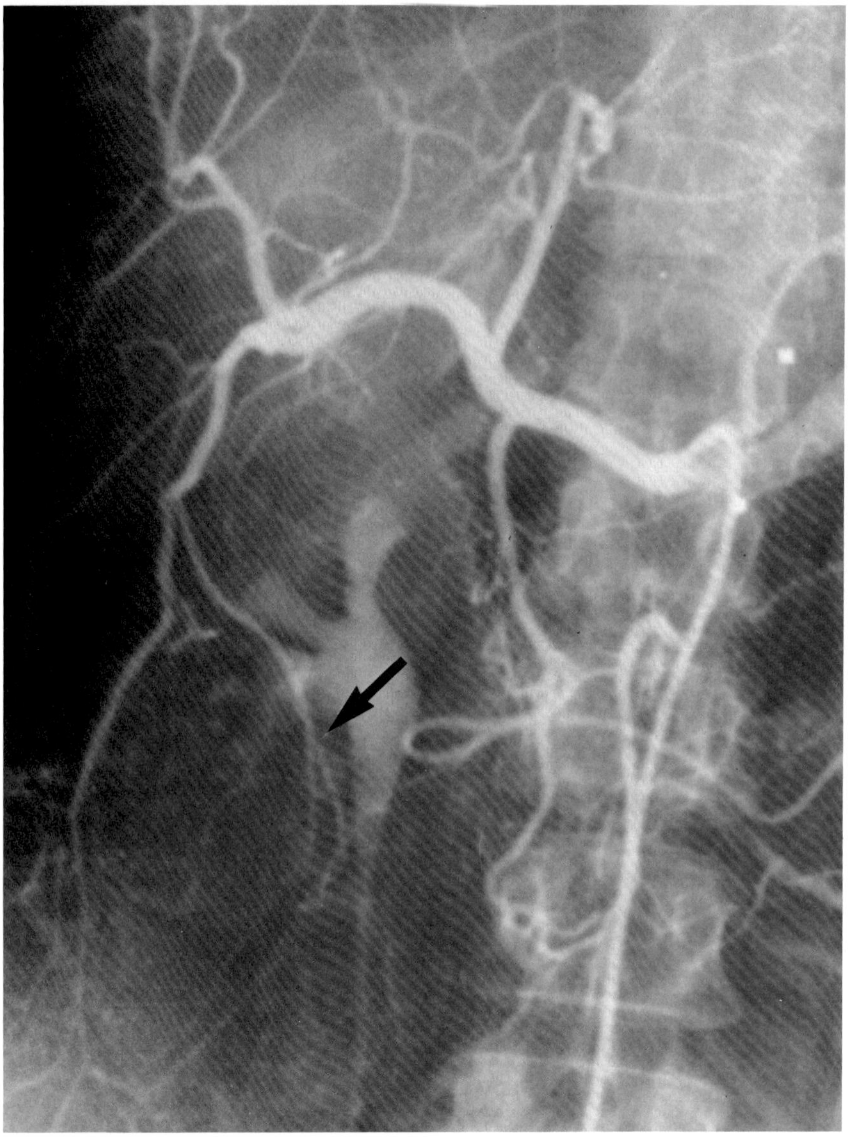

Figure 42A Histiocystic lymphoma. Hepatic arteriography defines a single focus of lymphomatous involvement in the right lobe of the liver. There is a fine feathery pattern of neovascularity.

greater selectivity of catheterization, newer chemotherapeutic agents, and a higher dose-time relationship, intra-arterial infusion has been resurrected and is improving the survival of patients with selected hepatic neoplasms.

Arterial embolization and occlusion have been effective in the treatment of primary and secondary hepatic neoplasms. The indications for transcatheter embolizations of neoplasms are (1) to control hemorrhage; (2) preoperatively, to facilitate resection by

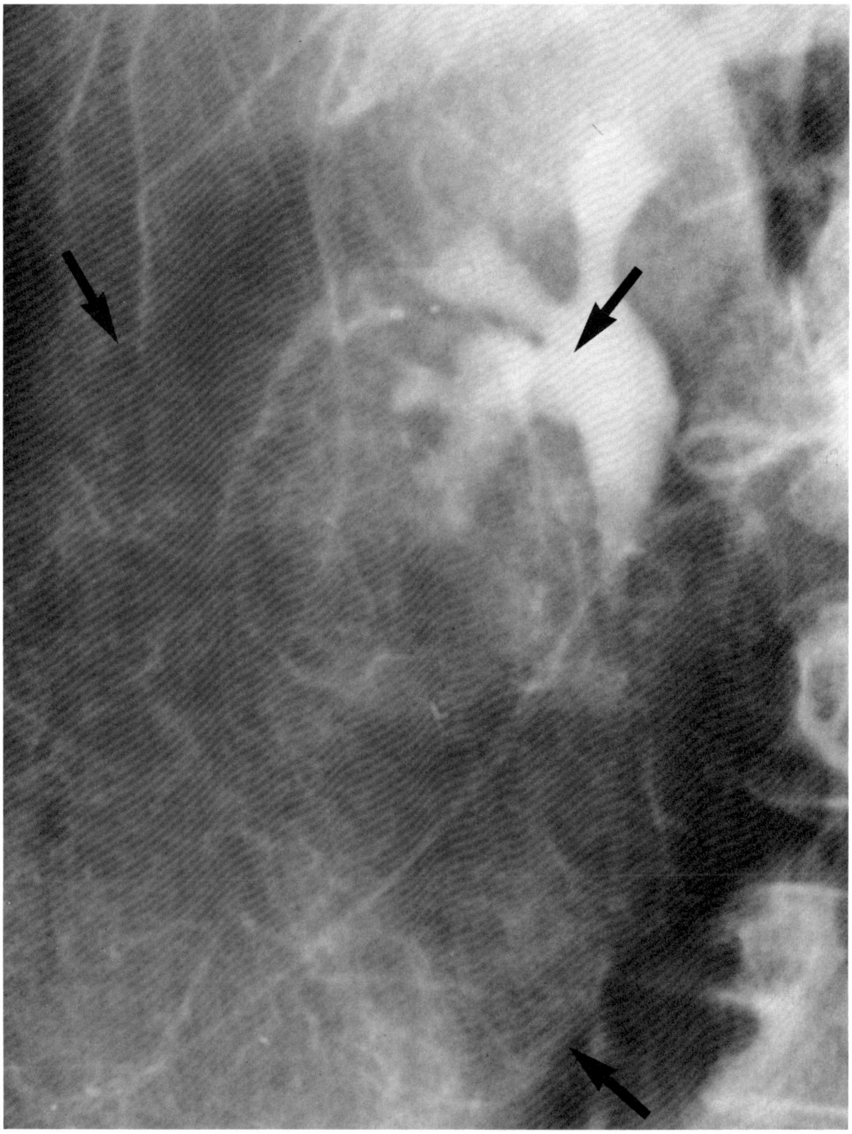

Figure 42B Late arterial phase, view of the lymphoma infiltrate (arrows).

decreasing blood loss and time of the surgical procedure; (3) to inhibit tumor growth; (4) to relieve pain; and perhaps (5) to stimulate an immune response to the ischemic neoplasm.

Hepatic arterial infusion (HAI) of chemotherapeutic agents is a viable alternative approach in patients whose disease is localized to the liver, especially after failure of systemic therapy by intravenous administration. Because of the variations of the normal arterial supply to the liver, optimal delivery of chemotherapy may necessitate

Table 7 Transcatheter Management of Hepatic Neoplasms

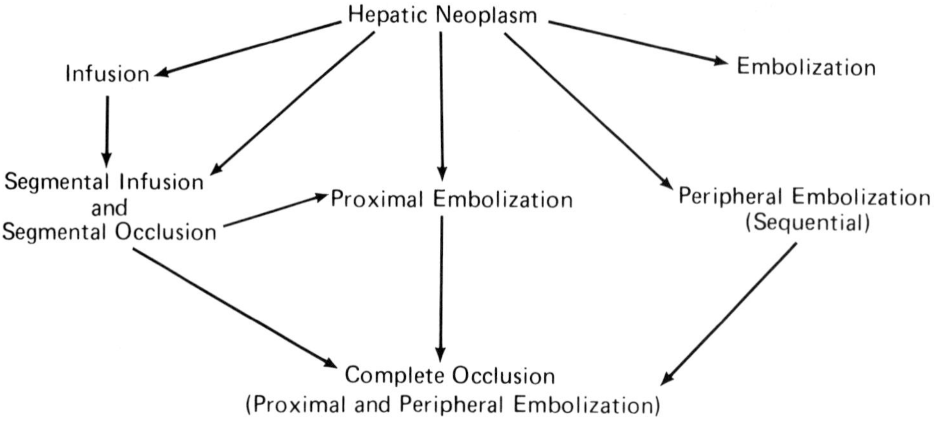

redistribution of hepatic artery flow by purposeful occlusion of certain vessels. Failure to respond to HAI or the absence of drugs effective in certain tumors frequently leads to peripheral *embolization* alone or in combination with central occlusion of the hepatic artery. Our interventional angiographic approach is summarized in Table 7. It must be stressed that, if an hepatic neoplasm is localized to a resectable segment, *surgery* is still the treatment of choice.

Hepatic Arterial Infusion (HAI)

Patients with hepatic metastases from colorectal carcinoma have a median survival of 5 months from the time of diagnosis (51). Intravenous chemotherapy may extend that survival to 8 months (126–130). Liver metastases refractory to systemic chemotherapy may respond to HAI (126–136). The rationale for HAI is based on the observation that most antitumor agents have a steep dose-response curve; the higher the concentration of the drug, the higher the antitumor effect (131). Since 90–95% of the blood supply to the hepatic neoplasm, primary or secondary, is derived from the hepatic artery (21,123,137–139), administration by HAI will expose the tumor to higher drug concentrations while keeping the side effects to a minimum.

Catheterization Technique

High brachial or femoral artery approaches are utilized for an infusion continuing for 5–10 days or longer. The brachial route allows greater mobility for the patient. The femoral approach is technically easier and more familiar for the angiographer but is somewhat more cumbersome and limiting to the patient. For an infusion of up to 24 hr, the femoral route is utilized. From a high brachial artery puncture, a 90- to 100-cm No. 5 French polyethylene catheter is placed into the hepatic artery; from the femoral artery, a 65-cm (No. 5 or 6.5 French) catheter is used. A down-going celiac artery, frequently found with an enlarged liver, is more readily catheterized from the brachial route, while an up-going celiac artery is best approached from a femoral puncture. The proper hepatic artery is the ideal site for catheter placement when anatomically and technically feasible.

When there is hepatopetal flow in the gastroduodenal artery, seen more frequently with hypervascular metastases, placement of the catheter in the common hepatic artery is adequate. Superselective catheterization of the desired vessel is accomplished in at least 95% of patients.

Infusion Technique

The catheter is connected to a pump (McGraw, Sigmamotor, Extracorporeal, etc.) for continuous infusion of chemotherapeutic agents. To minimize thrombotic complications, 10,000 to 25,000 units of aqueous sodium heparin are given each day by HAI or intravenously to achieve and maintain a 1.5-fold prolongation of the partial thromboblastin time (PTT) or activated clotting time (ACT). Heparin is incompatible with certain chemotherapeutic agents (e.g., Adriamycin) and the heparin must then be administered separately by intravenous route; otherwise, heparin is given concomitantly by HAI together with the chemotherapeutic drug. Aspirin, 650 mg, may be dispensed orally twice a day beginning 24 hr prior to catheterization. Fixation of the catheter to the skin is accomplished by plastic tape (Op-Site) covered by soft millipore adhesive tape (3M).

In the event of catheter displacement (5–10%) during the course of treatment, the catheter is bathed with antiseptic solution, replaced, and secured. Antibiotics are then instituted prophylactically.

Selection of Drugs

Mitomycin C (MTC), 15 mg/m^2 over a 2- to 24-hr period, and floxuridine (FUDR), 100 mg/m^2 per day for a 5-day continuous infusion, comprise the present protocol for hepatic metastases from colorectal carcinoma. Both drugs are metabolized by the liver. Adriamycin, 60–75 mg/m^2 given over the course of 5 days in three pulses of 20–25 mg/m^2, is added to the above for the treatment of a primary hepatoma and metastatic carcinoma from an unknown primary site (132–135). For metastases from breast carcinoma, soft tissue sarcoma, and melanoma, cis-diammnedichloroplatinum (CDDP), 120 mg/m^2, is infused over 2 hr (134). Other agents have also been employed for HAI, including 5-fluorouracil (5-FU), vincristine, vinblastine, imidazole carboximide (DTIC), and so on. Prior to the use of a new agent, the effects on the intima (vasculitis) with possible subsequent stenosis and/or occlusion must be investigated in laboratory animals. The treatment course is repeated every 4–6 weeks for three courses depending on the patient's tolerance and then reevaluated.

Results of HAI

Selective hepatic arteriography is performed prior to each infusion to delineate the vascular supply and its patency, and to establish and document the diagnosis. It is repeated after the entire treatment to record the tumor response (Fig. 40). Tumor response is evaluated by the change in the product of the two maximum perpendicular dimensions. Computed tomography and ultrasonography are used at times to assist in the evaluation. Tumor response is classified as CR (complete response) and PR (partial response of 50% or greater).

Of the patients with metastatic colorectal carcinoma to the liver treated with FUDR and MTC for at least three courses and followed up for as long as 2 years, there was a 55% rate of PR and a 12% CR rate. The median survival from the initiation of HAI was 8 months, and 15 months when the HAI was associated with occlusion of the hepatic artery either by intention or inadvertently as a complication of HAI (135).

Improved results are necessary to warrant the increased risk and expense to the patient. These are pursued by (1) meticulous and persistent efforts in selective catheter placement, (2) higher drug concentration over a shorter time interval, and (3) repeated HAI. One patient received 17 treatment courses during his 2-year survival, and several other patients were subjected to 10 courses.

The radiation exposure to the radiologist, the time and energy required, and the radiologic facilities available become serious considerations. Because of these, treatment is limited to a cycle of three courses of HAI at monthly intervals and, for responders, three additional courses. Usually, a response can be detected after the first course if the neoplasm is sensitive to the treatment. Failure to respond has precipitated the investigation of interventional alternatives, including hepatic artery embolization.

Redistribution of Hepatic Flow in HAI

An aberrant hepatic artery, which occurs in every other person in the general population (21,22), becomes a significant obstacle to HAI. A decrease of tumor size in one lobe following HAI with a simultaneous increase in the noninfused lobe was observed repeatedly. The use of two catheters, one in the celiac-hepatic and the other in the replaced hepatic from the superior mesenteric artery, increases the time of the procedure, radiation exposure, and patient discomfort. Transcatheter occlusion of the aberrant hepatic artery was therefore performed to redistribute the hepatic arterial flow to a single vessel (138–143). This was accomplished by the placement of a stainless steel coil at the origin of the replaced hepatic artery (Figs. 43, 44).

Complications

Vascular trauma is associated with superselective catheterization, higher concentrations of agents, shorter infusion time, or a combination of these factors. This resulted in a 15% incidence of occlusion, stenoses, aneurysm, and so on. (132,133,135,138) (Fig. 45). Greater experience in the technical aspects, careful drug administration, and adequate anticoagulation have minimized these complications.

Gastrointestinal complications Symptomatically, complications predominantly involve the gastrointestinal system. The arterial blood supply to the stomach, duodenum, gallbladder, and pancreas can originate from the hepatic artery. Unavoidable infusion into the gastroduodenal and left and right gastric arteries has resulted in symptoms of dyspepsia, gastritis, duodenitis, and/or the development of gastric ulcers in 11.6% (138) (Fig. 46). On occasion, cholecystitis and pancreatitis may occur.

The *gastroduodenal artery*, in approximately half the population, arises midway between the origin of the common hepatic artery from the celiac and its division into the right and left hepatic arteries; a proper hepatic artery is then present. In one-fourth of the population, the gastroduodenal artery arises either at the bifurcation of the common hepatic artery (i.e., a trifurcation with right and left hepatic arteries) or distal to the hepatic bifurcation (i.e., direct from either the right or left hepatic arteries). In the last one-fourth of the population, the gastroduodenal artery comes from replaced hepatic arteries or from other sources. Thus, only 50% of people have a proper hepatic artery (22). Placement of the infusion catheter beyond the gastroduodenal artery will decrease unintentional infusion of chemotherapeutic agents to the duodenum, stomach, and pancreas. Occasionally, the

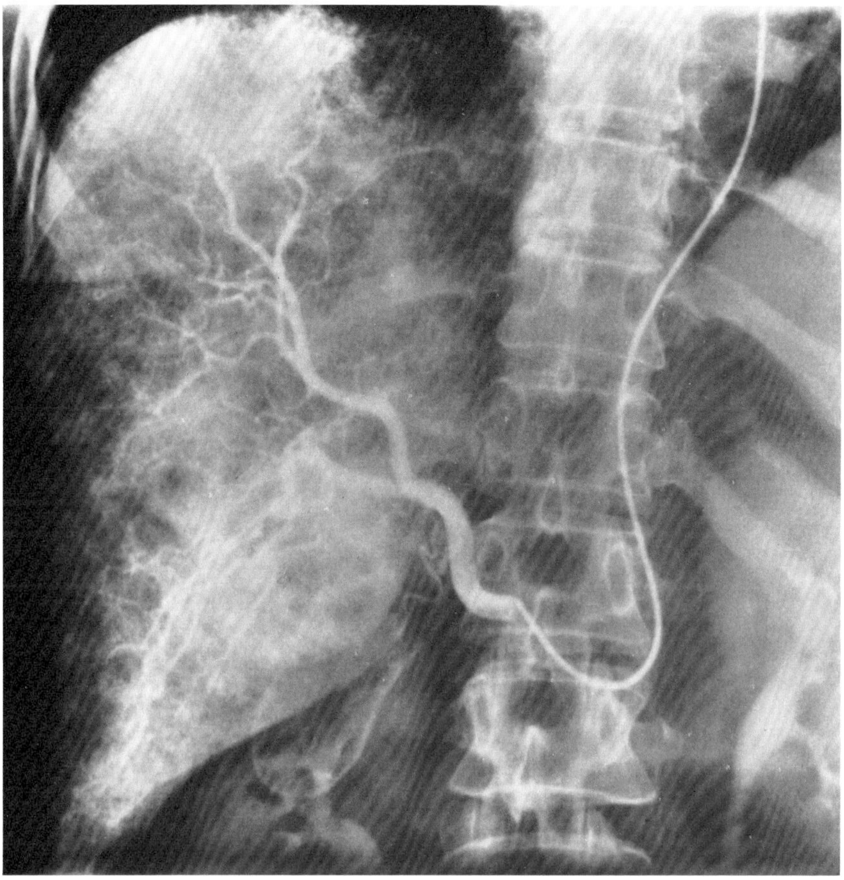

Figure 43A Colon carcinoma with liver metastases. Hepatic artery redistribution for chemotherapy. Replaced right hepatic artery originating from the superior mesenteric.

gastroduodenal artery has hepatopetal flow allowing safe placement in the common hepatic artery. Otherwise, occlusion of the gastroduodenal artery with a coil has been performed in selected patients who have developed serious gastrointestinal symptoms.

The right gastric artery originates from the proper hepatic artery or the left hepatic artery in some 80% of people (22). It is small (2 mm or less) and frequently unnoticed in a celiac arteriogram, but can be identified in most selective hepatic studies. In a series of 18 patients with gastrointestinal symptoms following HAI, problems could be attributed primarily to the infusion of the right gastric artery (138).

Hepatic Arterial Occlusion

Primary and secondary hepatic neoplasms receive their blood supply almost exclusively from the hepatic artery (90%), while normal liver parenchyma has a dual supply, the hepatic artery (25%), and the portal vein (75%), with 50% of the oxygen coming from each source (144). (See also Chapter 27.) The concept of treating hepatic neoplasms by

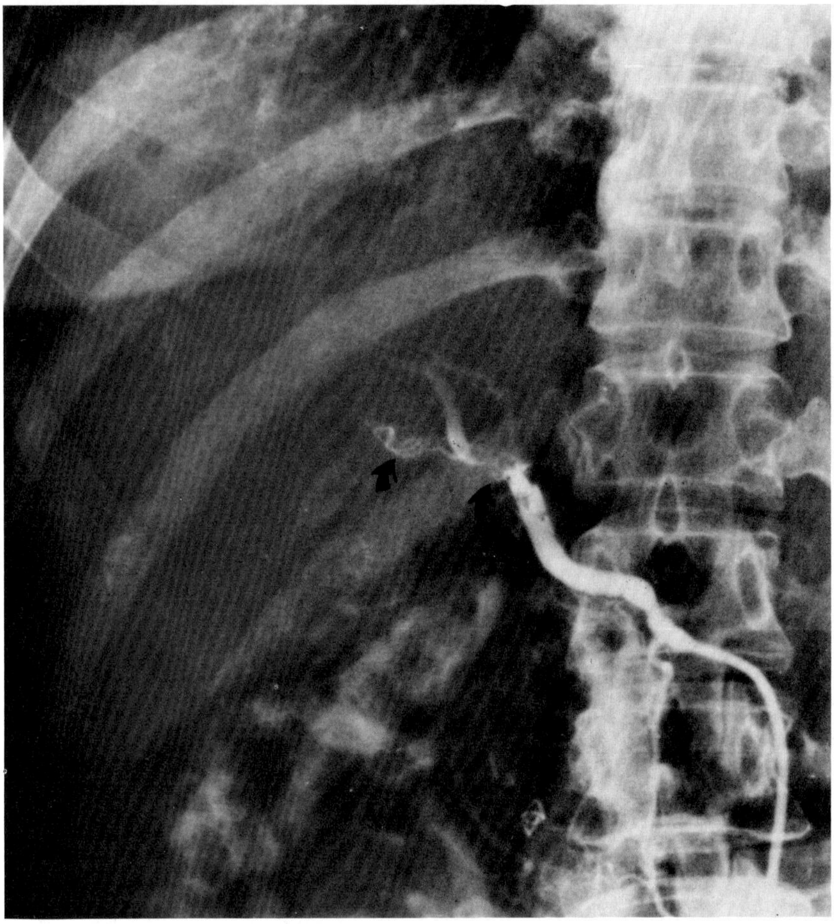

Figure 43B Occlusion of the replaced hepatic artery with coils (arrows).

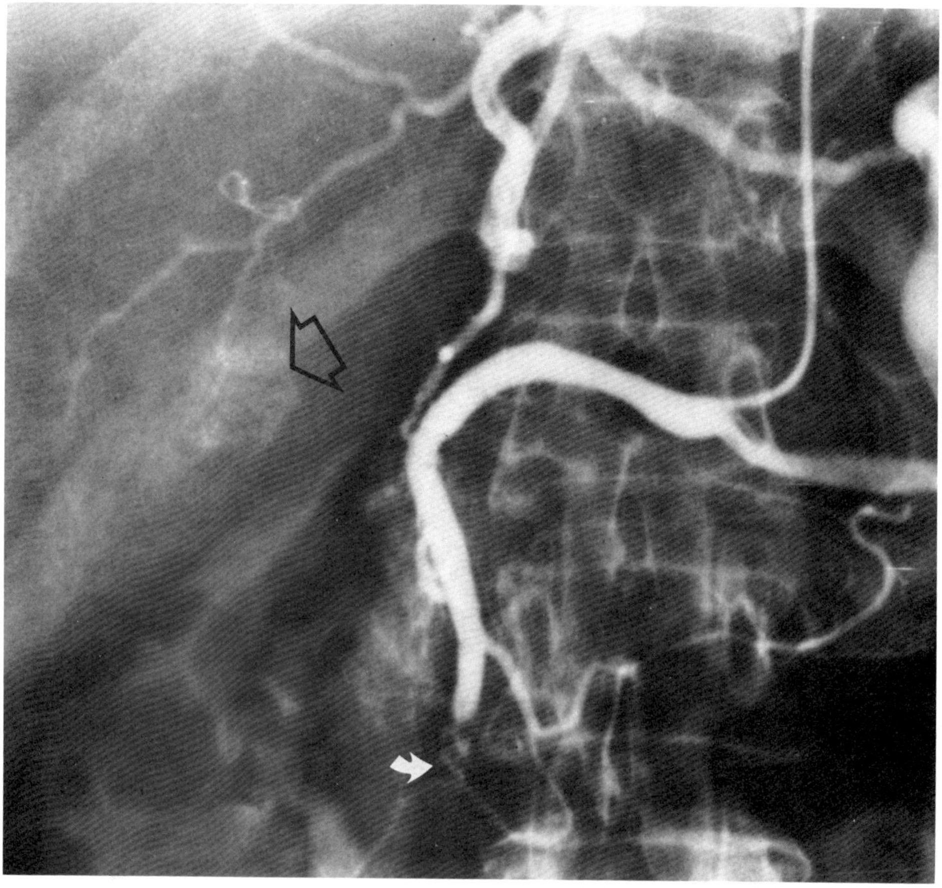

Figure 43C Occlusion of the gastroduodenal artery with a coil (arrow). Note calcified right hepatic metastasis (open arrow).

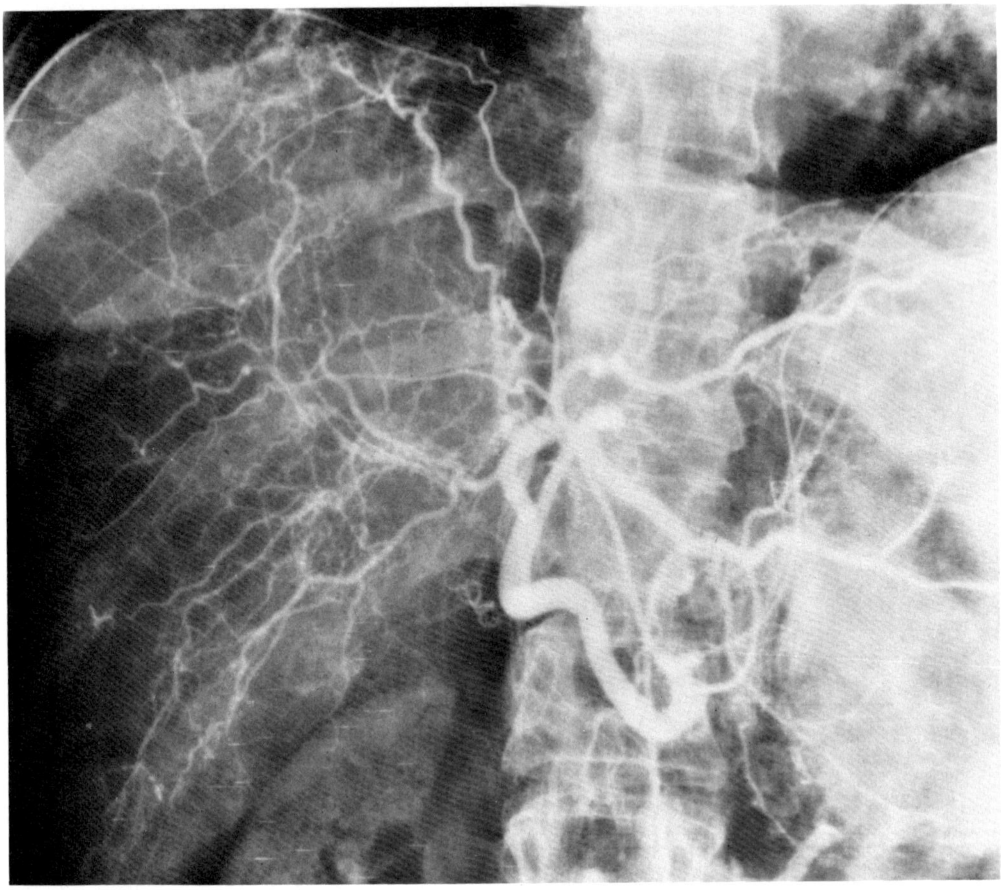

Figure 43D The entire liver could then be infused via the left hepatic artery. Note the intrahepatic collaterals.

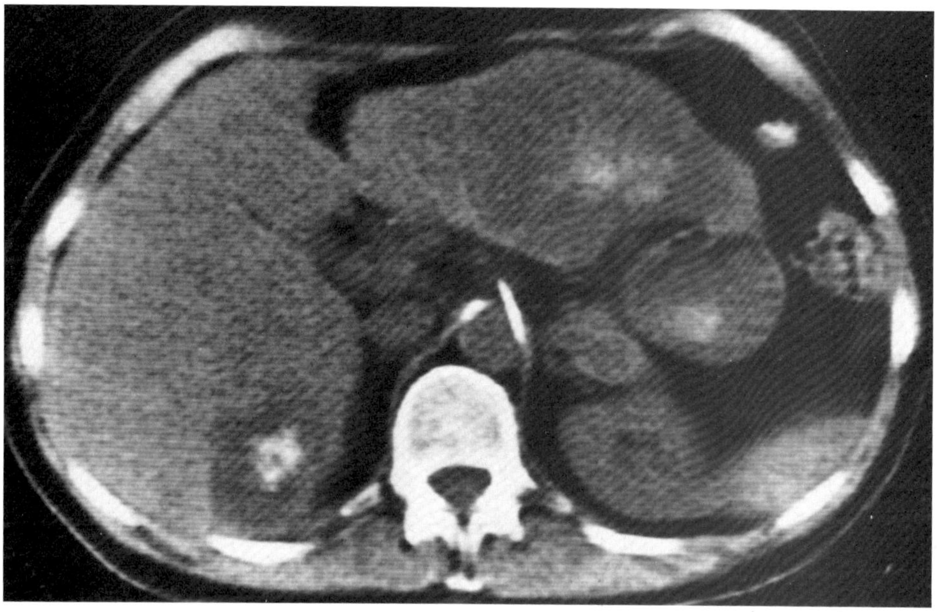

Figure 43E CT scan prior to infusion and redistribution.

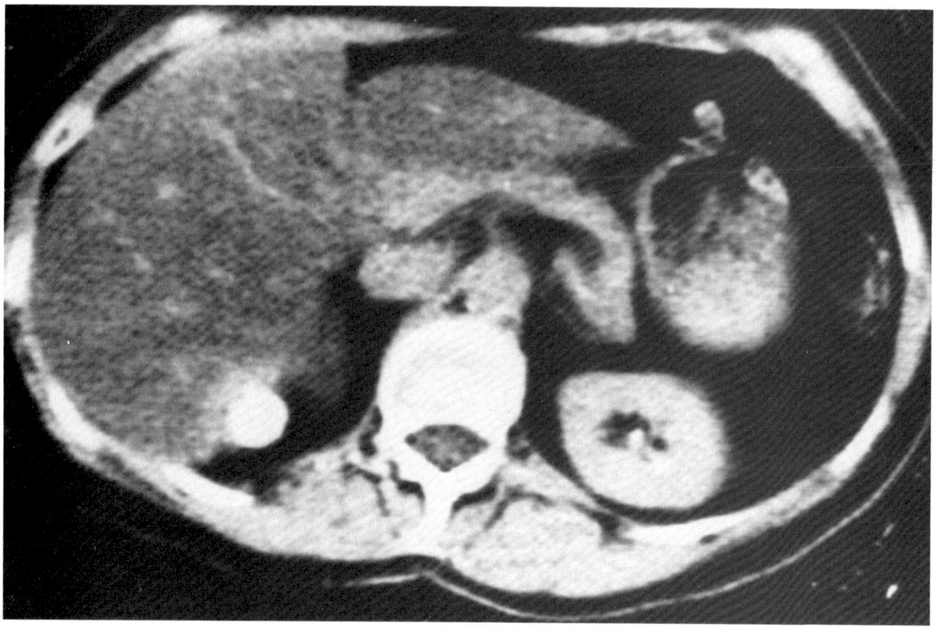

Figure 43F CT scan showing marked response to treatment 9 months later. Note the decreased size of the lateral segment of the left lobe and the replacement of the metastases in the posterior portion of the right lobe by dense calcification as well as the overall decreased attenuation of the liver, perhaps fatty replacement secondary to chemotherapy.

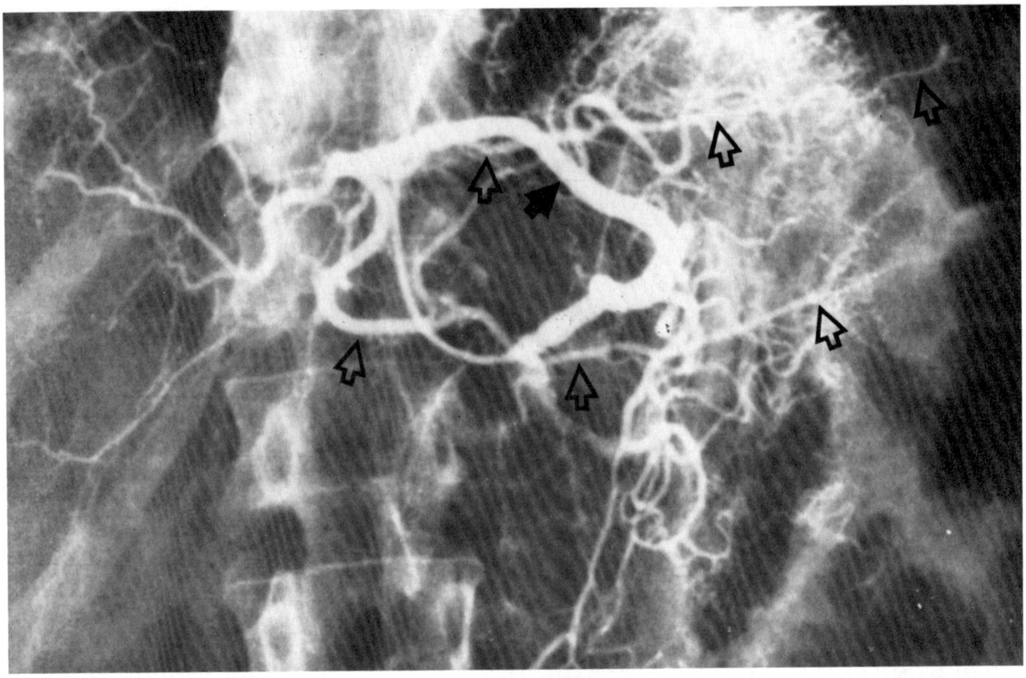

(A)

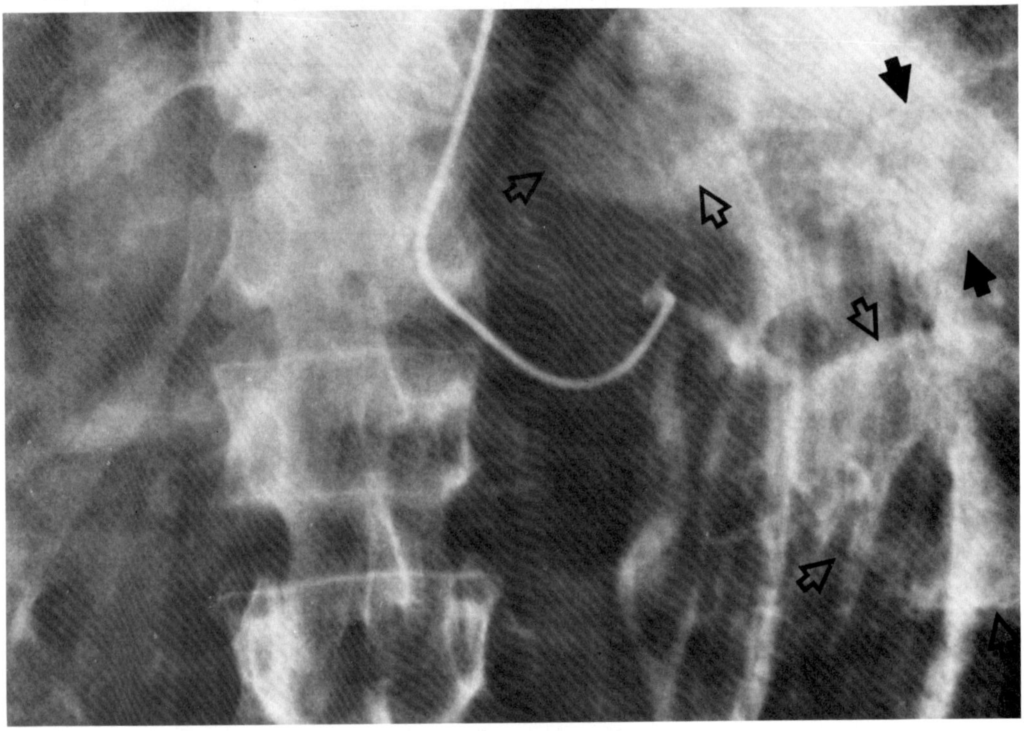

(B)

Figure 44 Colon carcinoma metastases. Redistribution of flow for chemotherapy. (A) The left hepatic artery originates from the left gastric artery (closed arrow). Open arrows indicate left lateral subsegmental branches. (B) Parenchymal phase. The metastatic lesions in the left lobe are optimally defined (arrows). (C) The catheter was advanced beyond the left gastric into the left hepatic artery to occlude it with coils. (D) The common hepatic artery now supplies the entire liver. Note the intrahepatic collaterals to the left lobe (arrows).

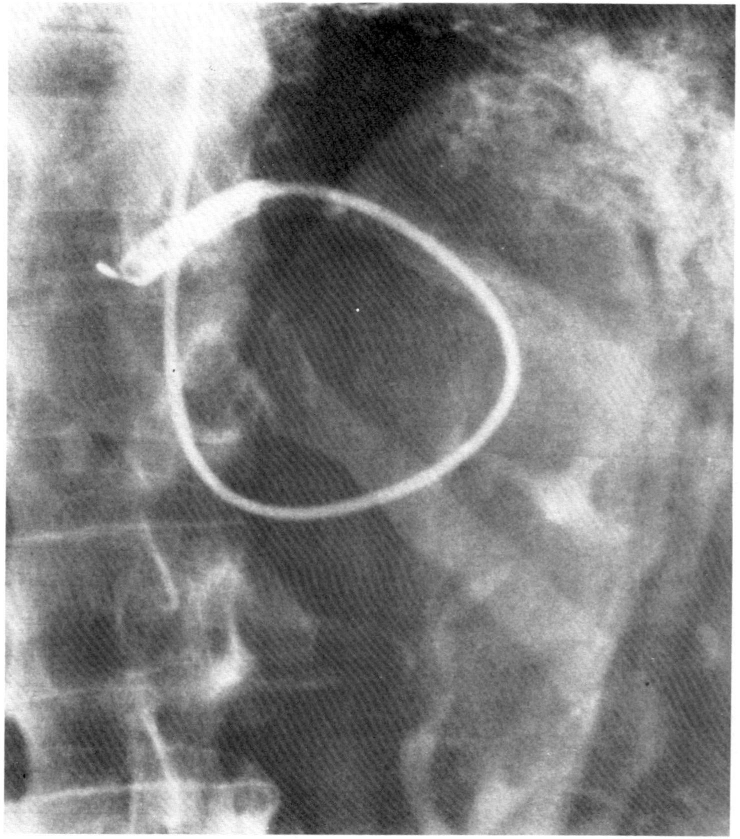
(C)

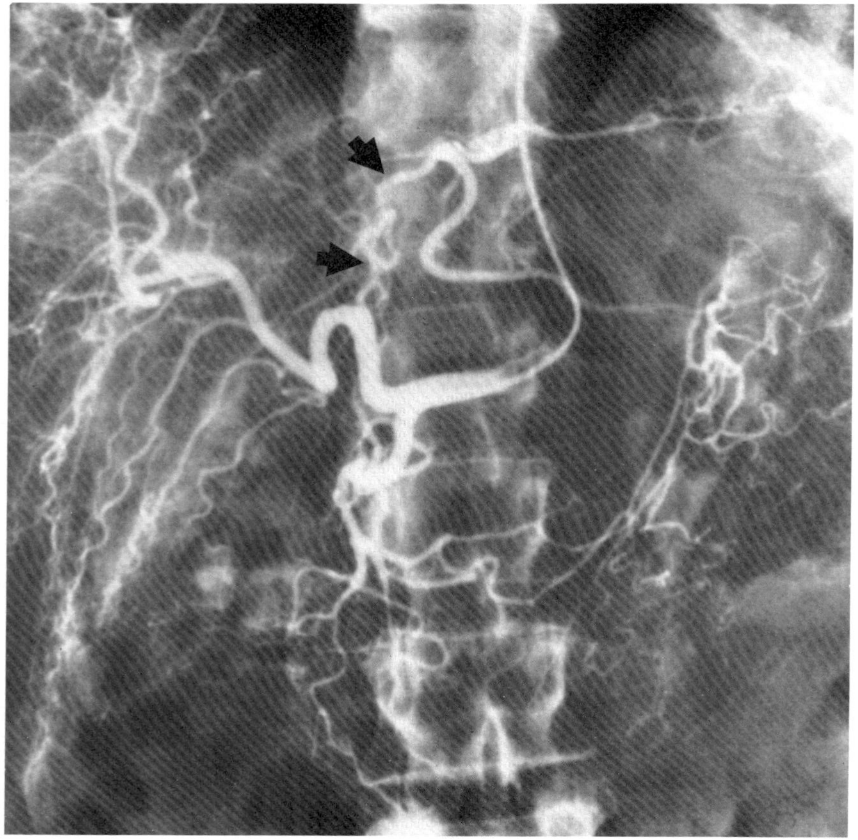
(D)

Figure 44 (continued)

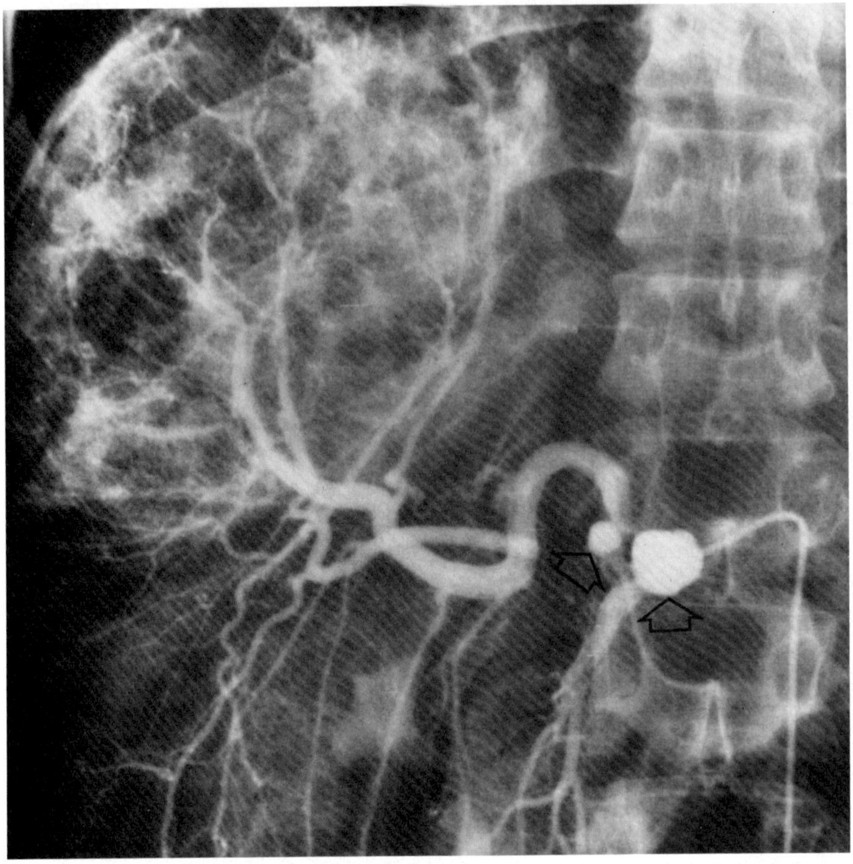

(A)

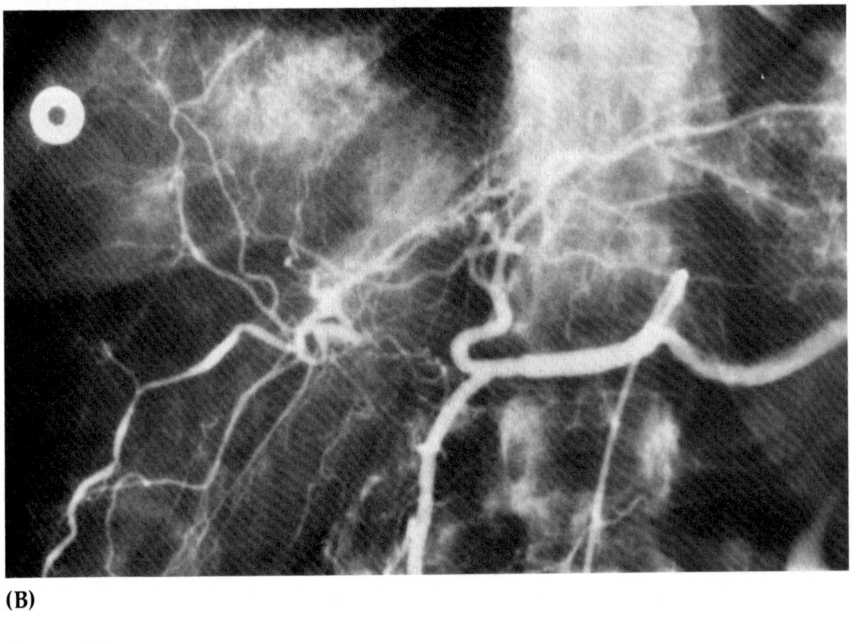

(B)

Figure 45

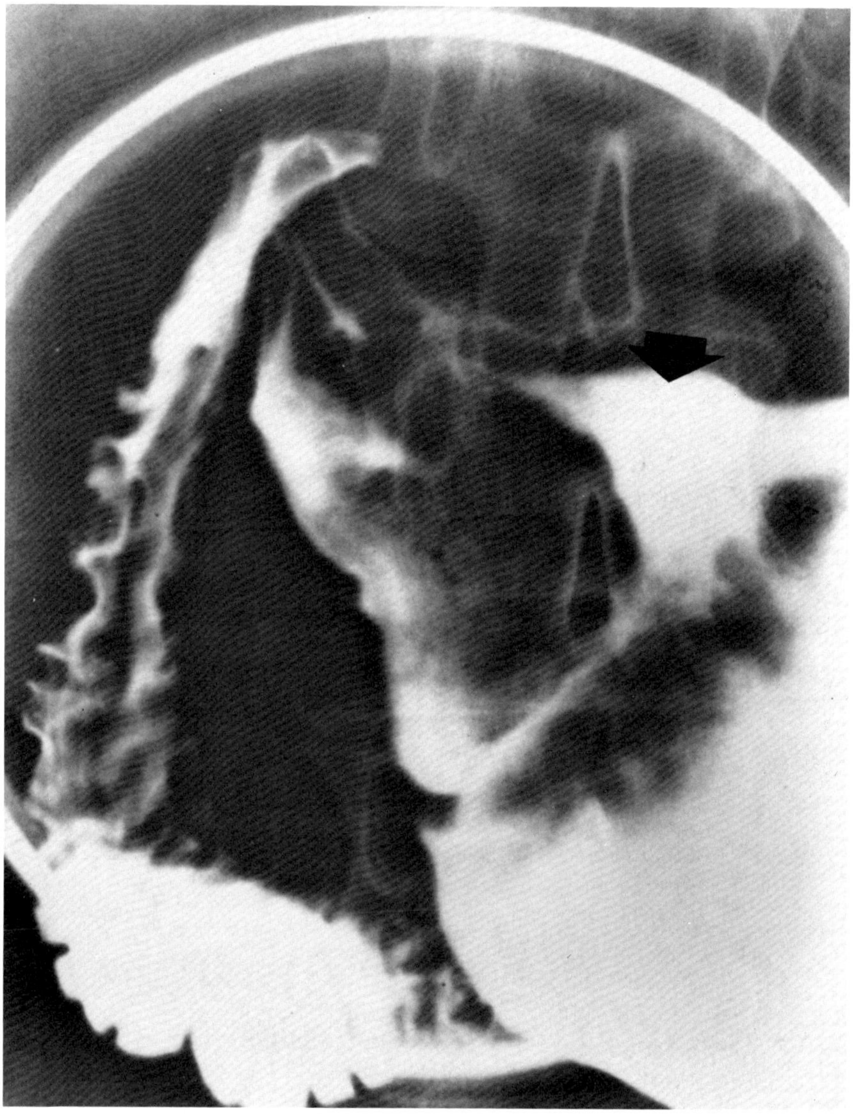

(A)

Figure 46

Figure 45 Vascular complications of hepatic artery infusion. (A) Aneurysms (arrows) as the result of the prior catheterization, the infusion, or both. (B) Occlusion of the right hepatic artery seen 1 month following the infusion chemotherapy. Note the considerable reduction of the extent of metastatic disease. Note also the opacification of the right hepatic artery branches via intrahepatic collaterals.

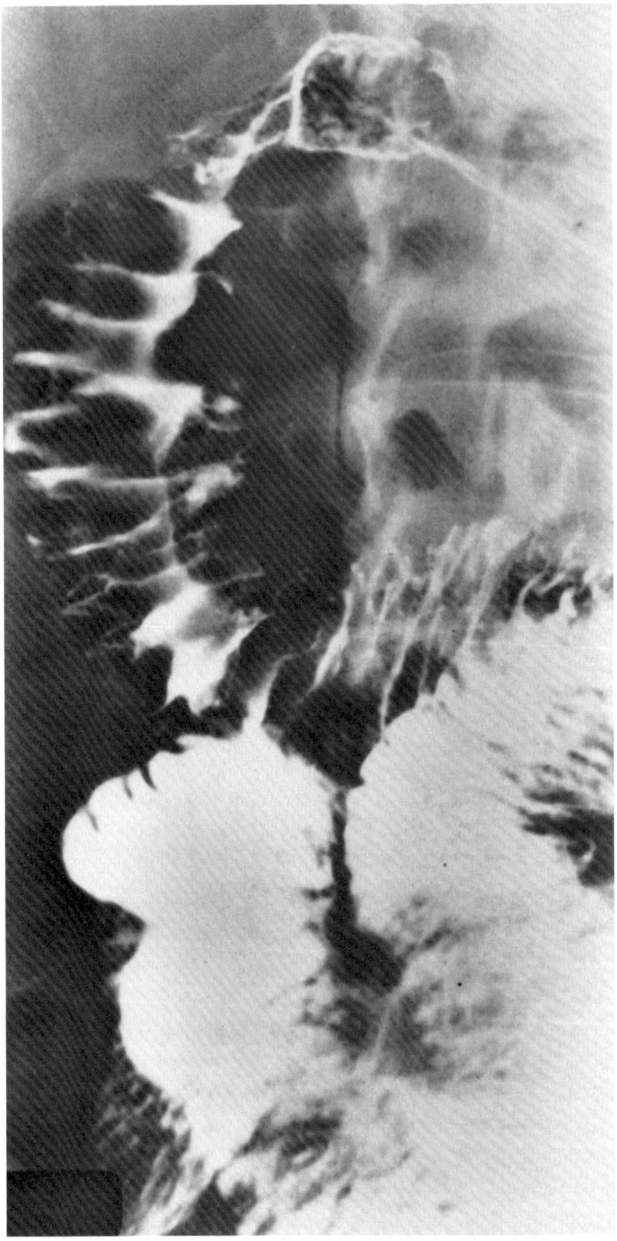

(B)

Figure 46 Gastroduodenal complications of HAI. (A) Gastric ulcer (arrow). It is frequently atypical, linear, and in the distribution of the right gastric artery. (B) Duodenitis and pancreatitis.

hepatic artery ligation was suggested by Markowitz in 1952 (145). Physiologic blood flow studies in patients using radioactive xenon demonstrated a 90% decrease in tumor blood flow after hepatic artery ligation, compared with 35–40% decrease in normal liver parenchyma (146,147). Mori et al. reported a selective destruction of the tumor without damage to the normal liver after ligation of the hepatic artery for metastatic gastric carcinoma (148). The response to surgical ligation is temporary, due in part to the formation of collateral circulation which may occur instantaneously, as illustrated following proximal coil occlusion of the hepatic artery for redistribution of hepatic flow (46,136,139,149) (Figs. 43, 44).

Method of Embolization

More lasting devascularization of an hepatic neoplasm can be achieved percutaneously by peripheral embolization with particulate material [Gelfoam alone, Gelfoam plus a sclerosing material such as sotradecol, polyvinyl alcohol foam (Ivalon), etc.] or a combination of peripheral embolization and central occlusion with a stainless steel coil (140–143). Prior to hepatic arterial embolization, the hepatic arteries, portal veins, and at times the hepatic veins and inferior vena cava are visualized (Fig. 47). Initially, complete embolization with Gelfoam and steel coils was undertaken if up to 70% (estimated) of the liver was replaced by tumor. More recently, peripheral embolization at monthly intervals for 3 months has been employed and better tolerated. If there is over 70% (estimated) replacement by neoplasm, partial sequential embolization is performed with great caution and care.

Indications

Embolization can be used in patients (1) with unresectable primary hepatic neoplasms; (2) preoperatively, to facilitate surgery of a resectable neoplasm; (3) with metastatic neoplasms that fail to respond to chemotherapy; (4) as the initial management of certain metastases known to be refractory to chemotherapy; and (5) to control pain and/or hemorrhage from an hepatic neoplasm.

Contraindications

In the presence of cirrhosis where a greater proportion of the nutritive supply to the normal parenchyma depends on the hepatic artery, the risks of hepatic artery embolization are greater, especially when there is reversal of flow in the portal vein. In these circumstances embolization is contraindicated. In contrast to this, reversal of flow or shunt due to the neoplasm itself may readily be ameliorated by embolization. Extrinsic compression of the portal vein, especially in the absence of collateral venôus opacification, may be successfully approached by occlusion; intrinsic compression with visualization of collateral venous drainage contraindicates embolization. Jaundice, if due to extrinsic compression of the biliary tract, might be available by occlusion. The indications for embolization still require further elucidation, which undoubtedly will evolve with greater experience (150).

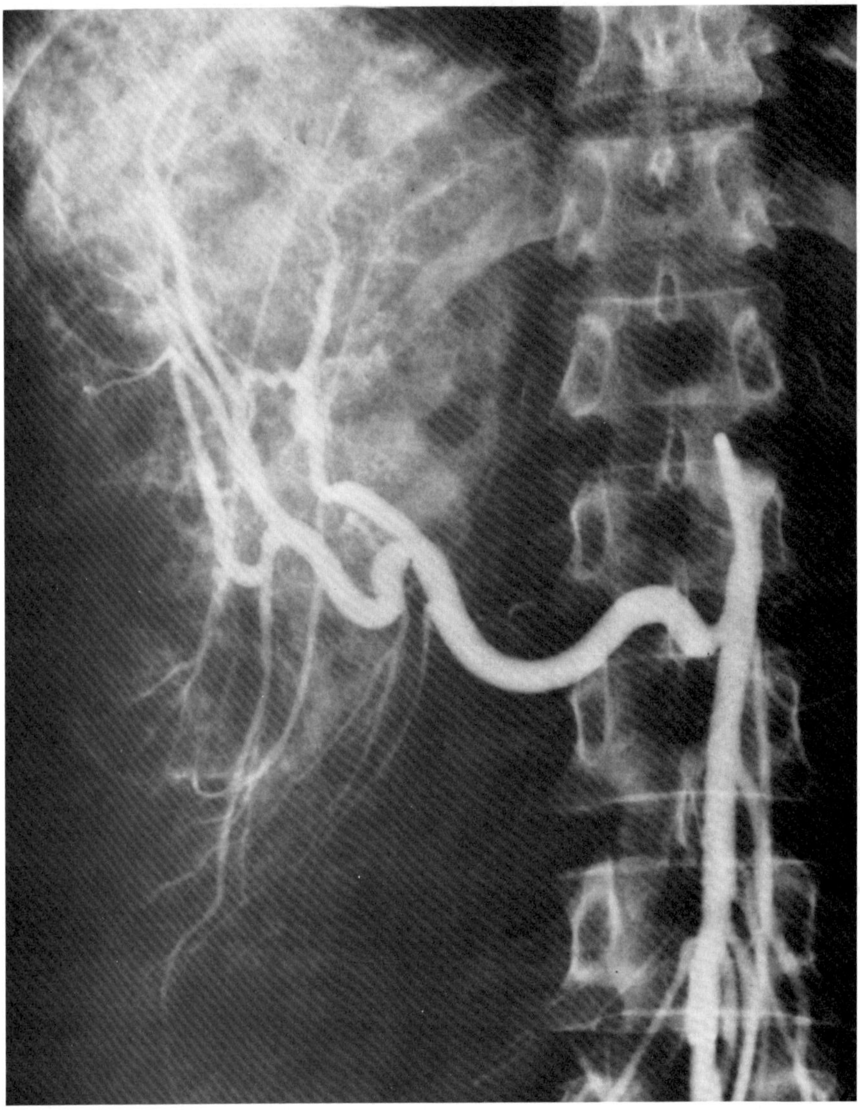

Figure 47A Metastatic disease. Extrinsic compression of the portal vein. Management by hepatic arterial devascularization. Arteriography. Replaced right hepatic artery from the superior mesenteric. Metastases are seen in the right lobe of the liver.

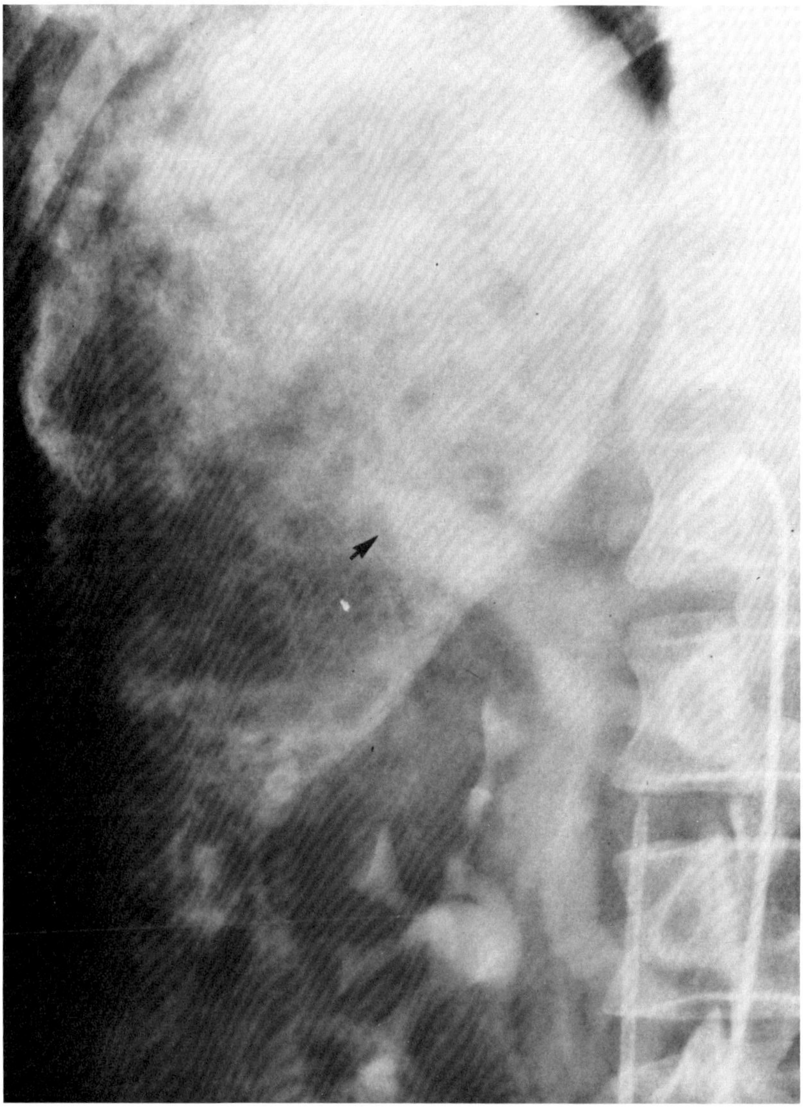

Figure 47B The superior mesenteric and portal veins are outlined in the venous phase. The portal vein is obstructed (arrow), the configuration suggesting an extrinsic etiology. Because of the obstruction the radiologist refused to embolize the hepatic artery. However, in view of the lack of collateral venous opacification and the absence of reversal of flow in the portal vein, the surgeon chose to ligate the hepatic artery.

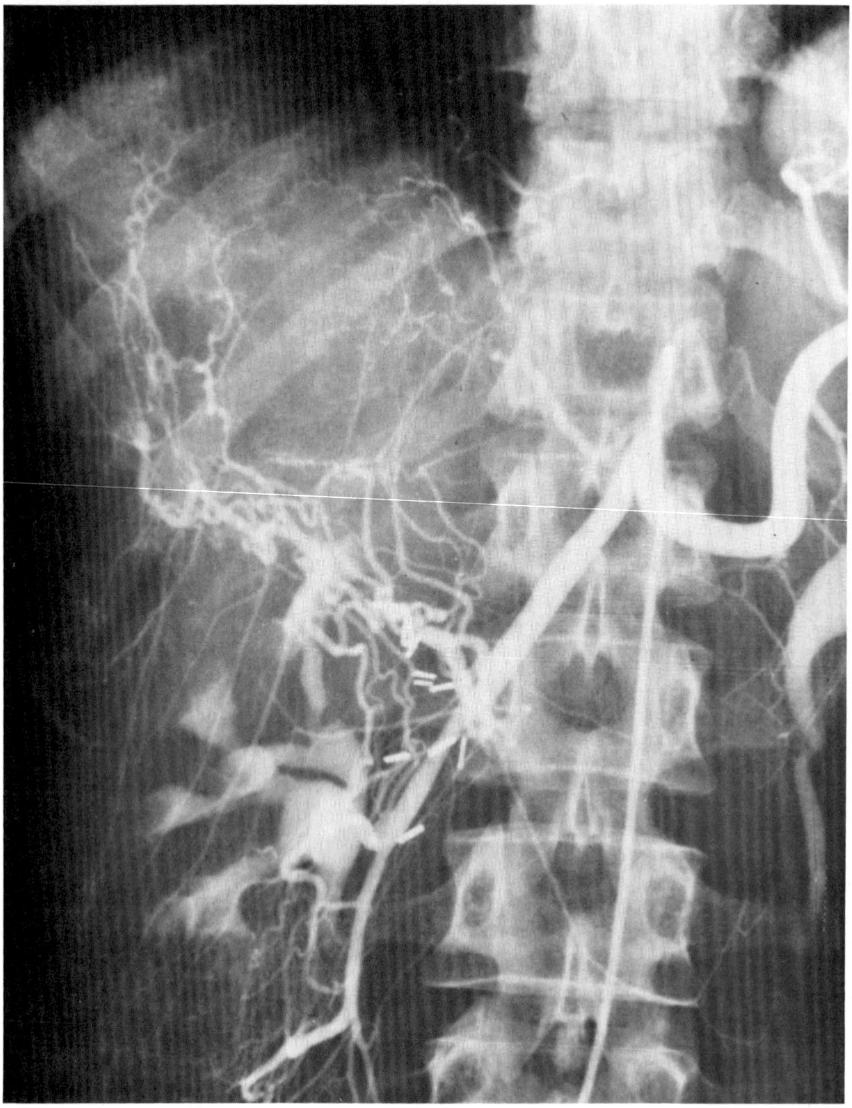

Figure 47C Celiac arteriography 1 year later demonstrates collateral flow to the liver from the gastroduodenal artery. (Note the clips from previous surgical ligation.) The gastroduodenal artery was now occluded. The patient survived a further 10 months.

Collateral Circulation and Sequential Embolization

Peripheral embolization of the hepatic artery was undertaken to minimize collateral circulation and to create a more ischemic tumor. Collateral circulation, both intra- and extrahepatic, develops almost instantaneously (46,136,150,151). Table 8 summarizes the many real and potential collateral pathways. Despite an apparent complete occlusion, the almost universal occurrence of a collateral circulation creates the necessity for sequential embolization. This is readily accomplished by repeated episodes of peripheral embolization usually utilizing Ivalon (250- to 500-μm particles) or Ivalon and Gelfoam (3-mm cubes) at intervals varying from 1 to 3 months depending on the patient's tolerance (Fig. 48). In the event of complete occlusion of the major hepatic arteries, purposeful by surgery, or with Ivalon, Gelfoam, and steel coils, or unintentional as a technical complication, access to the liver for embolization is accomplished through collateral

Table 8 Real and Potential Collateral Pathways

A. Intrahepatic collaterals
   1. Perivascular
   2. Interlobar or intersegmental
   3. Intralobar or intrasegmental

B. Extrahepatic collaterals
   1. Pancreaticoduodenal arcades
      a. Inferior pancreaticoduodenal artery
      b. Dorsal pancreatic artery
      c. Arc of Buhler
   2. Periportal route
      a. Common bile duct collaterals
      b. Retroduodenal or supraduodenal artery
      c. Cystic artery
      d. Right branches of dorsal pancreatic artery
      e. Multiple unnamed branches in the porta hepatis
   3. Left gastric route
      a. Left gastric to right gastric anastomosis
      b. Left gastric to left hepatic via lesser omentum
   4. Inferior phrenic route
      a. Right inferior phrenic artery
      b. Left inferior phrenic artery
   5. Right paracolic gutter route
      a. Branches from middle or right colic artery
      b. Direct adhesion to hepatic flexure
   6. Omental branches
   7. Internal mammary and superior epigastric artery
   8. Intercostal or lumbar artery
   9. Capsular branches of the right renal artery

Source: Charnsangavej C, Cheung VP, Wallace S, personal communication.

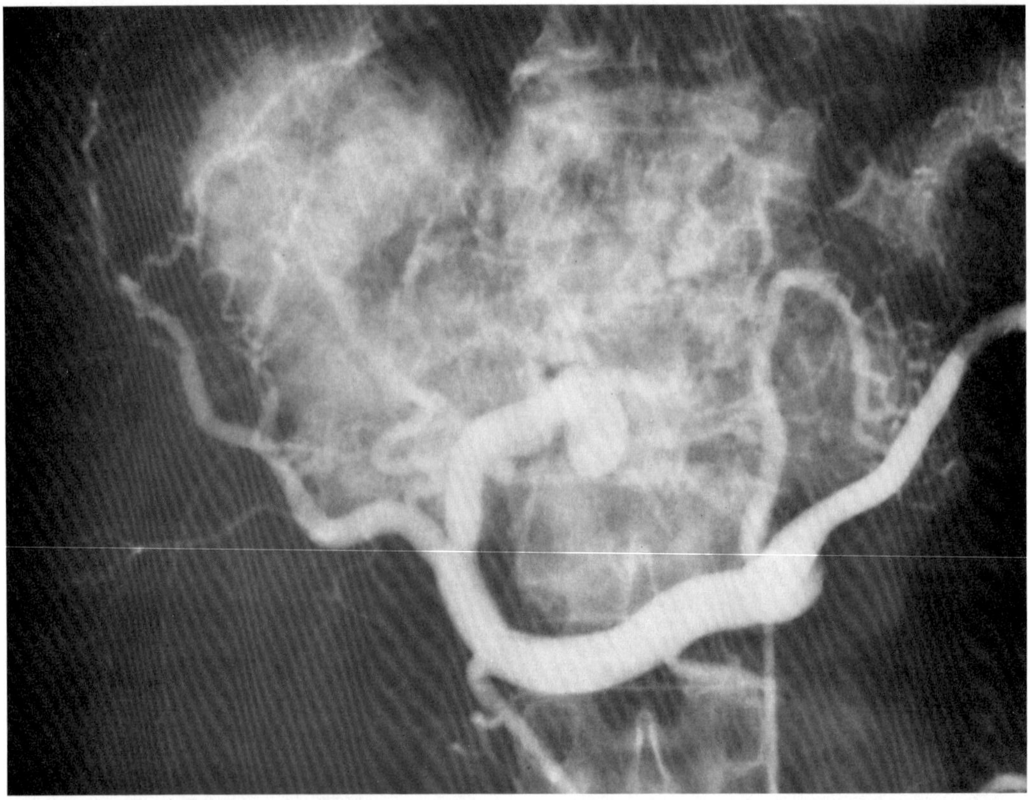

(A)

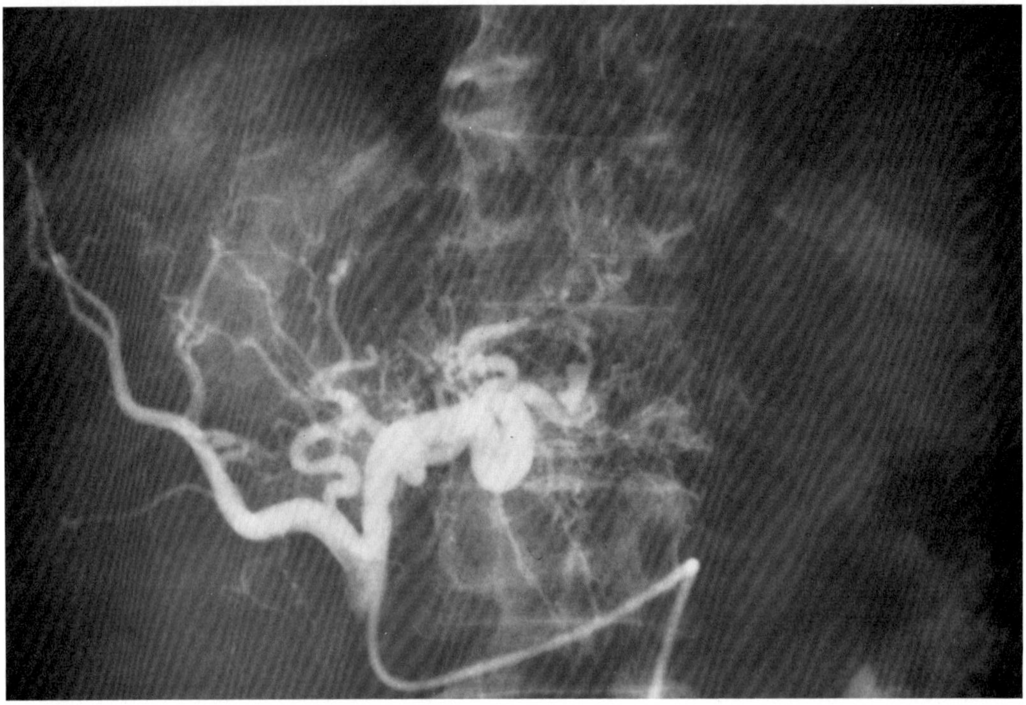

(B)

Figure 48

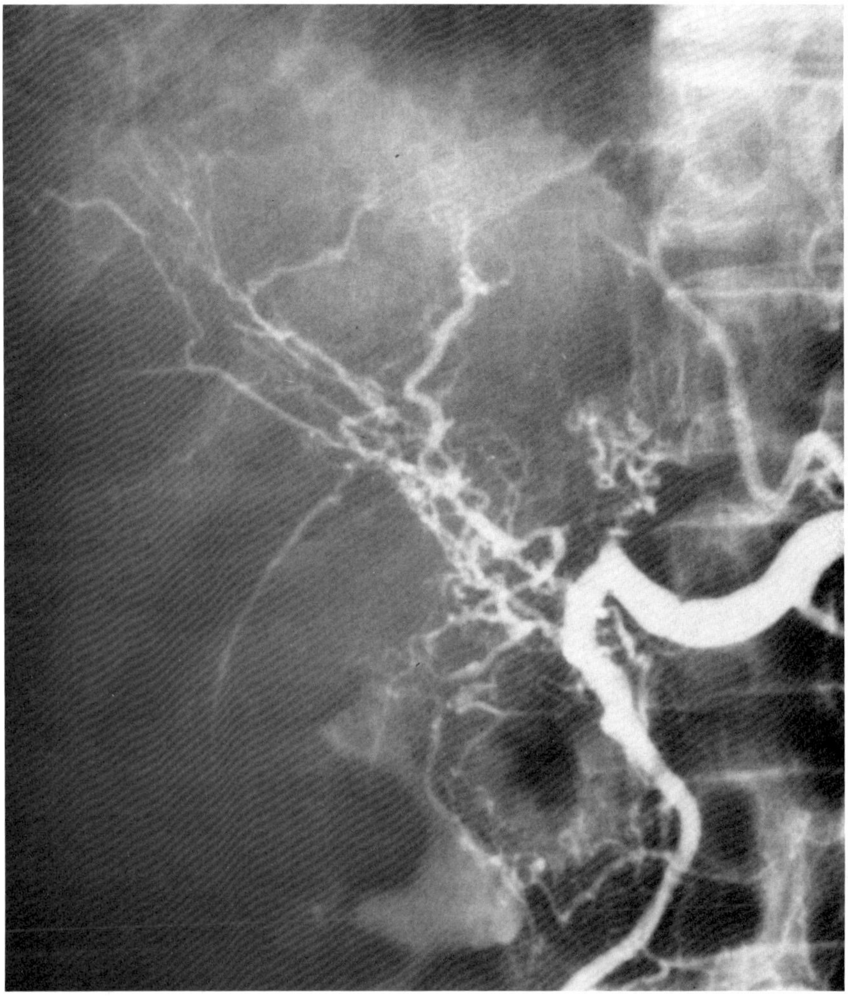

(C)

Figure 48 Cholangiocarcinoma managed by sequential hepatic devascularization. (A) Biopsy proven hypervascular cholangiocarcinoma involving the left lobe and extending into the right. (B) Marked improvement after sequential embolization of the left hepatic artery utilizing Gelfoam fragments. Three episodes of embolization were done at 2-week intervals. This was followed by surgical ligation of the hepatic artery. (C) One year later, hepatic arteriography opacifies collateral vessels to the liver which originate from the gastroduodenal artery. (D) In the capillary phase, the hypervascular cholangiocarcinoma is seen to be markedly reduced in size (arrows). (E) Reexamination 5 years later revealed progression of the vascular tumor. (F) At this time embolization was accomplished with the use of Ivalon particles (250–500 μm), Gelfoam, and steel coils. The patient is asymptomatic at the present time, 1 year later.

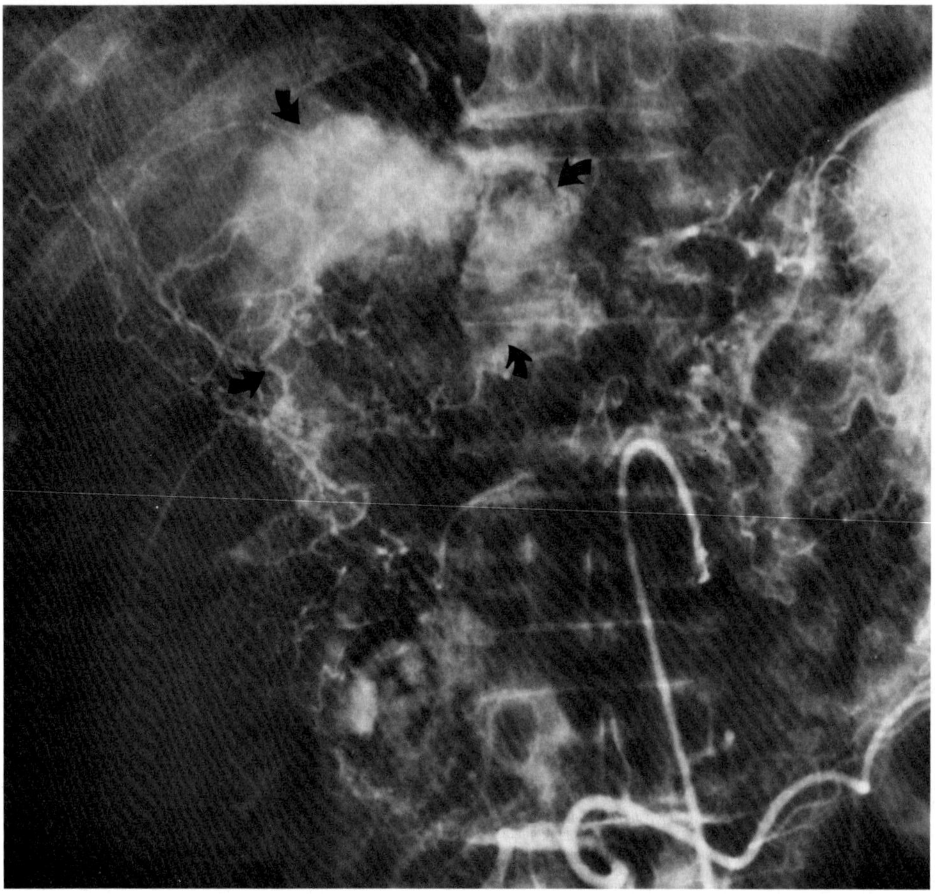

(D)
Figure 48 (continued)

vessels: the left gastric to the right gastric and the hepatic arteries (Fig. 49); the inferior pancreaticoduodenal to the superior pancreaticoduodenal to the gastroduodenal and the hepatic arteries; the inferior phrenic to hepatic capsular arteries and the hepatic arteries; and so on.

Sequential unilobar embolization is the preferred approach at present. Unilobar embolization leaves the other lobe to ensure normal metabolic function. Unilobar embolization is better tolerated by the patient, causing a less severe postembolization syndrome. However, several patients who had complete embolization at one sitting tolerated the procedure equally well (Fig. 41).

Side Effects

The posthepatic embolization syndrome was defined in 34 patients who received 46 embolic episodes (152). Liver function studies were monitored daily for the first week and

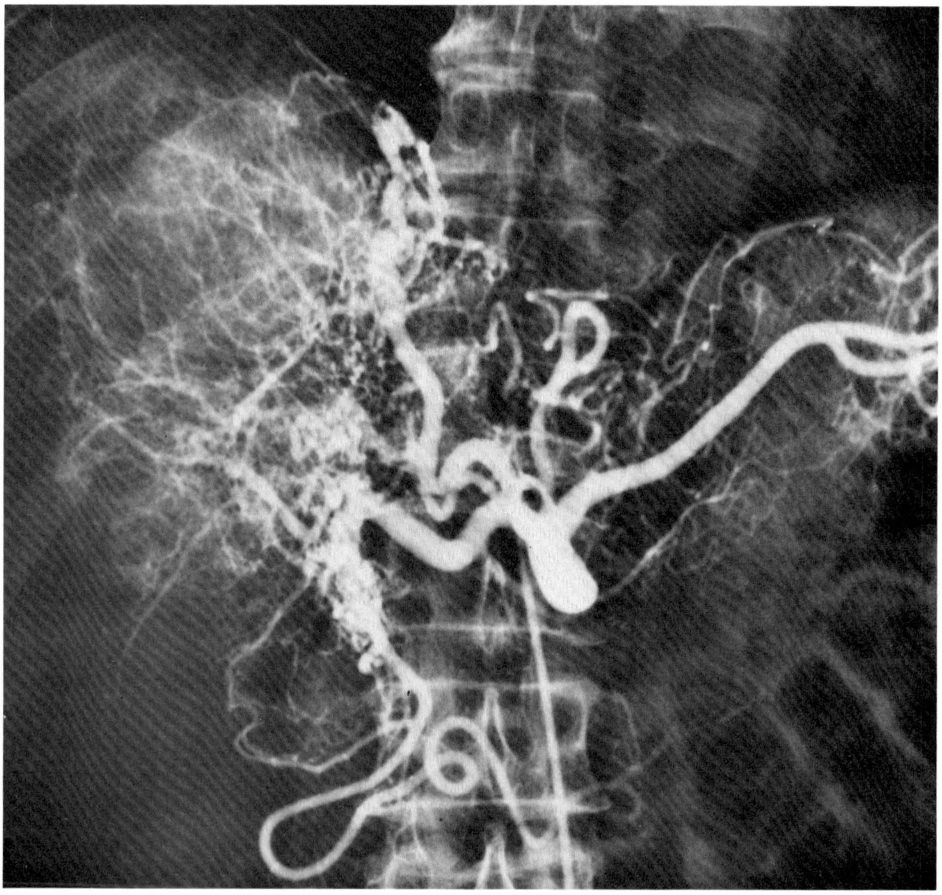

(E)
Figure 48 (continued)

then at least once a week for the next 4–5 weeks. These studies included the levels of serum bilirubin, alkaline phosphatase, serum transaminase, and prothrombin time. Eleven of the 46 patients had bilirubin elevations greater than twice the baseline value within 24 hr, normalizing to the preembolization level in 4–7 days. Three had elevations of bilirubin beyond 1 week and developed transient hepatic encephalopathy. In all patients, less than a twofold elevation above baseline of alkaline phosphatase was demonstrated, which returned to preembolization levels within 4–21 days. Forty-four of the 46 had serum transaminase elevation within 24 hr, usually 10- to 20-fold above baseline, returning to preembolization levels usually in 5 days or at the most in 21 days. Prothrombin time changed less than 2 sec in 33, 2–3 sec in 5, and 3 sec or more in 8. In three patients, failure to normalize within 1 week was associated with hepatic failure.

The incidence of nausea and vomiting was 50%. Six had abdominal distention lasting for 24–48 hr. All had temperature spikes to 100–102°F. In two embolic episodes,

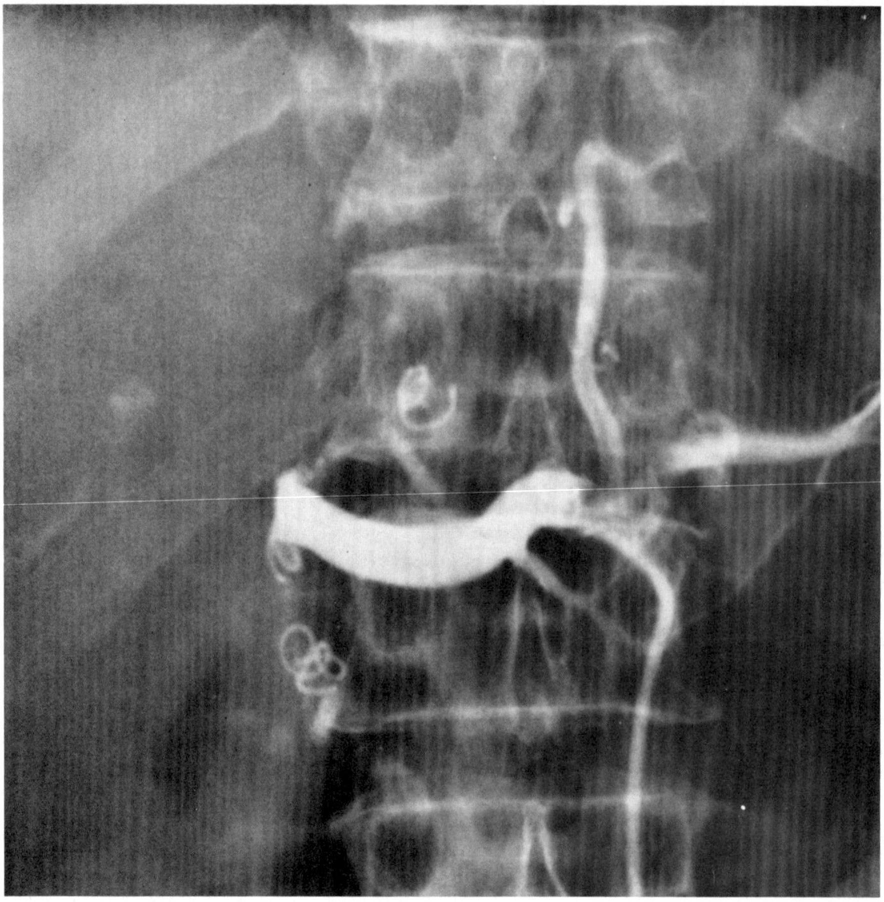

(F)

Figure 48 (continued)

the patients experienced hiccoughs. Forty-one of 46 embolizations were associated with varying degrees of right upper quadrant pain requiring narcotics. Almost every patient was given narcotics during the embolic procedure in aliquots of 25 mg of Demerol on demand. All of the symptoms noted above resolved in 3–4 days except in 3 patients with temperature spikes for 10 days and 2 with severe pain for 7 days.

Severe Complications

Of the 100 patients treated by 150 embolization, there were 7 deaths, which occurred within 1 month of the embolization. Three deaths were most probably related to embolization and the result of hepatic failure and/or the "hepatorenal" syndrome; 4 patients probably died of extensive metastases. The "hepatorenal" syndrome was seen in a total of 4 patients, 1 of whom failed to respond to therapy. This was associated with inappropriate secretion of antidiuretic hormone (ADH) and usually responded to hydration, electrolytes, and corticosteroids. Additional experience with hepatic embolization is presented in Chapter 27.

Results

The median survival duration for patients with untreated liver metastases of all types has been reported as 2.5 months (51) and 4.5 months (153). If liver metastasis from colorectal tumor only is considered, the median survival duration ranges from 5 to 6.5 months (51,154,155). The median survival duration from the diagnosis of liver metastases in patients with colorectal carcinoma who have undergone systemic chemotherapy has been reported to be 8.5 months (156) and was found to be 10 months at the M. D. Anderson Hospital and Tumor Institute (Y. Patt et al., unpublished data). The median survival duration in metastatic colorectal carcinoma of the liver treated with hepatic artery infusion ranges from 7.3 (126,127) to 11 months (Y. Patt et al., unpublished data). Most of the

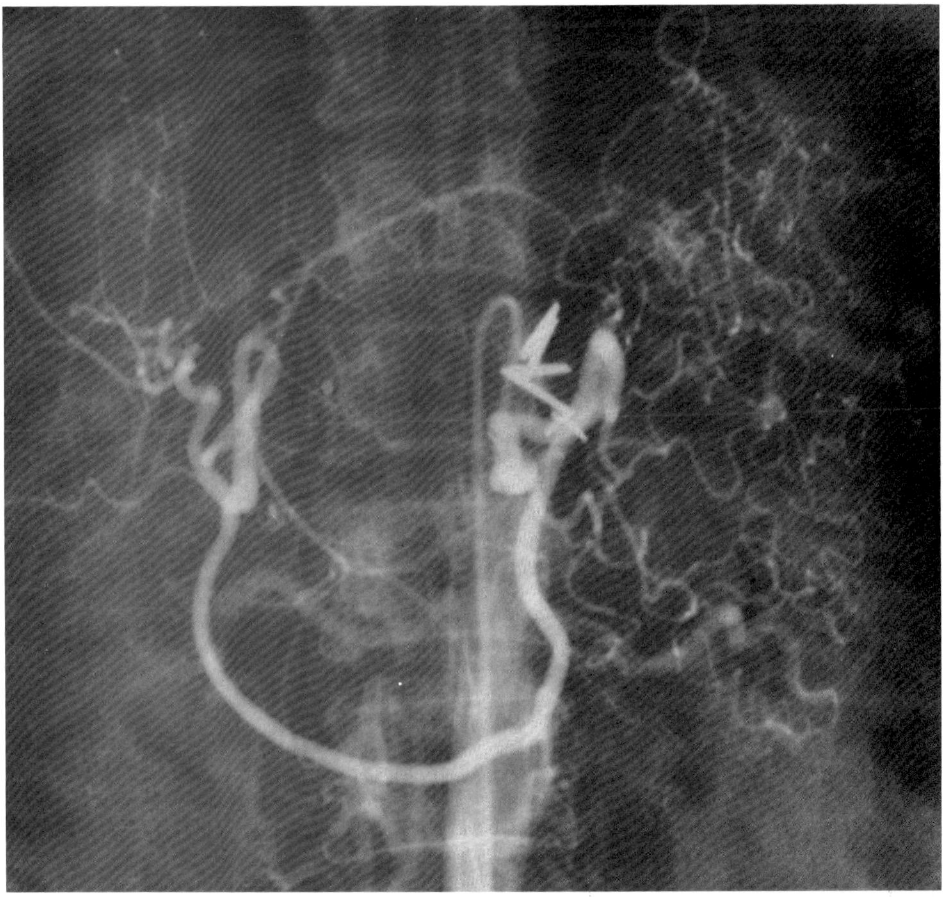

Figure 49A Common hepatic artery occlusion occurred following infusion therapy for metastatic colon carcinoma. With progression of metastatic disease, the left gastric to right gastric arterial arcade was found to provide access to the proper hepatic artery.

data above were calculated from the time of diagnosis of liver metastases. To evaluate the effect of a treatment modality, it is best to calculate the survival duration from the time of treatment. Our results of a median survival duration of 11.5 months (Fig. 50) *from the time of hepatic artery embolization* in patients with both primary and metastatic neoplasms show a significant improvement over any other currently available modality, especially in view of the fact that most patients in this series had failed to respond to prior systemic or hepatic infusion chemotherapy. Furthermore, in 55 patients with liver metastases from colorectal carcinoma treated with HAI of FUDR and MTC, the group of 31 patients treated with HAI alone had a median survival of 8 months from the initiation of treatment, as opposed to a group of 24 patients with HAI and hepatic artery occlusion, who had a median survival of 15 months (135).

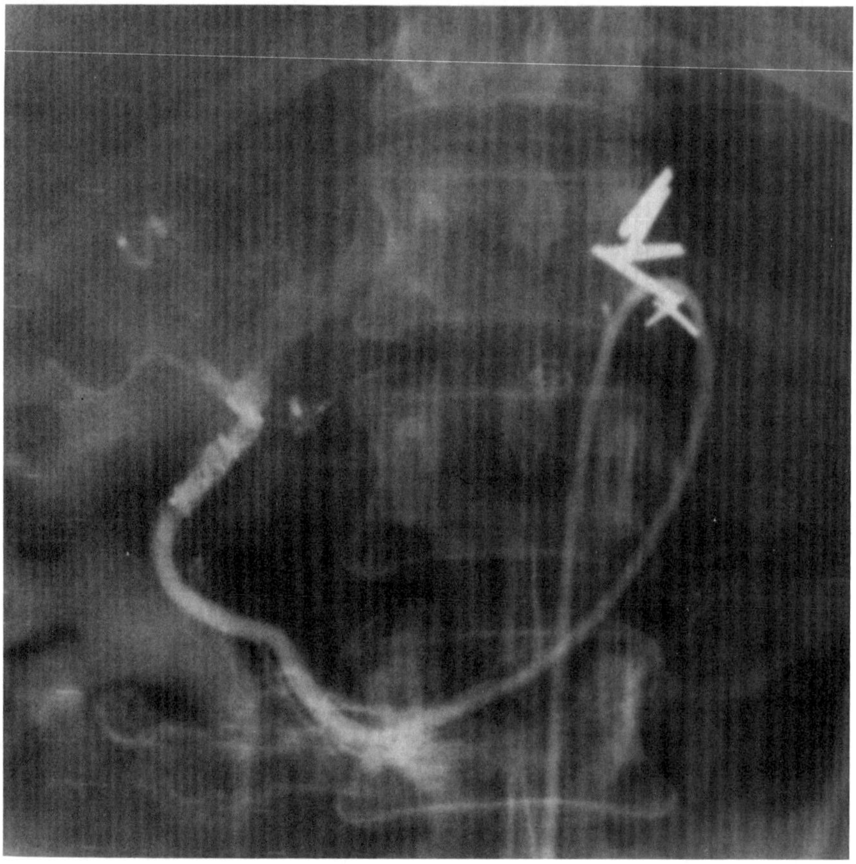

Figure 49B Catheterization of the arterial arcade could be followed by embolization of the liver with Ivalon and the placement of stainless steel coils.

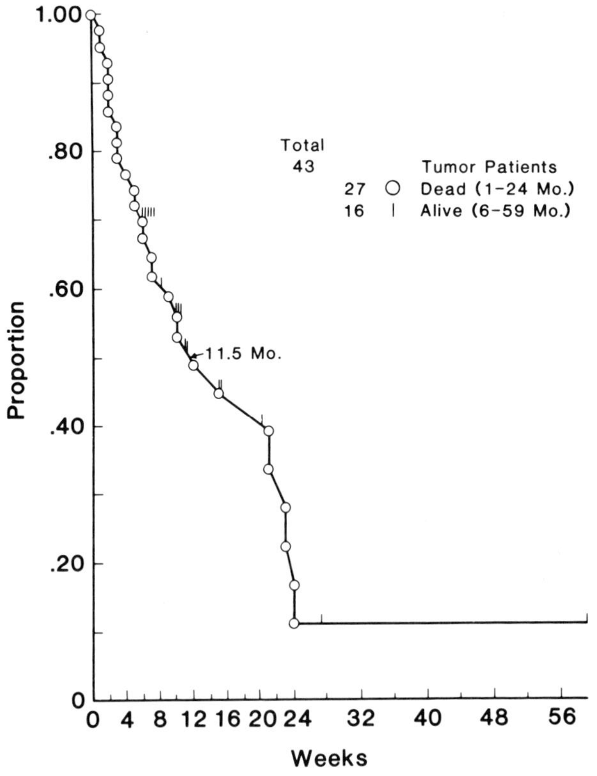

Figure 50 Results of hepatic artery embolization. Evaluation was possible in 43 of 47 patients embolized. The median survival *from the time of embolization* was 11.5 months.

Radiation Treatment

Therapeutic levels of irradiation to the liver may be the primary intent, but happen more often in the *management of adjacent malignancies* (157–174). This occurs during the treatment of retroperitoneal lymph nodes for Hodgkin's disease and non-Hodgkin's lymphoma, carcinoma of the testicle, dysgerminoma of the ovary, extended field radiation therapy for metastatic carcinoma from the cervix, and so on. Total abdominal irradiation for peritoneal carcinomatosis, usually associated with ovarian carcinoma, will affect the liver. Radiation directed to the thoracolumbar spine almost invariably includes a portion of the liver. Occasionally, in the management of the patient with neoplasm of the kidney, adrenals, stomach, pancreas, spleen, and so on, the liver may be included in the radiation portal.

The liver may be the *primary* object of radiation therapy in leukemia and lymphoma, primary and secondary hepatic neoplasms, hemangiomas of the liver, and so on (160,165–169). The intravascular infusion of radioactive isotopes has been attempted in the liver and will also induce radiation changes (166).

Pathologic Changes

An appreciation of the histologic findings helps the full understanding of the radiologic picture (163–174). The histologic changes consist of a progression of events which are partially reversible dependent on the extent of damage as well as the condition of the liver prior to therapy (165,169–171). The hallmark of radiation hepatitis is fibrinous occlusion of the central hepatic vein with sinusoidal congestion and parenchymal atrophy. These may progress to dense fibrous occlusion of the central vein and hepatic fibrosis (164,167,170,172).

Congestion of the sinusoids is most intense near the center of the hepatic lobule. When severe, necrosis of the liver cells and local atrophy frequently follow. Congestion may also extend to involve the portal bed with secondary splenomegaly and occasionally hypersplenism. The hepatic veins may recover by recanalization or the development of a collateral circulation. Congestion then subsides and, in mild cases, complete cellular repair may follow (164,167,170).

With severe injury, the irradiated portion becomes contracted and firm, and the surface of the liver granular. Histologically, there is central lobular fibrosis, sublobular venous fibrosis, and venous occlusion. Fibrosis also extends to the portal triads, with involvement of the portal vein radicles, hepatic arteries, and bile ducts (162,164,165,167,170,172).

Roentgen Appearance of Radiation Changes

The effects of ionizing radiation on the liver depend on the volume of liver irradiated, the time/dose of radiation, the quality of irradiation, and the condition of the hepatic cells at the time of irradiation. Clinically, the effects may be obscured because of the functional reserve and regenerative capacity of the liver (162,165,170). There is a significant difference in the clinical manifestations of radiation hepatitis when one compares the effects of partial with those of total irradiation.

Most patients with radiation injury to the liver have received a total dose in excess of 3500 rad during 3–4 weeks (159,160). The characteristic manifestations usually occur 2–6 weeks following completion of radiation therapy (172). The acute phase lasts for several months, gradually merging into the subacute and finally, after 3–6 months, into the chronic stage (159,160,164,172).

Partial Hepatic Irradiation

Irradiation of a portion of the liver with a time/dose relationship of 800–1000 rad/week for 4–5 weeks usually occurs as a side effect of radiation therapy to adjacent structures. The patient is usually hepatically asymptomatic, provided that the unirradiated portion of the liver is healthy. A minimum of 15% of normal nonirradiated liver is probably sufficient to maintain normal liver function and allow for compensatory hypertrophy (162,165).

Roentgen appearance of acute changes The acute phase lasts approximately 3–6 months. Repair and regeneration are initiated almost immediately (156,162,164). The

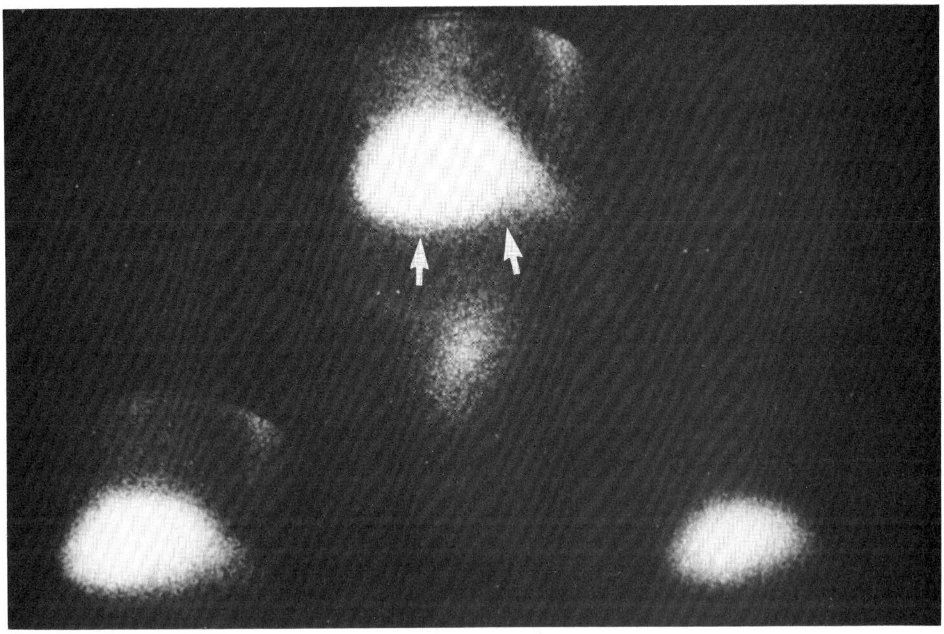

(A)

Figure 51 Partial hepatic irradiation (acute). (A) Scintigraphy 3 months after radiation therapy with cobalt, 2500 rad, in 3.5 weeks to the liver in a patient with Hodgkin's disease. There is normal uptake in the dome of the liver in comparison to diminished activity in the inferior portion of the right lobe. The sharp line of demarcation (arrows) coincided with the radiation portal. (B) In the dome, which was shielded, hepatic venography shows normal venous distribution and configuration. (C) The venogram in the irradiated portion of the right lobe revealed a "pruned tree" appearance. (D) A normal hepatic venogram obtained in another patient is shown for comparison.

decrease of normally functioning hepatic parenchymal and reticuloendothelial cells is reflected in the isotopic scan, which reveals a reduction in uptake in the treated area (173). Acute radiation changes most obviously affect the hepatic venous radicles. Hepatic venography would demonstrate a decrease in the number of peripheral branches, a "pruned tree" appearance (174) (Fig. 51). Enlargement of the irradiated portion of liver is represented by elongation and increased separation of the branches of the hepatic artery. The sinusoidal congestion in the distribution of the radiation portal may be manifested by a sharply defined zone of hypervascularity (Fig. 52). Occlusion of intralobar hepatic veins may occur and cause an obstruction to outflow, which is reflected in shunting from the hepatic artery to the portal vein with retrograde filling toward the nonirradiated areas. Under normal circumstances, there are communications between the hepatic artery and portal vein, but these seldom opacify unless there is obstruction to hepatic vein outflow, as is seen in venous occlusive disease or in hepatoma (93,102,174).

Roentgen appearance of chronic changes With progressive damage, chronic changes become obvious in approximately 6 months. Fibrosis and contraction of the

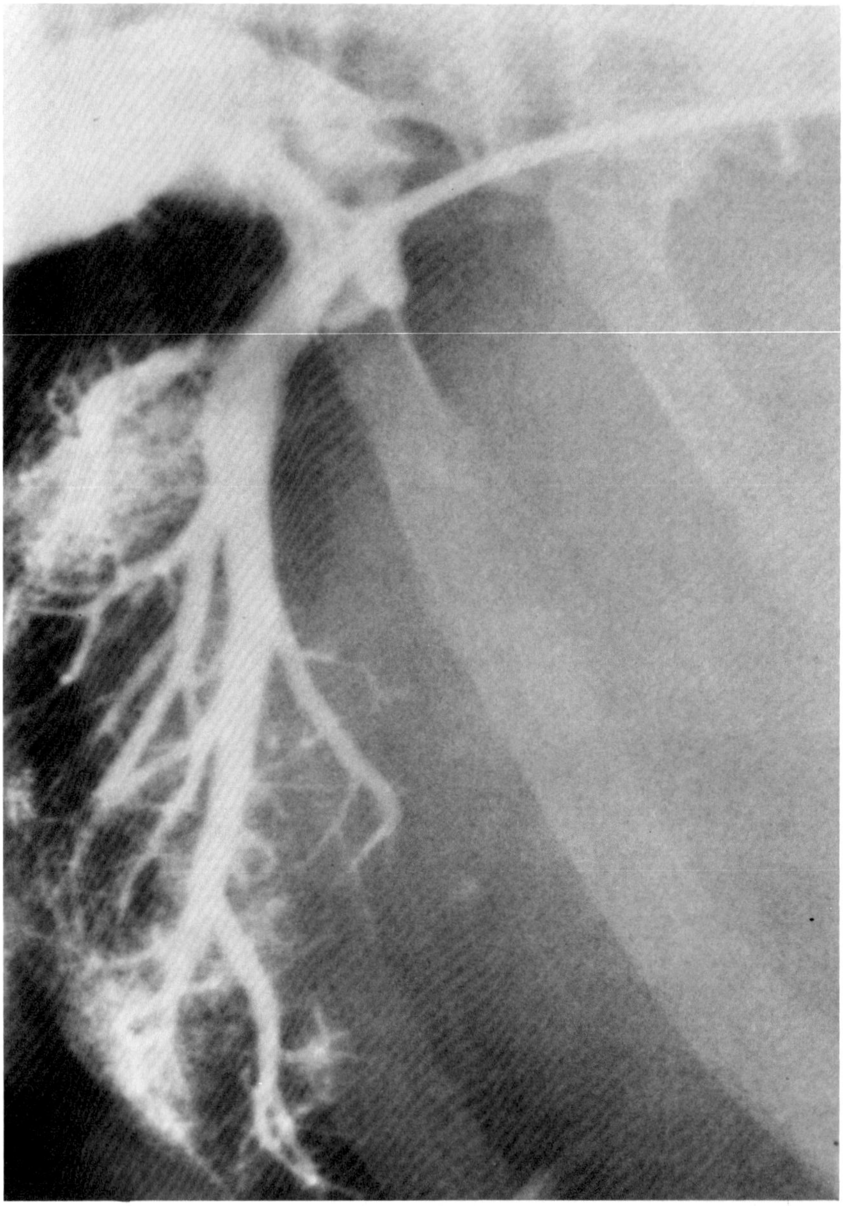

(B)

Figure 51 (continued)

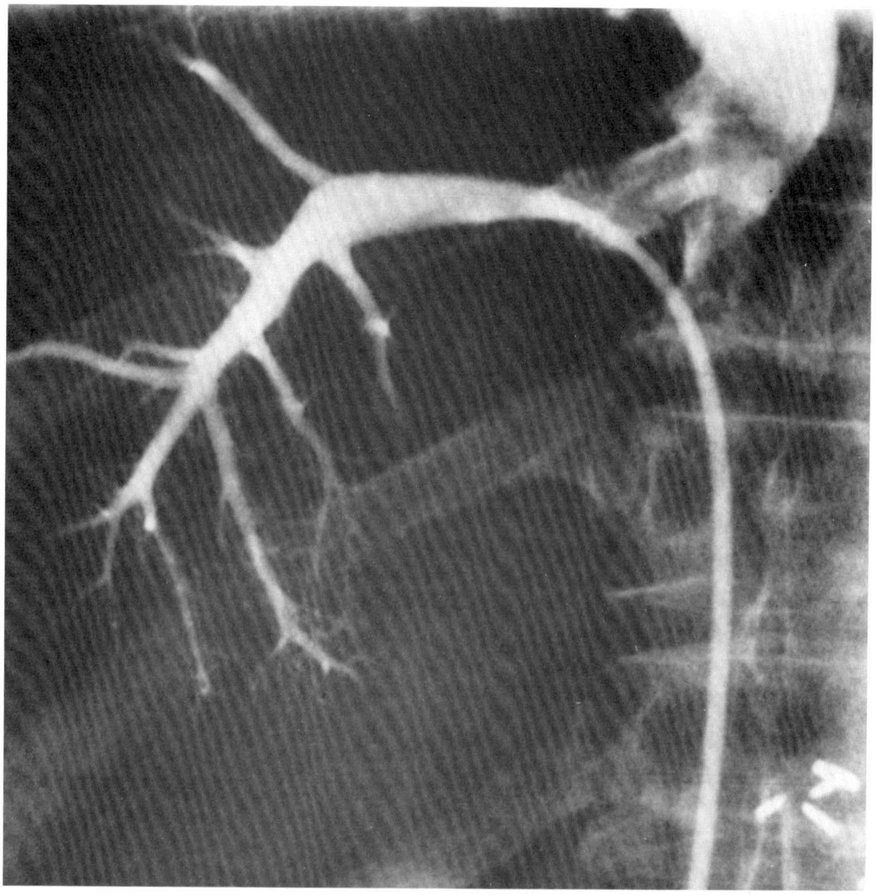

(C)

Figure 51 (continued)

irradiated portion of the liver are associated with tortuosity of branches of the hepatic artery, in contrast to the elongation and separation of the branches seen in the nonirradiated liver as evidence of compensatory hypertrophy (Fig. 53). Shunting to the portal vein is no longer seen. The portal venous flow is of normal direction, although diverted to the veins of the nonirradiated areas (157,162,172).

Total Hepatic Irradiation

Total liver irradiation is fraught with greater danger and is encountered most often with total abdominal radiation therapy. In a group of 65 patients with ovarian carcinoma treated at the M. D. Anderson Hospital and Tumor Institute between 1965 and 1967, by the moving-strip technique with ^{60}Co, ranging from 2450 to 2920 rad in 12 days, 14 patients apparently cured of cancer were noted to have the clinical features of radiation hepatitis. Eleven of the 14 patients died either directly or indirectly of radiation injury (164).

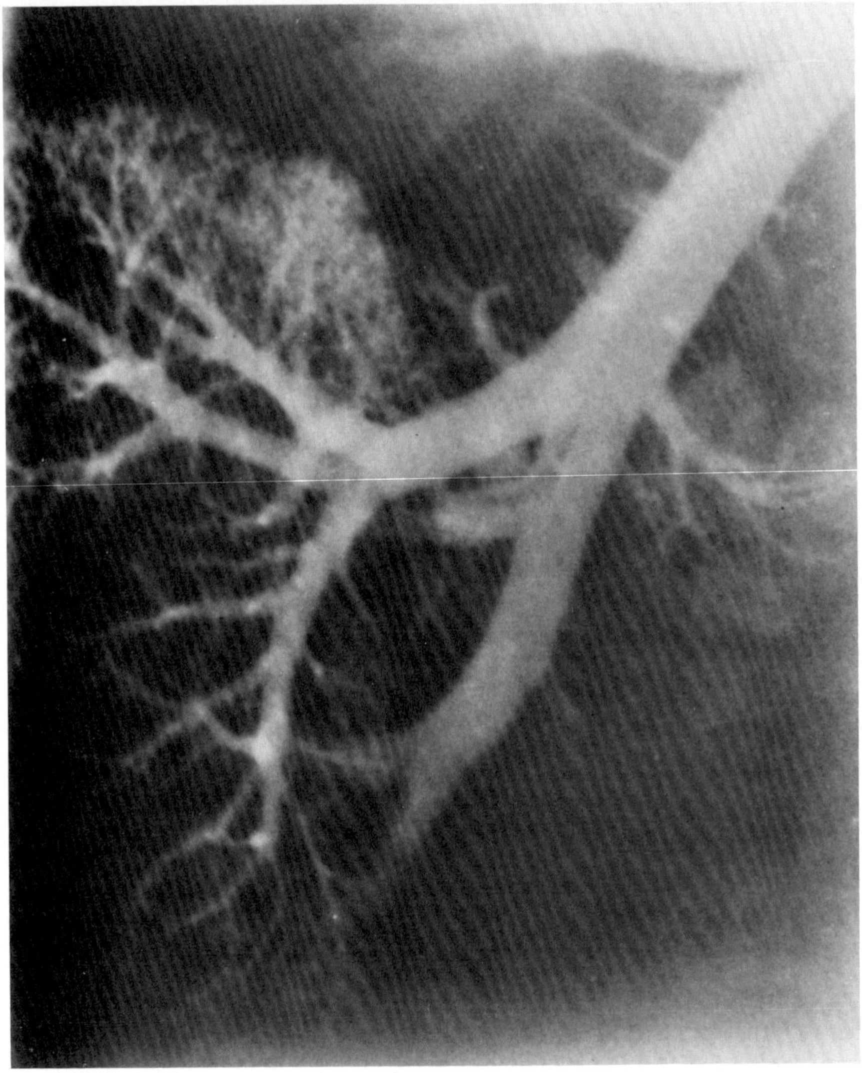

(D)

Figure 51 (continued)

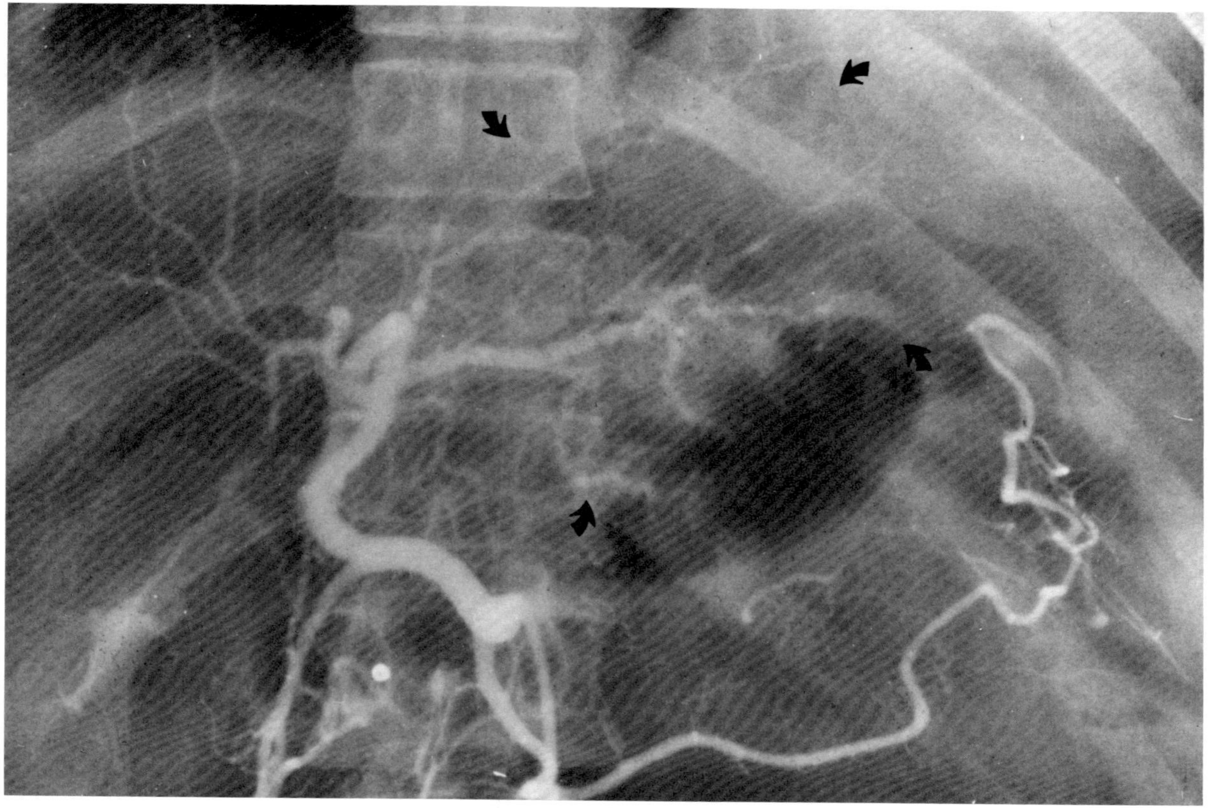

Figure 52A Partial hepatic irradiation (acute). This 39-year-old man with a carcinoma of the left kidney and pulmonary metastases was treated to the kidney for palliation with cobalt to a dose of 5500 rad in 6.5 weeks. The radiation portal included a portion of the left lobe of the liver. The branches of the left hepatic artery (arrows) were enlarged and separated probably due to edema and congestion.

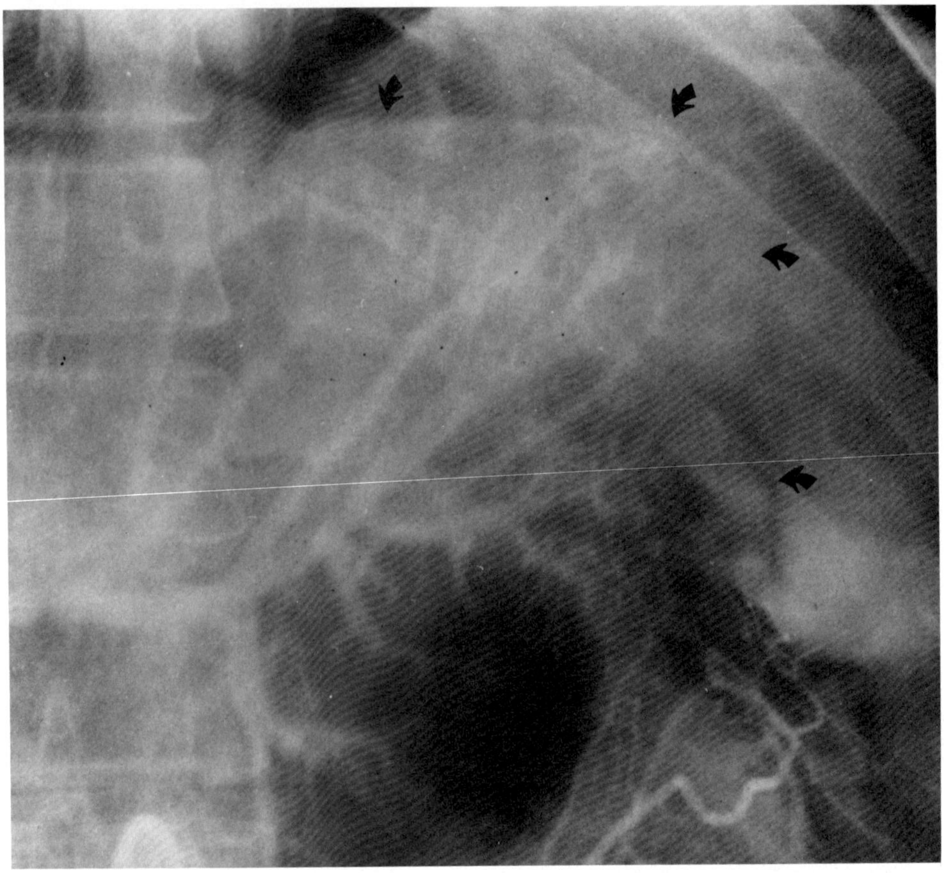

Figure 52B There was opacification and retrograde flow in the portal venous radicles of the left lobe of the liver. The radiation portal (arrows) is delineated by the hypervascularity.

In contrast to the patients given partial hepatic irradiation, those treated to their entire liver manifested the clinical features of radiation hepatitis. Based on the onset of clinical symptoms, length of survival, and histologic changes, the cases of radiation hepatitis could be divided into three groups: acute, subacute, and chronic.

During the acute stage, patients presented with hepatomegaly, ascites, and pleural effusion. In the chronic phase, the liver was contracted in addition to showing ascites and pleural effusion. Liver function studies were abnormal in all parameters. Liver failure and/or hematemesis were the usual causes of death (164).

Roentgen appearance Total hepatic irradiation results in the same sequence of histologic changes as previously described. With doses ranging from 2500 to 3000 rad in 2.5 weeks, the effects are slowly progressive, ultimately terminating in extensive hepatic fibrosis (164). The hepatic arteries are tortuous, reflecting the increase in peripheral vascular resistance (Figs. 54, 55). The direction of flow in the portal circulation is initially normal, even though hepatic fibrosis is considered responsible for the tortuosity of the intrahepatic branches of the portal vein. Eventually, with progressive intrahepatic disease, reversal of portal flow takes place, leading to opacification of collateral venous channels and the appearance of esophageal varices.

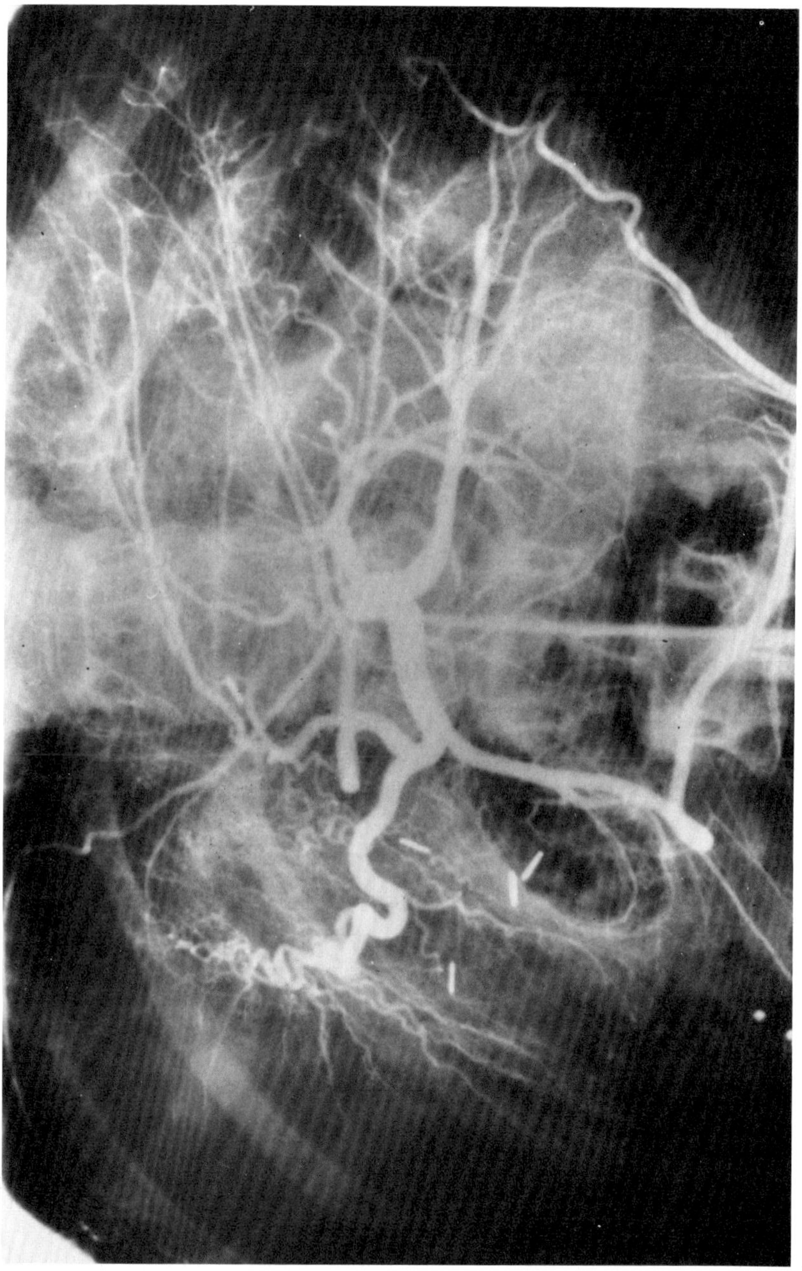

Figure 53

(A)

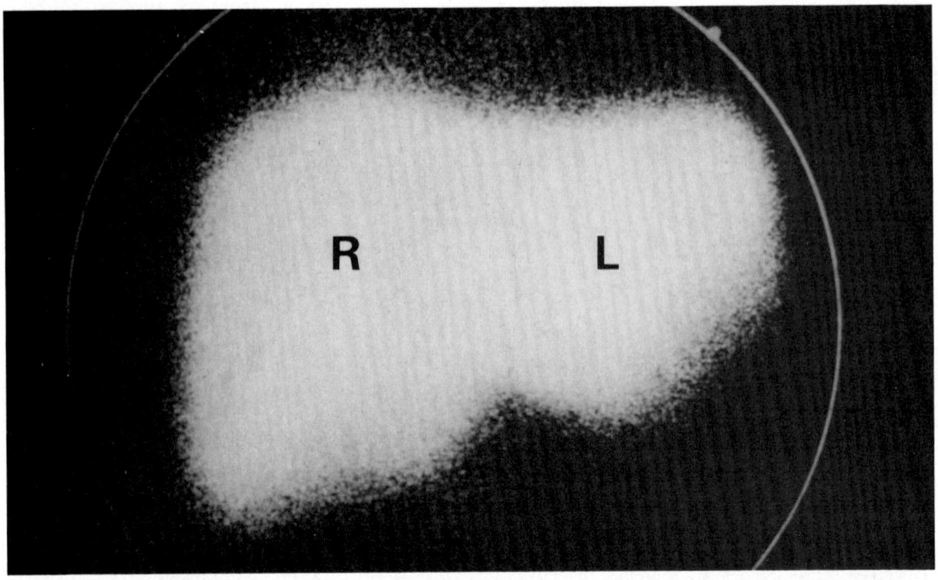

(B)

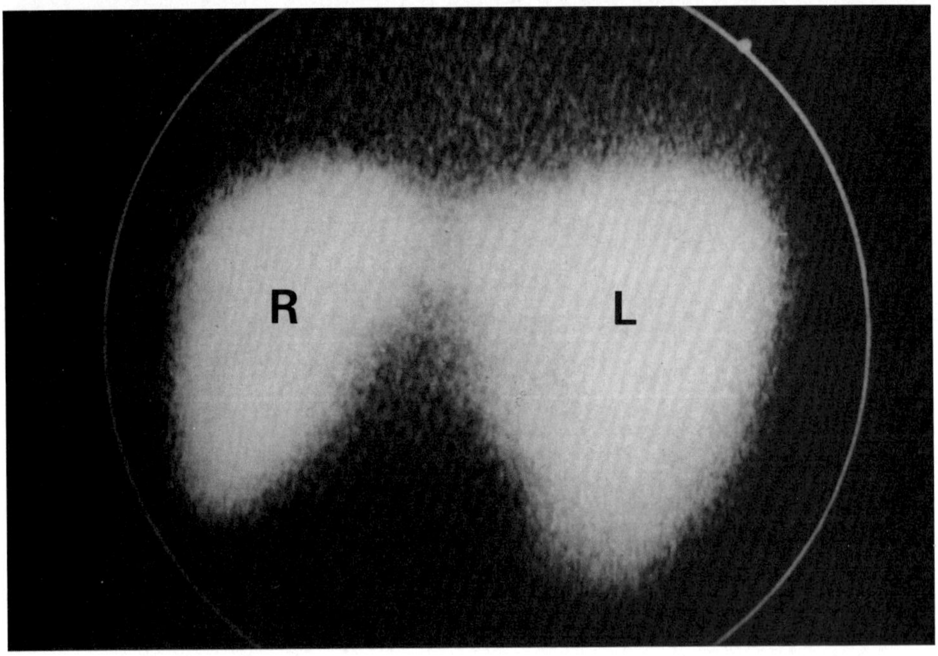

(C)

Figure 53 Partial hepatic irradiation (chronic). A 13-year-old female patient with carcinoma of the left adrenal gland developed a paracaval mass, probably metastases to the right adrenal. This mass and a portion of the right lobe of the liver were treated by cobalt therapy to 5000 rad in 5 weeks. (A) One year after irradiation a celiac arteriogram demonstrated marked tortuosity of the arteries, in the contracted area of the right lobe. The stretching of the left hepatic arterial branches reflected hypertrophy of the left lobe. The direction of venous flow was normal. (B) Scintiscan before irradiation. (C) Scintiscan 1 year later.

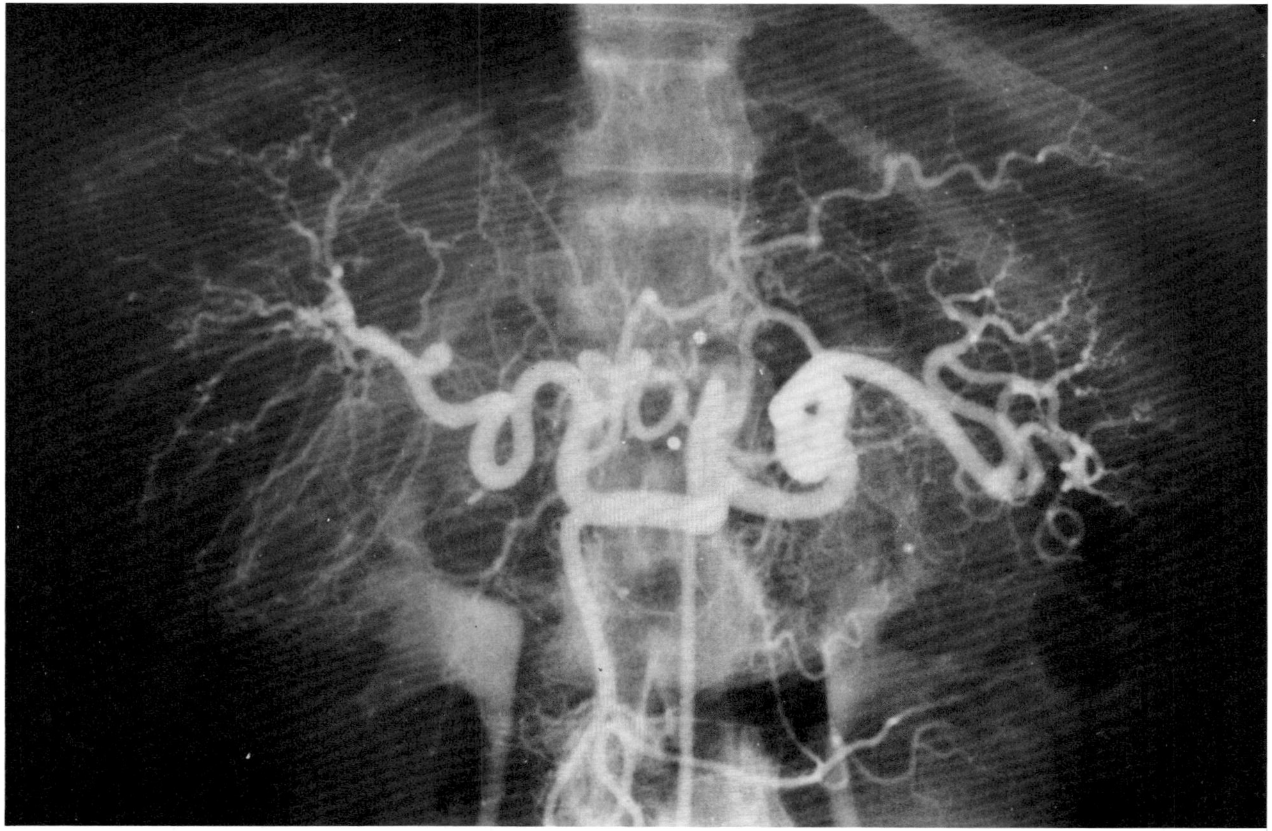

Figure 54A Total hepatic and splenic irradiation (chronic). This patient with carcinoma of the ovary was treated by cobalt to the entire abdomen with the moving-strip technique to a dose of 2800 rad in 12 days. Three years after treatment the patient had ascites and abnormal liver function studies compatible with cirrhosis. Celiac arteriogram reveals tortuous vessels in the spleen and liver.

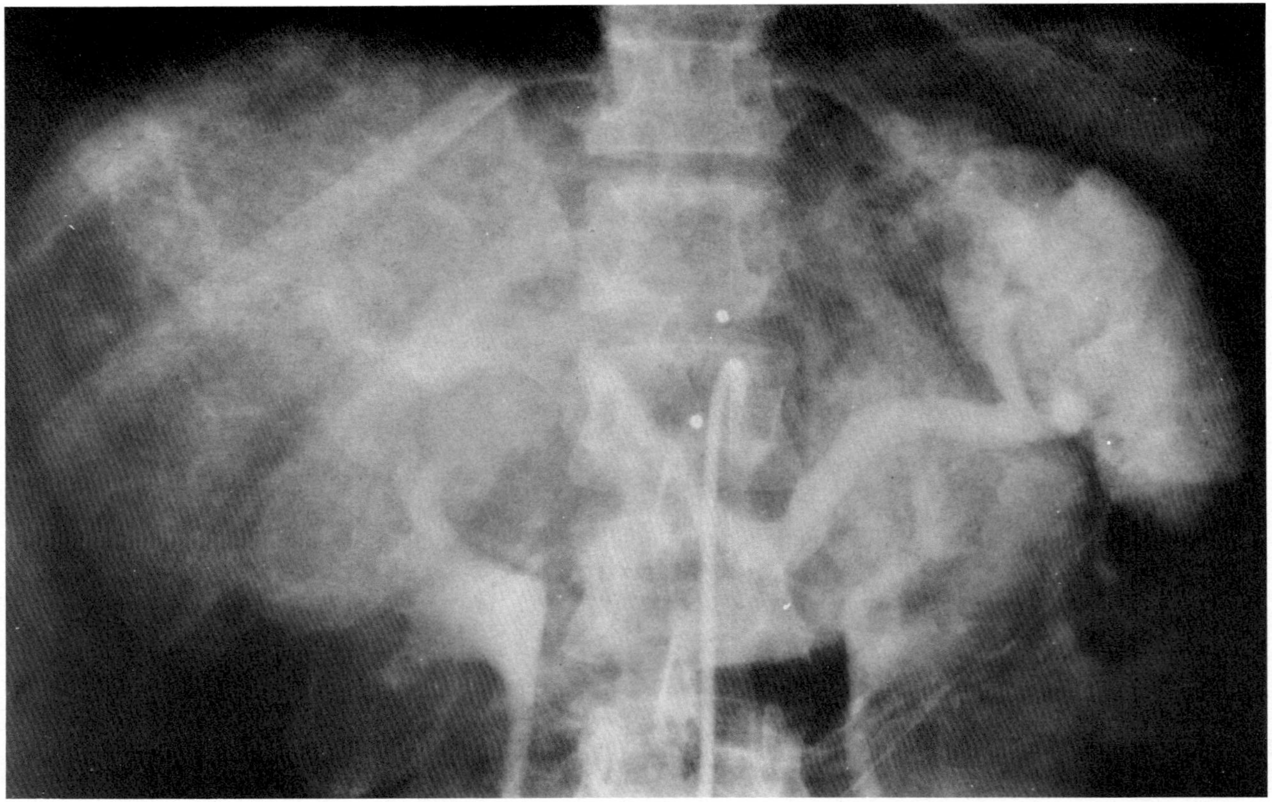

Figure 54B The venous phase disclosed that the spleen and liver were small. The venous flow was normal. The patient died 3 months later of liver failure with hepatic fibrosis and esophageal varices.

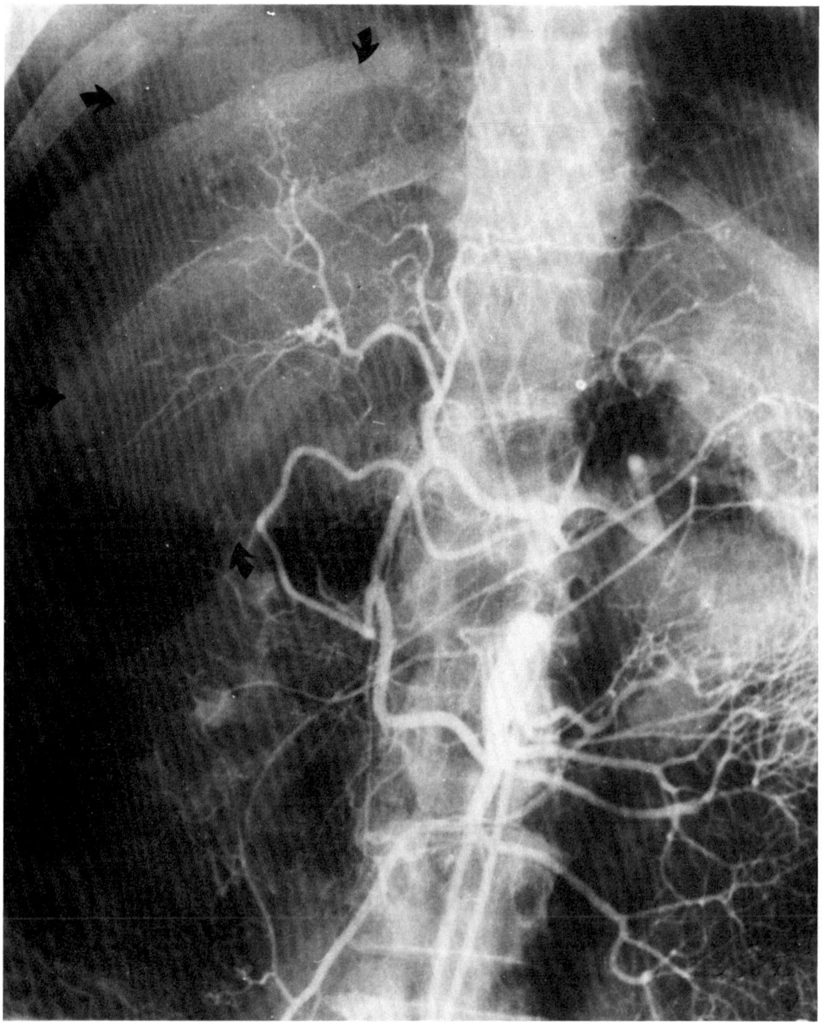

Figure 55A Total hepatic irradiation (chronic). This 43-year-old woman with ovarian carcinoma was treated by total abdomen irradiation by the moving-strip technique to 2800 rad in 12 days. Three and one-half years later she was admitted with ascites which on paracentesis revealed no tumor cells; BSP 60%; alkaline phosphatase 170; SGOT 165. Arterial phase: superior mesenteric injection revealed a small liver with tortuous arteries suggesting fibrosis (arrows).

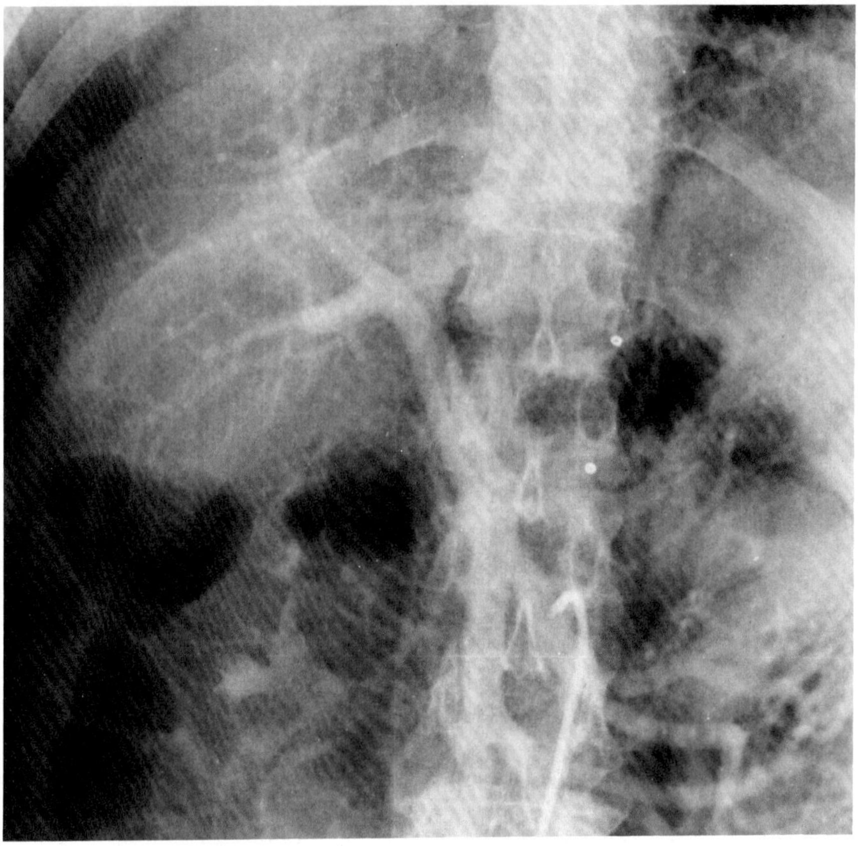

Figure 55B Venous phase: the portal veins were well opacified and slightly tortuous. The liver is small, 50–60% of normal, and displaced from the abdominal wall by the ascites. The direction of flow was normal.

References

1. Snow JH, Goldstein HM, Wallace S: Comparison of scintigraphy, sonography, and computed tomography in the evaluation of hepatic neoplasms. *Am J Roentgenol 132*:915, 1979.
2. Bryan PJ, Dinn WM, Grossman ZD, Wistow BW, McAffee JG, Kiefer SA: Correlation of computed tomography, gray scale ultrasonography, and radionuclide imaging of the liver in detecting space-occupying processes. *Radiology 124*:387, 1977.
3. Vermess M, Adamson RH, Doppman JL, Girton M: Computed tomographic demonstration of hepatic tumor with the aid of intravenous iodinated fat emulsion. *Radiology 125*:711, 1977.
4. Green B, Bree RL, Goldstein HM, Stanley C: Grey scale ultrasound evaluation of hepatic neoplasms: patterns and correlations. *Radiology 124*:203, 1977.
5. Taylor K, Carpenter D, Hill C, McCready V: Grey scale ultrasound imaging. *Radiology 119*:415, 1976.
6. Wooten WB, Green B, Goldstein HM: Ultrasonography of necrotic metastases. *Radiology 128*:447, 1978.
7. Bernardino ME, Thomas JL, Mayes GB: An initial experience with post-data processing in hepatic sonography. *Am J Roentgenol 136*:521, 1981.
8. McCready VR: Scintigraphic studies of space occupying liver disease. *Semin Nucl Med 2*:108, 1972.
9. Garrett W, Kossoff G, Uren R, Carpenter D: Grey scale ultrasonic investigation of focal defects on ^{99m}Tc sulphur colloid liver scanning. *Radiology 119*:425, 1976.
10. Lomonaco A, Kline P, Halpern S, Leopold G: Nuclear medicine and ultrasound: correlation in diagnosis of disease in liver and biliary tract. *Semin Nucl Med 5*:307, 1975.
11. Lunia S, Parthasarathy K, Bakshi S, Bender M: An evaluation of ^{99m}Tc sulphur colloid liver scintiscans and their usefulness in metastatic workup: a review of 1424 studies. *J Nucl Med 16*:62, 1974.
12. Rosenthal S: Are hepatic scans overused? *Am J Dig Dis 21*:659, 1976.
13. Margulis AR, Nice CM Jr, Rigler LG: The roentgen findings in primary heptaoma in infants and children. *Radiology 66*:809, 1956.
14. Wallace S: Primary liver tumors. In *Pediatric Oncologic Radiology*, Parker BR and Castellino RA (Eds). C. V. Mosby, St. Louis, 1977, p 301.
15. Pear BL and Boline JE: Teratoma of the liver. *Cancer Semin 4*:229, 1972.
16. Teng CT, Daeschner CW, Singleton EB, Rosenburg HS, Cole VN, Hill LL, Brennan JC: Liver disease and osteoporosis in children. *J Pediatr 59*:684, 1961.
17. Hansen AE, Palmer LS, Nelson JW: Composition of bone in extreme osteoporosis associated with hepatoma. *Proc Soc Exp Biol Med 43*:206, 1940.
18. Berdon W: Opacification of retrosternal lymph nodes following barium peritonitis. *Radiology 106*:171, 1973.
19. Prando A, Wallace S, Bernardino ME, Lindell MM: Computed tomographic arteriography of the liver. *Radiology 130*:697, 1979.
20. McBride CM and Wallace S: Cancer of the right lobe of the liver: a variety of operative procedures. *Arch Surg 106*:725, 1973.
21. Healy JE Jr, Schroy PC, Sorenson RJ: The intrahepatic distribution of the hepatic artery in man. *J Int Col Surg 20*:133, 1953.
22. Michels NA: *Blood Supply to the Upper Abdominal Organs with a Descriptive Atlas*. J. B. Lippincott, Philadelphia, 1955.

23. Couinaud C: Hepatectomies gauches lobaires et segmentaires (étude des conditions anatomiques). *J Chir 68*:697, 1952.
24. Rossi P and Goud HR: Angiography and scanning in liver disease. *Radiology 96*:553, 1970.
25. Rösch J: Liver, gallbladder, biliary ducts, pancreas, and spleen. In *Diagnosis and Staging of Cancer: A Radiologic Approach*, Steckel RJ and Kagan AR (Eds). W. B. Saunders, Philadelphia, 1976.
26. Reuter SR and Redman HC: *Gastrointestinal Angiography*, 2nd ed. W. B. Saunders, Philadelphia, 1977.
27. Goldstein HM, Thaggard A, Wallace S, Neiman HL: Priscoline—augmented hepatic angiography. *Radiology 119*:275, 1976.
28. Goldstein HM and Miller M: Angiographic evaluation of carcinoid tumors of the small intestine: the value of epinephrine. *Radiology 115*:23, 1975.
29. Goldstein HM, Zornoza J, Wallace S, Anderson JH, Bree RL, Samuels B, Lukeman J: Percutaneous film needle aspiration biopsy of pancreatic and other abdominal masses. *Radiology 123*:319, 1977.
30. Zornoza J, Wallace S, Ordonez N, Lukeman J: Fine needle aspiration biopsy of the liver. *Am J Roentgenol 134*:331–334, 1980.
31. Zornoza J: *Percutaneous Biopsy*. Williams & Wilkins, Baltimore, 1981.
32. Lundquist A: Fine needle aspiration biopsy for cytodiagnoses of malignant tumor in the liver. *Acta Med Scand 188*:465, 1970.
33. Holm HH, Rasmussen SN, Kristensen JK: Ultrasonically guided percutaneous puncture technique. *J Clin Ultrasound 1*:27, 1973.
34. Haaga JR and Alfidi RJ: Precise biopsy localization by computed tomography. *Radiology 118*:603, 1976.
35. Haaga JR and Vanek J: Computed tomographic guided liver biopsy using Menghini needle. *Radiology 133*:405, 1979.
36. Pereiras RV, Meiers W, Kunhardt B, Troner M, Hutson D, Barkin DS, Viamonte M: Fluoroscopically guided thin needle aspiration biopsy of the abdomen and retroperitoneum. *Am J Roentgenol 131*:197, 1978.
37. Zamcheck N and Klausenstock O: Liver biopsy II. The risk of needle biopsy. *N Engl J Med 249*:1062, 1953.
38. Ovlisen B and Baden H: Liver biopsy by the method of Menghini. *Nord Med 83*:297, 1970.
39. Rasmussen SN, Holm HH, Kristensen JK, Barlebo H: Ultrasonically-guided liver biopsy. *Br Med J 2*:500, 1972.
40. Johansen P and Svendsen KN: Scan-guided needle aspiration biopsy in malignant hepatic disease. *Acta Cytol 22*:292, 1978.
41. Madden RE: Complications of needle biopsy of the liver. *Arch Surg 83*:778, 1961.
42. Rosch J, Laken PC, Antonovic R, Dotter CT: Transjugular approach to liver biopsy and transhepatic cholangiography. *N Engl J Med 289*:227, 1973.
43. Sherlock P, Kim YS, Koss LG: Cytologic diagnosis of cancer from aspirated material at liver biopsy. *Am J Dig Dis 12*:396, 1967.
44. Ishak KG and Glunz PR: Hepatoblastoma and hepatocarcinoma in infancy and childhood: a report of 47 cases. *Cancer 20*:396, 1967.
45. Nikardoh H, Bogg J, Swenson O: Liver tumors in infants and children. *Arch Surg 101*:245, 1970.
46. Lin T-Y: Tumors of the liver, Part 1: Primary malignant tumors. In *Gastroenterology*, Bockus HL (Ed). Vol 3, 3rd ed, W. B. Saunders, Philadelphia, 1976, p 522.
47. Dehner LP and Ishak KG: Vascular tumors of the liver in infants and children. *Arch Pathol 92*:101, 1971.
48. Pack GT and Miller TR: The treatment of hepatic tumors. *NY State J Med 134*:59, 1953.
49. Bloomenthal ED and Spellberg MA: Therapy for carcinoma of the liver. *Am J Gastroenterol 56*:334, 1971.

50. Ariel IM and Pack GT: Intra-arterial chemotherapy for cancer metastatic to liver. *Arch Surg 91*:851, 1965.
51. Jaffe BM, Donegan WL, Watson F, Spratt JS Jr: Factors influencing survival in patients with untreated hepatic metastases. *Surg Gynecol Obstet 127*:1, 1968.
52. Edmondson HA: Tumors of the liver and intrahepatic bile ducts. In *Atlas of Tumor Pathology*, fasc 25, Washington, DC, AFIP, 1958.
53. Ishak KG and Rabin L: Benign tumors of the liver. *Med Clin North Am 59*:995, 1975.
54. Edmondson HA: Differential diagnosis of tumors and tumor-like lesions of the liver in infancy and childhood. *Am J Dis Child 91*:168, 1956.
55. Desser PL and Smith S: Non-parasitic liver cysts in children. *J Pediatr 49*:297, 1956.
56. Henson SW Jr, Gray HK, Dockerty MB: Benign tumors of the liver IV. Polycystic disease of surgical significance. *Surg Gynecol Obstet 104*:63, 1957.
57. Federle MP, Filly RA, Moss AA: Cystic hepatic neoplasms: complementary roles of CT and sonography. *Am J Roentgenol 136*:345, 1981.
58. Caroli J and Covinaud C: Une affection nouvelle sans doute congénitale des voies biliaires: unilobulaire des canaux hépatiques. *Sem Hop Paris 34*:136, 1958.
59. Mujahed Z, Glenn F, Evans JA: Communicating cavernous estasia of the intrahepatic ducts (Caroli's disease). *Am J Roentgenol 113*:21, 1971.
60. Watts DR, Lorenzo GA, Beal JM: Congenital dilatation of the intrahepatic biliary ducts. *Arch Surg 108*:539, 1971.
61. Doppmann JL, Dunnick NR, Girton M, Fance AS, Popovski MA: Bile duct cysts secondary to liver infarcts: report of a case and experimental production by small vessel hepatic artery occlusion. *Radiology 130*:1, 1979.
62. Wooten WB, Bernardino ME, Goldstein HM: Computed tomography of necrotic hepatic metastases. *Am J Roentgenol 131*:839, 1978.
63. Novy S, Wallace S, Goldman AM, Ben-Menachem Y: Pyogenic liver abscess. Angiographic diagnosis and treatment by closed aspiration. *Am J Roentgenol 121*:338, 1974.
64. Gerzof SG, Robbins AH, Birkett DH, JohnsonWC, Pugatch RD, Vincent ME: Percutaneous catheter drainage of abdominal abscesses guided by ultrasound and computed tomography. *Am J Roentgenol 133*:1, 1979.
65. Haaga JR, Alfidi RJ, Havrilla TR, Cooperman AM, Seidelman RE, Reich NE, Weinstein AJ, Meaney TR: CT detection and aspiration of abdominal abscess. *Am J Roentgenol 128*:465, 1977.
66. Lawson TL: Hepatic abscess: ultrasound as an aid to diagnosis. *Am J Dig Dis 22*:33, 1977.
67. Kuwar B, Alderson PO, Geisse G: The role of Ga-67 citrate imaging and diagnostic ultrasound in patients with suspected abdominal abscess. *J Nucl Med 18*:534, 1977.
68. Silber DL, Soper RT, Kent TH: Life threatening mesenchymal hamartoma of the liver. *J Pediatr Surg 5*:471, 1970.
69. Somppi E, Niemi K, Rumskanen O, Arajarvi P, Lauslahti K: Cavernous hepatic hemangioma in the newborn infant: case report of a successful resection. *J Pediatr Surg 9*:239, 1974.
70. Johnson CM, Sheedy PF, Stanson AW, Stephens DH, Hattery RR, Adson MA: Computed tomography and angiography of cavernous hemagiomas of the liver. *Radiology 138*:115, 1981.
71. Slovis TL, Berdon WE, Haller JO, Casarella WJ, Baker DH: Hemangioma of the liver in infants: review of diagnosis, treatment and course. *Am J Roentgenol 123*:791, 1975.
72. Adam YG, Huvos AG, Hadju SI: Malignant vascular tumors of liver. *Ann Surg 175*:375, 1972.
73. Pliskin M: Peliosis hepatis. *Radiology 114*:29–30, 1975.
74. Baghieri SA and Boyer JL: Peliosis hepatis associated with androgenic anabolic steroid therapy; a severe form of hepatic injury. *Ann Intern Med 81*:610, 1974.

75. Lande A, Bedford A, Schechter LS: The spectrum of arteriographic findings in Osler-Weber-Rendu disease. *Angiology 27*:223, 1976.
76. Jonsson K: Personal communication.
77. Moss AA, Clark RE, Palubinskas AJ, de Lormer AA: Angiographic appearance of benign and malignant hepatic tumors in infants and children. *Am J Roentgenol 113*:61, 1971.
78. Albritton DR, Tompkins RK, Longmire WP: Hepatic cell adenoma: a report of four cases. *Ann Surg 180*:14, 1973.
79. Goldstein HM, Neiman HL, Mena E, Bookstein JJ, Appelman HD: Angiographic findings in benign liver cell tumors. *Radiology 110*:339, 1974.
80. Salvo AF, Schiller A, Athanasoulis CA, Galdabini J, McKusick KA: Hepatoadenoma and focal nodular hyperplasia: pitfalls in radiocolloid imaging. *Radiology 125*:451, 1977.
81. Mays ET, Christopherson WM, Mahr MM, Williams HC: Hepatic changes in young women ingesting contraceptive steroids. Hepatic hemorrhage and primary hepatic tumors. *JAMA 235*:730, 1976.
82. Motsay GJ and Gamble WG: Clinical experience with hepatic adenomas. *Surg Gynecol Obstet 134*:415, 1972.
83. Baum JK, Holtz F, Bookstein JJ, Klein EW: Possible association between benign hepatomas and oral contraceptives. *Lancet 2*:926, 1973.
84. Sherlock S: Hepatic adenomas and oral contraceptives. *Gut 16*:753, 1976.
85. Casarella WJ, Knowles DM, Wolff M. Johnson PM: Focal nodular hyperplasia and liver cell adenoma: radiologic and pathologic differentiation. *Am J Roentgenol 131*:393, 1978.
86. McLoughlin MK, Colapinto RF, Gilday DL, Hobbs BB, Korobkin MT, McDonald P, Phillips MJ: Focal nodular hyperplasia of the liver. *Radiology 107*:257, 1973.
87. Rogers JV, Mack LA, Freeny PC, Johnson ML, Sones PJ: Hepatic focal nodular hyperplasia: angiography, CT, sonography and scintigraphy. *Am J Roentgenol 137*:983, 1981.
88. Whelan TJ, Baugh JH, Chandor S: Focal nodular hyperplasia of the liver. *Ann Surg 177*:150, 1973.
89. Stauffer JQ, Lopenski MW, Harold DJ, Myers JK: Focal nodular hyperplasia of the liver and intrahepatic hemorrhage in young women on oral contraceptives. *Ann Intern Med 83*:301, 1975.
90. Kew MC, Dos Santos HA, Sherlock S: Diagnosis of primary cancer of the liver. *Br Med J 4*:408, 1971.
91. Editorial: Foetoglobin and primary liver cancer. *Lancet 2*:93, 1968.
92. Kido C, Sasaki T, Kaneko M: Angiography of primary liver cancer. *Am J Roentgenol 113*:70, 1971.
93. Gregg PF, Goldstein HM, Wallace S, Casey JH: Arteriographic demonstration of intravenous tumor extension. *Am J Roentgenol 123*:100, 1975.
94. Clatworthy JJ, Boles ET Jr, Kottmeier PK: Liver tumors in infancy and childhood. *Ann Surg 154*:745, 1961.
95. McDonald P: Hepatic tumors in childhood. *Clin Radiol 18*:74, 1967.
96. Alcade VM, Traesman HS, Baffles T: Primary carcinoma of the liver in infancy and childhood. *Am J Dis Child 104*:245, 1962.
97. Bartley O, Edlund Y, Helander CG: Angiography in primary hepatic carcinoma. *Acta Radiol (Diagn) 6*:81, 1967.
98. Fredens M: Angiography in primary hepatic tumors in children. *Acta Radiol (Diagn) 8*:193, 1969.
99. Sorsdahl OA and Gay B: Roentgenologic features of a primary carcinoma of the liver in infants and children. *Am J Roentgenol 100*:172, 1967.
100. Novy S, Wallace S, Medellin H, McBride CM: Angiographic evaluation of primary malignant hepatocellular tumors in children. *Am J Roentgenol 120*:353, 1974.

101. Marks WM, Jacobs RP, Goodman PC, Lim RC Jr: Hepatocellular carcinoma: clinical and angiographic findings and predictability for surgical resection. *Am J Roentgenol 132*:7, 1979.
102. Okuda K, Obata H, Jinnouchi S, Kubo Y, Nagasaki Y, Shimokawa Y, Motoike Y, Moto H: Angiographic assessment of gross anatomy of hepatocellular carcinoma: comparison of celiac angiograms and liver pathology in 100 cases. *Radiology 123*:21, 1973.
103. Kunslinger F, Federle MP, Moss AA, Marks W: Computed tomography of hepatocellular carcinoma. *Am J Roentgenol 134*:431, 1980.
104. Itai Y, Nishikawa J, Tasaka A: Computed tomography in the evaluation of hepatocellular carcinoma. *Radiology 131*:165, 1979.
105. Inamoto K, Sugiki K, Yamasaki H, Miura T: CT of hepatoma: effects of portal vein obstruction. *Am J Roentgenol 136*:349, 1981.
106. Moss AA, Schrumpf J. Schnyder P, Korobkin M, Shimshak R: Computed tomography of focal hepatic lesions: a blind clinical evaluation of the effect of contrast enhancement. *Radiology 131*:427, 1979.
107. Biello DR, Levitt RG, Siegel BA, Sagel SS, Stanley RJ: Computed tomography and radionuclide imaging of the liver: a comparative evaluation. *Radiology 127*:159, 1978.
108. McNulty JR: *Radiology of the Liver*. W. B. Saunders, Philadelphia, 1977, p 368.
109. McDermott WV Jr, Greenberger NJ, Isselbacher KJ, Weber AL: Major hepatic resections; diagnostic techniques and metabolic problems. *Surgery 54*:56, 1963.
110. McDermott WV: Surgery of the liver and portal circulation. *Adv Surg 1*:247, 1967.
111. Foster JH: Survival after liver resection. *Cancer 26*:493, 1970.
112. Balasegaram M: Management of primary liver cell carcinoma. *Am J Surg 130*:33, 1975.
113. Linder GT, Crook JN, Cohn I Jr: Primary liver carcinoma. *Cancer 33*:1624, 1974.
114. Lin TY: Results of 107 hepatic lobectomies with preliminary report on the use of a clamp to reduce blood loss. *Ann Surg 177*:413, 1973.
115. Stanley RJ, Dehner LP, Hesker AE: Primary malignant mesenchymal tumors (mesenchymoma) of the liver in childhood; an angiographic-pathologic study of three cases. *Cancer 32*:973, 1973.
116. Margolis M and Homcy C: Systemic manifestations of hepatoma. *Medicine (Baltimore) 51*:381, 1972.
117. Jordan GL: Neoplasms in the liver. In *Textbook of Surgery*, Subiston DC Jr (Ed). W. B. Saunders, Philadelphia, 1977, p 1225.
118. Pack GT and Islami AH: Metastatic cancer to and from the liver. In *Tumors of the Liver*, Pack GT and Islami AH (Eds). Springer-Verlag, New York, 1970, p 293.
119. Heaston DK, Chuang VP, Wallace S, de Santos LA: Angiographic features of portal vein involvement from metastatic hepatic neoplasms. *Am J Roentgenol 136*:897, 1981.
120. Wirtanen G: A new angiographic technique in the diagnosis of liver tumor. *Radiology 108*:51, 1973.
121. Rösch J, Freeny P, Antonovic R, Gutierrez OH: Infusion hepatic angiography in diagnosis of liver metastases. *Cancer 38*:2278, 1976.
122. Priest RJ and Berk JE: Metastatic and other tumors, Part 2: Tumors of the liver. In *Gastroenterology*, Bockus HL (Ed). W. B. Saunders, Philadelphia, 1976, p 535.
123. Healy JE: Vascular patterns in human metastatic liver tumors. *Surg Gynecol Obstet 120*:1187, 1965.
124. Ginaldi S, Bernardino ME, Jing B-S, Green B: Ultrasonographic patterns of hepatic lymphoma. *Radiology 136*:427, 1980.
125. Zornoza J and Ginaldi S: Computed tomography in hepatic lymphoma. *Radiology 138*:405,1981.

126. Ansfield FJ, Ramirez G, Davis HL Jr, Wirtanen GW, Johnson RO, Bryan GT, Manalo FB, Borden EC, Davis TE, Esmaili ME: Further clinical studies with intrahepatic arterial infusion with 5-fluorouracil. *Cancer 36*:2413, 1975.
127. Oberfield RA, McCaffrey JA, Polio T, Clouse ME, Hamilton T: Prolonged and continuous percutaneous intra-arterial hepatic infusion chemotherapy in advanced liver adenocarcinoma from colorectal primary. *Cancer 44*:414, 1979.
128. Petreck JA and Minton JP: Treatment of hepatic metastases by percutaneous hepatic arterial infusion. *Cancer 43*:2182, 1979.
129. Grafe TB, Vassilopoulos PP, Shingleton WW, Jubert AB, Elias EG, Aust JB, Moss SE: Results of prospective randomized study of hepatic artery infusion with 5-fluorouracil versus intravenous 5-fluorouracil in patients with hepatic metastases from colorectal cancer. A Central Oncology Group study. *Surgery 86*:550, 1979.
130.. Sullivan RD: Rationale of protracted arterial infusion therapy and conduct of treatment. In *Clinical Cancer Chemotherapy Including Ambulatory Infusion*, Sullivan RD, (Ed). Charles C Thomas, Springfield, Ill, 1970.
131. Ensminger WD, Rosowsky A, Raso V, Levin DC, Glode M, Come S, Steele G, Frei E III: A clinical-pharmacological evaluation of hepatic arterial infusions of 5-fluoro-2 deoxyuridine and 5-fluorouracil. *Cancer Res 38*:3784, 1978.
132. Patt Z, Wallace S, Hersh EM, Hall SW, Ben Menachem Y, Granmayel M, McBride CM, Benjamin RS, Mavligit GM: Hepatic arterial infusion of corynebacterium parvum and chemotherapy. *Surg Gynecol Obstet 147*:897, 1978.
133. Patt YZ, Mavligit GM, Chuang VP, Wallace S, Johnston S, Benjamin RS, Valdivieso M, Hersh EM: Percutaneous hepatic arterial infusion (HAI) of mitomycin C and floxuridine (FUDR): an effective treatment for metastatic colorectal carcinoma in the liver. *Cancer 46*:261–265, 1980.
134. Calvo DB, Patt YZ, Wallace S, Chuang VP, Benjamin RS, Pritchard JD, Hersh EM, Bodey GP Sr, Mavligit GM: Phase I-II trial of percutaneous intra-arterial cis-diamminedichloro platinum(II) for regionally confined malignancy. *Cancer 45*:1278, 1980.
135. Patt YZ, Wallace S, Freireich EJ, Chuang VP, Hersh EM, Mavligit GM: The palliative role of hepatic arterial infusion and arterial occlusion in colorectal carcinoma metastatic to the liver. *Lancet*, 1980.
136. Chuang VP and Wallace S: Hepatic arterial redistribution for intra-arterial infusion of hepatic neoplasms. *Radiology 135*:295, 1980.
137. Ackerman NB, Lien WM, Kondi ES, et al: The blood supply of experimental liver metastases. The distribution of hepatic artery and portal vein blood to small and large tumors. *Surgery 66*:1067, 1969.
138. Chuang VP, Wallace S, Stroehlein J, Yap H-Y, Patt YZ: Hepatic artery infusion chemotherapy: gastric duodenal complications. *Am J Roentgenol 137*:347, 1981.
139. Nilsson LAC and Zettergren L: Blood supply and vascular pattern of induced primary hepatic carcinoma in rats. *Acta Pathol Microbiol Scand 71*:179, 1967.
140. Gianturco C, Anderson JH, Wallace S: Mechanical device for arterial occlusion. *Am J Roentgenol 124*:428, 1975.
141. Wallace S, Gianturco C, Anderson JH, Goldstein HM, Davis LJ, Bree RL: Therapeutic vascular occlusion utilizing steel coil technique: clinical applications. *Am J Roentgenol 127*:381, 1976.
142. Anderson JH, Wallace S, Gianturco C, Gerson RP: ''Mini'' Gianturco stainless steel coils for transcatheter vascular occlusion. *Radiology 132*:301, 1979.
143. Chuang VP, Wallace S, Gianturco C: A new improved coil for tapered tip catheter for arterial occlusion. *Radiology 135*:507, 1980.
144. Madding GF and Kennedy PA: Hepatic artery ligation. *Surg Clin North Am 52*:719, 1972.
145. Markowitz J: The hepatic artery. *Surg Gynecol Obstet 95*:644, 1952.

146. Gelin LE, Lewis DH, Nilsson L: Liver blood flow in man during abdominal surgery. *Acta Hepato-splenol 15*:21, 1968.
147. Lee YTN: Nonsystemic treatment of metastatic tumors of the liver—a review. *Med Pediatr Oncol 4*:185, 1978.
148. Mori W, Masuda M, Miyanaga T: Hepatic artery ligation and tumor necrosis in the liver. *Surgery 59*:359, 1966.
149. Koehler RE, Korobkin M, Lewis F: Arteriographic demonstration of collateral flow of the liver after hepatic artery ligation. *Radiology 117*:49, 1975.
150. Chuang VP and Wallace S: Hepatic artery embolization in the treatment of hepatic neoplasms. *Radiology 140*:51, 1981.
151. Charnsangavej C, Chuang VP, Wallace S: Collateral circulation after hepatic artery occlusion. *Radiology*. (In press.)
152. Shivshanker K, Soo CS, Chuang VP, Wallace S: Post hepatic embolization syndrome: review of 34 cases. (Submitted for publication.)
153. Donnegan WL, Harris HS, Spratt JS: Prolonged continuous hepatic infusion. *Arch Surg 99*:149, 1969.
154. Pestana C, Reitemeier RJ, Moertel CG, Judd ES, Dockerty MB: The natural history of carcinoma of the colon and rectum. *Am J Surg 108*:826, 1964.
155. Fischerman K, Petersen L, Jensen LS, Christensen KC, Epsen F: Survival among patients with liver metastases from carcinoma of colon and rectum. *Scand J Gastroenterol Suppl 37*:111, 1976.
156. Rappaport AH and Burleson RL: Survival of patients with systemic fluorouracil for hepatic metastases. *Surg Gynecol Obstet 130*:773, 1970.
157. Wallace S: Liver, spleen, and pancreas. In *Diagnostic Roentgenology of Radiotherapy Changes*, Libshitz H (Ed). Williams & Wilkins, Baltimore, 1979, p 101.
158. Case JJ and Warthin AS: The occurrence of hepatic lesions in patients treated by intensive deep roentgen irradiation. *Am J Roentgenol 12*:27, 1924.
159. Ingold JA, Reed GB, Kaplan HS, Bagshaw MA: Radiation hepatitis. *Am J Roentgenol 93*:200, 1965.
160. Kaplan HS and Bagshaw MA: Radiation hepatitis: possible prevention by combined isotopic and external radiation therapy. *Radiology 91*:1214, 1968.
161. Lansing AM, Davis WM, Brizel HE: Radiation hepatitis. *Arch Surg 96*:878, 1968.
162. Tefft M, Mitus A, Das L, Filler RM: Irradiation of the liver in children: review of experience in acute and chronic phases, and in the intact normal and partially resected. *Am J Roentgenol 108*:365, 1970.
163. Warren S: Effects of radiation on normal tissue. *Arch Pathol 34*:749, 1942.
164. Wharton JT, Delclos L, Gallager S, Smith JP: Radiation hepatitis induced by abdominal irradiation with cobalt 60 moving strip technique. *Am J Roentgenol 117*:73, 1973.
165. Filler RM, Tefft M, Vawter GF, Maddock C, Minus A: Hepatic lobectomy in childhood: effect of x-rays and chemotherapy. *J Pediatr Surg 4*:31, 1969.
166. Nolan TR, Grady ED, Crumbley AJ, LaRose JH, Cheek WV: Internal hepatic radiotherapy: I and II. *Am J Roentgenol 124*:590, 1975.
167. Ackerman LV: The pathology of radiation effect of normal and neoplastic tissue. *Am J Roentgenol 144*:447, 1972.
168. Witcofski RL, Pizzarello DJ, Everhart H: Repair and latent injury in rat liver after x-irradiation. *Radiology 105*:1975, 1972.
169. Anyama K, Fausto N, Tamvakopoulos E, VanLancker JL: Effects of x-irradiation on amino acid incorporation into regenerating liver proteins. *Radiat Res 42*:528, 1970.
170. Dettmer CM, Kramer S, Driscoll DH, Aponte GE: A comparison of the chronic effects of irradiation upon the normal, damaged and regenerating rat liver. *Radiology 91*:993, 1968.

171. Fabrikant JI: Radiation response in relation to the cell cycle in vivo. *Am J Roentgenol 105*:734, 1969.
172. Nebesar RA, Tefft M, Vawter GF, Filler RM: Angiography in radiation "hepatitis." *Br J Radiol 47*:588, 1974.
173. Spencer RP and Kligerman MM: Scan evidence of hepatic "refunction" after tumor irradiation. *J Nucl Med 11*:140, 1970.
174. Okuda K and Iio M: *Radiologic Aspects of the Liver and Biliary Tract*. Year Book Medical Publishers, Chicago, 1976.

27

Additional Experience with Hepatic Embolization: Endocrine Metastases

David J. Allison
Hammersmith Hospital and Royal Postgraduate Medical School
London, England

Introduction

Therapeutic hepatic embolization is the deliberate occlusion of branches of the hepatic artery by emboli injected through a selectively sited catheter. Embolization often provides an alternative form of treatment to surgery and is particularly useful in the liver, where the surgical management of deeply placed lesions or those involving vascular structures may be exceedingly difficult and dangerous. Another factor making the liver an appropriate organ for embolic therapy is the fact that its dual blood supply (systemic arterial and portal venous) protects it from infarction following arterial occlusion. Portal venous blood accounts for approximately 70% of the total liver blood flow in humans, and normal liver cells can apparently survive on portal blood alone. It is a convenient fact that whereas tumor cells usually arrive in the liver via the portal circulation, they commonly obtain their blood supply for growth from the hepatic arterial circulation; this means that embolization of the hepatic artery can induce selective necrosis of metastatic hepatic tumors while leaving normal liver relatively unaffected.

Surgical Ligation or Embolization

It might be supposed that surgical ligation or division of the hepatic artery (1) would achieve the same end result as embolization and achieve this in a more permanent way. There are, however, several reasons why this is not the case.

1. In the treatment of acute hepatic bleeding or in the case of a vascular malformation in the liver, it is possible by means of arteriography to identify the vessels supplying the lesions before embolization and ensure that they have all been occluded together with any other potential collateral sources of blood supply. This is particularly important in the liver, where anomalies of the arterial supply are very common (2,3).

2. Even a simple surgical ligation will require general anesthesia and an abdominal incision; both carry increased risks, particularly in patients in whom massive hepatomegaly may compromise respiratory excursion and may lead to pulmonary collapse and infection in the postoperative period. Endocrine metastases producing hormones affecting the cardiovascular and respiratory systems pose a particularly difficult problem for the anesthetist.

3. Mainstem hepatic arterial ligation is not an effective means of producing vascular occlusion, owing to the large number of potential collateral arterial routes to and within the liver (3–5). Michels (3) has shown that at least 26 such collateral pathways exist, and these may continue to feed a vascular malformation or tumor in the liver following ligation of the hepatic artery. Embolization obviates this problem by showering the peripheral arterial tree with minute emboli so that no vascular bed exists for any potential collateral sources to supply.

4. Hepatic artery ligation usually precludes any subsequent attempt at devascularizing the liver either by surgery or embolization should metastases recur or new deposits appear. A successful surgical attack on all collateral blood vessels is out of the question, and renewed blood supply may well derive from unusual vessels which may be impossible to catheterize selectively in the presence of a ligated mainstem artery. With the embolization method the procedure can be repeated as often as is considered necessary to deal with recanalized vessels or with intrahepatic collateral channels supplying recurrent tumor or new deposits.

Indications for Hepatic Artery Embolization

There are three principal situations in which hepatic embolization may prove useful: (1) the treatment of hepatic arterial and arteriovenous malformations (congenital or acquired); (2) the management of hepatic trauma, and (3) the treatment of hepatic tumors (primary or secondary).

Vascular Malformations

Vascular malformations or aneurysms in the liver may cause bleeding, pain, space occupation, or cardiac failure due to arteriovenous shunting. Embolization can be used to prevent or treat these developments and is usually effective and safe. Figure 1 shows the embolization of a liver that was the site of massive arteriovenous shunting in a case of hereditary hemorrhagic telangiectasia. The embolization successfully alleviated symptoms of cardiac failure attributable to the hemodynamic effects of the hepatic shunting.

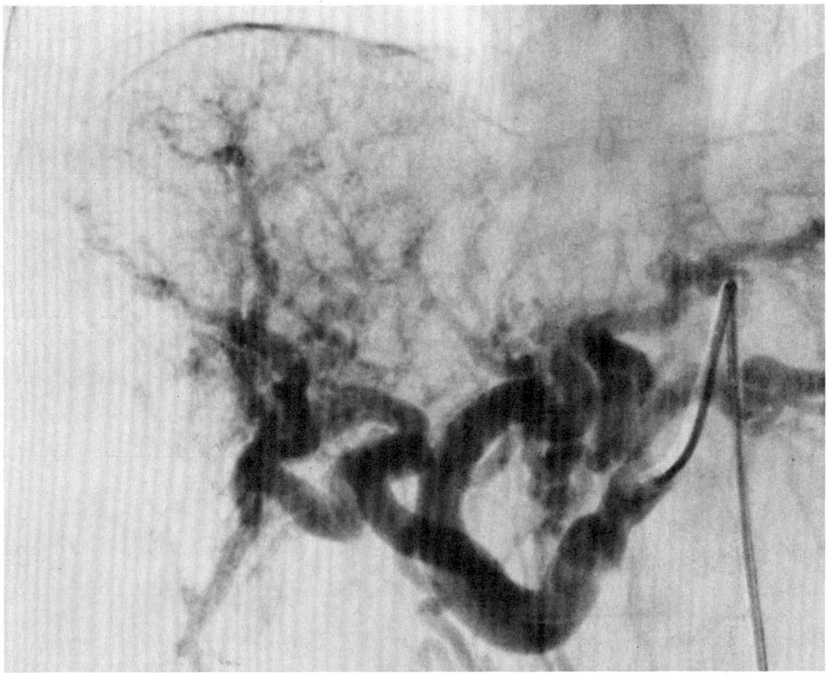

(A)

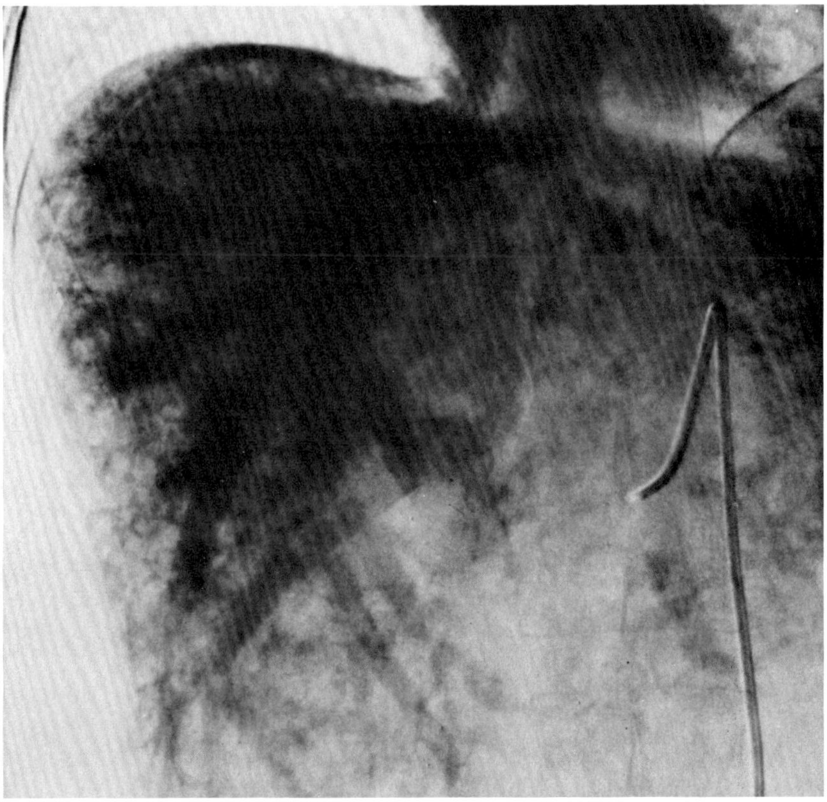

(B)

Figure 1

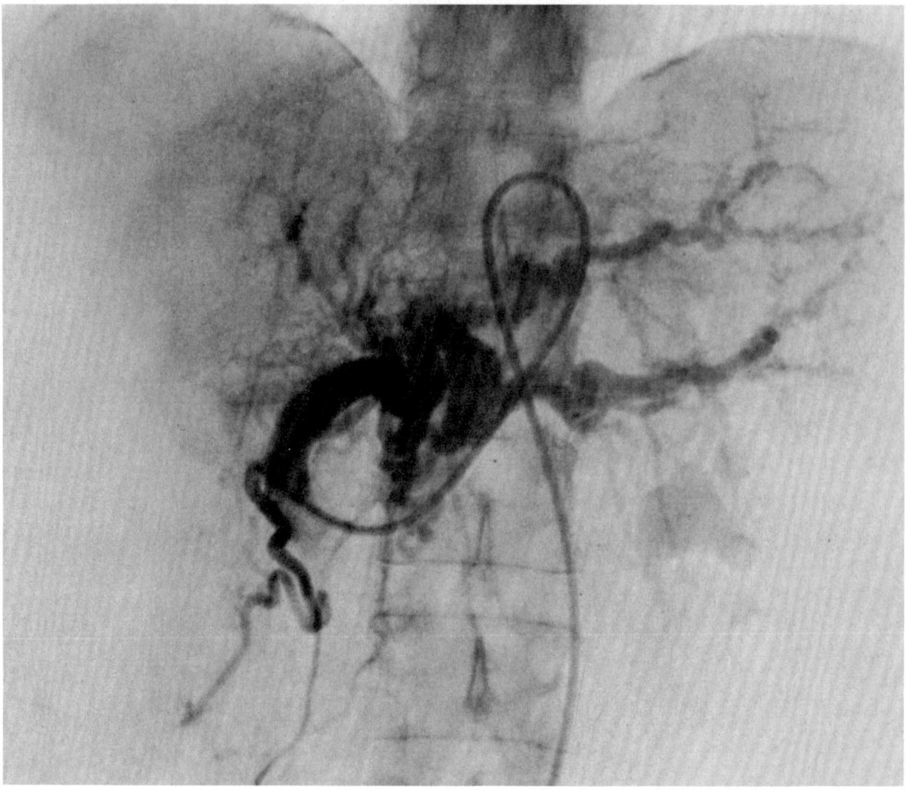

(C)

Figure 1 Embolization of hepatic arteriovenous communications in a patient in cardiac failure. (A) Selective hepatic arteriogram in a woman with multiple hereditary telangiectasia. The vessels are enlarged and tortuous. (B) Same study: later phase. Massive arteriovenous (AV) shunting in the liver; the hepatic veins are grossly enlarged and fill with contrast medium within seconds of the arterial injection. (C) The right hepatic artery has been embolized with gelatin sponge and human dura mater (Lyodura, David and Geck Ltd.). The AV shunting in the right lobe was abolished, with dramatic improvement in the condition of the patient.

Hepatic Trauma

Embolization can be used to control bleeding produced by blunt or penetrating injury to the liver (6,7), liver biopsy (8–10), or surgery (11,12). It is particularly useful in the management of bleeding from sites relatively inaccessible to the surgeon, in patients with associated diseases that would make hepatic surgery particularly undesirable (e.g., bleeding diatheses, cardiorespiratory disease, jaundice, etc.), and in centers where the services of an experienced hepatic surgeon are not available.

Figure 2 shows the embolization of an iatrogenic hepatic artery aneurysm. The artery had been damaged and repaired during hepatic surgery 6 weeks previously, and embolization successfully controlled a life-threatening hemorrhage that ensued when the artery ruptured at the site of aneurysm repair.

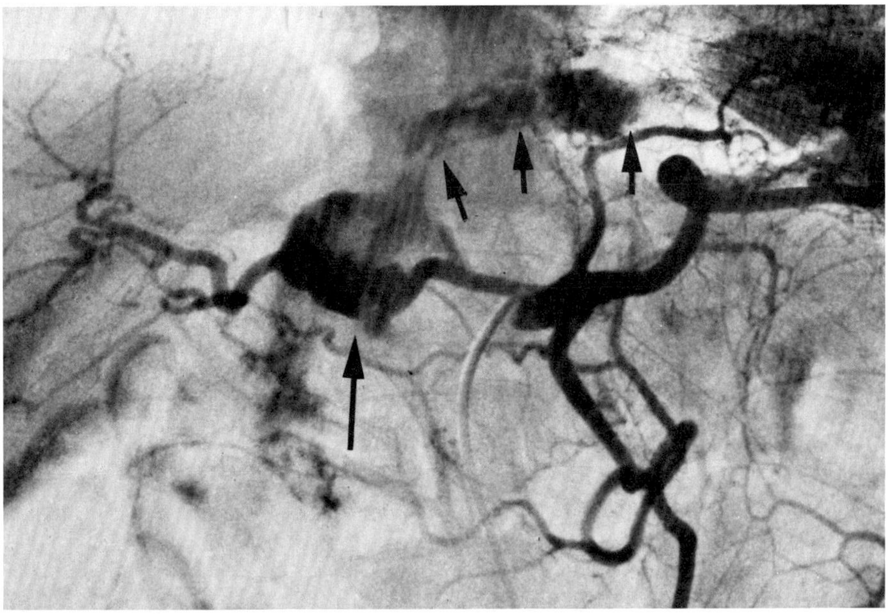

(A)

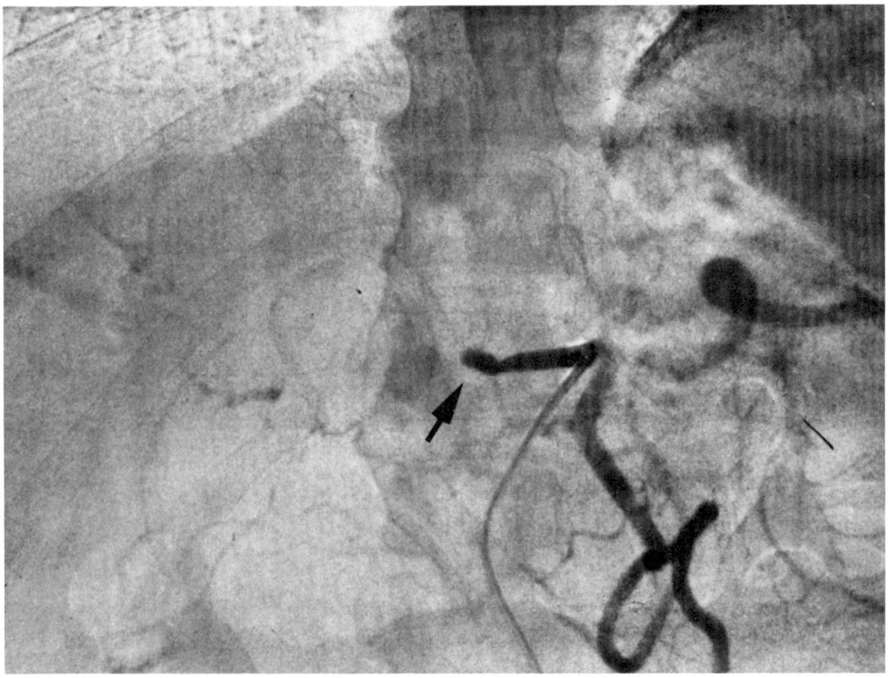

(B)

Figure 2 Embolization of a hepatic aneurysm. Left hepatic lobar resection for a solitary tumor 6 weeks previously, now life-threatening hematemesis. (A) Celiac arteriogram. Contrast medium is seen leaking from a false aneurysm (long arrow) and tracking along the bed of the liver to the fundus of the stomach (short arrows). (B) Postembolization arteriogram. The hepatic artery has been embolized with isobutyl-2-cyanoacrylate (arrow). No further bleeding occurred. The patient remains well 18 months later. (Reproduced with permission of the editor of the *British Journal of Hospital Medicine*.)

Hepatic Tumors

Embolization may be used in the management of benign and malignant primary liver tumors. It is, however, employed most commonly in the management of metastatic disease.

Embolization of Primary Tumors

Embolization is indicated where other methods of treatment, such as partial hepatectomy or radiotherapy, would be inappropriate or have already proved ineffective. Figure 3 illustrates the angiographic workup and the effect of embolization in a patient with a hepatic hemangioma.

The use and value of embolic therapy of primary malignant tumors of the liver are discussed fully in Chapter 26.

Embolization in Metastatic Disease

Not only will embolization alleviate pain or discomfort caused by the local effects of large deposits in the liver, but also, in the case of *functioning endocrine tumors*, it will reduce or abolish the adverse humoral effects associated with these neoplasms. The metastases arising from endocrine tumors, such as carcinoids, glucagonomas, insulinomas, and other apudomas, may be very slow growing and patients may survive for several years after secondary spread of such tumors is known to have occurred.

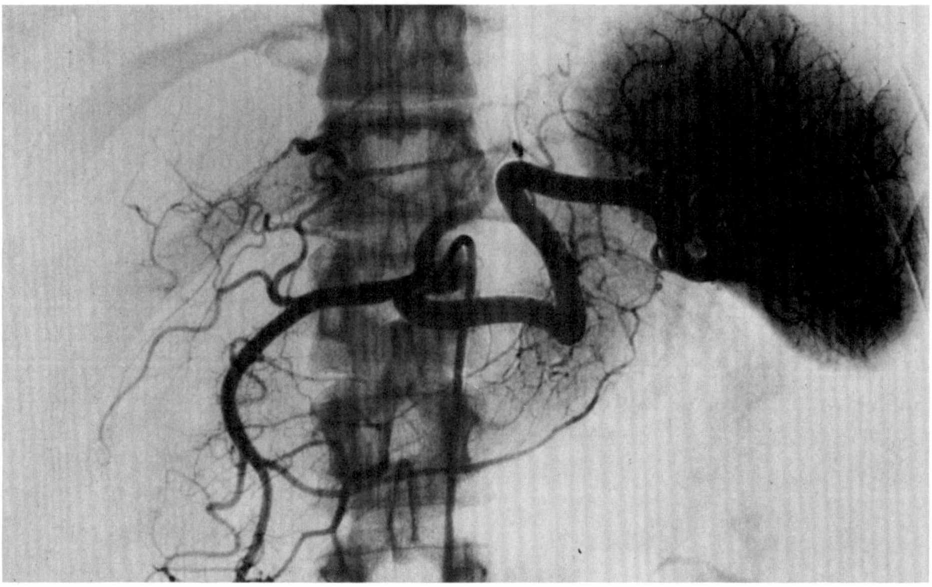

(A)

Figure 3 Embolization of hepatic hemangioma, previously diagnosed by laparotomy and biopsy. (A) Celiac angiogram shows a normal appearance of the liver, but the right hepatic artery is small, suggesting the existence of a dominant accessory artery. (B) Same study: late phase showing normal indirect splenoportogram. It is important to demonstrate a normal portal flow if arterial embolization is contemplated. (C) Same patient: the principal right hepatic artery arises from the superior mesenteric artery and supplies a large vascular tumor. (D) Same study: late phase showing abnormal vascular filling in the hemangioma. (E) The anomalous hepatic artery has been selectively catheterized and embolized with human dura mater (Lyodura, Davis and Geck Ltd.). The superior mesenteric supply to the gut is unimpaired.

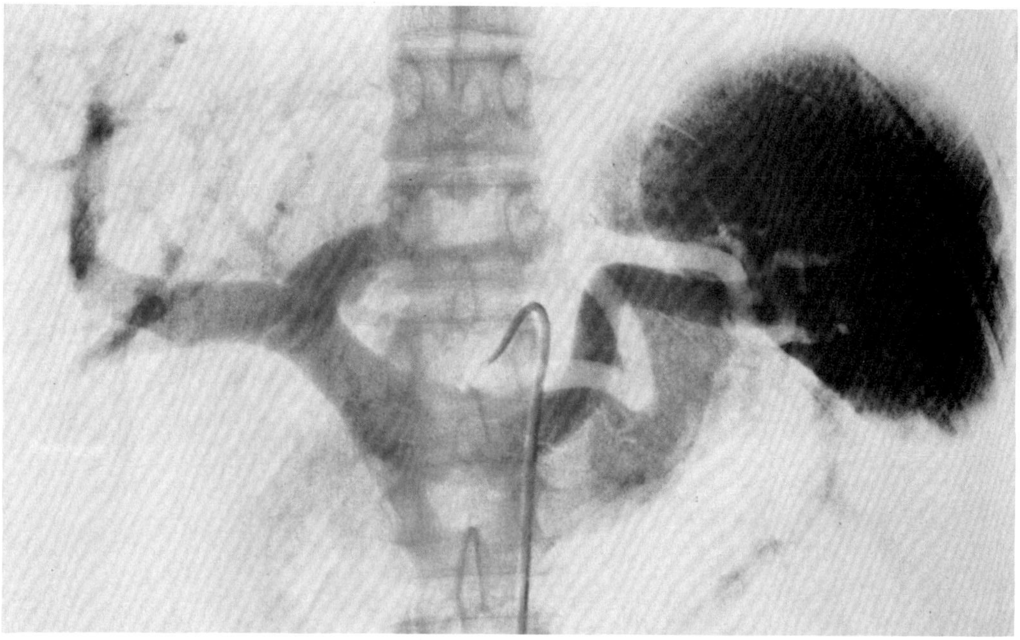

(B)

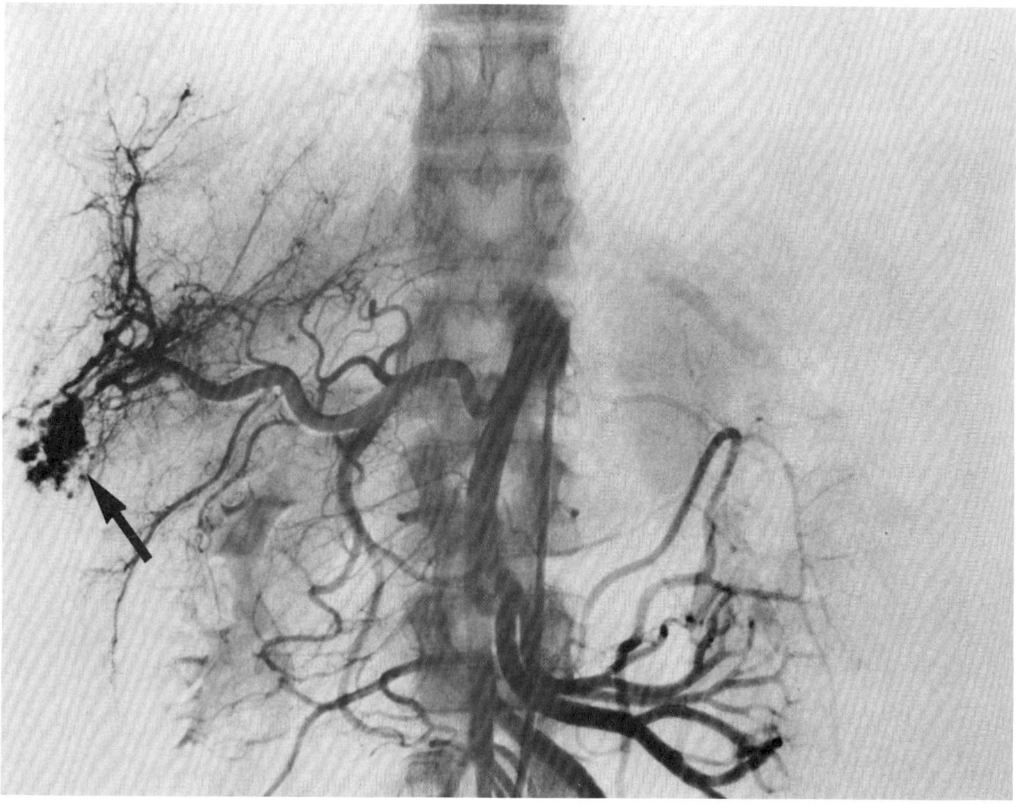

(C)

Figure 3 (continued)

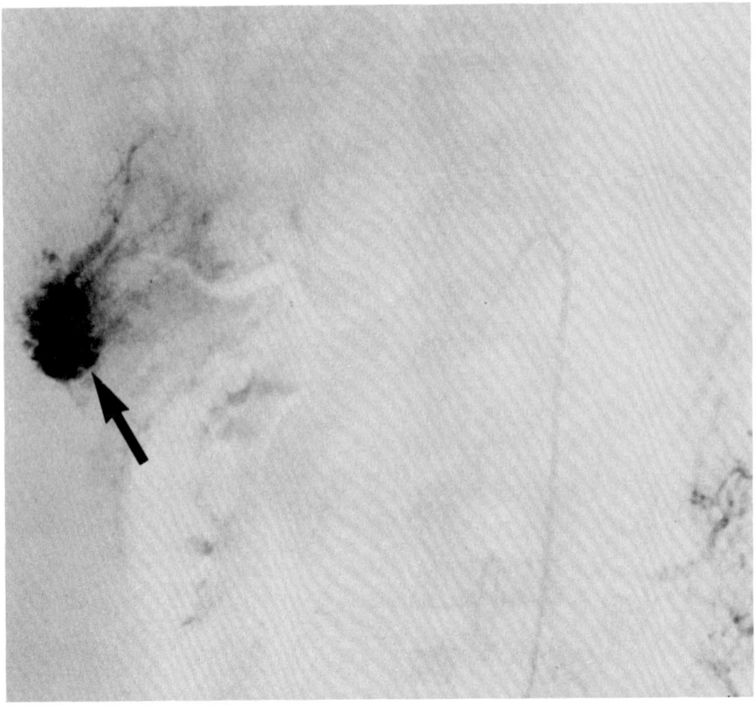

(D)

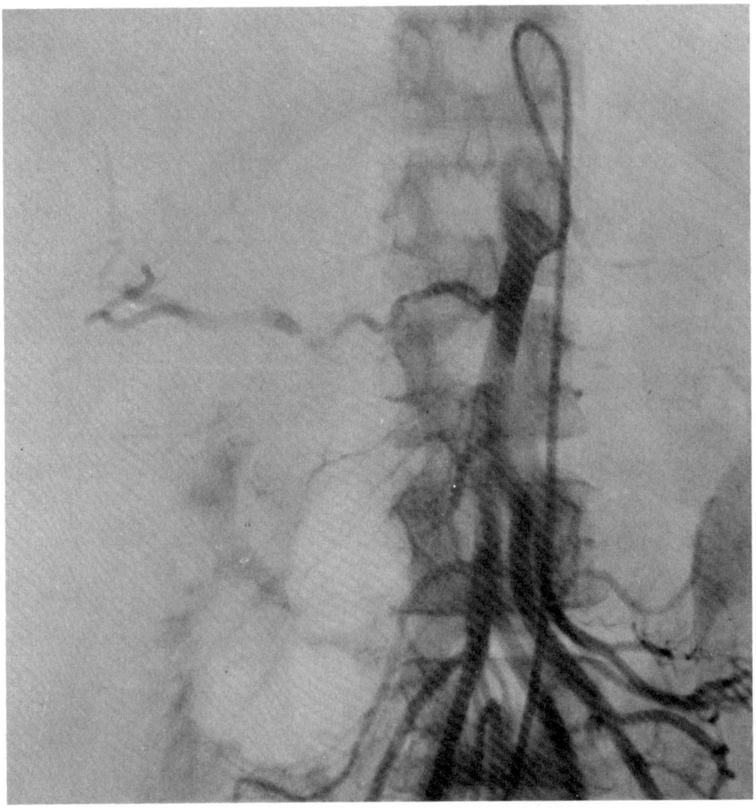

(E)

Figure 3 (continued)

Management of Functioning Endocrine Tumor Metastases

The patient may have to endure extremely unpleasant symptoms caused by the overproduction of hormone by the secondary tumor. The nature of these symptoms will depend on the predominant hormone produced by the tumor, but typical effects include severe flushing attacks, bronchospasm, cardiac dysfunction, marked fluctuation in blood pressure, skin rashes, diabetes, and diarrhea. In the later stages of the disease symptoms referable to the local effects of the hepatic tumor deposits occur. These include pain or abdominal discomfort, dyspnea due to splinting of the diaphragm by massive hepatomegaly, portal vein occlusion, and obstruction of the inferior vena cava. Although the ultimate prognosis is poor once the liver metastases have become established, palliation of symptoms is clearly important, particularly in the early stages of secondary disease, when increased hormonal activity may be the only adverse effect experienced by the patient.

Since the metastases from apudomas are usually multiple, partial hepatectomy (13) or tumor enucleation are not usually practicable; radiotherapy is also of limited value in the management of endocrine tumors, and at the present time palliation in inoperable cases is best achieved by the use of pharmacological antagonists to the tumor metabolites, chemotherapy (given either systemically or by local infusion), embolization of the vascular supply to the tumor (14,15), or a combination of these methods. Whether the primary tumor has been resected or not is a factor which does not usually influence the decision to embolize the liver, since the total mass of the liver deposits commonly exceeds considerably that of the primary tumor (which in some cases may never even have been located). It is preferable, on general therapeutic principles, to have histological proof of the nature of the liver deposits before proceeding to embolization; in many cases, however, the weight of circumstantial evidence from previous diagnostic tests will be sufficient to proceed with embolization on the basis of a clinical decision. Embolization may be used prior to, as an adjunct to, or following the use of pharmacological antagonists or chemotherapeutic agents, and there are as yet no controlled trials comparing the efficacy of these different possible regimens. Such trials would be exceedingly difficult to conduct and interpret due to the very variable degree of malignancy of endocrine tumors and the unpredictable nature of their clinical course. The precise way in which such drugs may be used in conjunction with hepatic embolization is therefore best decided in accordance with the particular circumstances of each case and the preference and expertise of the physician or surgeon concerned.

Technique of Embolization

Patient Preparation

The patient is starved on the morning of the procedure and informed consent is obtained. General anesthesia is necessary in children, but adequate premedication with a sedative and an analgesic is normally sufficient in adults. Depending on the tumor type, it may be necessary to treat the patient with an appropriate pharmacological antagonist to minimize the effects of sudden variations in hormone production during the process of embolization and the ensuing period of tumor necrosis. Carcinoid tumors are particularly liable to release vasoactive amines and patients with these neoplasms are pretreated with antagonists such as cyproheptadine and p-chlorophenylalanine, and this therapy is continued for a variable period following the embolization, depending on the clinical response. All patients should have estimates of pre- and postembolization blood levels (and/or urinary levels where appropriate), in order to assess the effect of the procedure on tumor function. A mixture of prophylactic antibiotics is given with the premedication and continued for at least 6 days after embolization; the drugs given will depend on current antibiotic practice, but a typical regime might include tobramycin, flucloxacillin, and metronidazole. At the start of the procedure, an intravenous infusion line is inserted for the rapid administration of drugs; an experienced physician should be in attendance to monitor systemic blood pressure, heart rate, and cardiac rhythm, and to take appropriate measures if fluctuations in hormone production should cause dangerous disturbances in these variables.

Angiography

The celiac axis is usually catheterized using a percutaneous femoral approach and the initial study consists of a general celiac injection with early- and late-phase films. This gives information concerning the site and vascularity of the tumor deposits, the arterial anatomy of the liver, and in the late films, the state of the portal circulation. If the intrahepatic branches of the portal vein are compressed by the metastases, it is probably wise not to proceed to embolization. This is because occlusion of the hepatic artery in the presence of portal obstruction might completely deprive the liver of its blood supply and lead to massive hepatic necrosis. Assuming that the portal circulation is adequate and the decision to embolize the liver has been made, the hepatic artery is selectively catheterized, the catheter tip being ideally sited distal to the origin of the gastroduodenal artery. It is important to ascertain that all the hepatic arterial supply has, in fact, been identified since there is a great deal of variation in the normal anatomy; if there is any doubt, a selective superior mesenteric angiogram must also be performed to demonstrate any accessory supply to the right lobe. If such a vessel exists and is supplying tumor deposits, it must be catheterized subselectively since emboli must not be allowed to enter the superior mesenteric artery (see Fig. 3).

Embolization

Any degree of embolization of the liver can be performed, from the selective embolization of a single deposit, to the complete embolization of one or both lobes. The extent of the embolization will depend on the general state of the patient, liver function, the size and distribution of the deposits, the vascular anatomy of the liver, the degree of patency of the portal circulation, and the confidence, experience, and skill of the embolist.

Embolic Materials

Many different agents are available: these include sterile absorbable gelatin sponge (sterispon), oxidized cellulose (Oxycel), lyophilized human dura mater (Lyodura), steel coils, Invalon, detachable balloons, and rapidly setting polymers such as isobutyl-2-cyanoacrylate. The appropriate application of these different materials to particular vascular situations or specific clinical circumstances has been examined by many investigators (16–19), but there have as yet been no comparative studies to indicate which embolic material would be most suitable for the management of liver metastases. The agent employed may be long-lasting in its effect, with the object of achieving permanent obliteration of the hepatic arterial bed. It is important that at least some of the emboli should be small enough to reach the very small arteries and arterioles that supply the tumor; simply occluding large vessels is not enough (5) because of the rich potential collateral circulation available. For this reason relatively large emboli such as steel coils are probably unsuitable unless used in combination with smaller embolic particles. Finely chopped human dura mater (Lyodura) is effective in blocking peripheral tumor vessels, and this can be followed if desired by a combination of dura mater with larger particles such as Gelfoam; the dura mater gives a more permanent quality to the mixture.

The embolizing mixture is suspended in contrast medium and a broad-spectrum antibiotic can be added to this mixture if desired to reduce the risk of subsequent infection. The suspension is then injected under continuous fluoroscopic control. As with all embolization procedures, it is extremely important to avoid the reflux of embolic areas outside the vascular bed under attack. This is best achieved by injecting the embolic suspension in the form of multiple small increments rather than in a few large boluses. An additional safety precaution is provided by video monitoring if this facility is available; each phase of the embolization can then be recorded and its effect immediately reviewed before proceeding to the next injection.

Postembolization

When the embolization procedure has been completed, angiography should be performed to record the extent of the vascular occlusion and to check that flow to neighboring vascular beds has been preserved intact. It is hardly necessary to point out that all embolic material must be cleared from the catheter before this angiography is performed. Figure 4 shows the pre- and postembolization hepatic arteriograms of a patient suffering from metastatic glucagonoma. Note that the tumor circulation has been abolished, but that the flow to other territories (e.g., gastroduodenal) remains uninterrupted. This embolization did produce a dramatic symptomatic improvement: the troublesome skin rash caused by the glucagonoma began to fade within 24 hr of the procedure.

Contraindications

Embolization of the liver should not be performed in the presence of significant jaundice or other evidence of severely disordered liver function, liver sepsis, or portal venous obstruction. It is also inappropriate to use the technique in terminally ill patients, in whom it may simply precipitate a final deterioration. Previous surgical ligation of the hepatic artery is not an absolute contraindication to attempted embolization, but it does make the procedure more difficult to perform and less complete in its effect. This is because the liver metastases in such cases will almost certainly be supplied by collateral vessels such as the phrenic and pancreaticoduodenal arteries, which may prove most difficult to catheterize selectively and embolize.

Complications

The complications of liver embolization may be immediate or delayed.

Immediate Effects

The immediate problems include the potential hazards associated with any catheter procedure, such as arterial dissection, arterial obstruction, hematoma formation, thrombosis, and adverse reactions to intravascular contrast agents. Immediate problems related to the embolization procedure include the inadvertent embolization of extrahepatic vessels, pain, and nausea. The accidental embolization of vessels outside the liver can be avoided by meticulous technique; if it does occur, the vessels most frequently involved are the gastroduodenal artery and the splenic artery. The accidental reflux of a few emboli into either of these territories is fortunately not usually associated with any untoward clinical effects, but this fact cannot be relied upon (particularly with regard to the splenic territory), and it in no way constitutes an excuse for careless technique. Pain or discomfort in the hepatic area frequently follows extensive embolization of liver vessels but is not usually severe, and is readily controlled by standard analgesics. Nausea is an almost inevitable consequence of extensive hepatic embolization and usually requires the parenteral administration of an antiemetic agent at the time of embolization. In the case of neoplasms producing vasoactive substances such as carcinoid tumors, sudden fluctuations in blood pressure and heart rate may occur during the embolization procedure and for several days thereafter as necrosis of the tumor proceeds. These problems can be minimized by appropriate premedication with blocking agents, by careful monitoring of cardiovascular variables during the procedure, and by having the appropriate drugs available to counteract any adverse reactions during the procedure.

Delayed Effects

Delayed effects of embolization may be observed in the days or weeks following the procedure. Most patients will show an elevation of liver enzyme levels during the first few postembolization days. Approximately 12% of patients develop a temporary paralytic ileus, requiring treatment by intravenous fluid and nasogastric aspiration. All these side effects usually subside in the course of the first postembolization week, and most patients make an uneventful recovery thereafter.

Gas in the liver is an occasional phenomenon which may appear in the first 48 hr following embolization. This will be apparent on the plain abdominal radiograph and does not necessarily indicate infection with gas-forming organism. Branching air collections within the embolized tumor could be shown by CT in 11 or 14 postinfarction studies; in no case was an abscess present (20). Although such infections can, of course, occur in embolized organs, it seems that in some cases gas may be released from degenerating blood cells trapped in occluded vessels, a mechanism similar to that which is believed to occur in the fetal circulation following death in utero.

Infection is the most serious delayed complication of liver embolization and may occur in the form of liver abscesses or as a generalized septicemia. Areas of relatively ischemic liver containing foreign particles obviously constitute a favorable culture medium for pathogenic microorganisms which may be introduced at the time of the embolization or may arrive there subsequently in the portal venous blood. The incidence of infection can be minimized by a good aseptic technique during the procedure, by the addition of antibiotics to the embolizing suspension, and by the use of prophylactic systemic antibiotics. The first of these factors is probably the most important.

Gallbladder infarction has been described following hepatic artery embolization (21,22) but is a rare complication; no case of gallbladder necrosis has been observed in over 40 hepatic embolizations performed by the author. In practice, it is not usually possible to avoid embolization of the cystic artery which may arise from the hepatic artery at a point which lies too distal to be spared if complete hepatic arterial occlusion is desired. It may, in many cases, be difficult to identify, particularly as more than one cystic artery is present in a significant proportion of patients (2).

Functioning Endocrine Tumor Metastases Treated by Embolization

Embolization is increasingly employed as a major component of the therapeutic regimen. The marked reduction in the levels of circulating hormone following embolization also attests to the therapeutic efficacy of the technique. What is much more difficult to assess in any quantitative fashion is the improvement in the quality of life that hepatic embolization may confer on patients suffering from this form of metastatic disease in the liver. Any such analysis must rely to some extent on the subjective opinion of the patients themselves, as well as the more objective evidence afforded by clinical examination and the results of biochemical and imaging tests. No adequate controlled trial comparing the benefits of embolization with other forms of treatment has yet been conducted, but the available evidence suggests that some objective improvement will occur in approximately 75% of patients embolized for symptomatic liver deposits, and that subjective improvement will be found in a slightly higher proportion.

Glucagonoma Metastases

Figure 4 has illustrated the prompt response of blood glucagon levels to the embolization of hepatic deposits from a malignant glucagonoma, with levels remaining normal and the patient symptom-free 5 months later. A similar clinical response was shown in another patient whose malignant glucagonoma metastases to the liver were supplied exclusively by an accessory right hepatic artery arising from the superior mesenteric (Fig. 5).

Carcinoid Metastases

A patient with severe flushing attacks and diarrhea and with extensive deposits of carcinoid in the liver has responded promptly to embolization and has remained asymptomatic over the last 18 months (Fig. 6).

Even when relatively short acting embolic materials (such as Gelfoam) have been used and recanalization of the hepatic artery has occurred, the marked reduction in the levels of urinary 5-hydroxyindoleacetic acid (5-HIAA) as well as the clinical improvement of the patient have continued. This favorable clinical response has been maintained even though repeat arteriography has demonstrated that metastases, although markedly reduced in size and vascularity, were still present in the liver (Figs. 7, 8). Any later deterioration of the clinical status of these patients will probably respond to further embolization through the recanalized hepatic artery.

The permanent occlusion of the hepatic artery by surgical ligation is undesirable, as it will be followed rapidly by the development of a collateral blood supply to the growing metastases and may render subsequent attempts at embolization difficult or impossible. Figure 9 illustrates the problems created by the surgical ligation of the hepatic artery.

Calcitonin-Producing Metastases

In a rare case of liver metastases from a calcitonin-producing thyroid tumor, presenting with severe diarrhea, embolization considerably improved the patient's symptoms (Fig. 10).

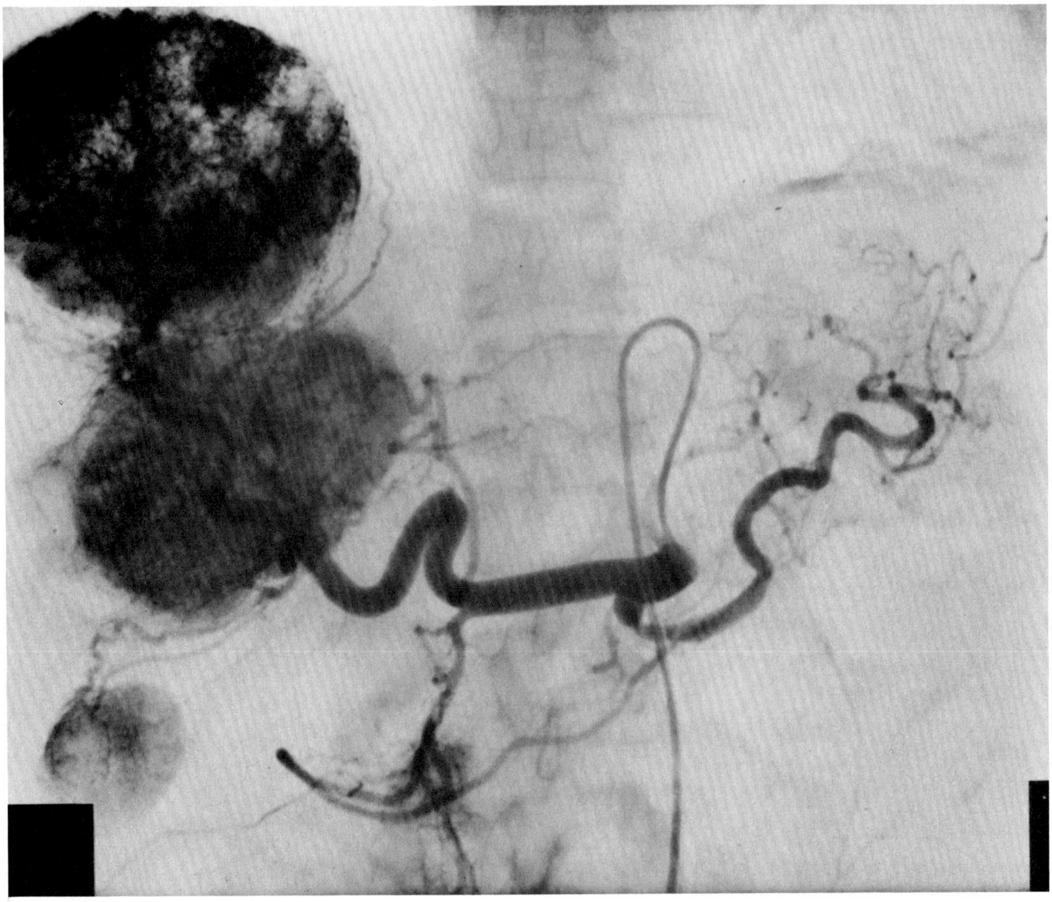

(A)

Figure 4 Embolization of malignant glucagonoma metastases. (A) Celiac arteriogram in patient with a malignant pancreatic glucagonoma and liver metastases. (B) Same study: the vascular deposits are very conspicuous in the capillary phase. (C) The hepatic arterial supply to the tumor deposits has been embolized with particles of human dura mater. (D) Graph showing the changes in blood levels of glucagon, gastrin, and pancreatic polypeptide following embolization of this and other endocrine metastases. Note that the blood glucagon level fell to the normal range within 12 hr of the procedure. It was still normal 5 months later, and the patient is symptom-free, having previously suffered from an intractable skin rash. (Reproduced with permission of Churchill Livingstone Ltd.)

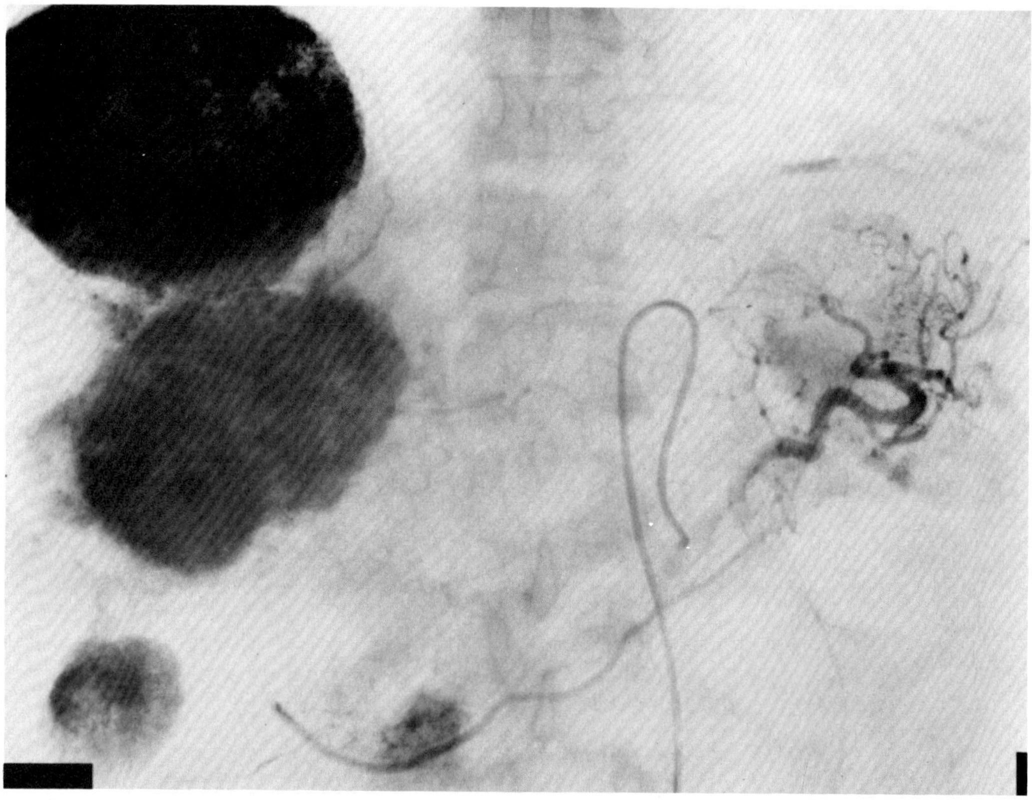

(B)

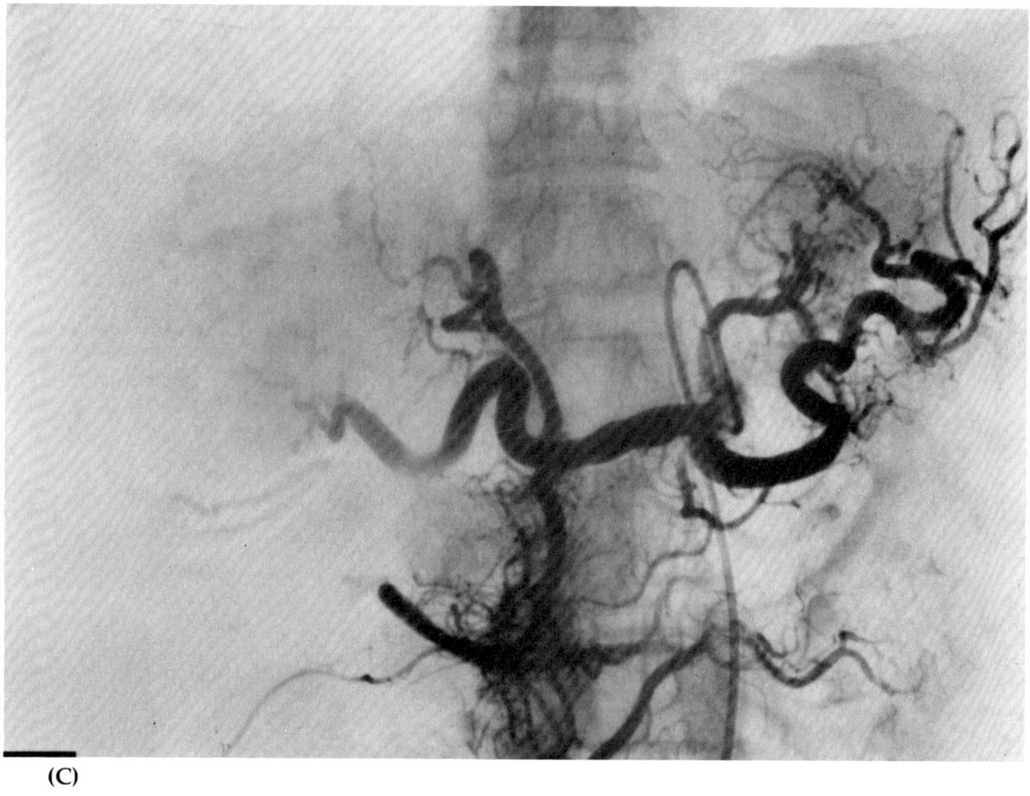

(C)

Figure 4

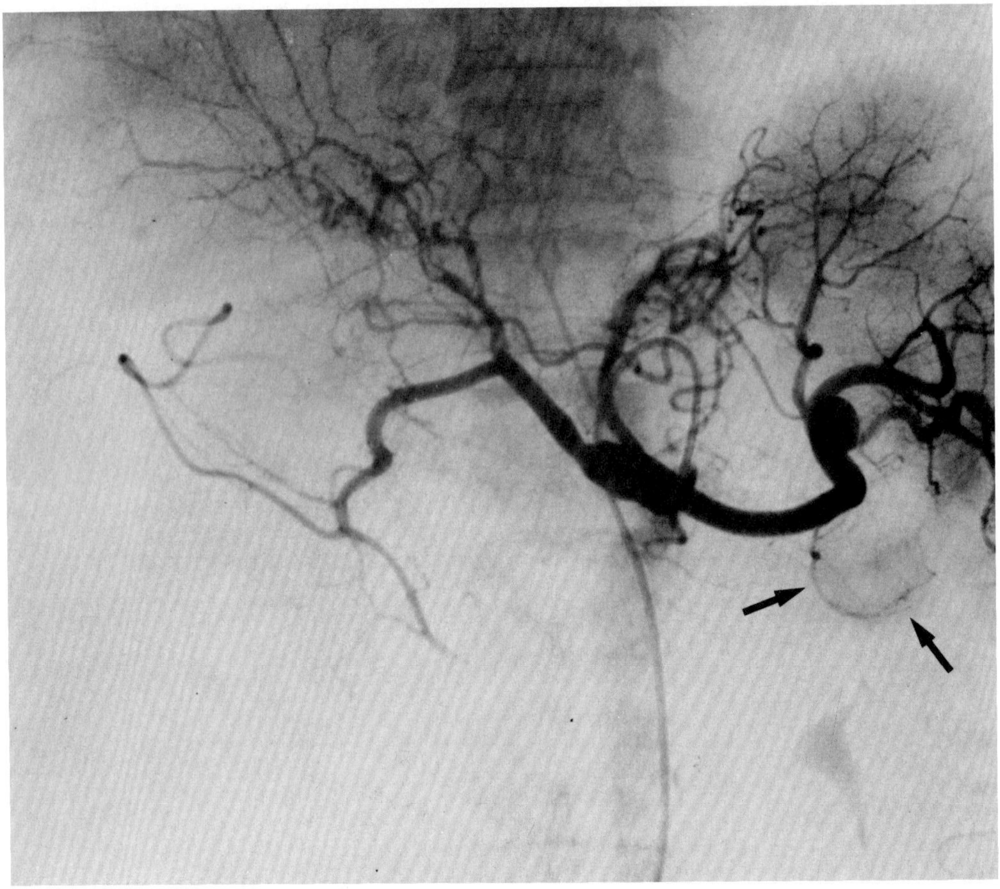

(A)

Figure 5 Embolization of malignant glucagonoma metastases. (A) Celiac arteriogram in a man with glucagonoma syndrome. The primary tumor is seen in the pancreatic tail (arrows). There are no obvious hepatic metastases but note that the right hepatic artery appears small, suggesting the presence of an unopacified accessory source of supply. (B) An accessory right hepatic vessel arises from the superior mesenteric artery, and supplies two large vascular metastases (arterial phase). (C) The metastases are more conspicuous in a later film in the sequence (capillary phase). (D) The accessory artery has been embolized with Sterispon and human dura mater. (Reproduced with permission of the editor of *World Medicine*.)

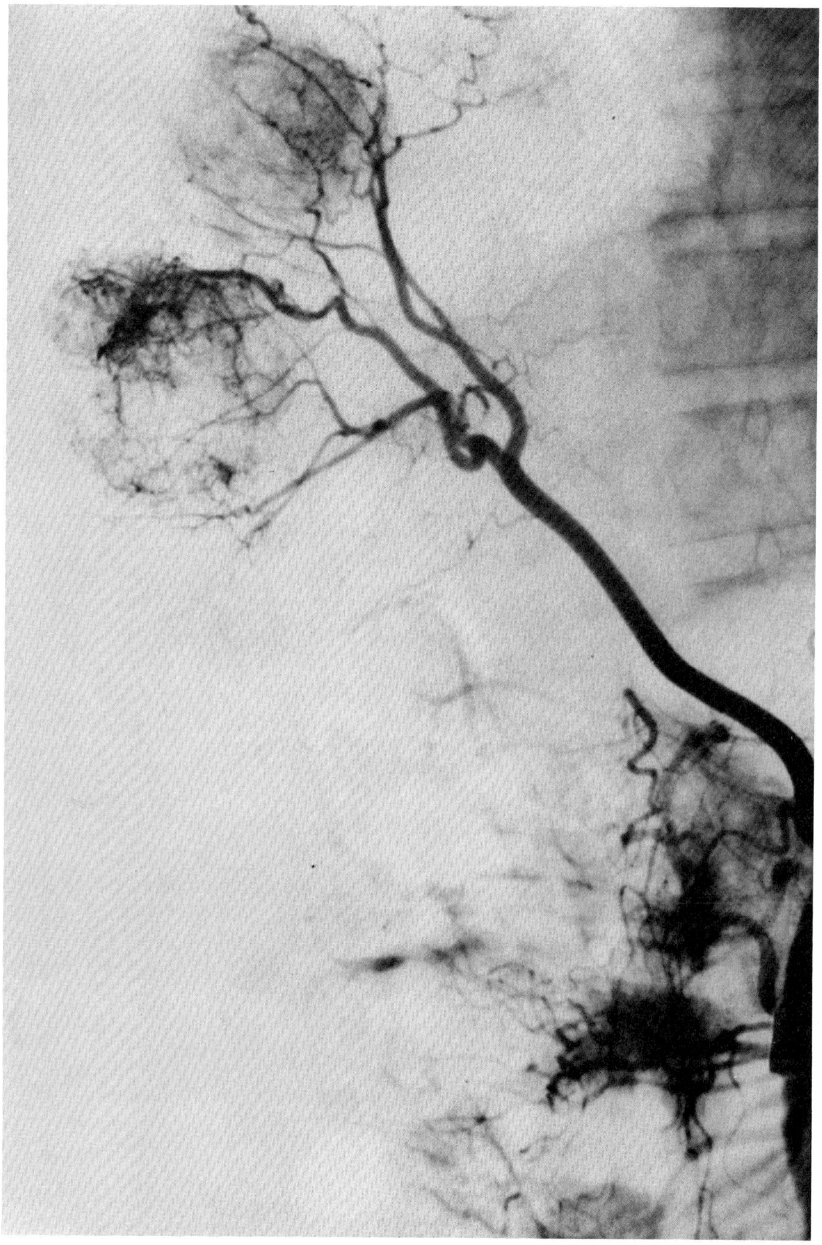

(B)

Figure 5 (continued)

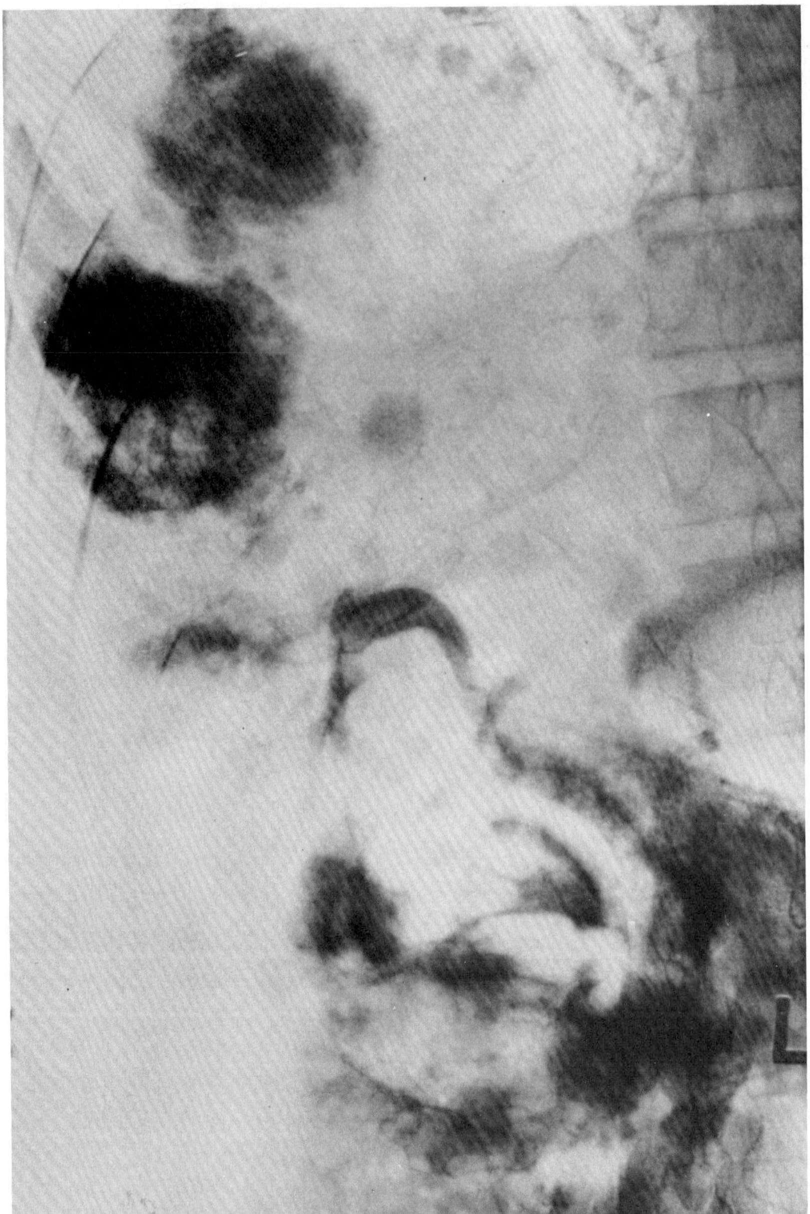

(C)

Figure 5 (continued)

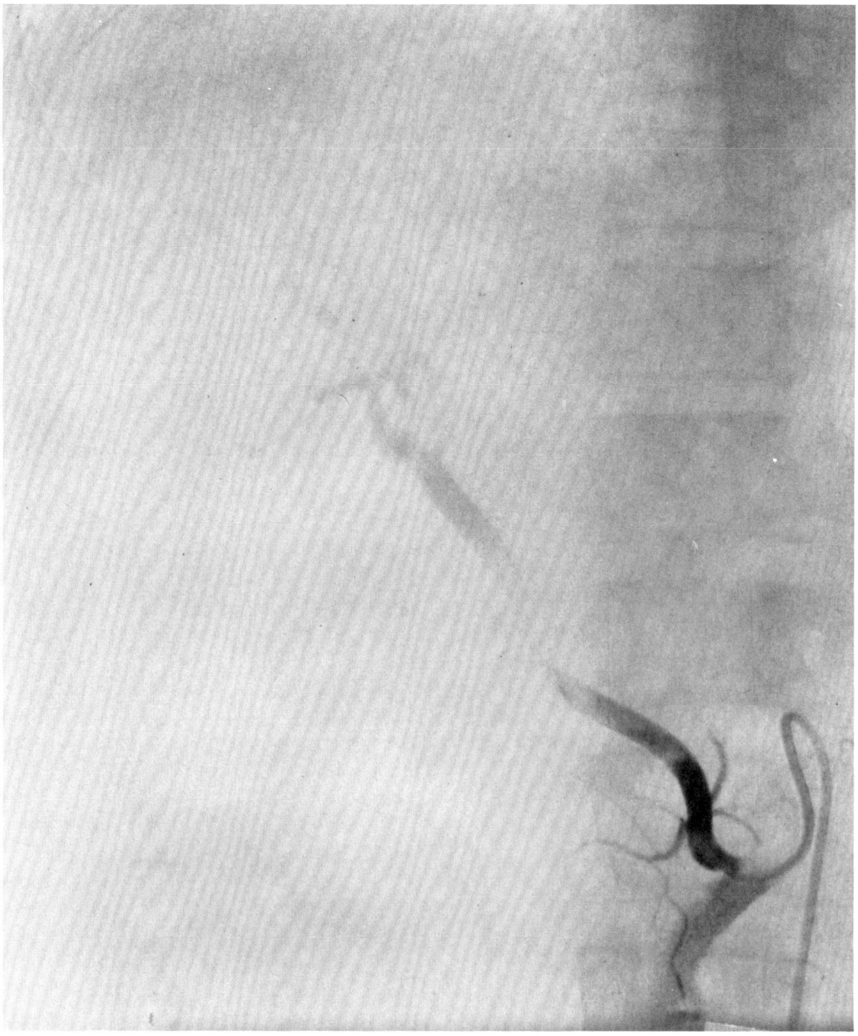

(D)

Figure 5 (continued)

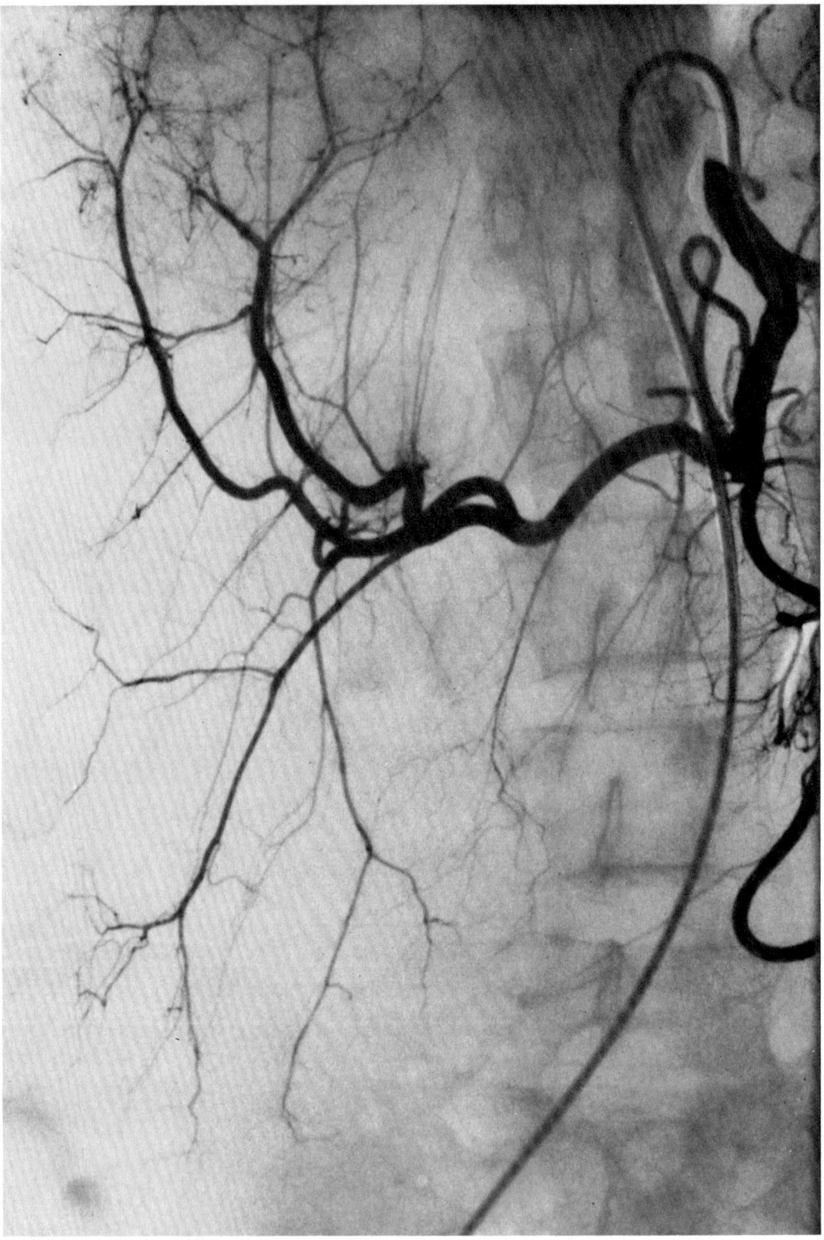

Figure 6A Embolization of carcinoid deposits in the liver. Hepatic arteriogram in a woman aged 50 with severe flushing and diarrhea.

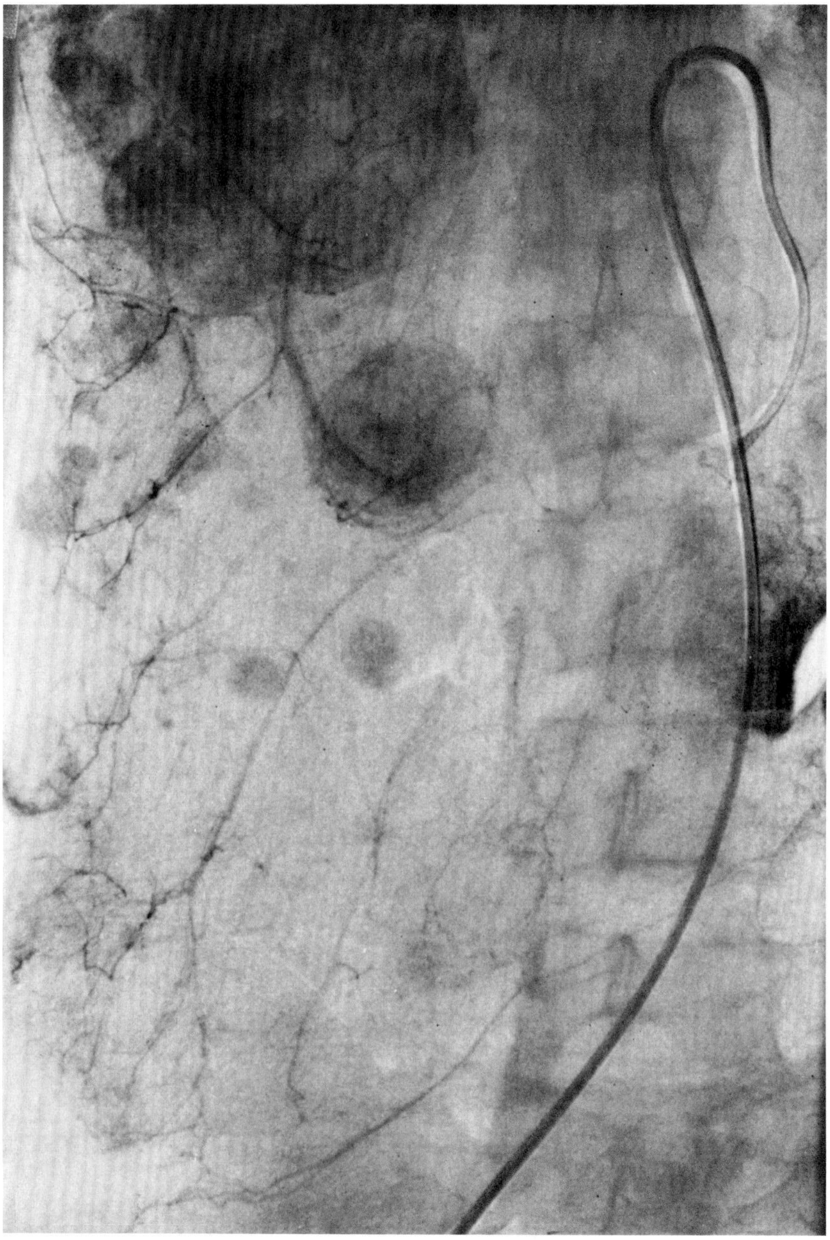

Figure 6B Capillary phase of study shows vascular carcinoid deposits in the liver.

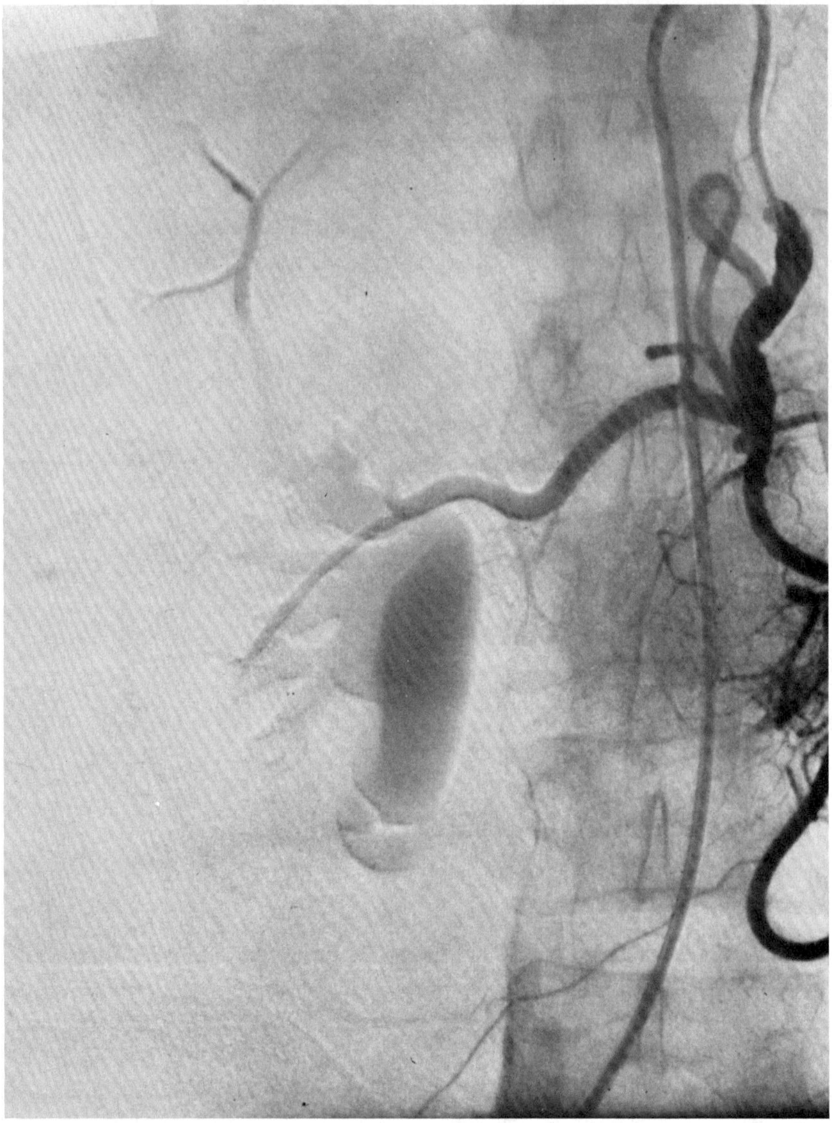

Figure 6C The hepatic artery has been embolized. This procedure produced complete remission of the carcinoid syndrome, and the patient remains symptom-free 18 months later. (Reproduced with permission of Churchill-Livingston Ltd.)

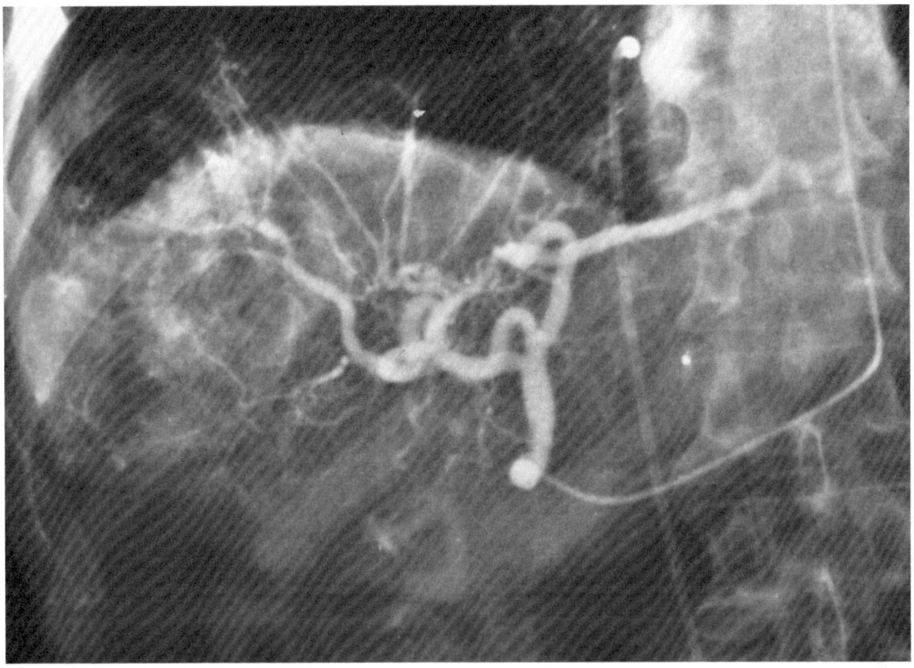

(A)

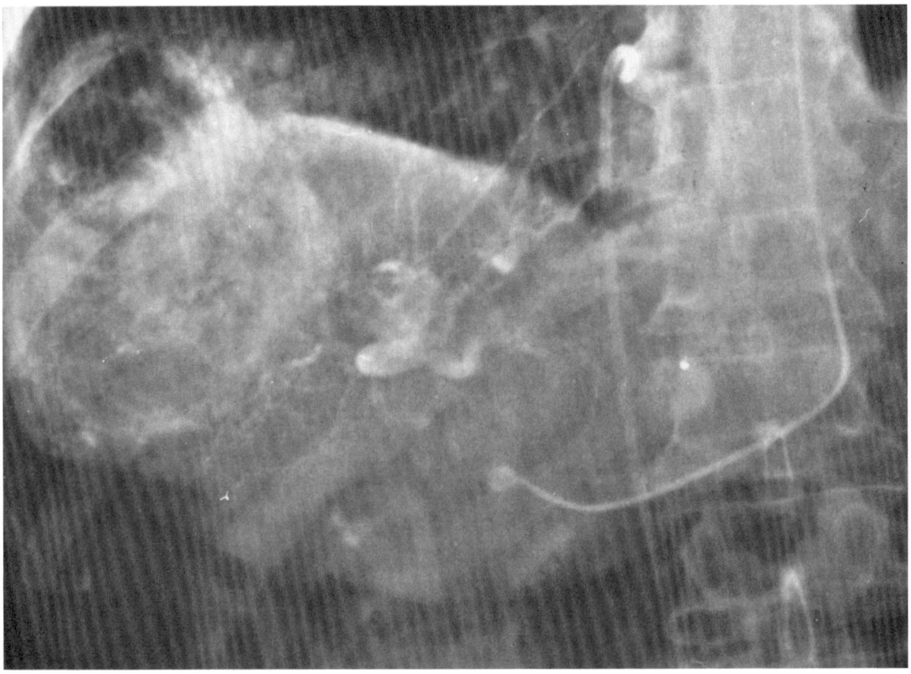

(B)

Figure 7 Embolization of carcinoid metastases: 64-year-old patient with carcinoid metastases to the liver and carcinoid syndrome. Previous resection of the right lobe to reduce tumor volume. Transbrachial catheterization of the proper hepatic artery. Highly vascular metastases in the medial segment of the left lobe. (A) Arterial phase. (B) Parenchymal phase.

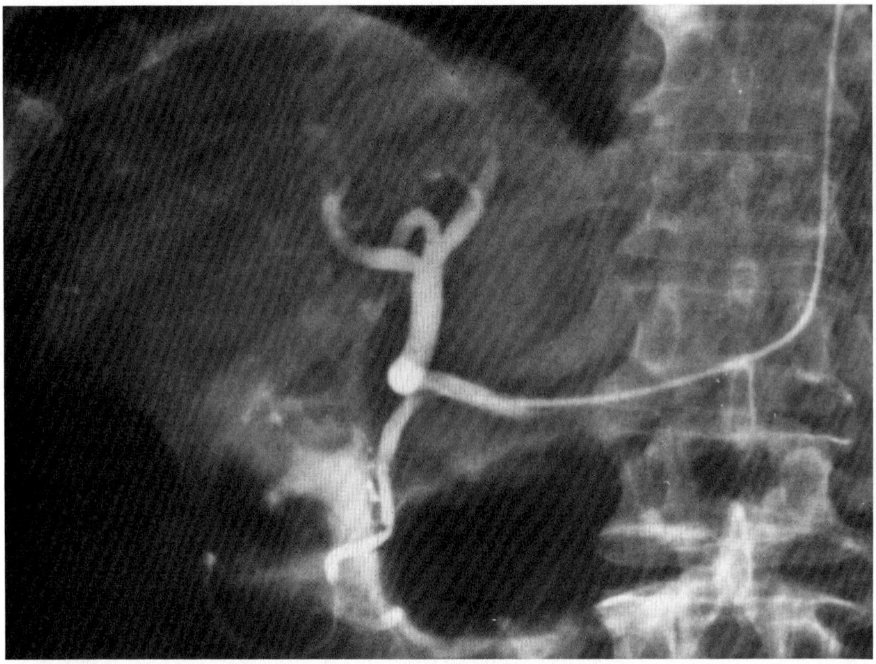

(C)

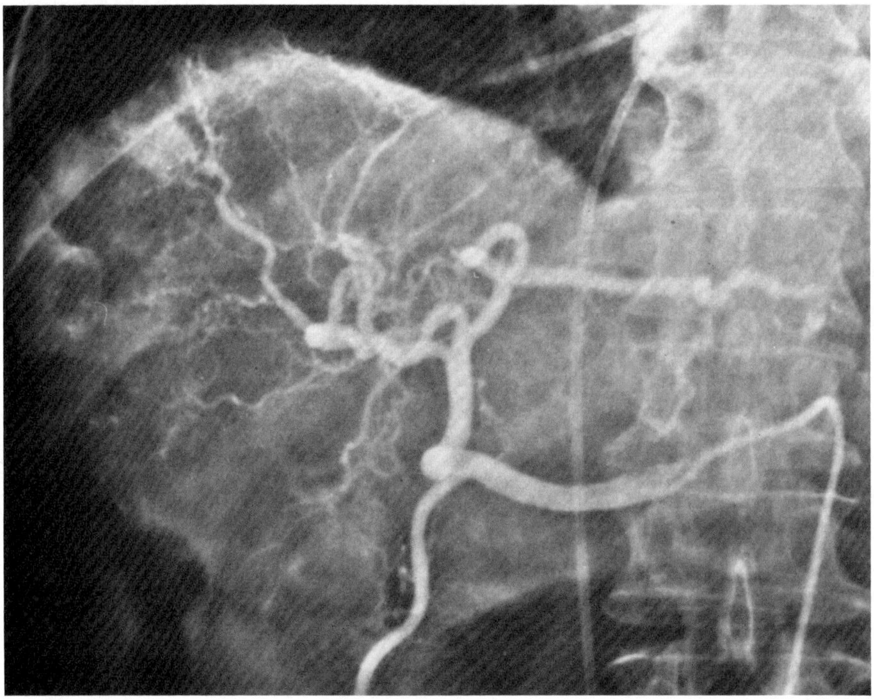

(D)

Figure 7 (continued)

(C) After embolization with 1 cc of Gelfoam powder, the flow to the liver is totally occluded. (D) One month after embolization all hepatic branches are recanalized. Reduced vascularization of the metastases.

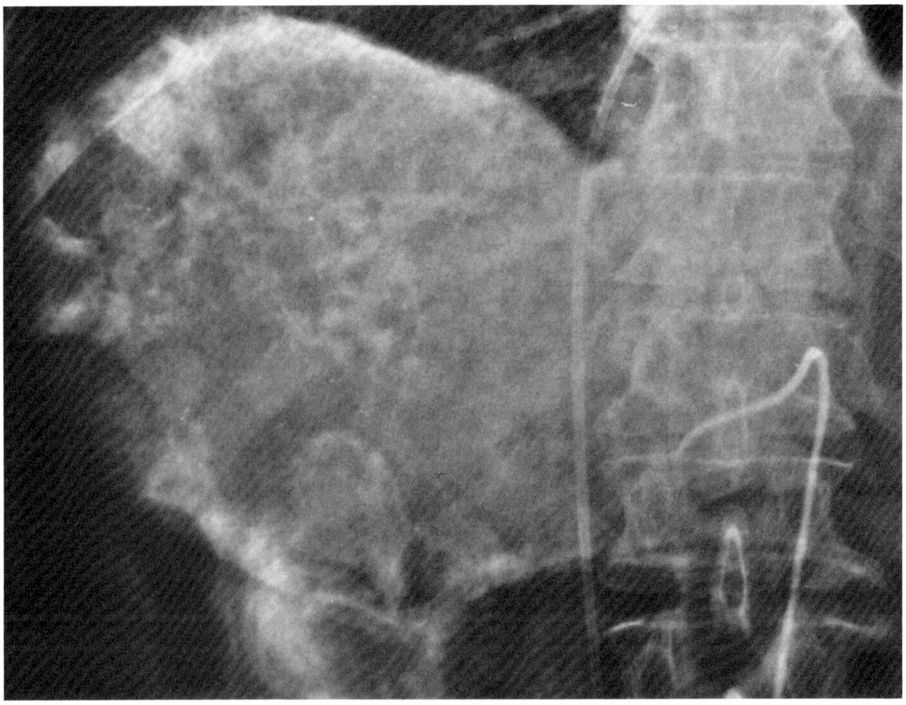

(E)

Figure 7 (continued)
(E) Parenchymal phase. Carcinoid symptoms had disappeared within a few days of the embolization and the patient is still free of symptoms 10 months later.

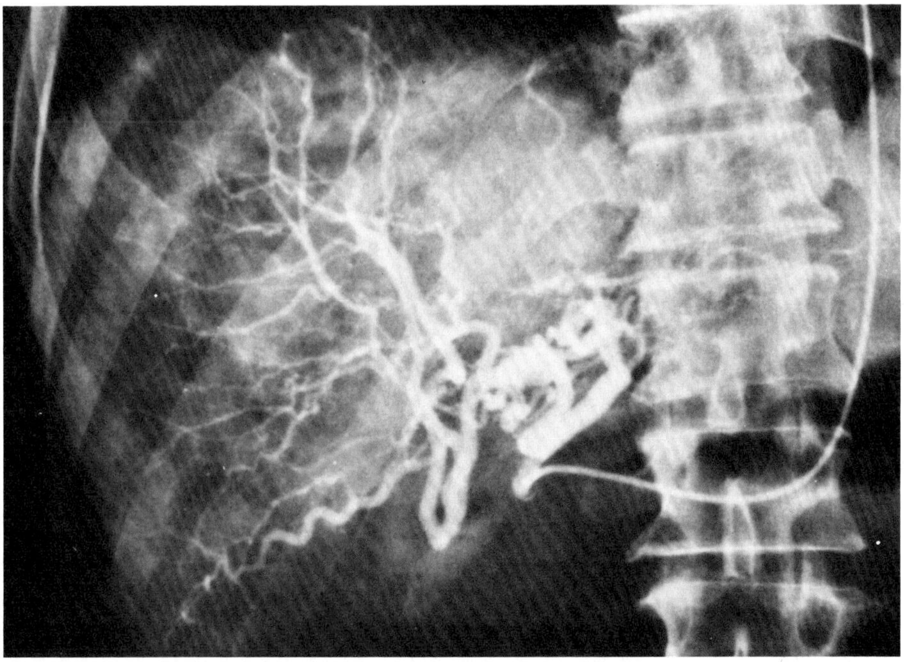

Figure 8A Embolization of carcinoid metastases: 74-year-old man with liver metastases from carcinoid tumor and severe carcinoid syndrome. Transbrachial catheterization of the proper hepatic artery shows an enlarged liver filled with metastases.

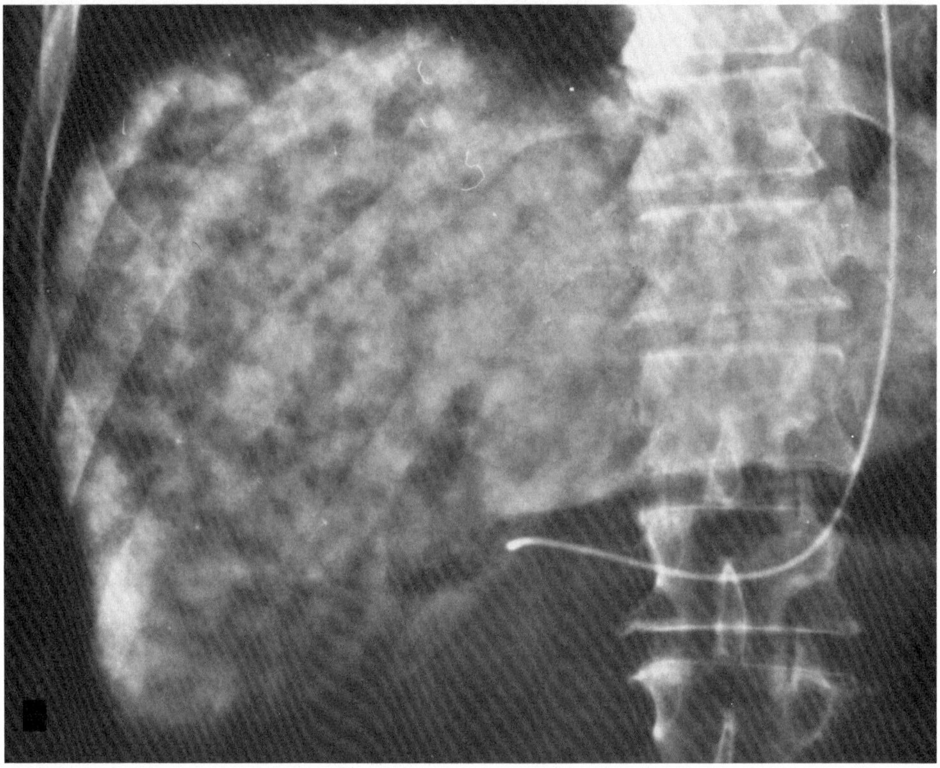

Figure 8B Parenchymal phase.

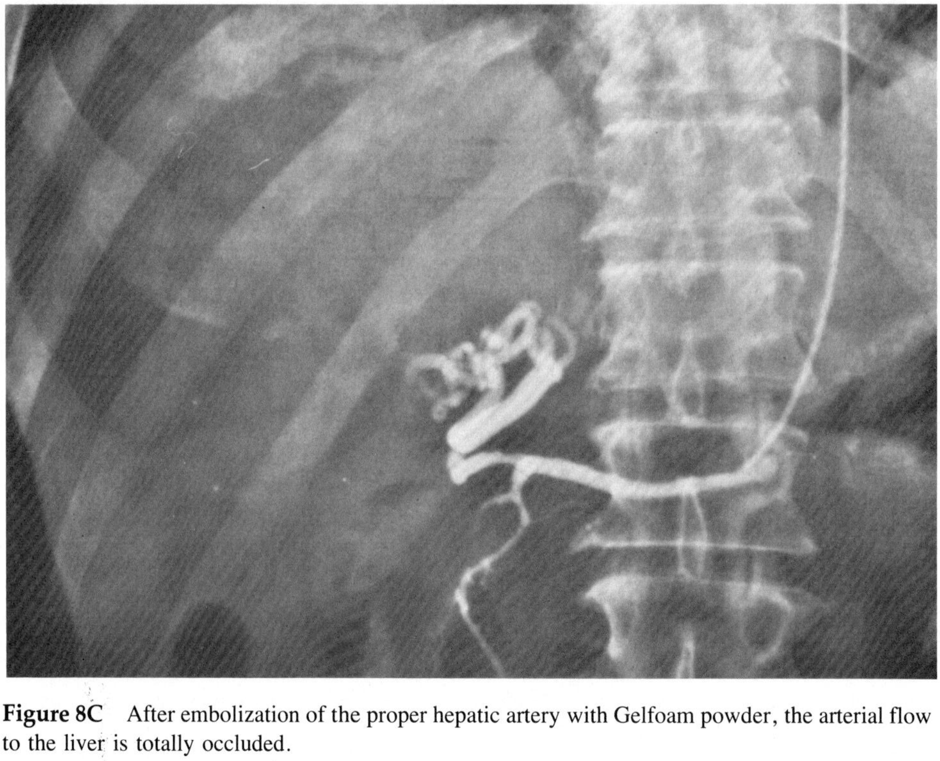

Figure 8C After embolization of the proper hepatic artery with Gelfoam powder, the arterial flow to the liver is totally occluded.

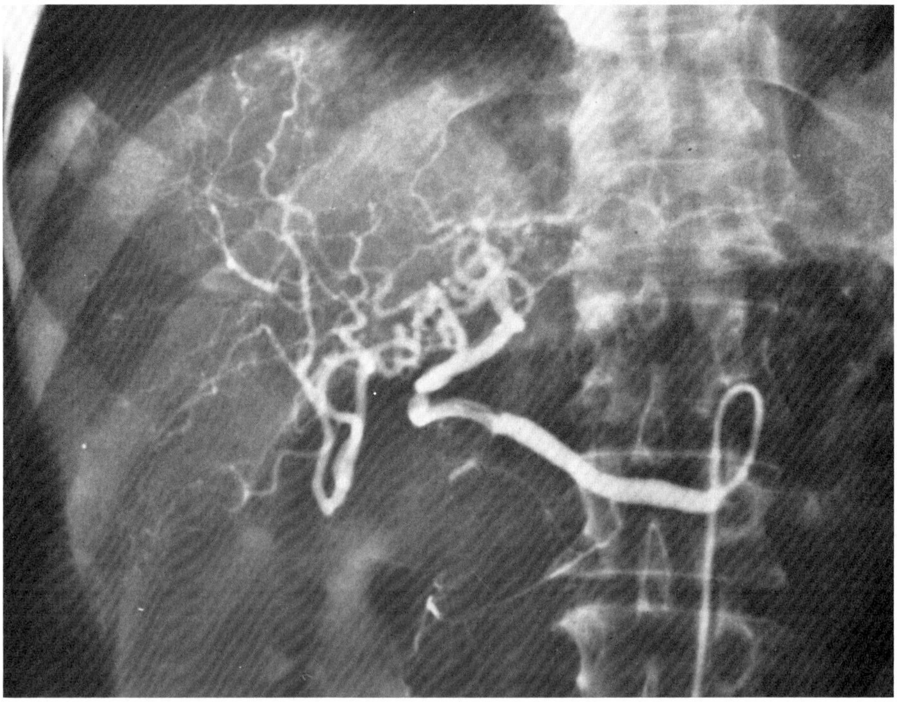

Figure 8D Control angiography 3 months after the embolization shows recanalization of all hepatic branches. Liver volume is reduced compared with the preembolization examination.

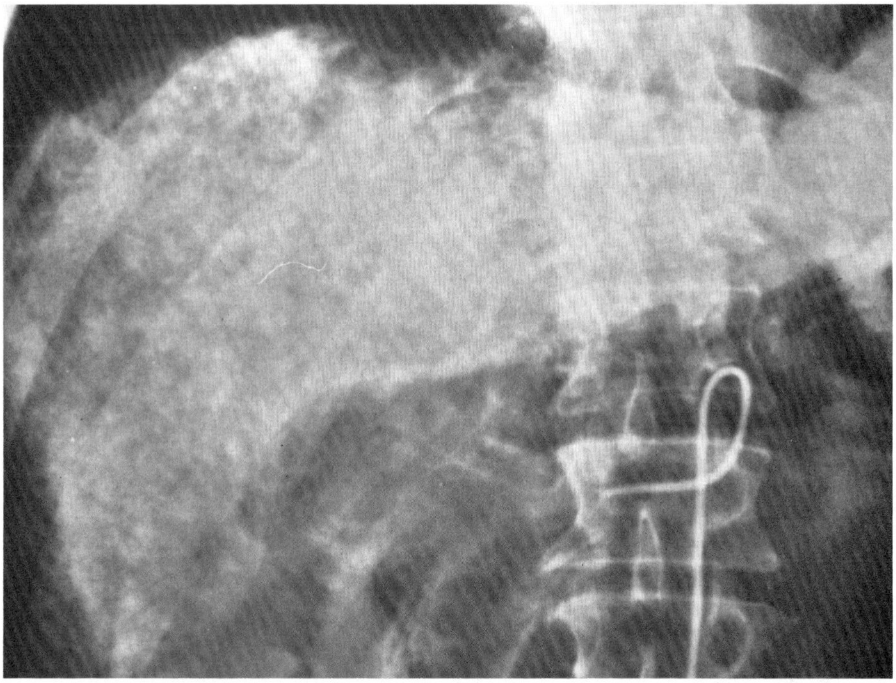

Figure 8E The parenchymal phase shows reduced vascularization of the metastases. Carcinoid syndrome had disappeared within a few days of the embolization and the patient is still free of symptoms 4 months later.

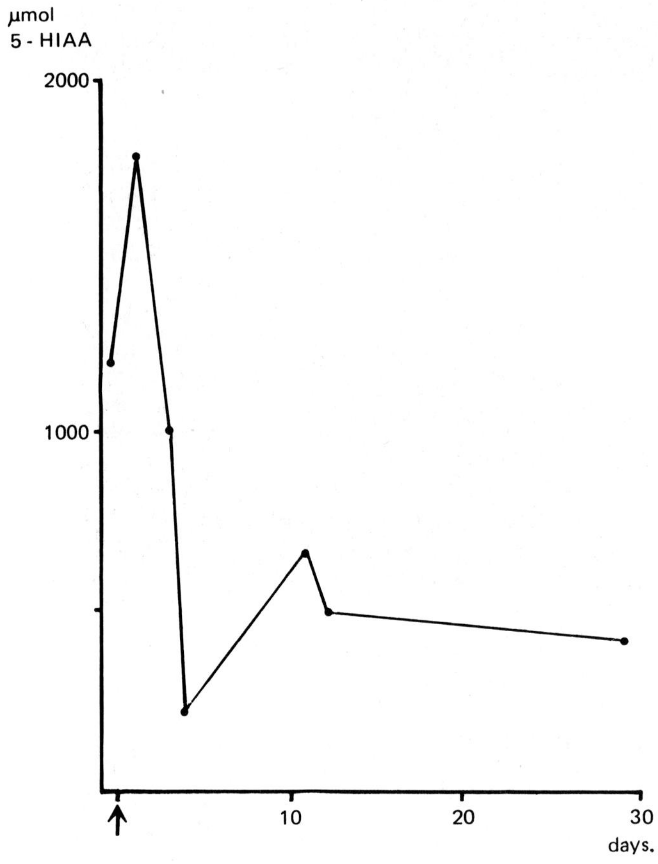

Figure 8F Concentration of 5-HIAA in urine (μmol/liter) before and after the embolization; marked reduction of excretion after the embolization.

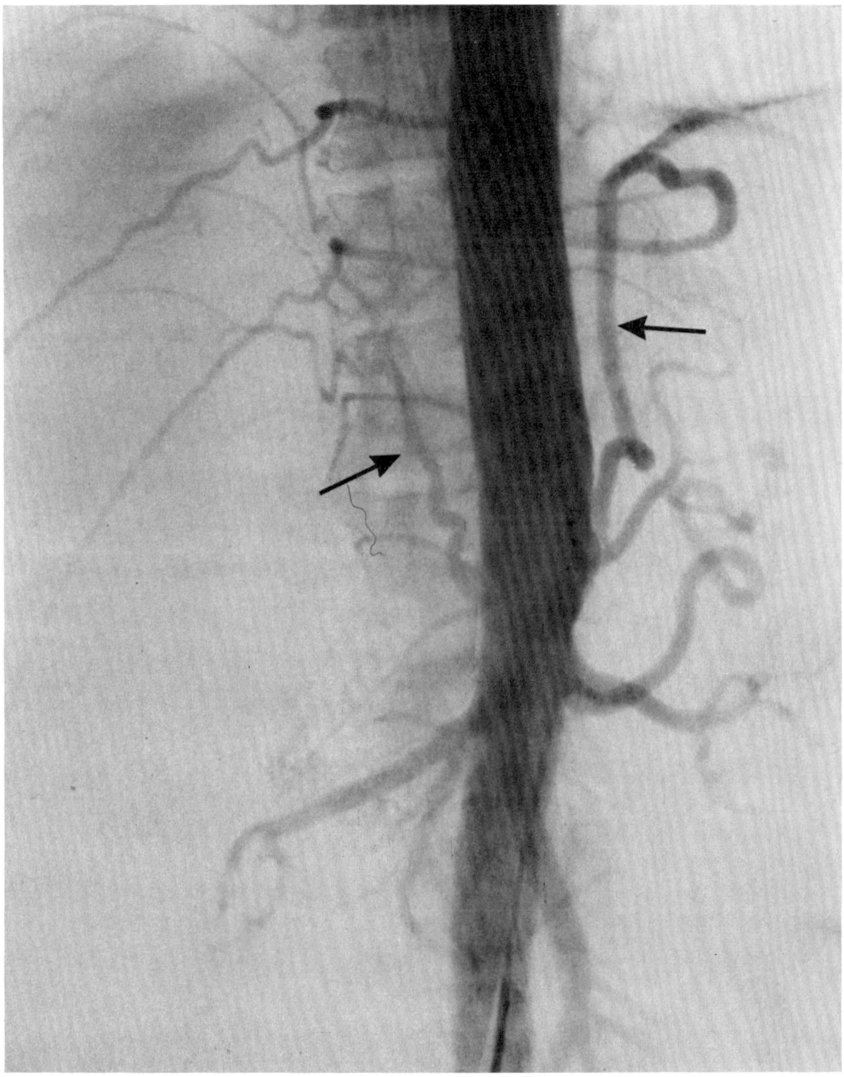

Figure 9A Embolization of carcinoid metastases in the liver. This case illustrates the futility of hepatic arterial ligation. Aortogram in a man with hepatic carcinoid metastases. The hepatic artery had been ligated surgically 1 year previously in an attempt to devascularize the tumor deposits. Note the enlarged phrenic collateral vessels (arrows).

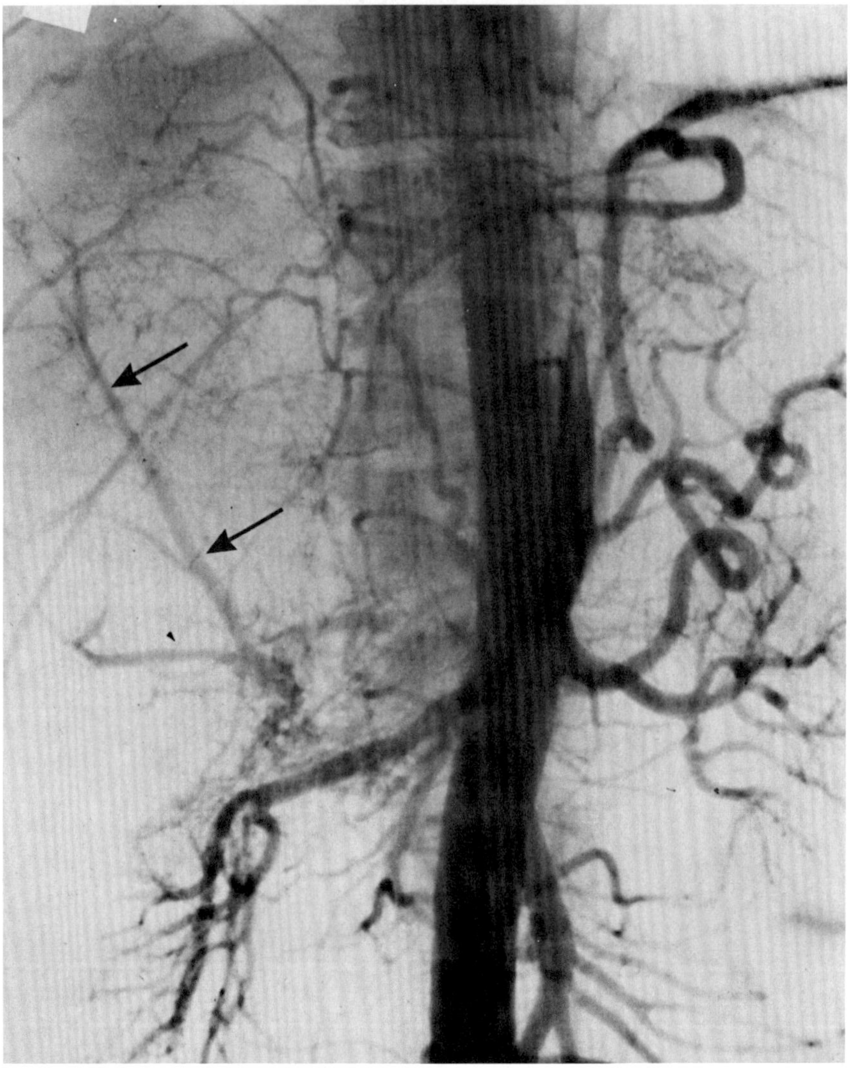

Figure 9B A later-phase film shows the hepatic artery (arrows) filling distal to the ligature via collateral vessels.

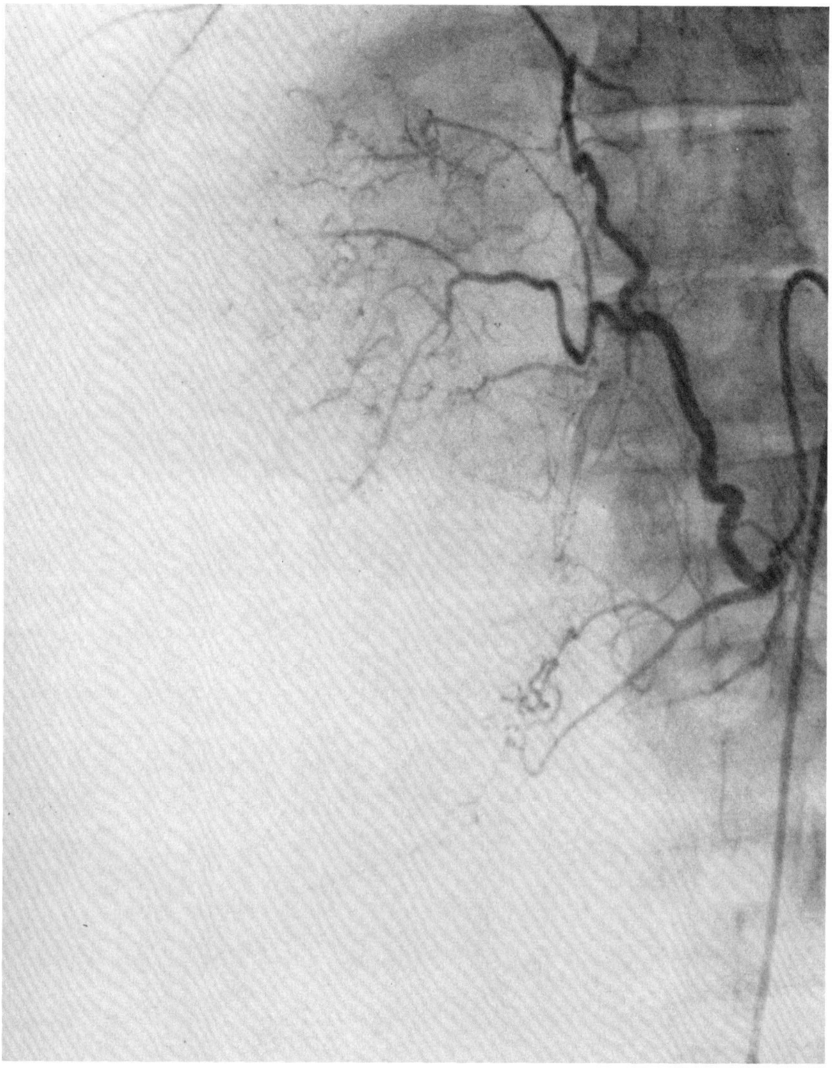

Figure 9C The enlarged right phrenic artery supplies massive tumor deposits.

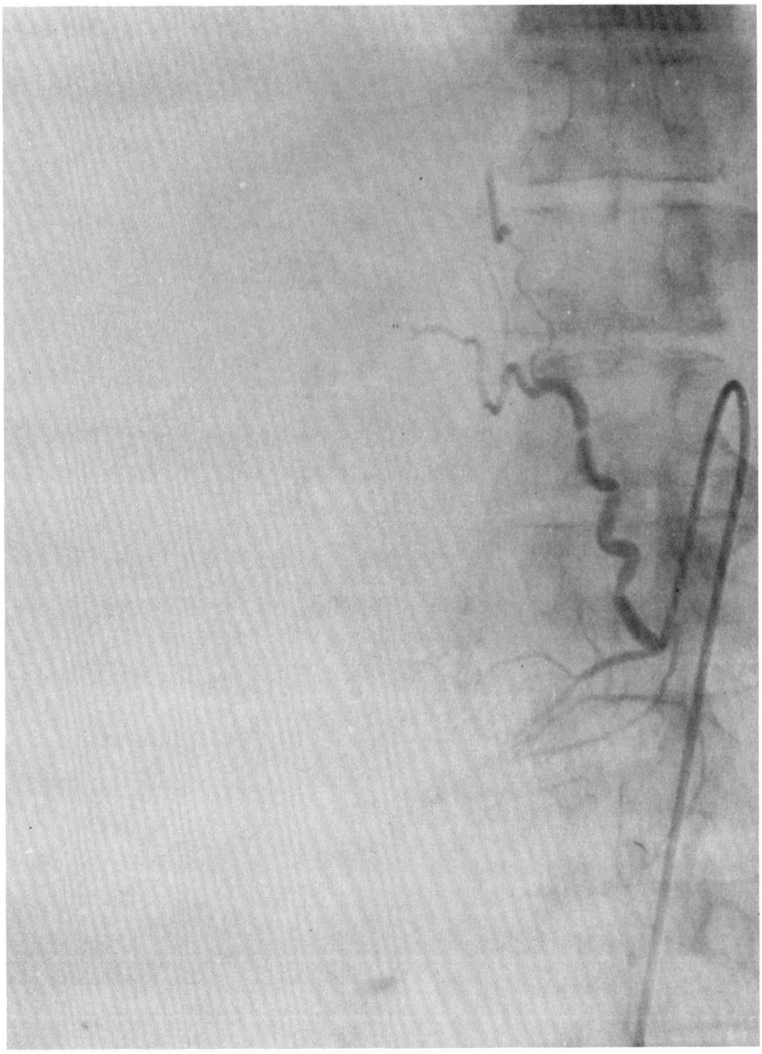

Figure 9D The phrenic artery has been embolized. It proved impossible to embolize all the collateral vessels to the hepatic deposits and the embolization was unsuccessful as a palliative procedure. This failure was largely due to the previous surgical ligation of the hepatic artery.

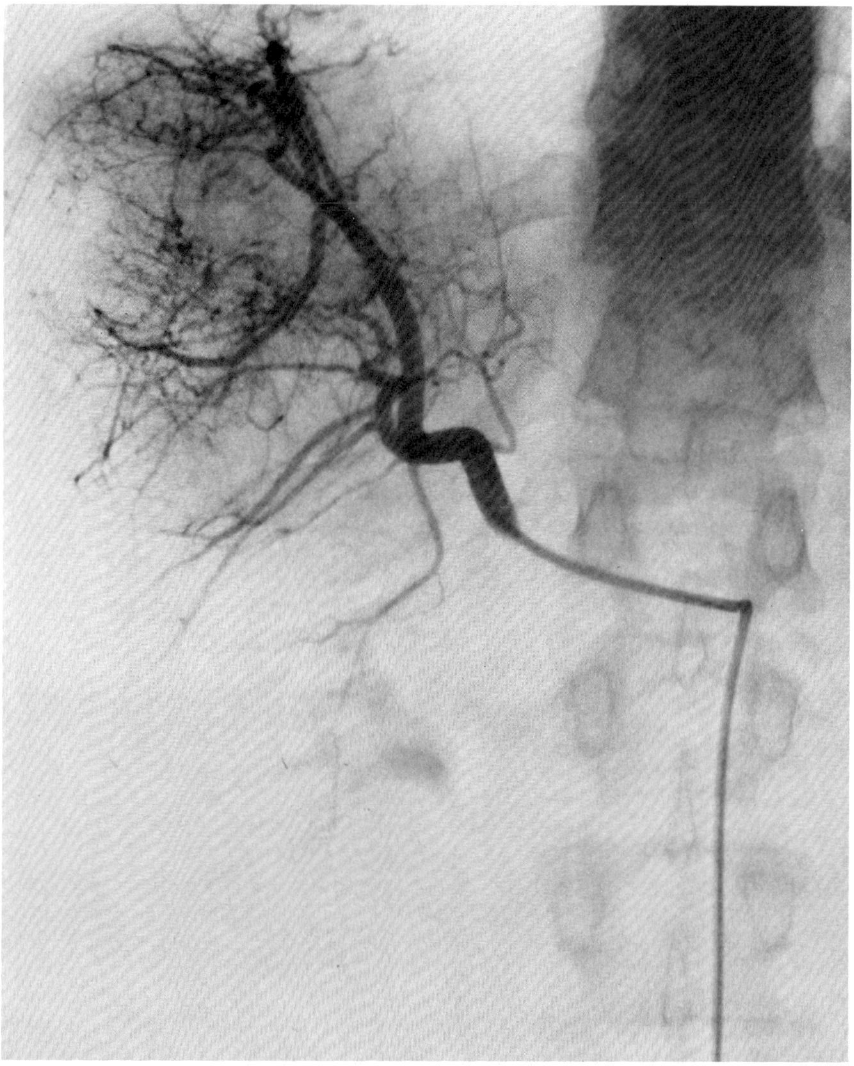

Figure 10A Embolization of calcitonin-producing hepatic metastases. Selective right hepatic arteriogram in a man with a calcitonin-producing thyroid tumor causing severe diarrhea. A hepatic metastasis was found on an isotope scan and the arteriogram shows displacement of vessels in the region of this tumor.

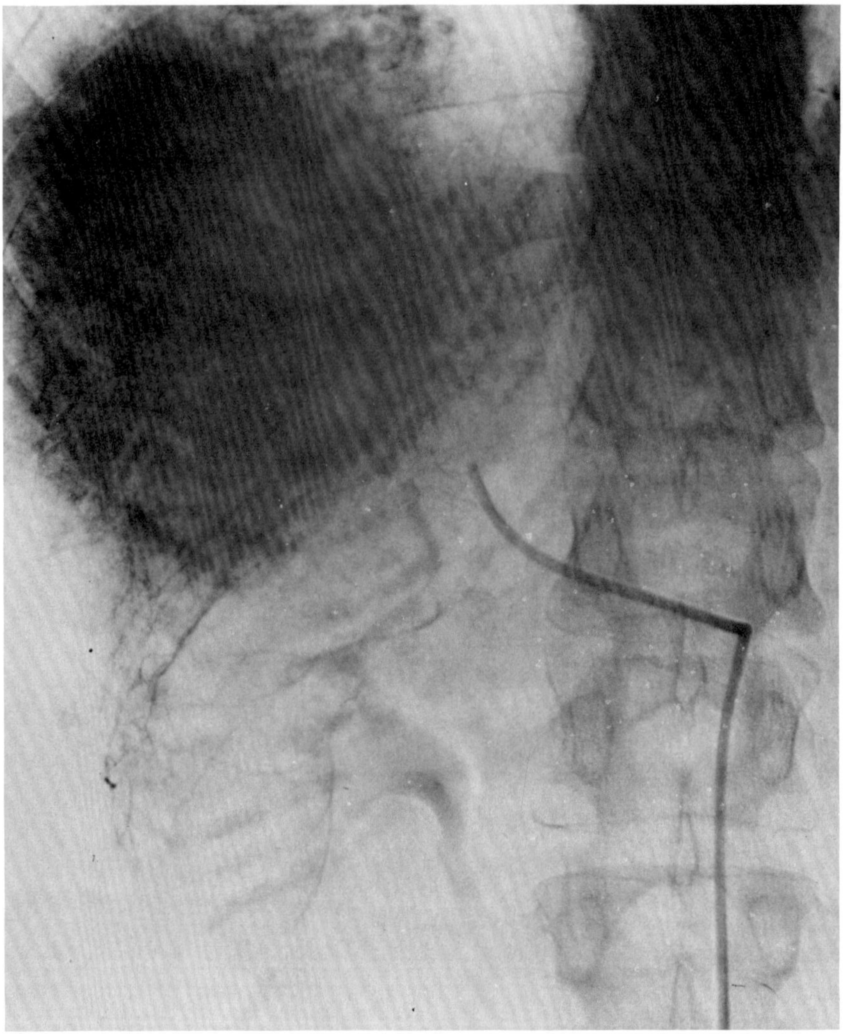

Figure 10B A dense pathological circulation is seen in the tumor during the capillary phase of the study.

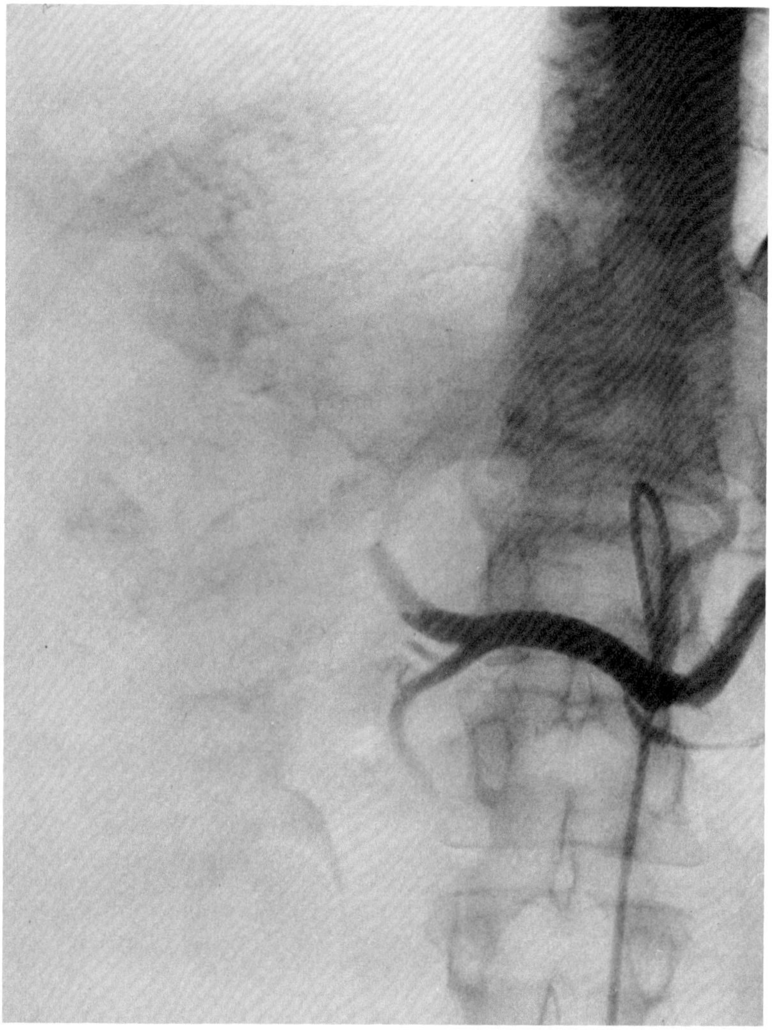

Figure 10C The tumor has been embolized with Sterispon and dura mater. This procedure produced considerable amelioration of the patient's symptoms.

Conclusion

The long-term efficacy of embolization for the control of the growth and humoral activity of the endocrine hepatic metastases is not yet known. It seems certain, however, from the encouraging results obtained in the relatively small number of patients treated to date, that therapeutic arterial embolization will be put to increasing use in the management of patients with hepatic tumors that exhibit an active endocrine function.

Acknowledgment

The author wishes to express his gratitude to Cordis UK Limited for their generous support.

References

1. Murray-Lyon IM, Dawson, JL, Parsons VA, Rake MO, Blendis LM, Laws JW: Treatment of secondary hepatic tumours by ligation of hepatic artery and infusion of cystoxic drugs. *Lancet* *2*:172, 1970.
2. Nebesar RA, Kornblith PL, Pollard JJ, Michaels NA: *Coeliac and superior mesenteric arteries*. J. A. Churchill, London, 1969.
3. Michels NA: Collateral arterial pathways to the liver after ligation of the hepatic artery and removal of the coeliac axis. *Cancer 6*:708, 1953.
4. Sivula A. and Sipponen P: The effect of hepatic dearterialization and re-dearterialization on carcinoid liver metastases. *Ann Chir Gynecol 65*:168, 1976.
5. Mays ET and Wheeler, CS: Demonstration of collateral arterial flow after interruption of hepatic arteries in man. *N Engl J Med 290*:993, 1974.
6. Jander HP, Laws HL, Kogutt MS, Mihas AA: Emergency embolization in blunt hepatic trauma. *Am J Radiol 129*:249, 1977.
7. Rubin BE, and Katz BT: Selective hepatic artery embolization to control massive hepatic hemorrhage after trauma. *Am J Radiol 129*:253, 1977.
8. Fagan EA, Allison DJ, Chadwick VS, Hodgson HJH: Treatment of haemobilia by selective arterial embolization. *Gut 21*:541, 1980.
9. Walter JF, Passo BT, Cannon WB: Successful transcatheter embolic control of massive hematobilia secondary to liver biopsy. *Am J Radio. 127*:847, 1976.
10. Merino-de Villasante J, Alvarez-Rodriguez RE, Hernandez-Ortiz J: Management of post biopsy hemobilia with selective arterial embolization. *Am J Radiol 128*:668, 1977.
11. Allison DJ: Therapeutic embolization and venous sampling. In *Recent Advances in Surgery*, Vol 10, Selwyn Taylor (Ed). Churchill Livingstone, Edinburgh, 1980.
12. Allison DJ and Nunnerley HB: Interventional radiology—therapeutic embolization. *Clin Radiol 31*:378, 1980.
13. Zeegen R, Rothwell-Jackson R, Sandler M: Massive hepatic resection for the carcinoid syndrome. *Gut 10*:617, 1969.
14. Allison DJ, Modlin IM, Jenkins WJ: Treatment of carcinoid liver metastases by hepatic-artery embolization. *Lancet 2*:1323, 1977.
15. Goldstein HM, Wallace S, Anderson JH, Bree RL, Gianturco C: Transcatheter occlusion of abdominal tumors. *Radiology 120*:539, 1976.
16. Giantaurco C, Anderson JH, Wallace S: Mechanical devices for arterial occlusion. *Am J Roentgenol Rad Ther Nucl Med 124*:428, 1975.

17. Dotter CT, Goldman ML, Rösch J: Instant selective arterial occlusion with isobutyl-2-cyanoacrylate. *Radiology 114*:227, 1975.
18. Dick R: Radiology now: therapeutic angiographic embolization. *Br J Radiol 50*:241, 1977.
19. Allison DJ: Therapeutic embolization. *Br J Hosp Med 20*:707, 1978.
20. Bernardino ME, Chuang VP, Wallace S, Thomas JL, Soo CS: Therapeutically infarcted tumors: CT findings. *Am J Roentgenol 136*:527, 1981.
21. De Jode LR, Nicholls RD, Wright PL: Ischaemic necropsos of the gall bladder following hepatic artery embolism. *Br J Surg 63*:621, 1976.
22. Jacob ET, Shapira Z, Morag B, Rubinstein Z: Hepatic infarction and gall bladder necrosis complicating arterial embolization for bleeding duodenal ulcer. *Dig Dis Sci 24*:482, 1979.

28

Radiology in Liver Trauma

Erik Boijsen
University Hospital
Lund, Sweden

Tryggve Aakhus
Rikshospitalet
Oslo, Norway

Ivar Enge
Akers Hospital
Oslo, Norway

Introduction

Blunt trauma to the right lower thorax or the upper abdomen is the most common cause of liver injury in Europe, while penetrating trauma due to gunshot or stabbing seems to be the most often observed form of liver trauma in the United States (1–6). The increasing use of percutaneous transhepatic cholangiography or portography and of percutaneous biliary drainage for diagnostic and therapeutic purposes has raised the incidence of iatrogenic injuries (7–15). Surgery is another, though infrequent cause of hepatic injury (7,16,17). Spontaneous rupture of the liver is rarely encountered (18–22).

Any kind of trauma to the liver region may cause bleeding or leakage of bile. In the immediate posttraumatic period blood or bile may accumulate in the peritoneal cavity, in the liver parenchyma or below the liver capsule, depending on the site and type of the lesion. Bleeding into the gastrointestinal tract, hemobilia, may occur as a later consequence of the injury.

The clinical diagnosis of a liver lesion resulting from trauma is often obvious. The case history and the clinical status give important information. Many patients, however, arrive in a state of shock and multiple organ lesions are often present. In those situations it may be impossible to define the exact nature of the lesions or determine which of them may need attention most urgently. Acute surgery is often required, but even then it may not be feasible to evaluate the full extent and degree of injury to the liver. Liver trauma carries a high mortality rate, particularly in the multiorgan-injured patients. The most serious lesions are those due to gunshot and blunt trauma.

Role of Surgery

There is no unanimity among surgeons concerning the method of treatment of hepatic rupture. In many centers it is not only the most severely injured patient who is taken directly to surgery; often, cases with only moderate or slight trauma to the liver region are scheduled for surgical exploration. Thus laparotomy seems to be undertaken whenever laparocentesis or peritoneal lavage revealed even traces of intra-abdominal blood. Angiography or other radiologic procedures are often regarded as unnecessary and of so little value that they are not even mentioned as diagnostic alternatives (1,4,5,23,24).

Various surgical procedures are recommended, from ligation of the hepatic artery or its branches (25–28) to hepatic resection (4,6,29–31). Although such aggressive forms of surgical intervention may be required in difficult circumstances, a more conservative approach to liver injuries has been recommended more recently (2,5). To the surgeon this could mean early diagnosis by surgical exploration, while avoiding extensive surgical intervention as far as possible. Approximately 80% of all injuries to the liver are amenable to rather simple surgical procedures, such as suturing of small superficial lacerations or merely drainage (1,2,4,5). In about one-fourth of the cases, bleeding had already ceased at the time of surgery, which could thus be regarded as an additional and unncessary form of trauma to the patient.

Stages of Injury

Four main stages of lesions of the liver are encountered with blunt as well as penetrating injuries:

1. *Contusion with or without a small laceration* of the parenchyma. A small capsular tear may be present with traces of blood in the abdominal cavity. Without a capsular tear, a small subcapsular hematoma may be found.
2. *Moderate laceration with active bleeding*. If the capsule of the liver is ruptured, bleeding will extend into the peritoneal cavity. With the liver surface intact, a large hematoma will form below the capsule.
3. *Intrahepatic hematoma* of varying size, at times combined with aneurysm formation, arterioportal or arteriobiliary fistula, or arterial or venous occlusion.
4. *Extensive lacerations* with transection of vessels and bile ducts. Hepatic vein disruption alone or in combination with other lesions is a serious consequence of hepatic trauma.

Complications following liver trauma occur postoperatively as well as in nonoperated patients. The most frequently recorded are pulmonary atelectases with pleural effusion, intrahepatic or subphrenic abscesses, jaundice, and hemobilia.

The Place of Radiology

At the present time, radiology has no place in the management of the shocked and severely injured patient. It is true that operation on such a patient carries a very high mortality rate and that the main reason for this is severe bleeding from transsected vessels. Acute percutaneous embolization might then be an alternative to operation. The time delay involved in this procedure, however, could be significant, and more experience is required before angiography with embolization can be recommended for the severely injured patient. (However, see Chap. 27.)

Radiologic procedures in the acute situation should, therefore, be applied only to patients whose clinical status permits further evaluation of the consequences of the trauma. Routine chest and abdominal survey films will give a limited indication of the extent and degree of the lesion. Pulmonary complications, pleural effusion, enlargement of the liver, rib fracture, blood in the abdominal cavity, and an elevated diaphragm are findings which, though nonspecific, nevertheless give important information on the extent of the injury (32). The upper margin of the liver may be mistaken for an elevated diaphragm, and this may cause the diagnosis of diaphragmatic rupture to be overlooked for a considerable time (33,34). The induction of pneumoperitoneum may demonstrate the rupture, the gas passing into the pleural cavity; however, this is not invariably so, as the rupture may have sealed off. The lateral chest film may show an increased distance between the anterior part of the diaphragm (or liver) and the anterior chest wall (35), an appearance not found with a normal, relaxed diaphragm (Fig. 1). The diagnosis can be confirmed by hepatic angiography when the liver parenchyma and its supplying vessels will be found to be compressed where they pass through the diaphragmatic tear (34)

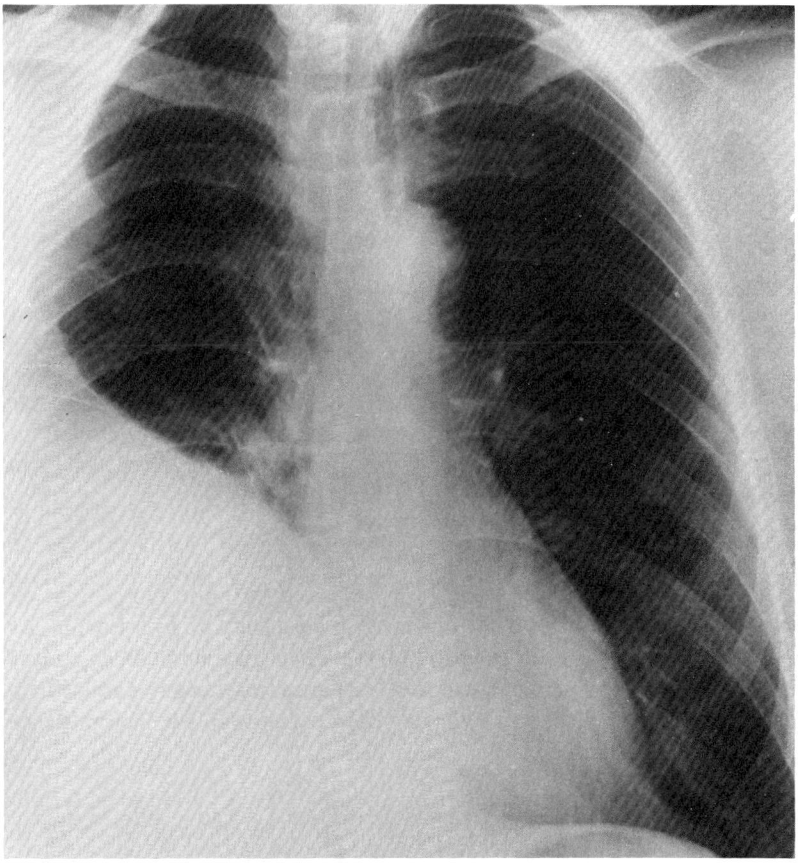

Figure 1A Rupture of right hemidiaphragm. Admitted because of multiple injuries following a car accident. Chest, posterior-anterior view. Persistent densities in the right hemithorax originally misinterpreted as due to pleural effusion.

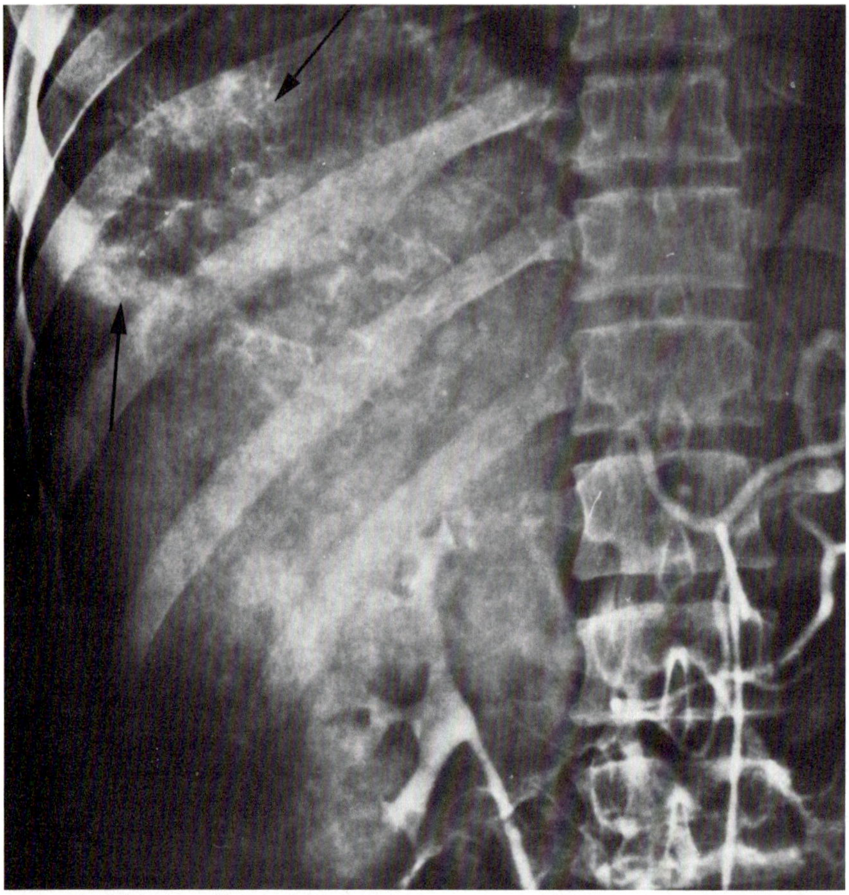

(B)

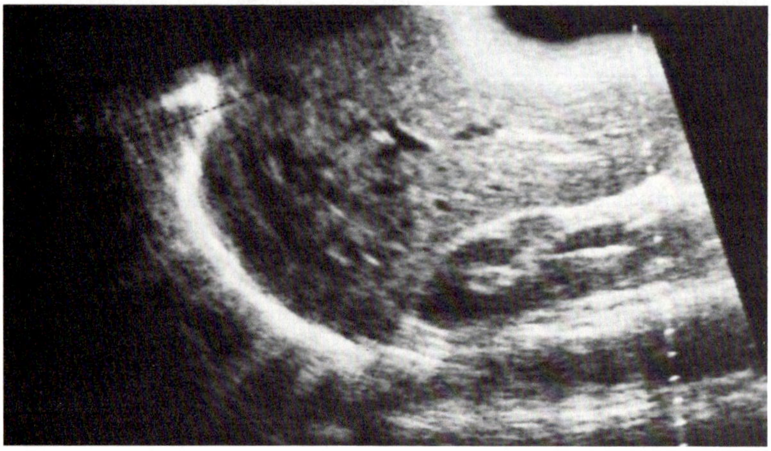

(C)

Figure 3 (continued)

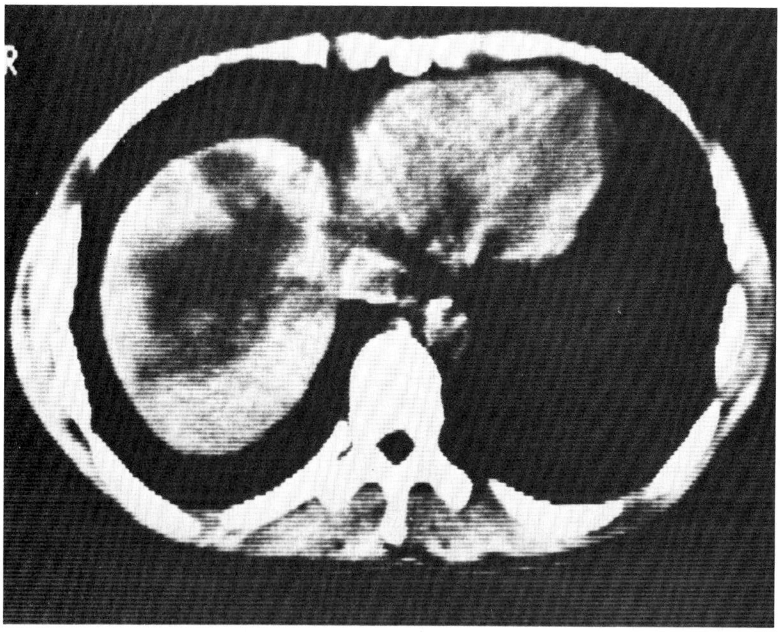

(D)

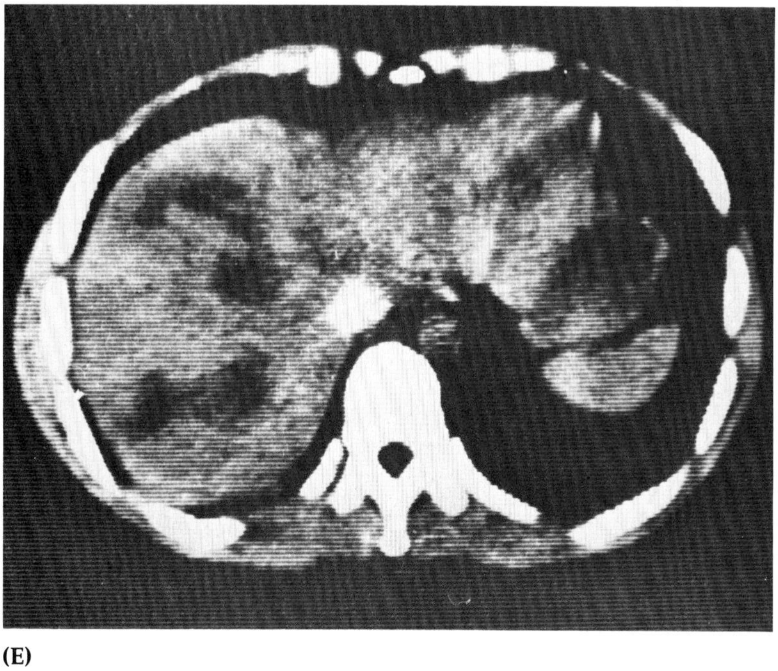

(E)

Figure 3 (continued)

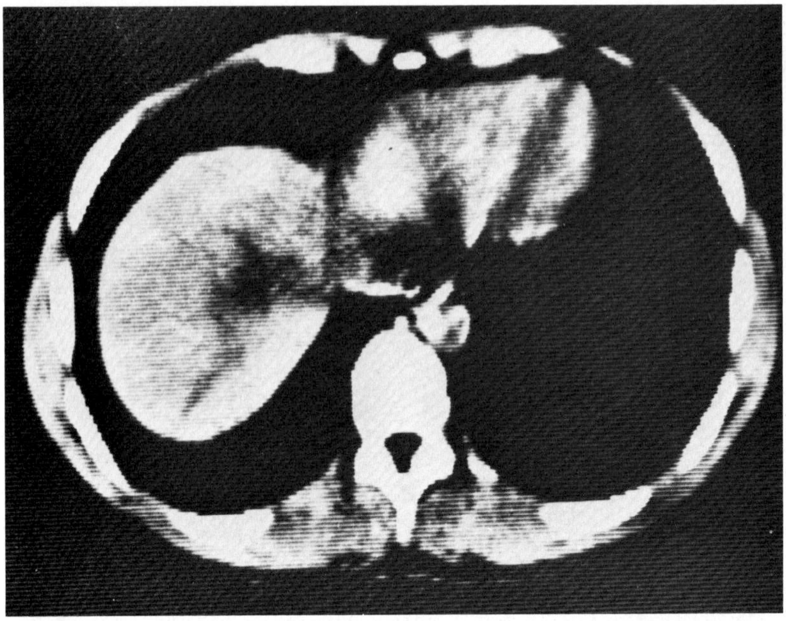

(F)

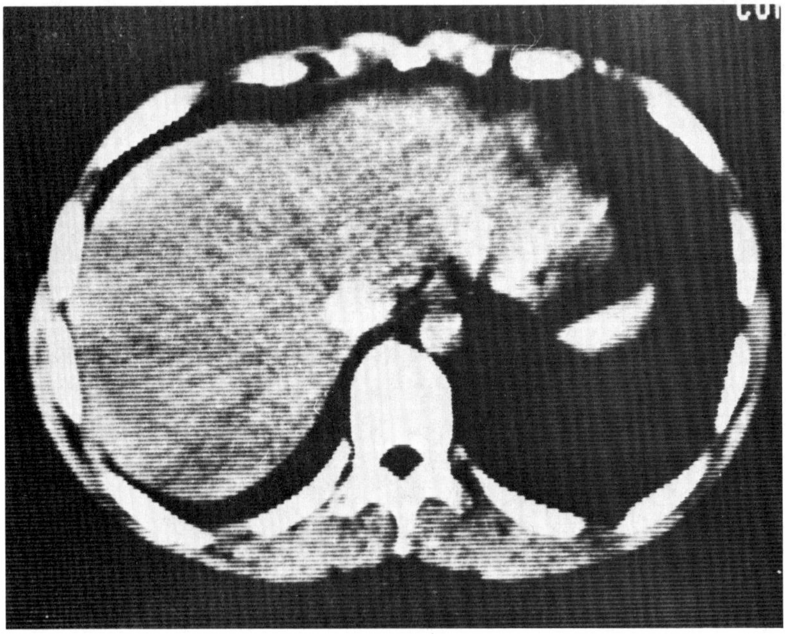

(G)

Figure 3 (continued)

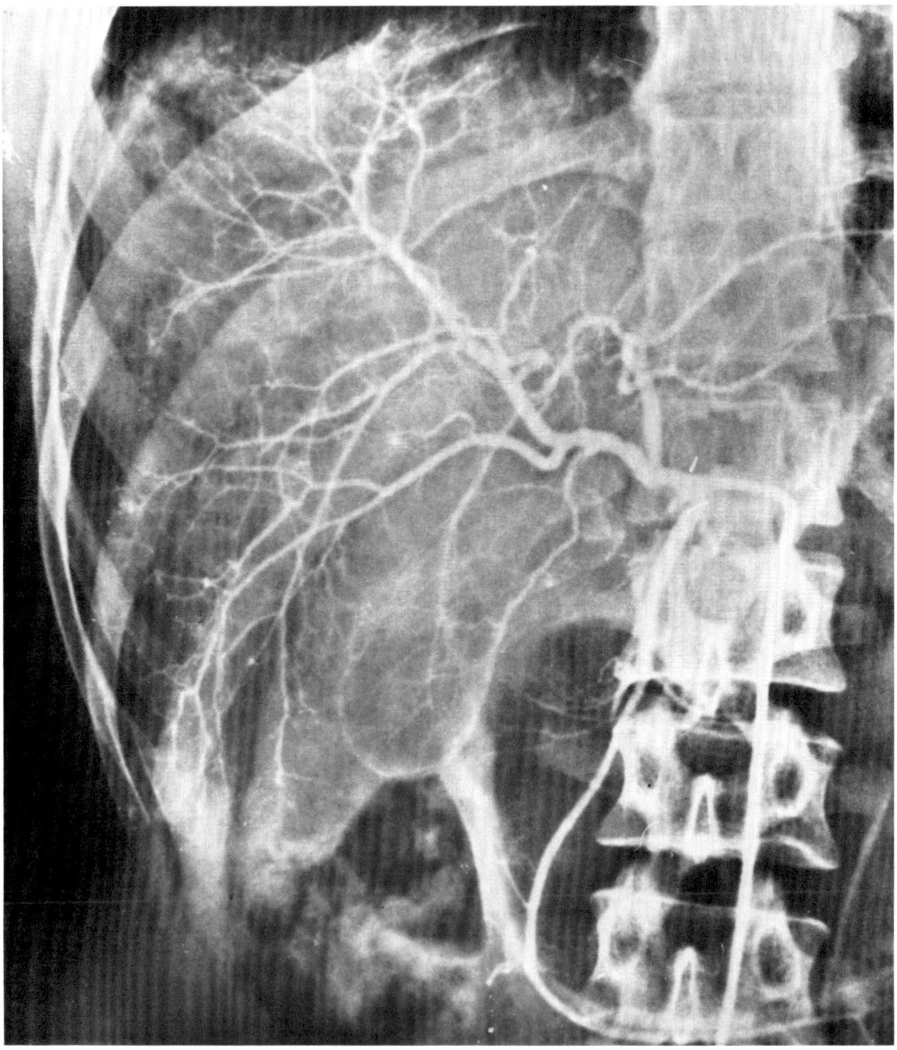

(A)

Figure 4 Blunt liver injury with rupture of the liver capsule and laceration of the parenchyma. (A,B) At hepatic angiography 6 hr after trauma there was marked hypervascularity, irregular mottled accumulation of contrast medium, and arterioportal connections. Observe the marked accumulation of contrast medium in the liver capsule, outlining the laceration and capsular tear (B) (between arrows) at the level of the fractured ribs. Small extravasations are observed close to the laceration (crossed arrows) with blood in the adjacent peritoneal cavity. (C) Renal angiography shows occlusion of a branch to the lower pole as well as constriction of the dorsal artery at its origin (arrow). (D,E) CT the following day revealed the capsular tear, a rather small hematoma, and the peritoneal blood on the surface of the liver. (F) Fourteen days later only small remnants of the hematoma were observed at CT. The patient made an uneventful recovery.

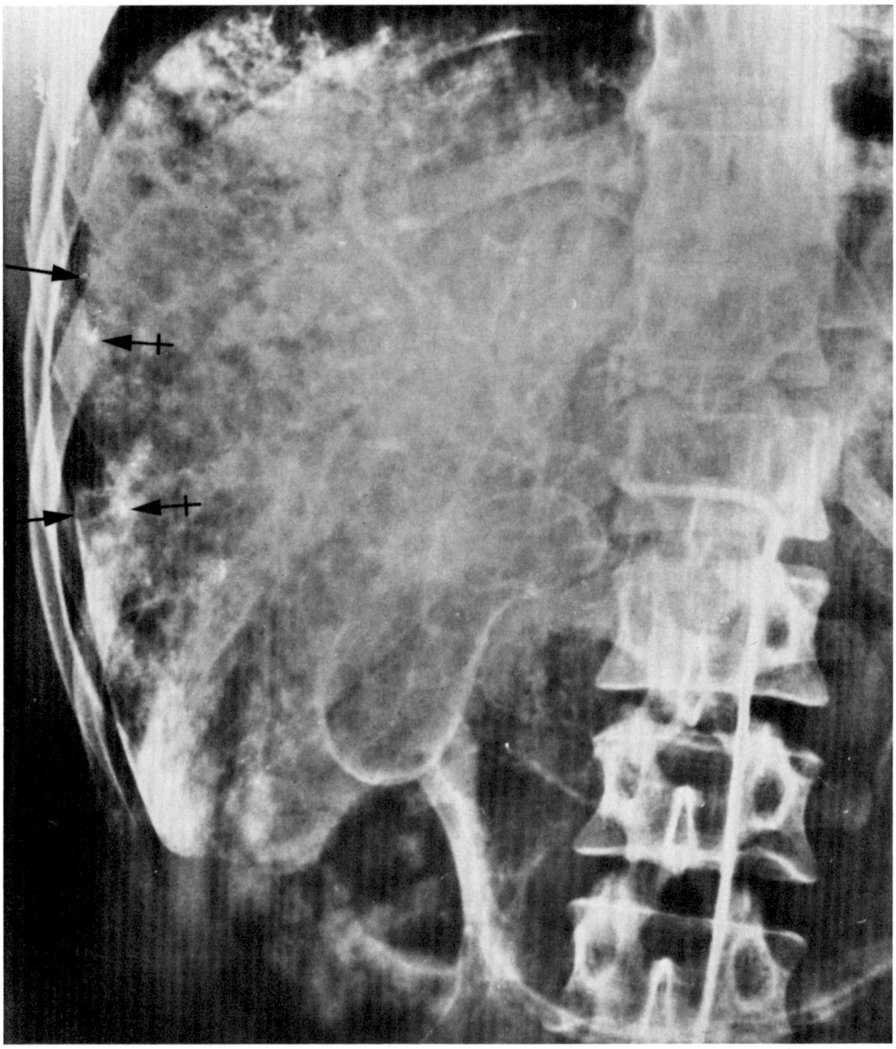

(B)

Figure 4 (continued)

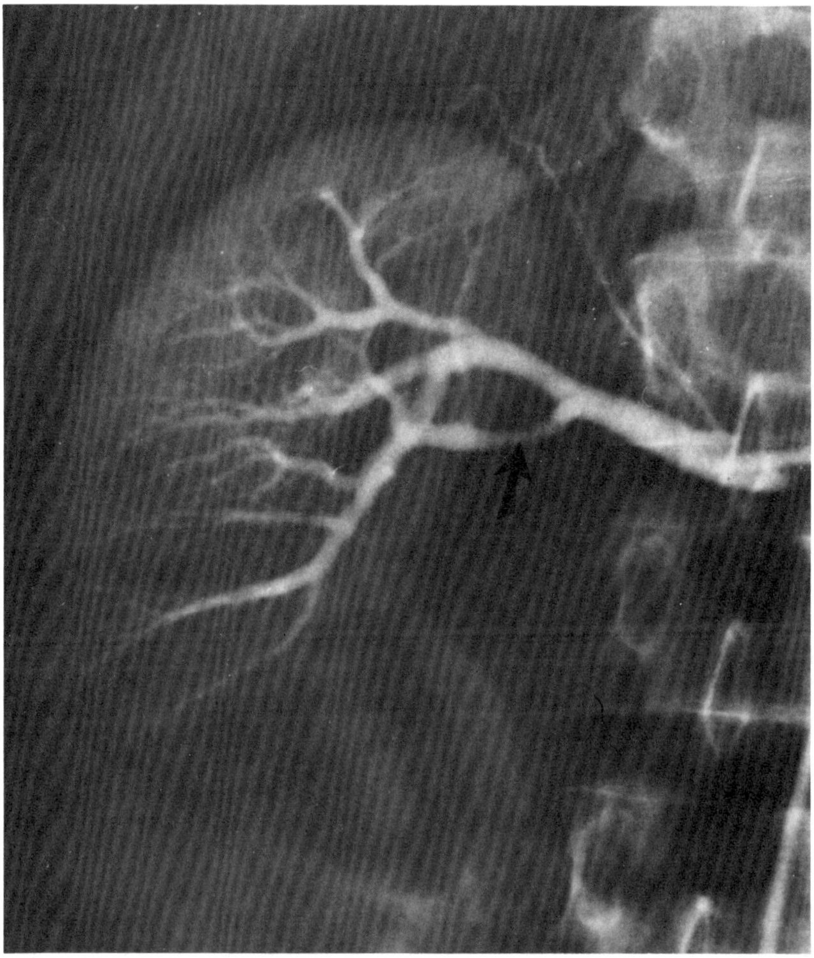

(C)

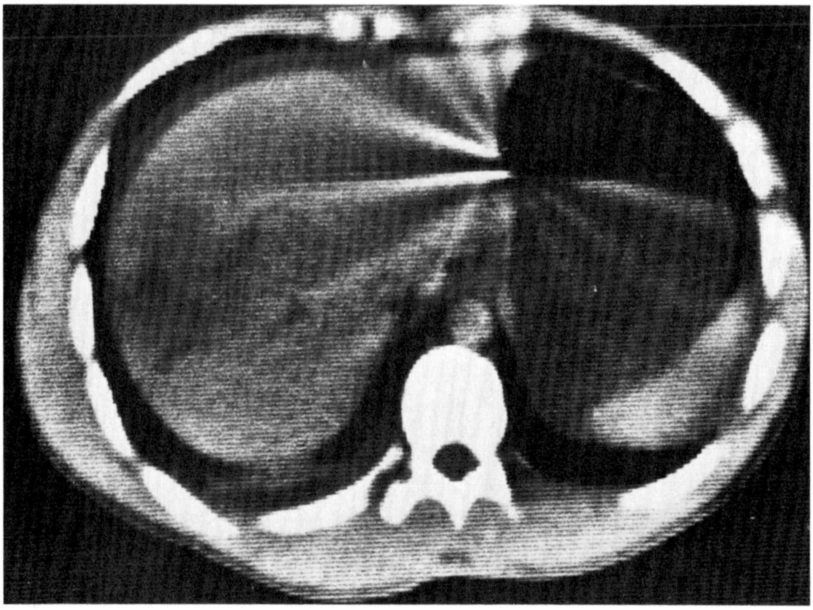

(D)

Figure 4 (continued)

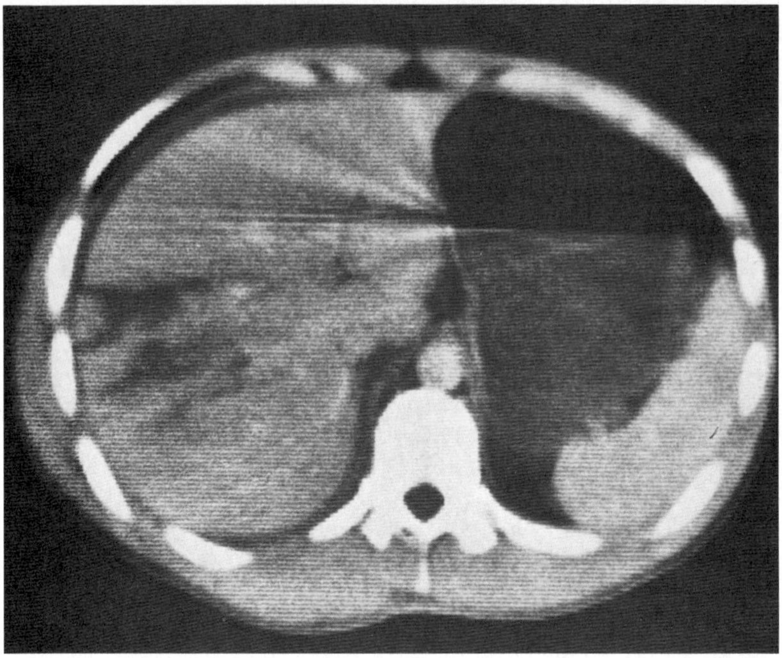

(E)

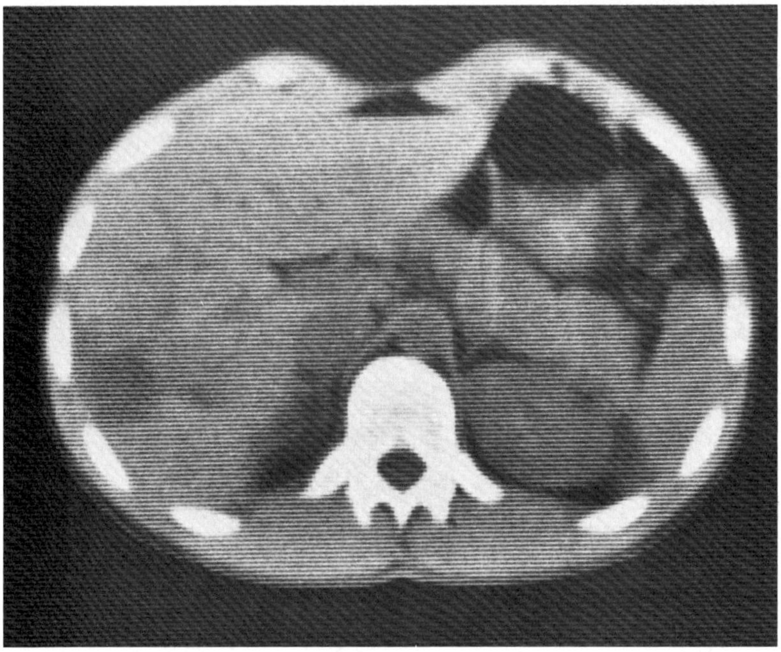

(F)

Figure 4 (continued)

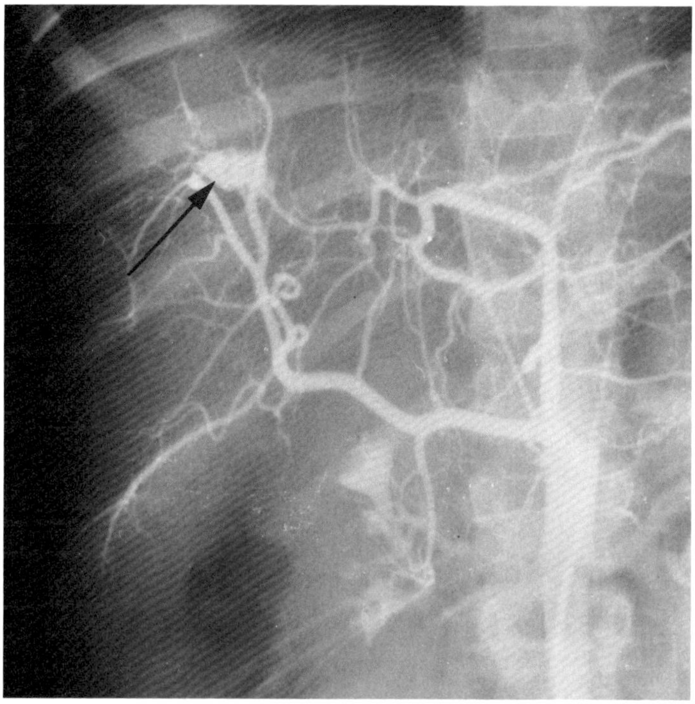

(A)

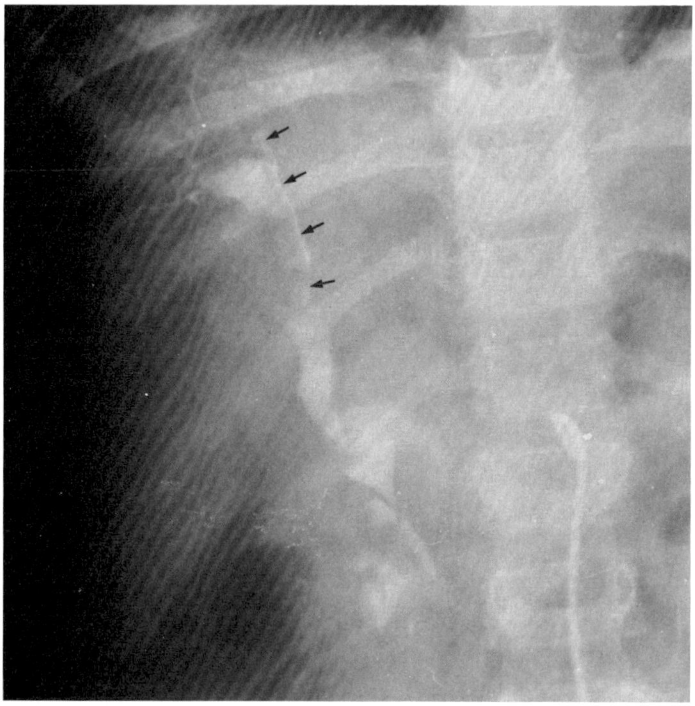

(B)

Figure 5

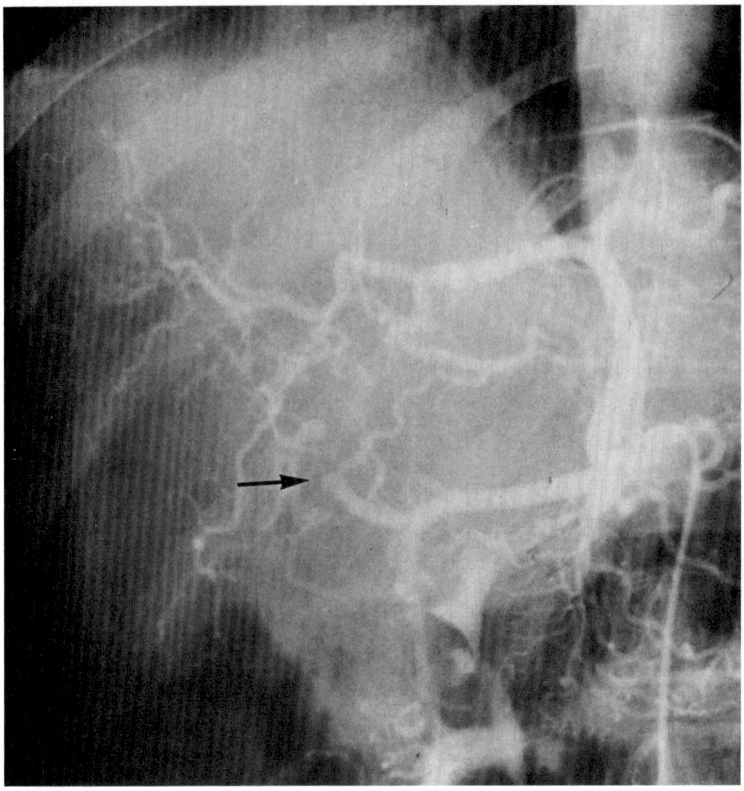

(C)

Figure 5 Blunt trauma of the upper abdomen in a child who collapsed 5 days later. Laparotomy was normal. Jaundice, hematemesis, and melena followed later. Two further laparotomies failed to reveal the cause. Angiography 3 months after the trauma showed (A) an aneurysm (arrow) and (B) an arteriobiliary fistula (small arrows). Repeat operation with ligature of the feeding artery. (C) Two months later the ligated right artery is shown (arrow), but now no aneurysm or fistula is visible.

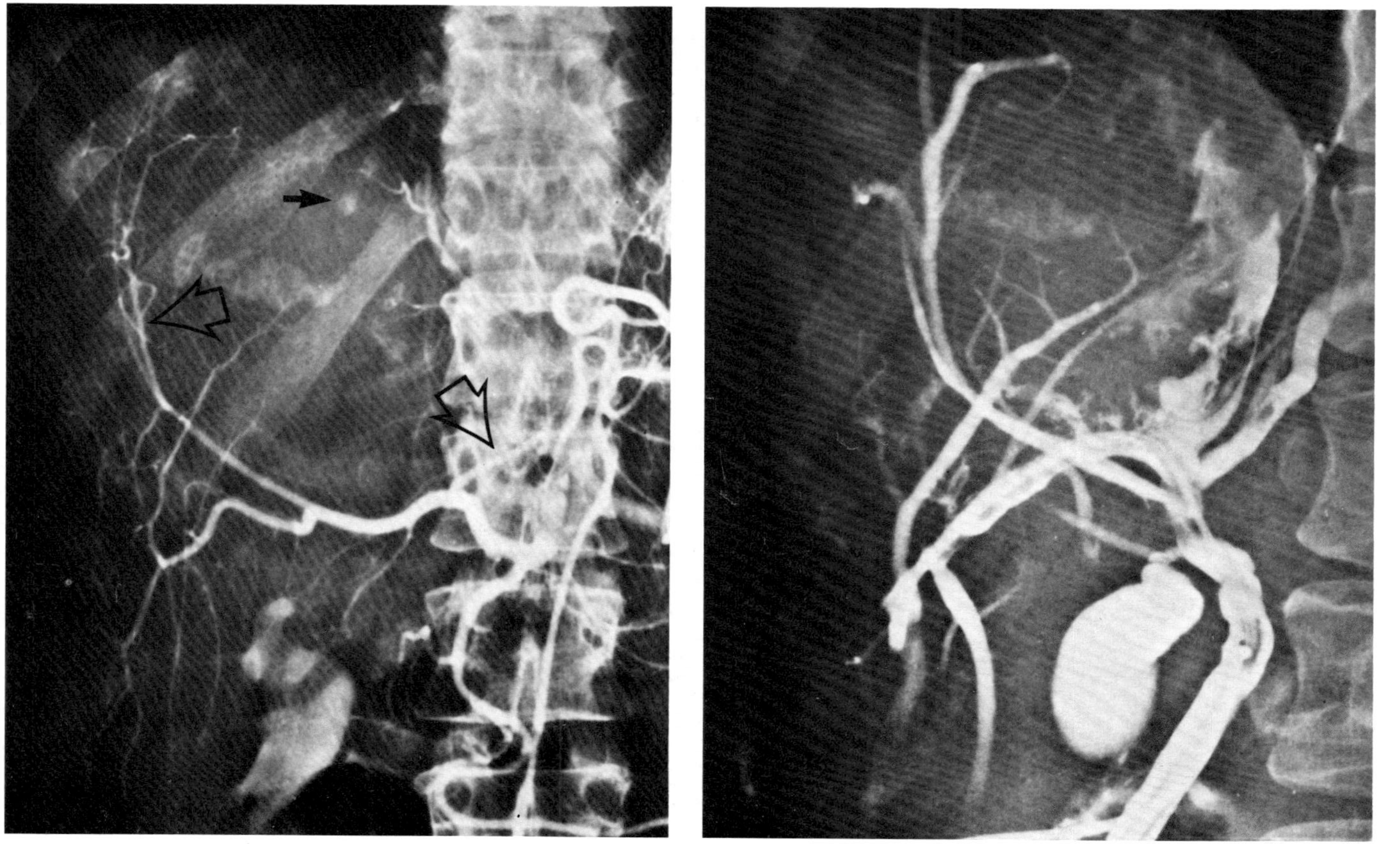

(A) (B)

Figure 6 (A) Blunt trauma with hematoma and arteriobiliary fistula. On admission the patient was in shock and immediate laparotomy revealed a superficial rupture of the liver, which was sutured. Two weeks later severe upper abdominal pain and gastrointestinal bleeding. At angiography a large intrahepatic hematoma is indicated by vessel displacement (open arrows) and by a small extravasation (arrow). (B) At operation, cholangiography revealed disruption of displaced bile ducts. After drainage for 3 months the course was uneventful.

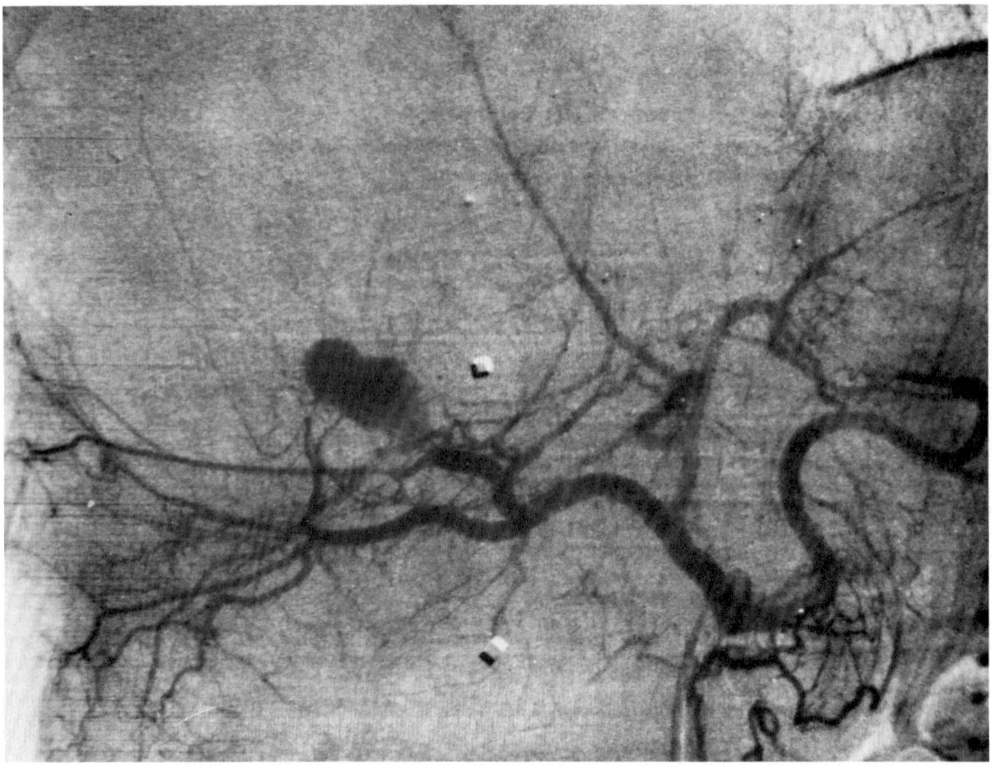

(A)

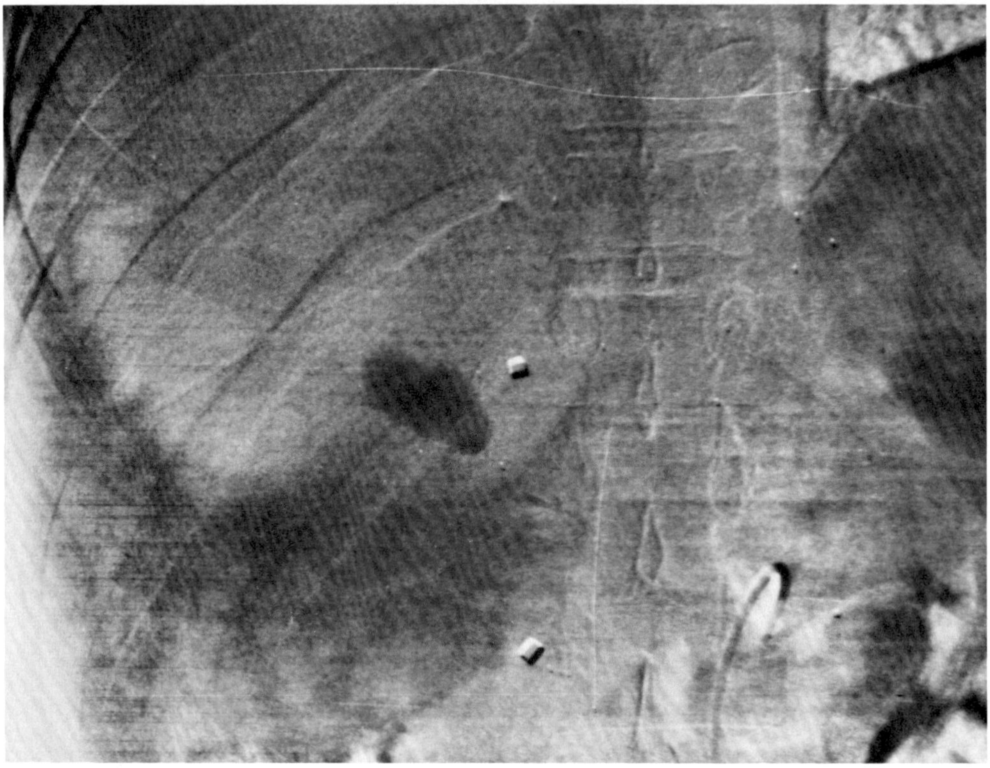

(B)

Figure 7

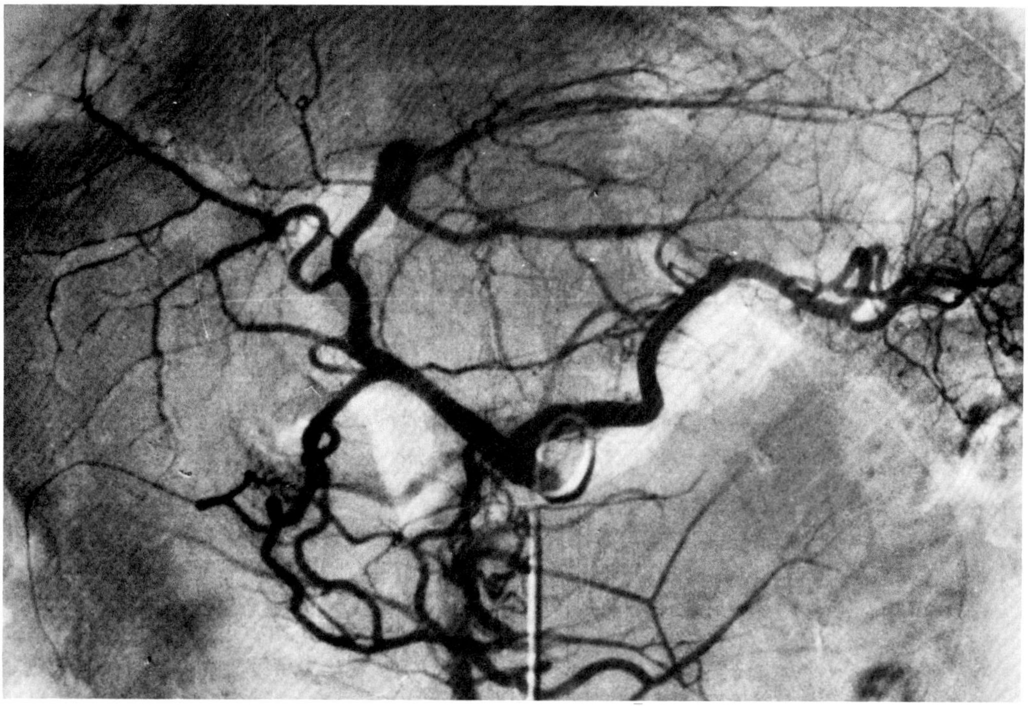

(C)

Figure 7 Blunt trauma to the upper abdomen requiring immediate operation, with deep sutures of the lacerated right lobe of the liver. In the postoperative period, increasing abdominal pain with liver enlargement. (A,B) Angiography 1 month later revealed a large hematoma with pseudoaneurysm. Right hepatic resection was followed by uneventful recovery. (C) This was confirmed by a control angiography 3 years later.

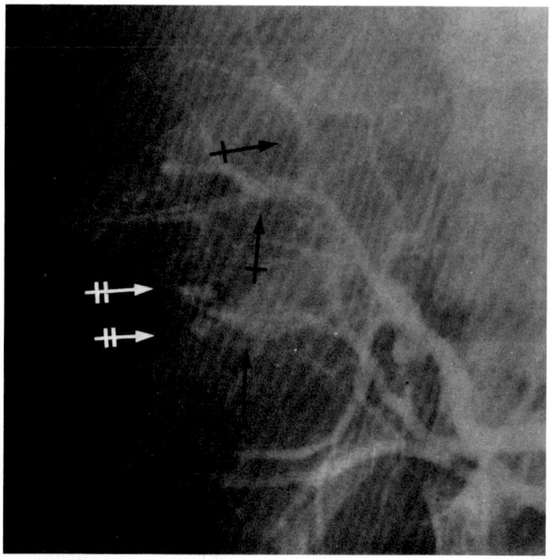

Figure 8 Blunt trauma to the upper abdomen. Operation a few hours after admission and suture of a rupture of the posterior part of the liver. Because of recurrent pain, angiography was performed 12 days later. Displacement and occlusion of an intrahepatic artery of the right lobe of the liver. Minor pseudoaneurysms (white arrows) and early appearance of portal vein radicles (crossed arrow).

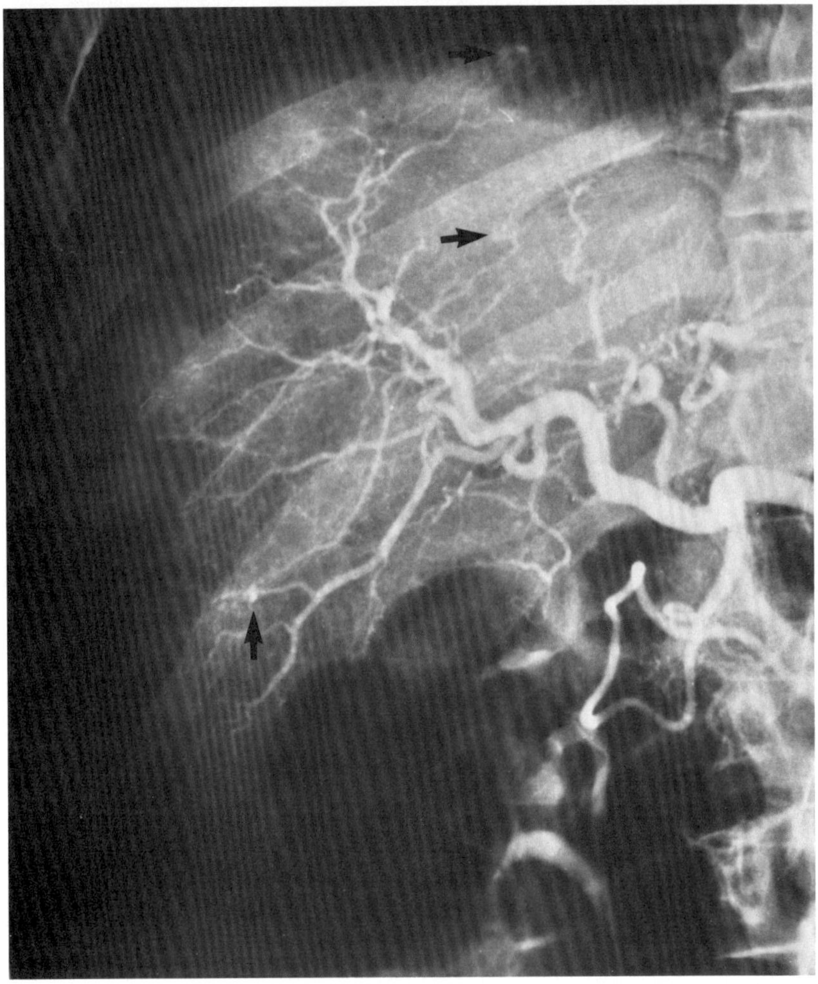

(A)

Figure 9 Blunt trauma to the lower right thorax with rib fractures. During the next days, slight elevation of bilirubin and transaminases. At scintigraphy, suggestion of an intrahepatic hematoma. (A) At angiography 3 days after injury an intrahepatic hematoma with multiple extravasations (arrows), hypervascularity, arterioportal shunting, and irregular accumulation of contrast medium are observed. Small amount of blood in the abdominal cavity. Uneventful recovery without operation. (B) Angiography and scintigraphy 1 month later were normal.

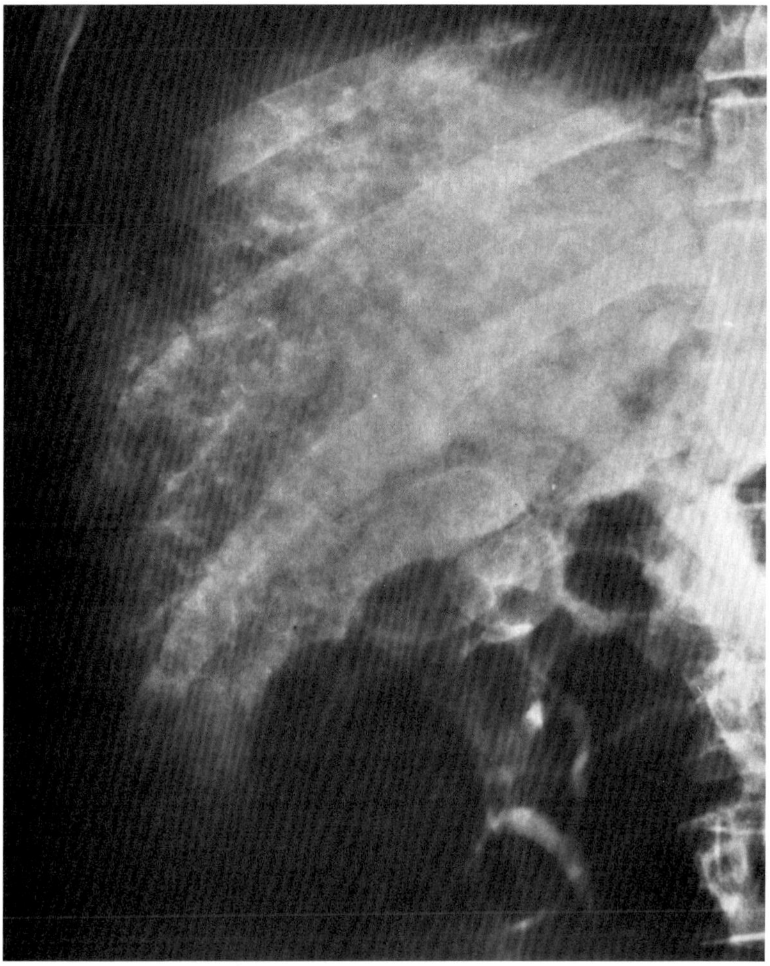

(B)

Figure 9 (continued)

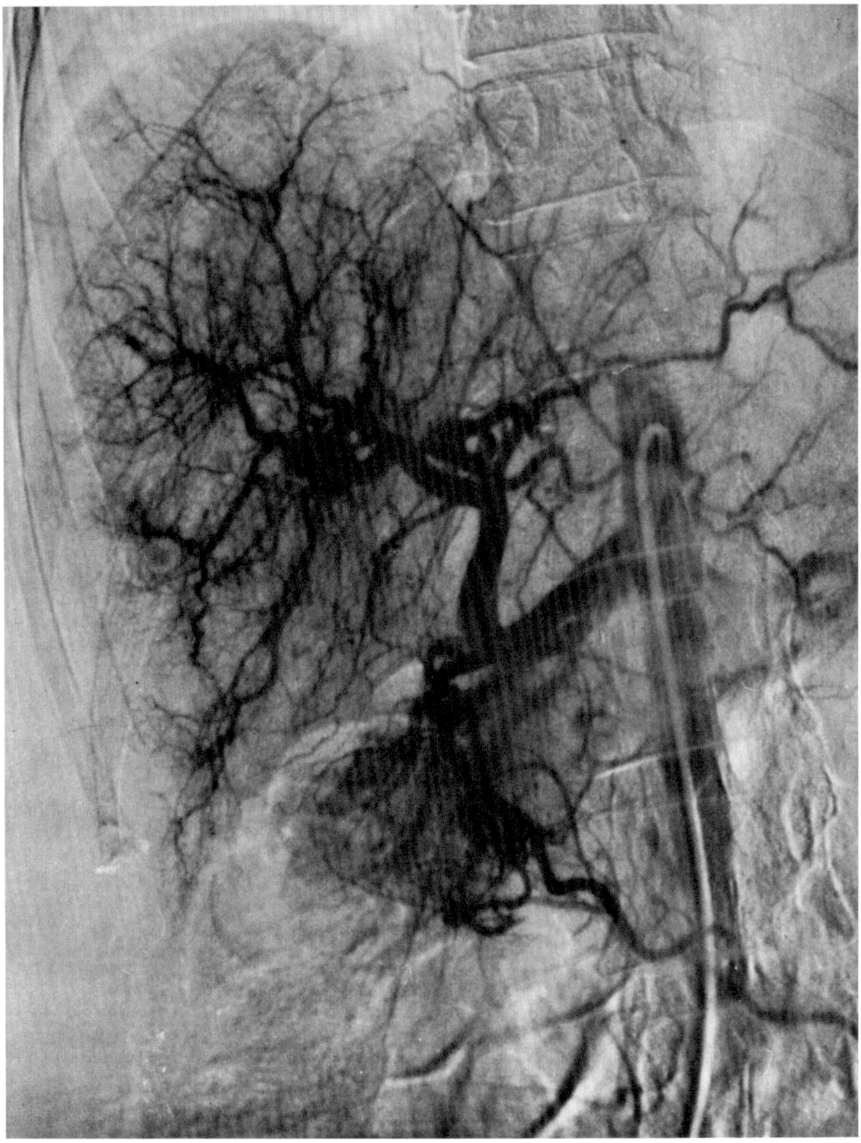

(A)

Figure 10 Blunt trauma to the upper abdomen with an insignificant amount of blood at peritoneal lavage. Angiography 24 hr after the trauma shows hypervascularity of the right lobe of the liver with irregular accumulation of contrast medium in the capillary phase and with small peripheral arterioportal shunts. Slight capsular hyperemia. The lesion was regarded as a contusion effect. Uneventful recovery without exploration.

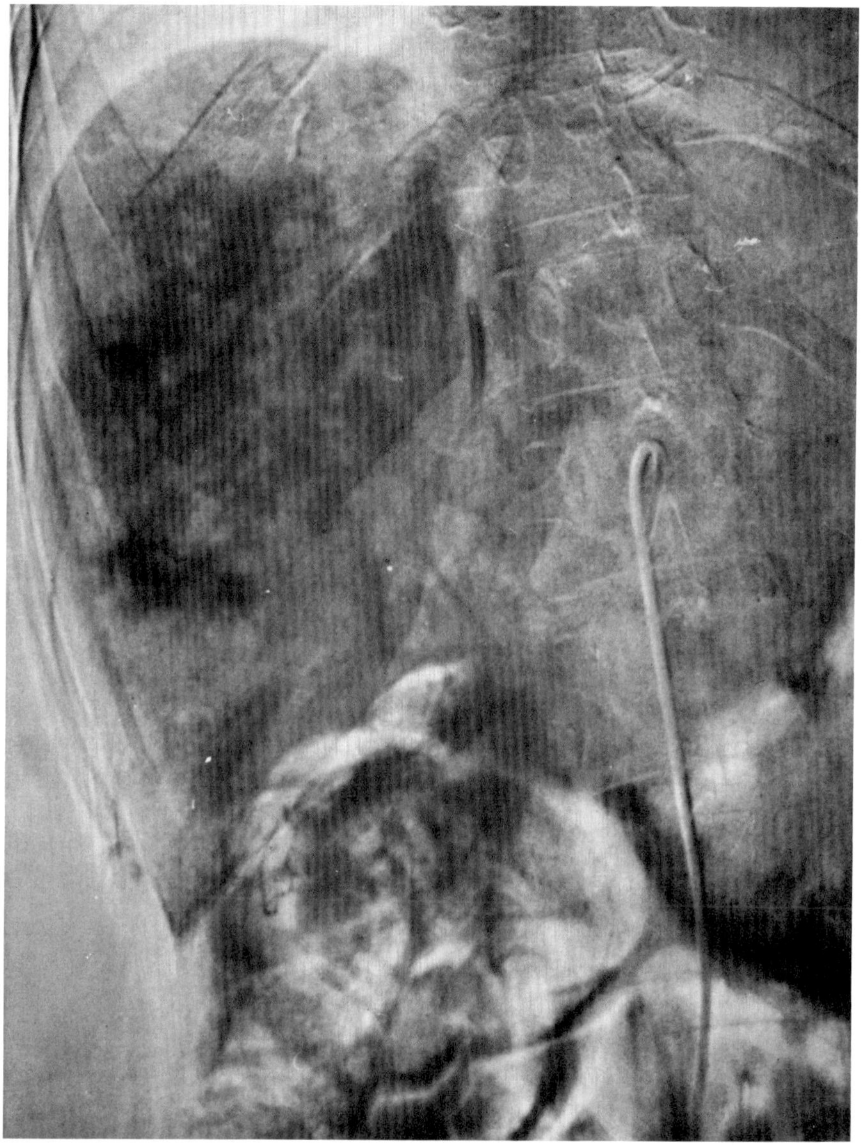

(B)

Figure 10 (continued)

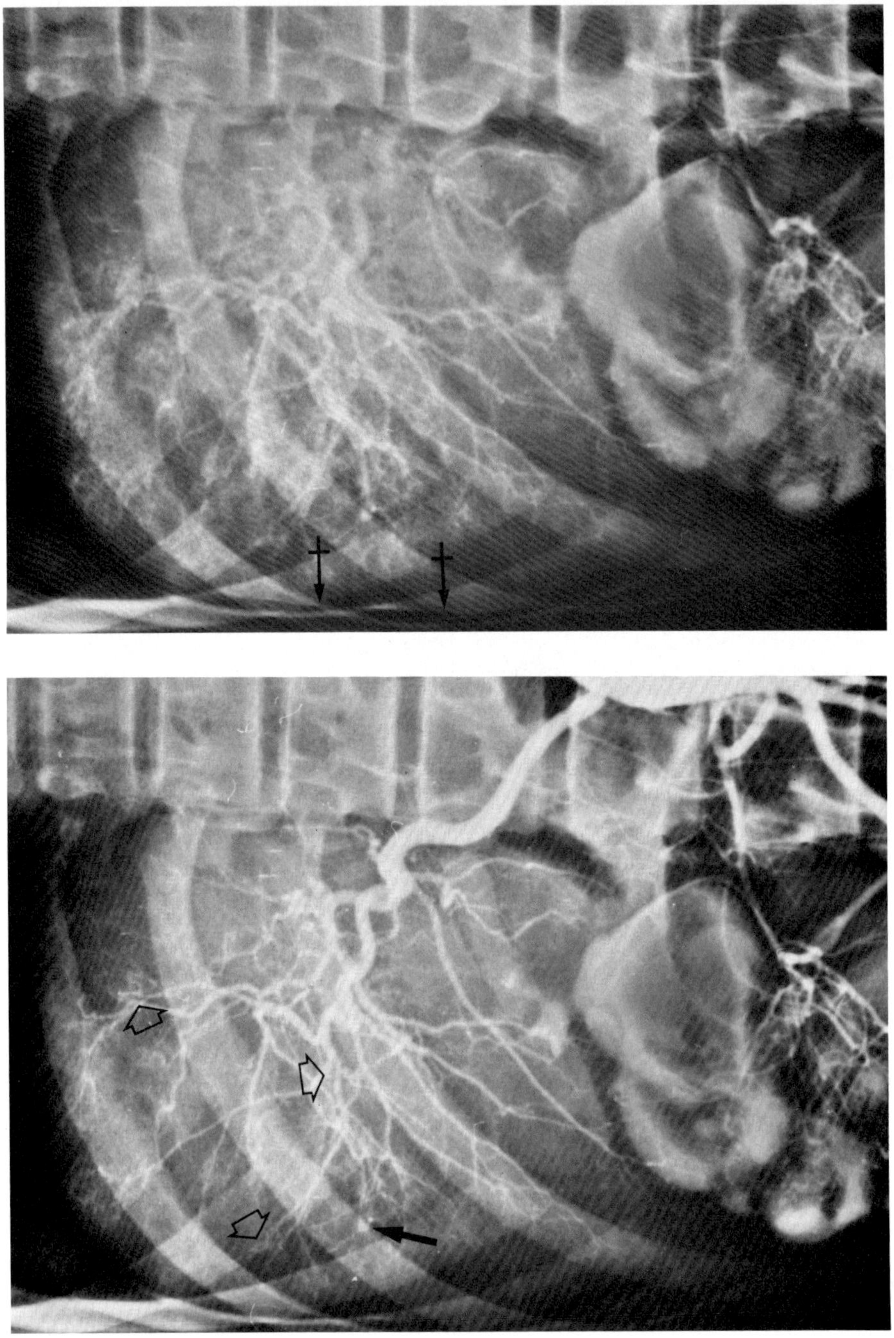

(A) (B)

Figure 11

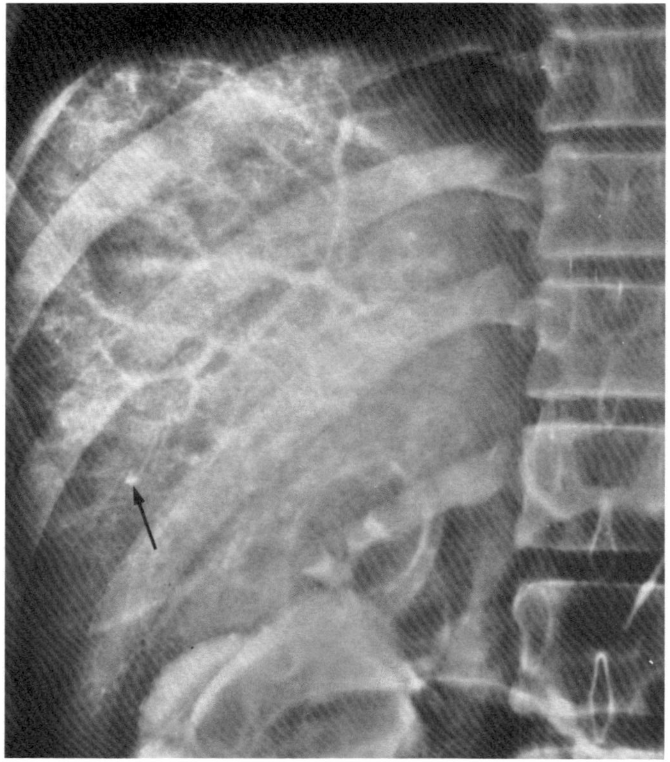

(C)

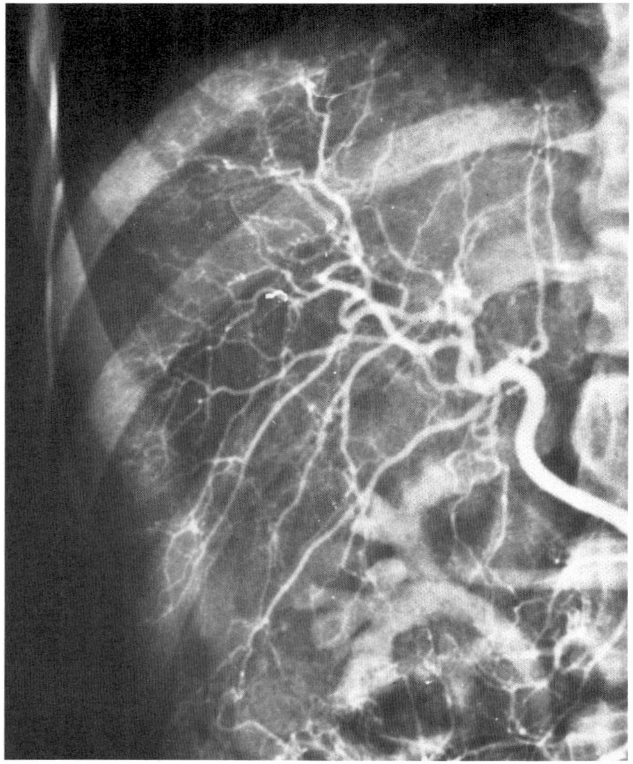

(D)

Figure 11 During soccer play blunt trauma sustained to the right upper abdomen followed by severe upper abdominal pain. (A–C) Angiography 24 hr after injury showed a hematoma (open arrows), also small punctate extravasations (arrows) and early filling of portal veins. Marked hypervascularization and capsular hyperemia (crossed arrows). Small amount of fluid in the abdominal cavity. At operation a 3-cm rupture was found and a hematoma was drained. Control angiography 1 month later appears normal (D).

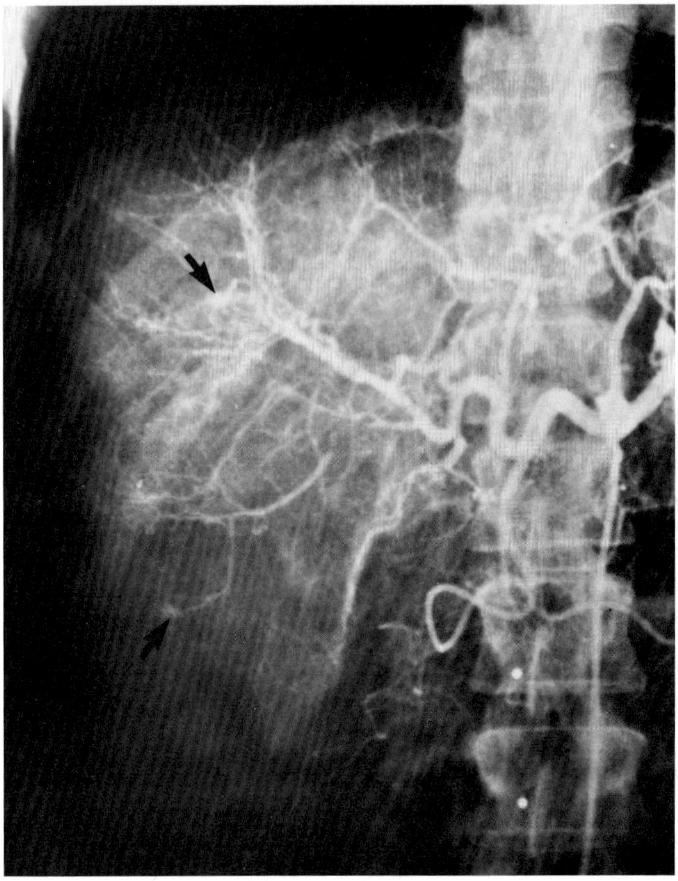

(A)

Figure 12 Celiac angiography a few hours after a car accident, with blunt trauma to the right upper abdomen. (A) Arterial phase. (B) Capillary phase. The liver is displaced medially by an extrahepatic hematoma. Hypervascularization and irregular accumulation seen in the capillary phase (A) Punctate extravasations (arrows) of contrast material close to an intrahepatic hematoma and to the ruptured surface. (B) Dense accumulation in the liver capsule to the level of the rupture (crossed arrows). Occlusion of portal veins and hepatic artery to the caudal segment, where an infarction has developed (white arrows). Findings were verified at operation. The lower part of the right lobe was necrotic and had to be resected.

Radiologic Findings in Blunt Trauma

Immediate Posttraumatic Period

The angiographic findings are unpredictable in patients with blunt trauma to the liver region. It is said that a normal hepatic angiogram of good quality rules out a liver injury that would require operation (42,47,48). Such angiographic information, together with peritoneal lavage showing only insignificant amounts of blood in the abdomen, should be sufficient reason for conservative, nonoperative treatment. However, since there have

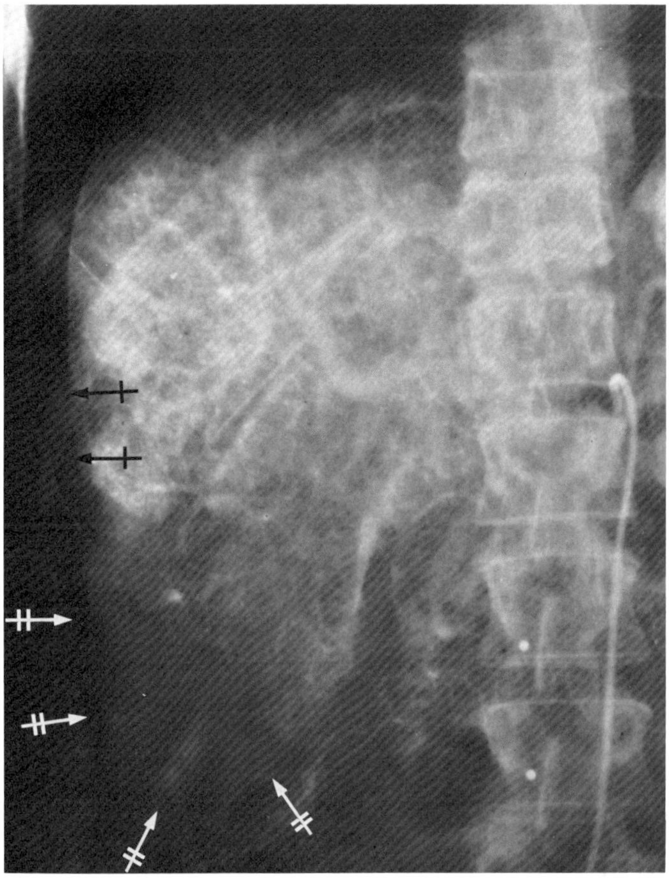

(B)

Figure 12 (continued)

been a few reports of negative angiograms in cases of significant hepatic ruptures, the presence of substantial amounts of blood in the abdominal cavity may be considered sufficient indication for surgical treatment (36). There is no doubt that small lacerations can pass unrecognized at hepatic angiography unless active bleeding is present.

The clinical symptoms may be quite alarming in the acute situation, particularly when contusion of the soft tissues of the abdominal wall has produced pain and tenderness. The liver may be uninjured and the angiogram normal or may merely demonstrate arterial spasm (Fig. 13).

Contusion of the liver parenchyma without hematoma formation will present at angiography with marked hypervascularity, with varying degrees of irregular contrast accumulation within the traumatized part of the liver (Figs 10, 14). Often peripheral portal branches are seen to opacify, giving the impression of arterioportal shunting. It may be difficult to decide whether *localized punctate or larger opacifications* within the liver represent the effects of contusion (Fig. 10), of extravasation (Figs. 4, 9, 12), or are due to

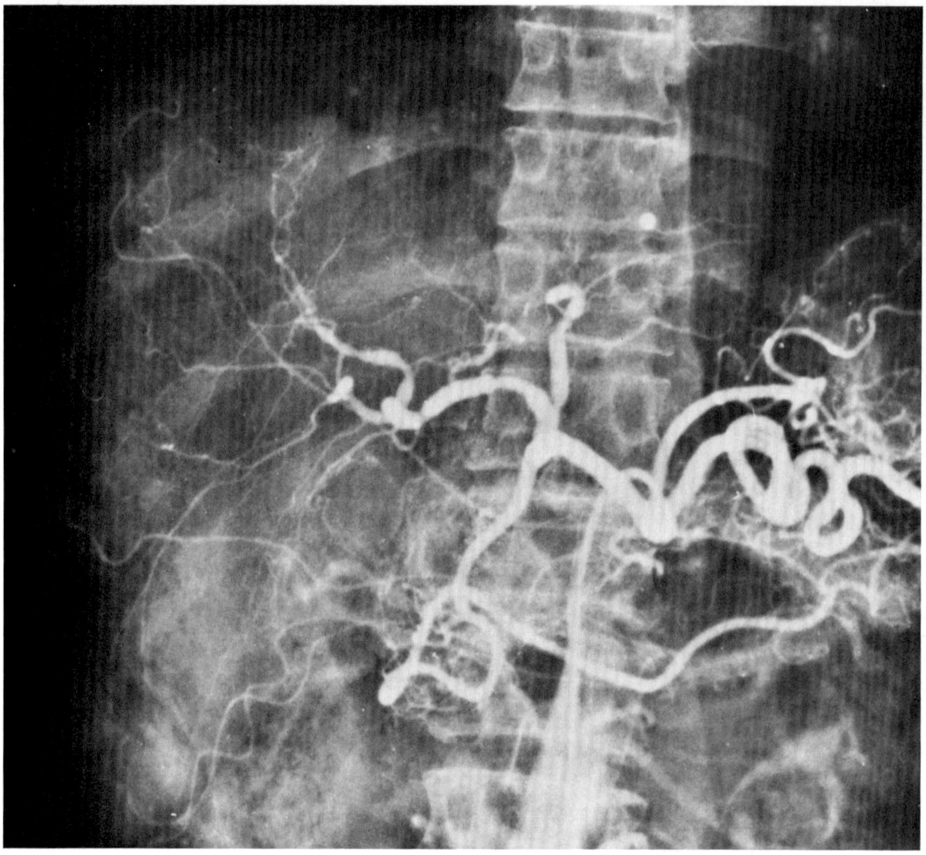

Figure 13 Blunt trauma to the liver region in a 4-m fall. Intense tenderness and pain below the right costal arch with multiple rib fractures. No hypovolemia. At celiac angiography 2 hr later, there are multiple constrictions of the hepatic arteries probably caused by a release of vasoconstrictors. Operation because of intense pain, but no liver damage was found.

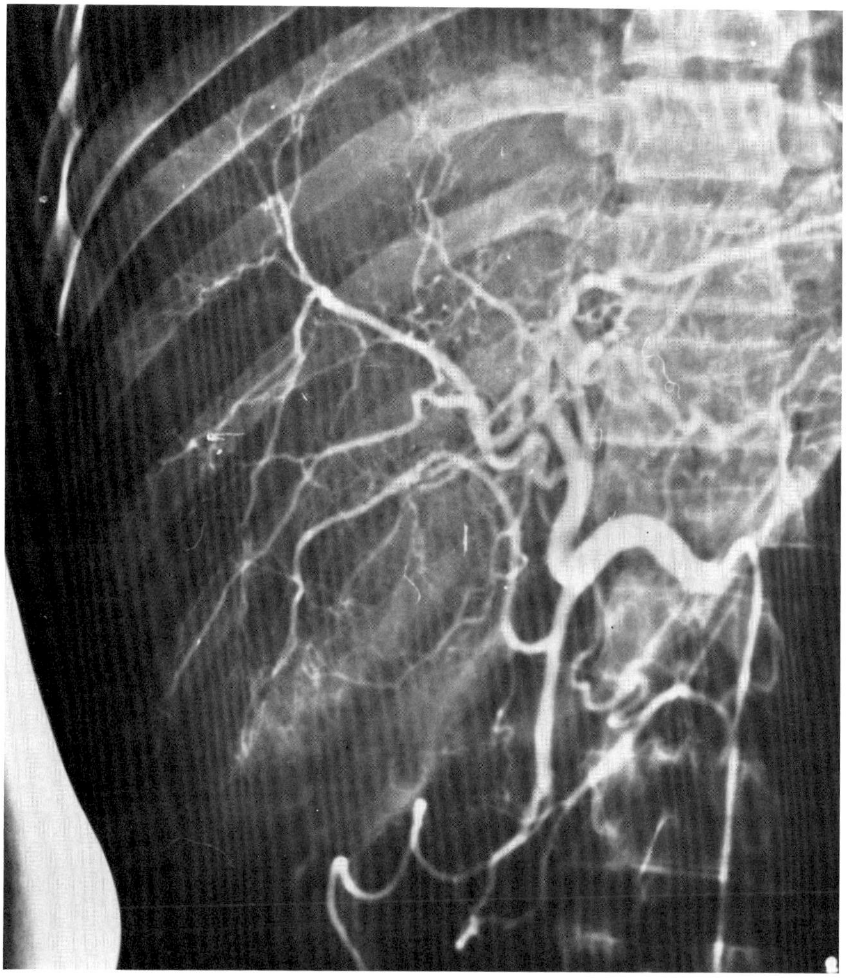

(A)

Figure 14

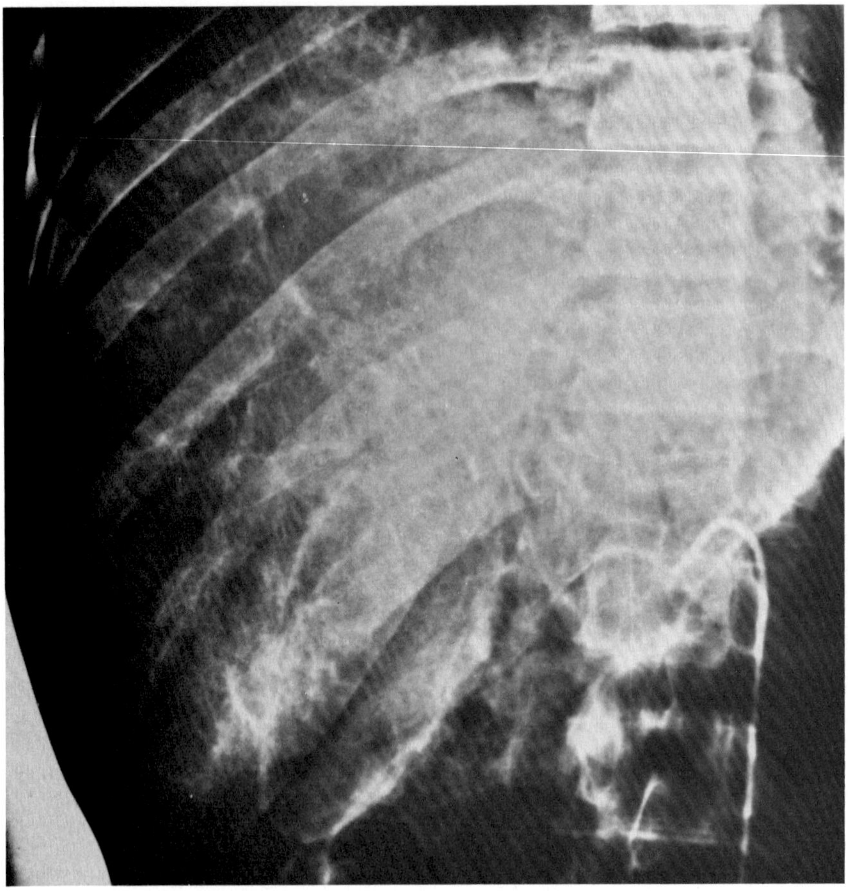

(B)

Figure 14 Severe cerebral contusion, vertebral fractures with paraplegia, fractures of the right tibia and fibula, hematuria, and right retroperitoneal hematoma after a car accident. (A,B) Because of upper abdominal tenderness and muscular defense, angiography is performed, revealing marked contusion effect in the left lobe of the liver extending to the lower part of the right lobe, but without indication of rupture. Marked hypervascularity in this area, whereas the remaining portion of the right lobe is normal.

dense accumulation within capsular veins (Figs. 15–17). The latter are well circumscribed and follow the liver surface when viewed tangentially. Any small extravasations are usually few in number, poorly outlined, and tend to persist into the late capillary phase. Contrast medium accumulations resulting from contusion are more diffusely spread throughout the injured lobe. Neither of these lesions shown by angiography require surgical treatment unless more extensive damage is present in addition. A period of observation possibly followed by control angiography will usually show a return to normal (Figs. 9, 16).

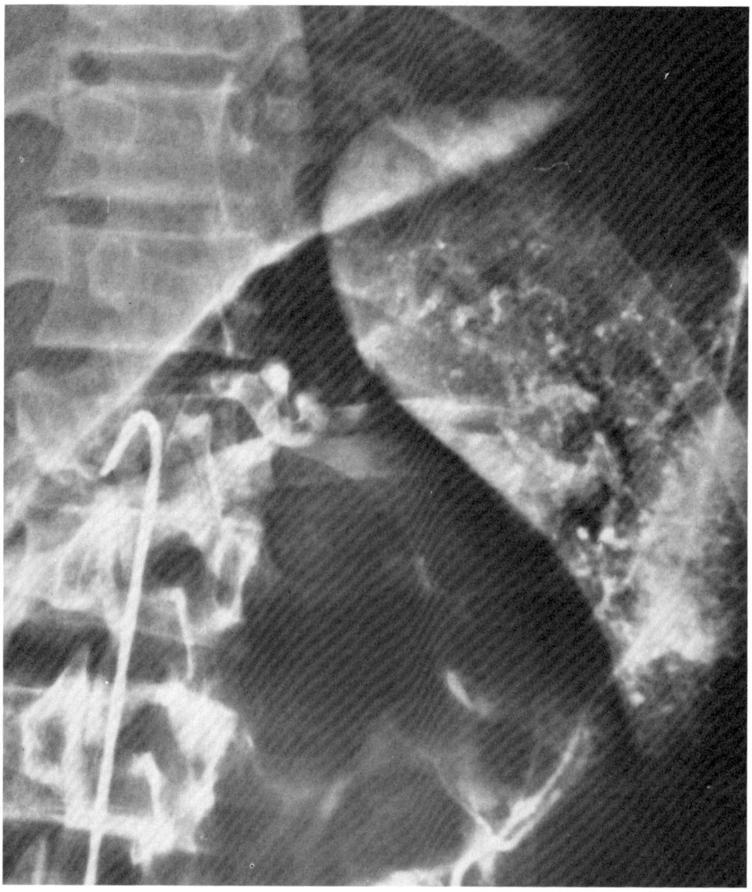

(C)

Figure 14 (continued)

(C) Splenic angiography showed punctate lesions typical for splenic contusion. At operation, no intra-abdominal blood. Spleen and liver appeared normal. Splenectomy was performed with morphological changes typical for contusion.

The angiographic features of contusion—*hypervascularization* with an *irregular distribution* of the contrast material in the capillary phase and the demonstration of *peripheral arterioportal communications*—are illustrated also in patients with intrahepatic or subcapsular hematomas (Figs. 3, 4, 9, 15–17). The arterioportal shunting is often more prominent in these cases (Figs. 8, 11, 12). The early appearance of peripheral portal veins does not mean that true fistulae are present, merely that the normal arterioportal connections have been opened up. In blunt trauma true arterioportal fistulae do occur but are rarely encountered in the acute situation (Fig. 18).

The *acute intrahepatic or subcapsular hematoma* (Figs. 3, 4, 8, 9, 11, 12, 15–17) may vary in size and appearance. *Displacement* and *compression of vessels* in relation to

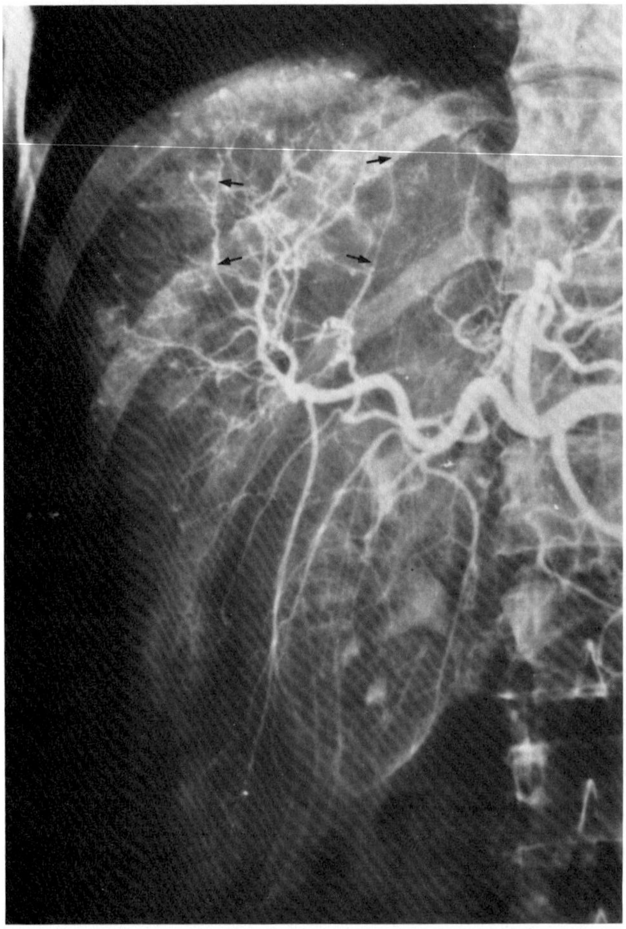

Figure 15 Blunt trauma to the upper abdomen. Intense upper abdominal pain and enlargement of the liver led to prompt operation. A subcapsular hepatic rupture was found and sutured. Due to continuous bleeding, hepatic angiography was performed 2 days later. There was intra-abdominal blood and displacement of branches in the right ventrocranial segment (arrows) due to hematoma. Punctate lesions in the same area, mainly located in the subcapsular space, probably representing subcapsular veins, but local extravasation may also be present. Patient recovered without further surgery.

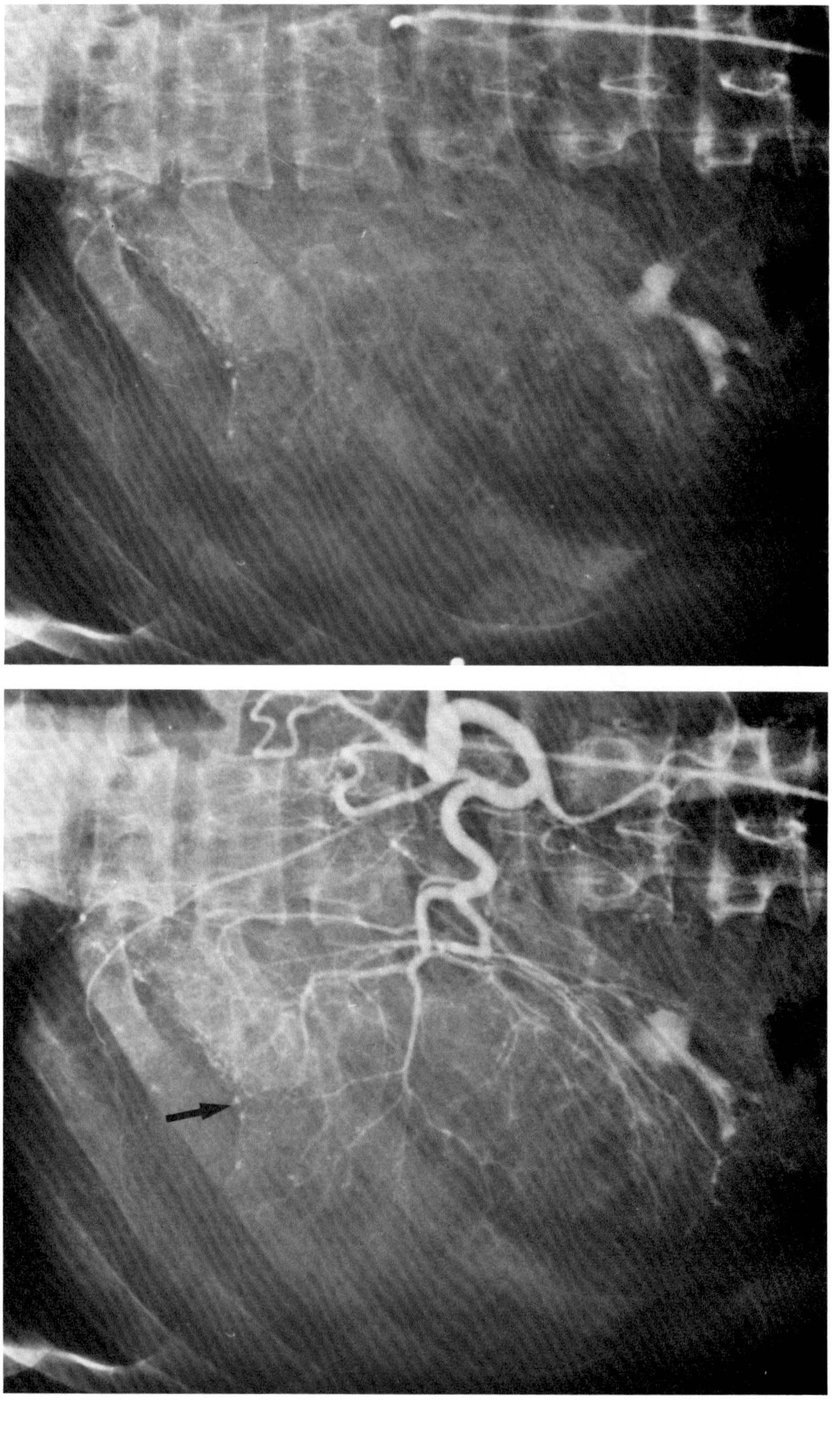

(A) (B)

Figure 16

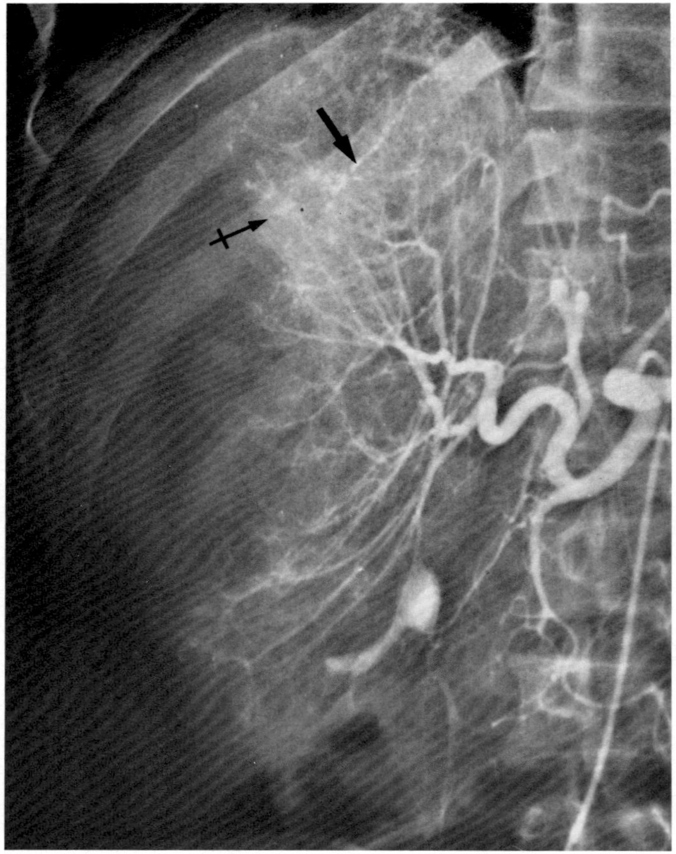

(C)

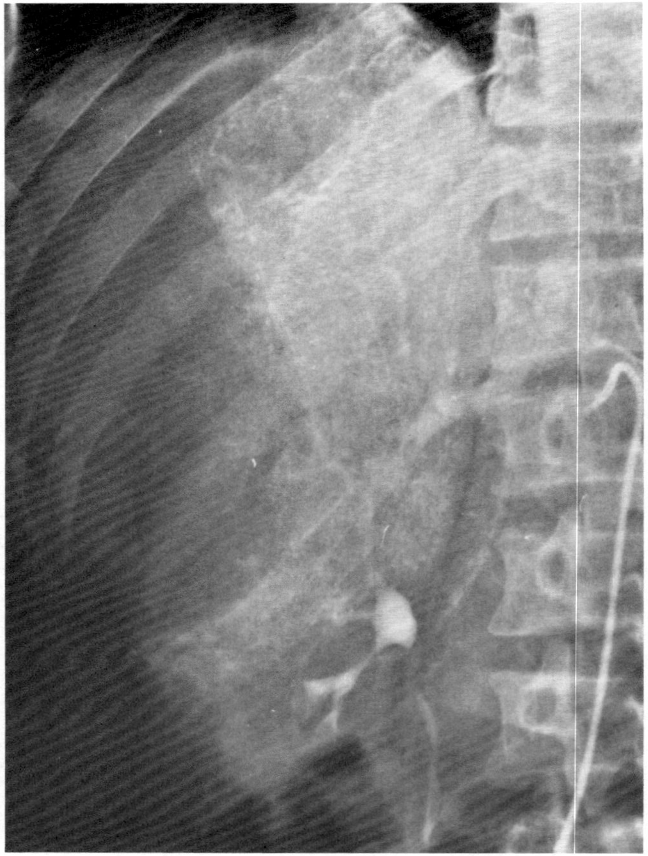

(D)

Figure 16

Blunt Trauma after fall from horseback. No fracture and no signs of bleeding at arrival, but 2 days later upper abdominal pain and rigidity. (A,B) Celiac angiography in anteroposterior position. (C,D) Angiography with patient right posterior oblique (RPO). A large subcapsular hematoma is shown with signs of liver contusion. The distinction between subcapsular and intrahepatic hematoma is made clear in the RPO position. Multiple fine punctate contrast densities seen on the liver surface mainly represent contrast medium and superficial veins (arrows); however, small extravasations are also present (crossed arrow).

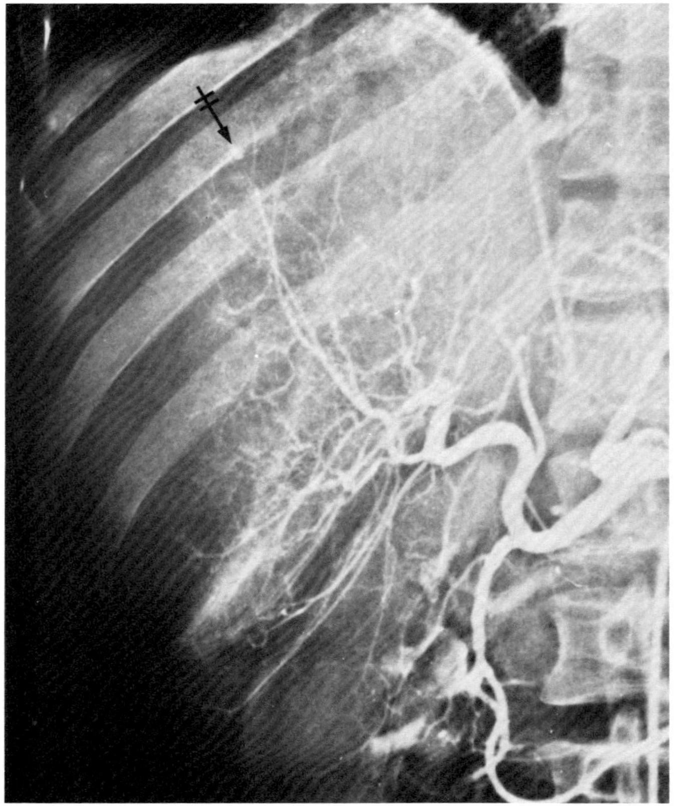

(E)

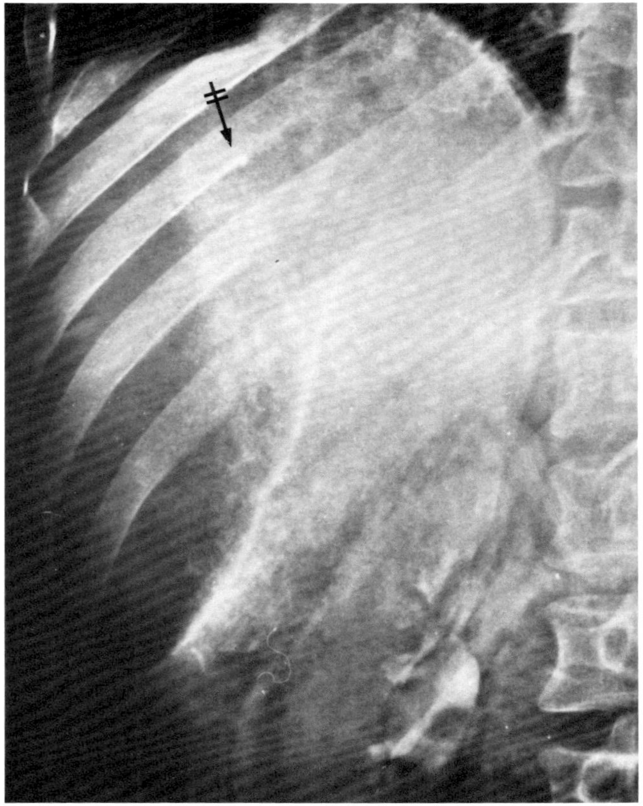

(F)

Figure 16 (continued)

(E,F) Follow-up angiography shows the size of the hematoma slightly reduced. A small extravasation is still present (crossed arrow), probably explaining the poor regression of the hematoma. Observe the dense opacification of the thickened liver surface. Further scintigraphic follow-up showed more regression, still incomplete 14 months after the injury.

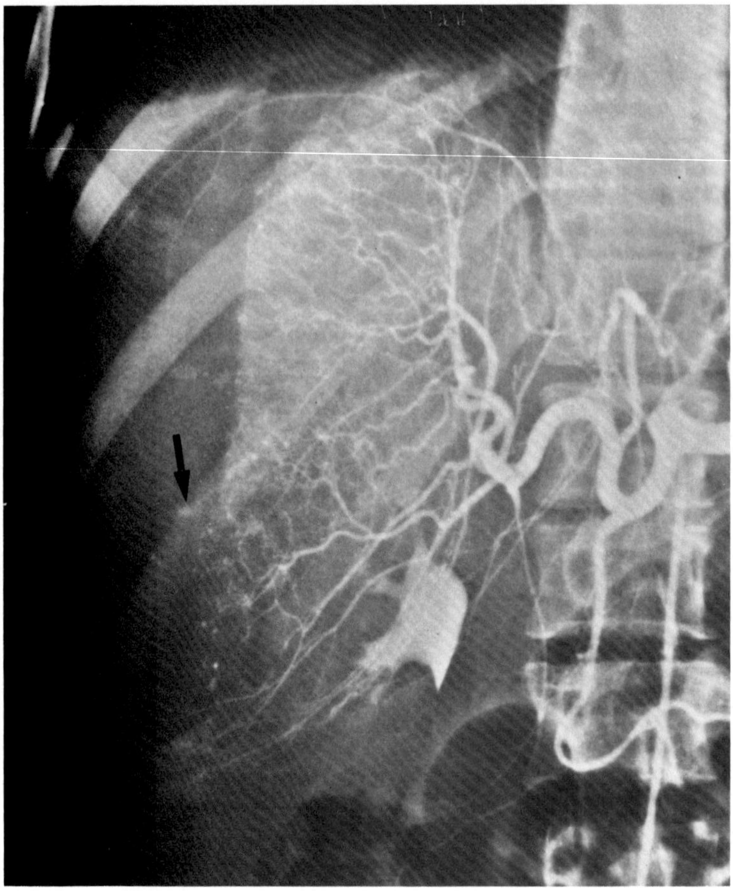

(A)

Figure 17 Blunt trauma to the upper abdomen. Increasing pain and falling hematocrit. (A) Celiac angiogram 2 days after injury. Large subcapsular hematoma with somewhat dense opacification of part of the underlying liver surface and with areas showing small punctate densities, probably representing opacified veins. A small extravasation (arrow) is also observed. At operation the large subcapsular hematoma was confirmed and evacuated. A small vessel on the liver surface was the only bleeding point seen. (B) A control angiogram 1 month later seemed normal.

an avascular area and *small extravasations* close to the hematoma are observed frequently. The hematoma is not found at surgery when positioned deep in the parenchyma (Figs. 6–8). In our case material some of the large hematomas have been drained surgically (Figs. 10–12, 17), whereas in others, of similar size, no operation was performed, yet recovery was uneventful. Scintigraphic scanning and CT offer a good opportunity to follow the uncomplicated hematoma (Figs. 3, 4, 16). Angiography is an alternative method to monitor the healing process of operated or nonoperated hematomas (41,68) (Figs. 7, 9, 11, 17).

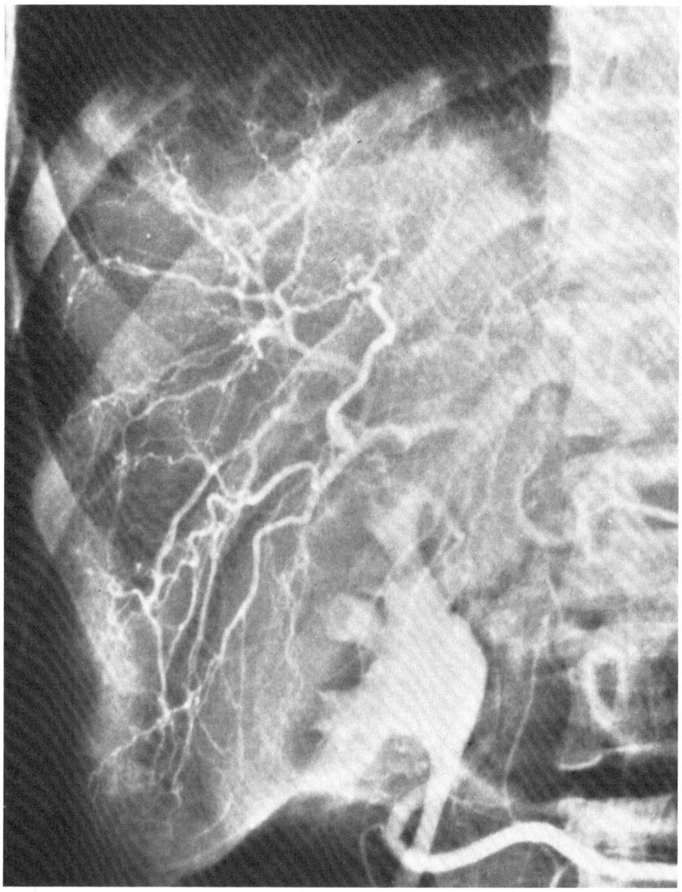

Figure 17B

The distinction between an intrahepatic and subcapsular hematoma by angiography can occasionally be difficult. Differential diagnosis will require film series to be taken in several different projections (Fig. 16).

Blood in the abdominal cavity close to the liver presents as an increased distance between liver and abdominal wall (Figs. 3, 4, 9, 11, 12). A subcapsular hematoma always causes a deformity of the adjacent liver surface, which is not present if the hematoma is outside the liver capsule. The exact site and extent of the bleed are best disclosed by CT (Fig. 3).

A previously not recorded but often encountered angiographic finding in hepatic trauma is the *early and dense opacification of the liver capsule* (69) (Figs. 4, 10–2, 17). The exact site of a capsular rupture can thus be demonstrated (Figs. 4, 12). The capsular tear can also be delineated by CT (Fig. 4). Angiography soon after hepatic trauma may also demonstrate pseudoaneurysms which are usually small (Figs. 8, 18). These heal, as a rule, but may occasionally rupture later and cause hemobilia or a large intrahepatic hematoma (Figs. 5, 7).

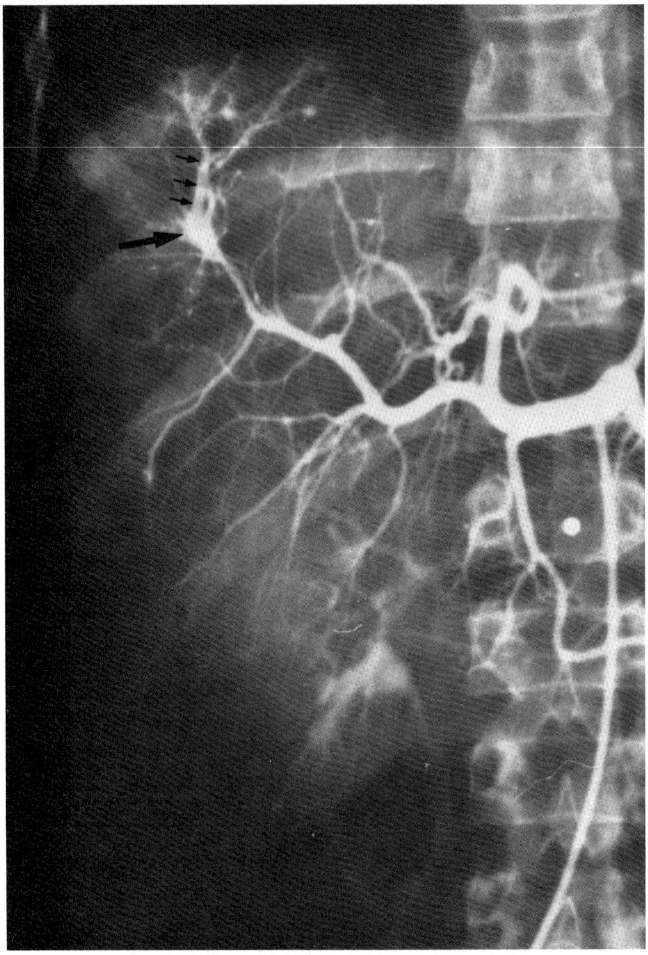

Figure 18 Blunt trauma to the liver in a young boy. Celiac angiography 9 days later because of progressive anemia. An arterioportal fistula (small arrows) and a small pseudoaneurysm (arrow) were observed. There was uneventful recovery.

Arterial and venous occlusions are sometimes observed (Figs. 8, 12). Intrahepatic arterial collaterals may bypass the occlusion, but when there is also occlusion of portal veins, the diagnosis of liver necrosis will become obvious (Fig. 12).

Computerized tomography will usually give information about the site and extent of a laceration or hematoma formation, but cannot provide sufficient detail about the many vascular lesions present in the acute situation. Furthermore, the attenuation values of a hematoma will alter (70–72), and may approximate those of the liver substance. Consequently, contrast enhancement by bolus technique is needed if CT is to rule out the presence of a hematoma in the liver.

Late Effects of Blunt Trauma

The late consequences of hepatic trauma can be assessed by scintigraphy, CT, or ultrasonography. The regression of a hematoma or the appearance of an *abscess as a complication* of hematoma can be monitored in this way. Although it is possible to detect an arteriovenous fistula by enhancement CT (51), more reliable information is obtained by angiography, particularly when an arteriobiliary fistula or a pseudoaneurysm is suspected (Figs. 5–7).

Arterioportal fistulae may persist or increase in size and may be located centrally in the liver (73–76). They are rarely of hemodynamic importance to the systemic circulation, because of a protecting regulatory effect of the liver, probably based on increased resistance in its capillary bed.

Cysts of enormous size, located below the liver capsule, are a rare consequence of blunt hepatic trauma and a residue of a subcapsular hematoma. Ultrasonography or CT will disclose the true nature of the lesion (Fig. 19).

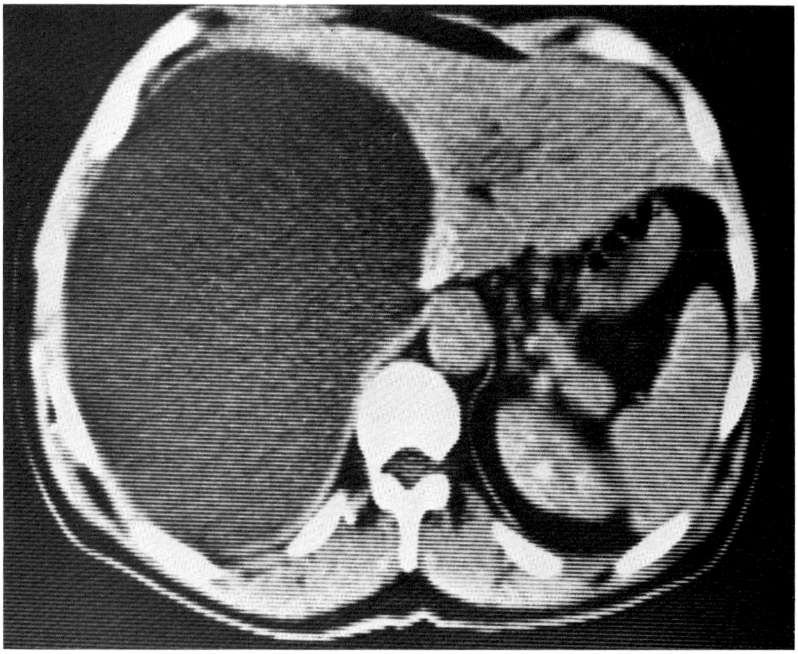

Figure 19 Blunt trauma to the right flank 2 years before. CT done because of hepatomegaly. A 15 × 20 cm cyst is present in the right lobe of the liver. Percutaneous drainage followed.

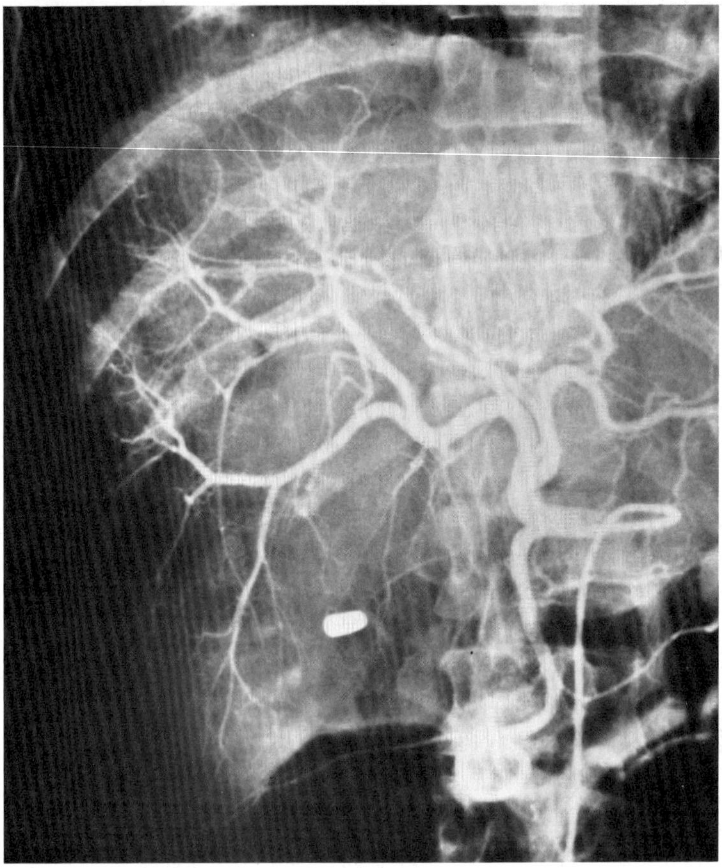

(A)

Figure 20 Gunshot wound, the bullet entering the thorax just below the right breast, passing through the liver and right kidney. Angiography was performed because of increasing abdominal pain and hematuria. (A,B) At hepatic angiography the entrance of the bullet into the liver could be identified because of accumulation of contrast medium in the capsule on either side of a capsular tear (arrows). Displaced hepatic arteries and hypervascularity outline an intrahepatic hematoma caused by the transit of the bullet. There is occlusion of a peripheral branch of the right hepatic artery (crossed arrow). (C) Renal angiography revealed an intrarenal hematoma with abnormal tapering of anterior intermediate branches. No surgery was done.

Radiologic Findings in Penetrating Trauma

Penetrating hepatic injury due to gunshot has a poor prognosis and angiography is seldom performed in the acute phase. The findings resemble those in blunt trauma, with capsular rupture, hematoma formation, fistulae, vessel occlusion, and others (Fig. 20). Late complications include abscess formation and arterioportal and arteriobiliary fistulations and can be demonstrated by angiography (77–81).

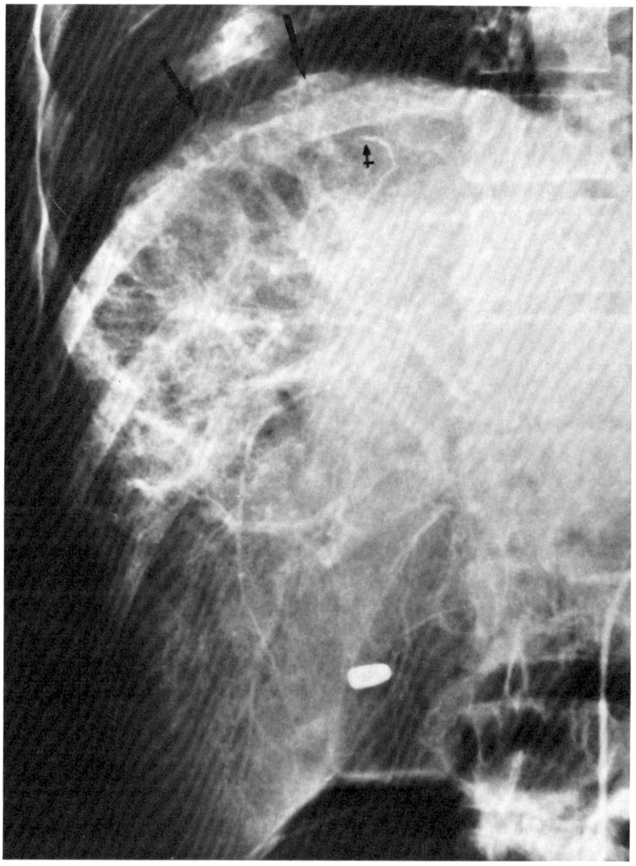

(B)

Figure 20 (continued)

Iatrogenic Trauma

Percutaneous liver biopsy for histology, percutaneous transhepatic cholangiography, or portography, as well as percutaneous biliary drainage, are today probably the most common forms of penetrating liver injury. Serious intra-abdominal bleeding (see Fig. 13 in Chap. 15), bile leakage, and intrahepatic or subcapsular hematoma formation (Fig. 21) have been revealed by arteriography or CT (8–10,12–15,55,82–85). Both experimentally and clinically it has been shown that these lesions can heal spontaneously, and their high incidence did, therefore, not become obvious until angiography was performed after the causative procedure. Serious complications are rare and occur particularly when wide-bore tubings are used for puncture or drainage. Liver injury has also been found to occur during wedged hepatic venography (86).

Iatrogenic lesions secondary to gallbladder surgery (7,16,17,87) may cause severe trauma to the liver, as could be observed in one of our patients in whom hepatic artery

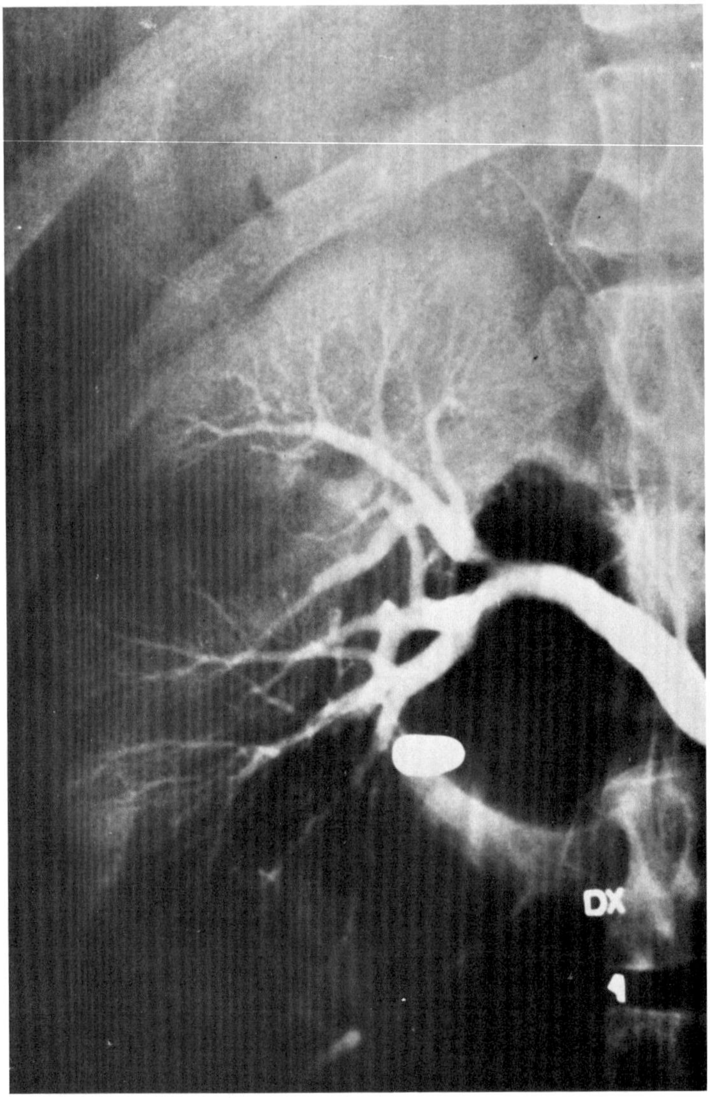

(C)

Figure 20 (continued)

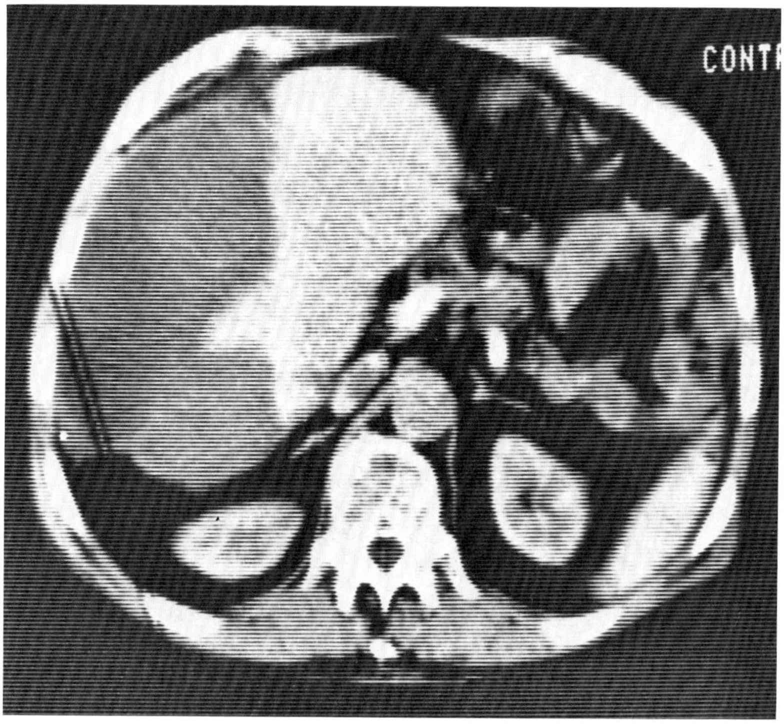

Figure 21 Palpable abdominal tumor and hepatomegaly led to liver biopsy, after which the patient became hypovolemic and had severe abdominal pain. Referred for CT 2 months later, when a large subcapsular hematoma was still present (contrast enhancement).

ligation was ineffective (Fig. 22). Aneurysm formation and hemobilia can be further consequences of complicated biliary surgery (Fig. 23).

Although ultrasonography, CT, and scintigraphy can have a primary diagnostic function, the main method for revealing hepatic lesions caused by trauma, whatever their origin, must still be angiography. The noninvasive imaging modalities find their best usage in the follow-up of lesions already documented by angiography. Cholangiography and portography (88) are methods for occasional use in diagnosis.

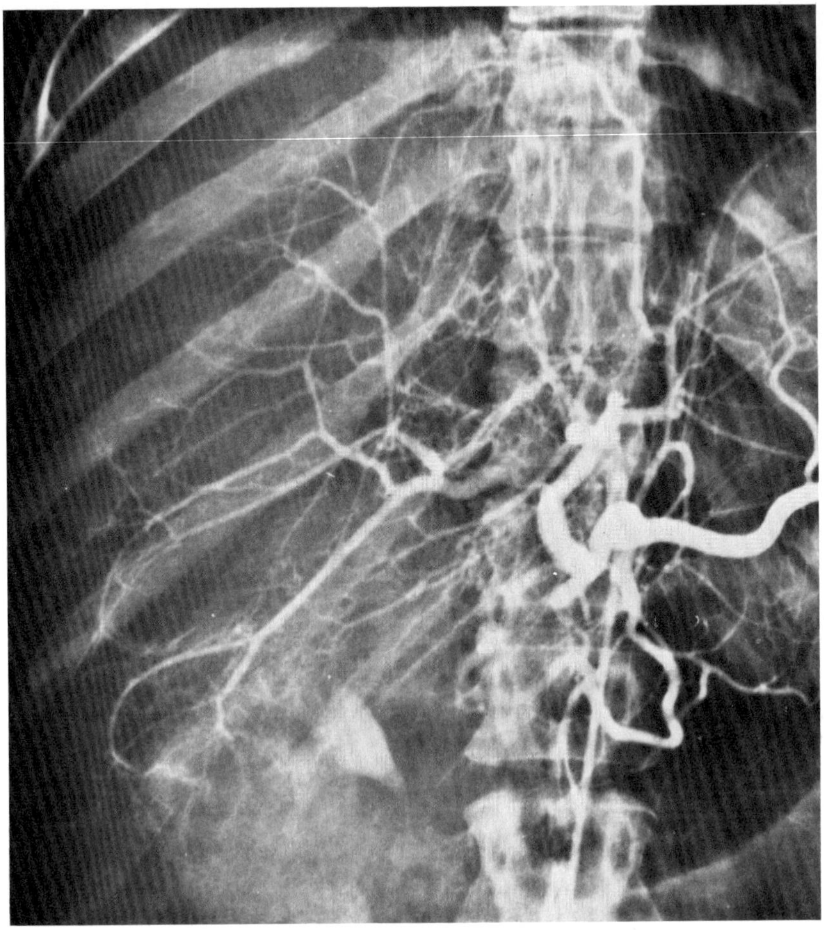

(A)

Figure 22 Severe hypovolemia followed cholescystectomy and was due to hepatic rupture close to the bed of the gallbladder, extending posteriorly. Suturing and tamponade were performed, but continuing blood loss required a third operation for ligation of the hepatic artery. Celiac angiography was done 7 days after the first operation. There is well-established collateral circulation via the left hepatic artery. In the caudal segment of the right lobe pronounced hypervascularity is associated with delayed circulation and with reverse flow into portal branches. A large- and extrahepatic (see arrows to liver surface) hematoma is present. Repeated follow-up scintigraphy showed slow regression with changes still present 10 months later.

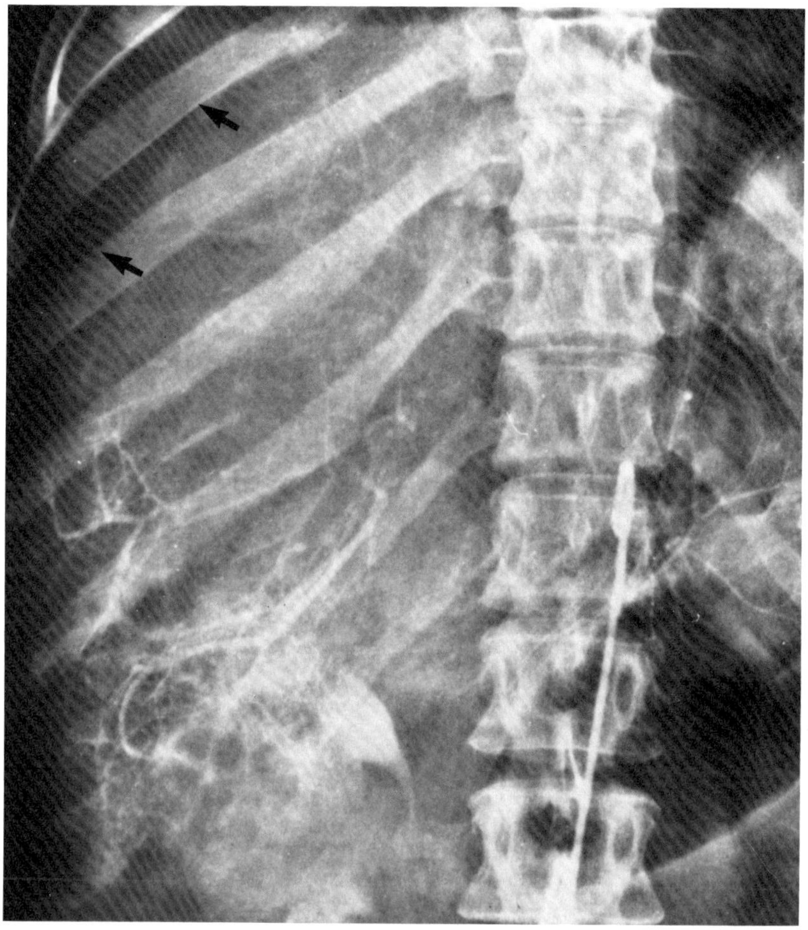

(B)

Figure 22 (continued)

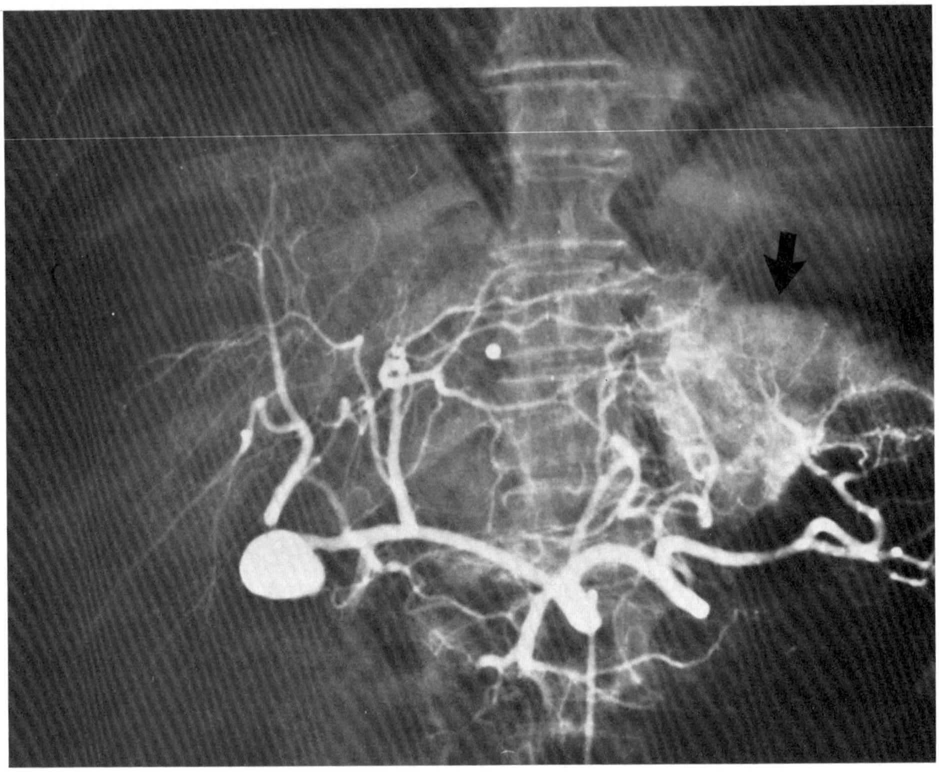

Figure 23 Aneurysm of the right hepatic artery after complicated biliary surgery. Two days after surgery blood passed through the choledochal drain, and during the following days severe bleeding required repeated blood transfusions. Arteriography 1 month later revealed a 20 × 30 mm aneurysm of the right hepatic artery. In addition, a subphrenic abscess was disclosed, displacing the spleen caudally (arrow). After ligation of the hepatic artery and drainage of the abscess there was no further bleeding.

Management of Arterial Bleeding

Ligation of the hepatic artery to stop bleeding has been used extensively by surgeons (25–27). The value of this technique is under debate. The immediate development of collaterals will usually abolish its effectiveness.

Embolization with Gelfoam has been found to be increasingly useful. By this means the occlusion is brought closer to the bleeding site and is therefore more effective and lasting than hepatic artery ligation at some distance (64, 89–96). Embolization is thus an alternative to operation and may be lifesaving in patients in poor clinical condition. The period of convalescence is much reduced and the complications, so far, are fewer than with surgery. Ischemic necrosis of the gallbladder has been reported as an occasional complication that may require operation (97). The advantage of embolization is of course that both diagnosis and therapy can be carried out together, by the same angiographic method (see Chap. 27).

Concomitant Lesions

Adjacent organ lesions should always be looked for in cases of trauma to the liver. Renal (Fig. 4) as well as splenic injuries (Fig. 14) are frequently observed. Angiography is the most reliable method to define concomitant lesions, and adjacent organs should, therefore, always be included in the angiographic field.

References

1. Aldrete JS, Halpern NB, Ward S, Wright JO: Factors determining the mortality and morbidity in hepatic injuries. Analysis of 108 cases. *Ann Surg 189*:466, 1979.
2. Defore WW Jr, Mattox KL, Jordan GL, Beall AC: Management of 1590 consecutive cases of liver trauma. *Arch Surg 111*:493, 1976.
3. Gillquist J, Martensson O, Wallenberg LR: Trauma mot buken—problem vid diagnostik och terapi. *Lakartidningen 69*:1616, 1972.
4. Trunkey DD, Shires GT, McClelland R: Management of liver trauma in 811 consecutive cases. *Ann Surg 179*:722, 1974.
5. Walt AJ: The mythology of hepatic trauma—or Babel revisited. *Am J Surg 135*:12, 1978.
6. Williams LF Jr, and Byrne JJ: Trauma to the liver at the Boston City Hospital from 1955 to 1965. *Am J Surg 112*:368, 1966.
7. Andersen PT: Traumatic false aneurysm of the right hepatic artery: an unusual complication of cholecystectomy. *Aust NZ J Surg 40*:273, 1971.
8. Hellekant C: Vascular complications following needle puncture of the liver: clinical angiography. *Acta Radiol (Diagn) 17*:209, 1976.
9. Hoevels J, and Nilsson U: Intrahepatic vascular lesions following nonsurgical percutaneous transhepatic bile duct intubation. *Gastrointest Radiol 5*:127, 1980.
10. Monden M, Okamura J, Kobayashi N, Shibata N, Horikawa S, Fujimoto T, Kosaki G, Kuroda C, Uchida H: Hemobilia after percutaneous transhepatic biliary drainage. *Arch Surg 115*:161, 1980.
11. Okuda K, Musha H, Nakajima Y, Takayasu K, Suzuki Y, Morita M, Yamasaki T: Frequency of intrahepatic arteriovenous fistula as a sequel to percutaneous needle puncture of the liver. *Gastroenterology 74*:1204, 1978.
12. Preger L: Hepatic arteriovenous fistula after percutaneous liver biopsy. *Am J Roentgenol 101*:619, 1967.
13. Seldinger SI: Percutaneous transhepatic cholangiography. *Acta Radiol (Suppl) 253*:1966.
14. Tylen U, Hoevels J, Vang J: Percutaneous transhepatic cholangiography with external drainage of obstructive biliary lesions. *Surg Gynecol Obstet 114*:13, 1977.
15. Wallace S, Medellin H, Nelson RS: Angiographic changes due to needle biopsy of the liver. *Radiology 105*:13, 1972.
16. Boijsen E, Göthlin J, Hallböök T, Sandblom PH: Preoperative angiographic diagnosis of bleeding aneurysms of abdominal visceral arteries. *Radiology 93*:781, 1969.
17. Eaton SB Jr, Wirtz RD, Teneyck JR, Richards JC: Iatrogenic liver injury resulting from ductal instrumentation with the Fogarty biliary balloon catheter. *Radiology 100*:581, 1971.
18. Ameriks JA, Thompson NW, Frey CF, Appelman HD, Walter JF: Hepatic cell adenomas, spontaneous liver rupture, and oral contraceptives. *Arch Surg 110*:548, 1975.
19. Benedict KT Jr, Chen PS, Janover ML, Farmelant MH, Howard JT, McDermott W: Contraceptive-associated hepatic tumor. *Am J Roentgenol 132*:452, 1979.
20. Borra S and Kleinfeld M: Subcapsular liver hematomas in a patient on chronic hemodialysis. *Ann Int Med 93*:574, 1980.
21. Davis TJ, and Berk RN: Benign hepatic lesions in women taking oral contraceptives. *Gastrointest Radiol 2*:213, 1977.

22. Slattery LR, Abrams RM, Berenbaum ER, Labow SB, Aron B: Spontaneous hematoma of liver during pregnancy. *Obstet Gynecol 32*:664, 1968.
23. Levin DC, Watson RC, Sos TA, Baltaxe HA: Angiography in blunt hepatic trauma. *Am J Roentgenol 119*:95, 1973.
24. Schorn L, and Coln D: Hepatic angiographic changes after trauma. *Am J Surg 134*:754, 1977.
25. Aaron S, Fulton RL, Mays ET: Selective ligation of the hepatic artery for trauma of the liver. *Surg Gynecol Obstet 141*:187, 1975.
26. Mays ET: Hepatic trauma. *N Engl J Med 288*:402, 1973.
27. Mays ET: Lobar dearterialization for exsanguinating wounds of the liver. *J Trauma 12*:397, 1972.
28. Mays ET, and Wheeler CS: Demonstration of collateral arterial flow after interruption of hepatic arteries in man. *N Engl J Med 290*:993, 1974.
29. Bengmark S, Almersjö O, Engevik L, Hafström LO: Kirurgisk behandling av levertrauma och dess komplikationer. *Lakartidningen 64*:33, 1967.
30. Engevik L, Almersjö O, Bengmark S: Hemihepatectomy in man. *Acta Chir Scand (Suppl) 357*:239, 1966.
31. Perry JF Jr, Root HD, Hauser CW, Keizer PJ: Treatment of hepatic injuries. *Surgery 62*:853, 1967.
32. McCort JJ: Rupture or laceration of the liver by non-penetrating trauma. *Radiology 78*:49, 1962.
33. Burrell M, Toffler R, Lowman R: Blunt trauma to the abdomen and gastrointestinal tract: plain films and contrast study. *Radiol Clin North Am 11*:561, 1973.
34. Enge I, and Froysaker T: Rupture of the right hemidiaphragm with herniation of the liver. *Radiology 92*:1273, 1969.
35. Enge I: To be published.
36. Aakhus T, and Enge I: Angiography in rupture of the liver. *Acta Radiol (Diagn) 11*:353, 1971.
37. Berk RN, Wholey MH, Stockade R: The angiographic diagnosis of splenic and hepatic trauma. *J Can Assoc Radiol 21*:230, 1970.
38. Freeark RJ, Shoemaker WC, Baker RJ: Aortography in blunt abdominal trauma. *Arch Surg 96*:705, 1968.
39. Nahum H, and Levesque M: Arteriography in hepatic trauma. *Radiology 109*:557, 1973.
40. Bocquet M, Gimbergues H, Josipovici JJ, Bosch A, Batisse R, Garreta L: L'intérêt de l'artériographie dans les contusions de l'abdomen. *Ann Radiol 15*:553, 1972.
41. Boijsen E, Judkins MP, Simay A: Angiographic diagnosis of hepatic rupture. *Radiology 86*:66, 1966.
42. Boijsen E, Kaude J. Tylen U: Angiography in hepatic rupture. *Acta Radiol (Diagn) 11*:363, 1971.
43. Delorme G, Tavernier J, Grelet PE, Diard F: L'angiographie dans les traumatismes des viscères abdominaux. Essai de sémilogie radiologie schématique. *Ann Radiol 15*:623, 1972.
44. Katz MC, and Meng CH: Angiographic evaluation of traumatic intrahepatic pseudoaneurysm and hemobilia. *Radiology 94*:95, 1970.
45. Lamarque JL, Ginestie JF, Prioton JM, Joyeux R, Lopez E: Arteriographic diagnosis of false traumatic aneurysms of the liver. Report of 2 cases. *Nouv Presse Med 1*:791, 1972.
46. Lim RC Jr, Glickman MG, Hunt TK: Angiography in patients with blunt trauma to the chest and abdomen. *Surg Clin North Am 52*:551, 1972.
47. Müller, JHA, and Reiher P: Die angiographische Diagnostik der stumpfen Leberverletzungen. *Dtsch Gesundheitwes 33*:2035, 1978.
48. Redman HC, Reuter SR, Bookstein JJ: Angiography in abdominal trauma. *Ann Surg 169*:57, 1969.
49. Reuter SR, and Redman HC: Hepatic trauma. In *Gastrointestinal Angiography*, 2nd ed. W. B. Saunders, Philadelphia, 1977, 189.

50. Olsen WR, Redman HC, Hildreth DH: Quantitative peritoneal lavage in blunt abdominal trauma. *Arch Surg 104*:536, 1972.
51. Axel L, Moss AA, Berninger W: Dynamic computed tomography demonstration of hepatic arteriovenous fistula. *J Comput Assist Tomogr 5*:95, 1981.
52. Brecht G, Lackner K, Janson R, Thurn P: Die Computertomographie in der Notfallsdiagnostik.*Fortschr Roentgenstr. 132*:272, 1980.
53. Druy EM, and Rubin BE: Computed tomography in the evaluation of abdominal trauma. *J Comput Assist Tomogr 3*:40, 1979.
54. Rossi P, Lamarque JL, Passariello R, Simonetti G, Gould H, Rovighi L: CT evaluation of hepatic trauma. In *Abdominal Computerized Tomography*, Lamarque JL and Brüel JM (Eds). Excerpta Medica, Amsterdam, 1979.
55. Tylen U, Hoevels J, Nilsson U: Computed tomography of iatrogenic hepatic lesions following percutaneous transhepatic cholangiography and portography. *J Comput Assist Tomogr 5*:15, 1981.
56. Arnesjö B, Dahl EP, Fredlund P, Hegedüs V, Ihse I: Diagnosis and treatment of traumatic hemobilia caused by intrahepatic pseudo-aneurysm. *Fortschr. Roentgenstr. 126*:268, 1977.
57. Bismuth H: L'hémobilie. *(Arch Fr) Mal Appar Dig 61*:793, 1972.
58. Doutre LP, Perissant J, Tavernier J, Hirigoyen P, Beaulieu JC: À propos des contusions de l'abdomen: intérêt et place de la ponction-lavage du péritoine et de l'artériographie sélective du tronc coeliaque dans le diagnostic de lésions hépato-splénique. *Chirurgie 97*:383, 1971.
59. Enge I, Knutrud O, Normann T: Central rupture of the liver with traumatic hemobilia. *Br J Radiol 41*:789, 1968.
60. Goerttler U, and Herfarth C: Arteriographischer Befund bei der traumatischen Hämobilie. *Dtsch Med Wochenschr 98*:2135, 1973.
61. Graff RJ: Considerations in the treatment of traumatic hemobilia. *Am J Surg 105*:662, 1963.
62. Halsband H, Rehbein F, Kerk L: Posttraumatische Hämobilie infolge intrahepatischer Aneurysma-Bildung. *Z Kinderchir (Suppl) 11*:534, 1972.
63. Sandblom P: *Hemobilia* (biliary tract hemorrhage). Charles C Thomas, Springfield, Ill, 1972.
64. Schmidt B, Bhatt GM, Abo MN: Management of posttraumatic vascular malformations of the liver by catheter embolization. *Am J Surg 140*:332, 1980.
65. Steichen FM, and Sheiner NM: Traumatic intrahepatic hemobilia. *Arch Surg 92*:838, 1966.
66. Whelan TJ, and Gillespie JT: Treatment of traumatic hemobilia. *Ann Surg 162*:920, 1965.
67. Wolf K-J, Bulle G, Shenk W: Präoperative Angiographie bei der traumatischen Hämobilie. *Fortschr Roentgenstr. 120*:488, 1974.
68. Hendren WH, Warshaw AL, Fleischli DJ, Bartlett MK: Traumatic hemobilia: nonoperative management with healing documented by serial angiography. *Ann Surg 174*:991, 1971.
69. Boijsen E, and Lunderquist A: To be published.
70. Bergström M, Ericson K, Levander B, Svendsen P, Larsson S: Variation with time of the attenuation values of intracranial hematomas. *J Comput Assist Tomogr 1*:57, 1977.
71. Hübener KH, and Schmitt WGH: Computertomographische Densitometrie des menschlischen Blutes. Einfluss auf das Absorptionsverhalten von parenchymatösen Organen und Ergussbildungen. *Fortschr Roentgenstr 130*:185, 1979.
72. New PFJ, and Aronson S: Attenuation measurements of whole blood and blood fractions in computed tomography. *Radiology 121*:635, 1976.
73. Creech O, Gantt J, Wren H: Traumatic arteriovenous fistula at unusual sites. *Ann Surg 161*:908, 1965.
74. Foley WJ, Turcotte JG, Brant RL, Ause RG, Hoskins PA: Intrahepatic arteriovenous fistulas between the hepatic artery and portal vein. *Ann Surg 174*:849, 1971.
75. Kaude J, Dudgeon DL, Talbert JL: The role of selective angiography in the diagnosis and treatment of hepatoportal arteriovenous fistula. *Radiology 92*:1271, 1969.
76. Malette WG, Griffen WO, Stivers JR, Berardi RS: Traumatic intrahepatic fistula of the hepatic artery and portal vein. *Am Surg 39*:164, 1973.

77. Berner CF, Cox EF, Buxton RW: Unusual arteriovenous fistulae involving hepatic artery, portal vein and internal iliac vessels: case reports and a review of the literature. *Am Surg 33*:276, 1967.
78. Chisholm TP, and Lenio PT: Traumatic injuries of the portal vein. *Am J Surg 124*:770, 1972.
79. Cohen A, and Debakey ME: Successful repair of traumatic arteriovenous fistulas between hepatic artery and portal vein and right renal artery and inferior vena cava. *Surgery 48*:548, 1960.
80. Grant RN, Gliedman ML, Deterling RA Jr: Coexisting traumatic arteriovenous fistulae between the aorta and vena cava, and the hepatic artery and portal vein, complicated by a "Goldblatt kidney." *Ann Surg 148*:286, 1958.
81. Ryan KG, and Lorber SH: Traumatic fistula between hepatic artery and portal vein. *N Engl J Med 279*:1215, 1968.
82. Hellekant C, and Olin T: Vascular complications following needle puncture of the liver. An angiographic investigation in the rabbit. *Acta Radiol (Diagn) 14*:577, 1973.
83. Hoevels J, Lunderquist A, Owman T: Complications of percutaneous transhepatic catheterization of the portal vein and its tributaries. *Acta Radiol (Diagn) 21*:593, 1980.
84. Hoevels J, Lunderquist A, Tylen U: Percutaneous transhepatic portography. *Acta Radiol (Diagn) 19*:643, 1978.
85. Tavernier J, Fagola M, Delorme G, Diard F, Labat JP: Fistules artério-portales intrahépatiques. *J Radiol Electrol 53*:783, 1972.
86. Castaneda-Zuniga WR, Jauregui H, Rysavy JA, Formanek A, Amplatz K: Complications of wedge hepatic venography. *Radiology 126*:53, 1978.
87. Guynn VL, and Reynolds JT: Surgical management of hemobilia. Spontaneous hemobilia of intrahepatic origin. *Arch Surg 83*:89, 1961.
88. Hankins JR, Ayella RJ, Gill W, Cowley RA: Umbilical vein portohepatography in hepatic trauma. *Surg Gynecol Obstet 137*:200, 1973.
89. Bass EM, and Crosier JH: Percutaneous control of posttraumatic hepatic hemorrhage by Gelfoam embolization. *J Trauma 17*:61, 1977.
90. Greenfield AJ: Transcatheter vessel occlusion: selection of methods and materials. *Cardiovasc Intervent Radiol 3*:222, 1980.
91. Heimbach DM, Ferguson GS, Harley JD: Treatment of hemorrhagic hemobilia with angiographic embolization. *J Trauma 18*:221, 1978.
92. Jander HP, Laws HL, Kogutt MS, Mihas AB: Emergency embolization in blunt hepatic trauma. *Am J Roentgenol 129*:249, 1977.
93. Jander HP, and Russinovich NAE: Transcatheter Gelfoam embolization in abdominal, retroperitoneal and pelvic hemorrhage. *Radiology 136*:337, 1980.
94. Perlberger RR: Control of hemobilia by angiographic embolization. *Am J Roentgenol 128*:672, 1977.
95. Rubin BE, and Katzen BJ: Selective hepatic artery embolization to control massive hepatic hemorrhage after trauma. *Am J Roentgenol 129*:253, 1977.
96. Walter JF, Paaso BT, Cannon WB: Successful transcatheter embolic control of massive hematobilia secondary to liver biopsy. *Am J Roentgenol 127*:847, 1976.
97. De Jode LR, Nichols RJ, Wright PL: Ischemic necrosis of the gallbladder following hepatic artery embolism. *Br J Surg 63*:621, 1976.

29

Vascular Disease of the Liver

Ernest J. Ring
Hospital of the University of Pennsylvania
Philadelphia, Pennsylvania

Introduction

Although many forms of hepatic parenchymal pathology cause striking changes in the arteries and veins of the liver, abnormalities intrinsic to these structures are relatively uncommon. The consequences of such primary hepatic vascular processes as occlusive disease, aneurysm, and arteriovenous (AV) fistula can lead to a spectrum of complicated problems which are often difficult to assess clinically. Noninvasive imaging procedures are not usually diagnostic for these conditions, although occasionally some abnormality may be suggested. Angiography remains the specific imaging modality to diagnose vascular pathology and precisely depict surgical anatomy. In the past few years the selective angiographic catheter has also been successfully developed as a vehicle for providing innovative forms of therapy for a variety of vascular diseases, including those involving the liver.

Most primary hepatic vascular lesions are surprisingly asymptomatic. However, when diminished hepatic arterial or portal venous perfusion deprives the liver of oxygenation and nutrition, parenchymal function can be affected. Obstruction of the hepatic veins causes congestion with ascites and portal hypertension. Aneurysms may obstruct adjacent bile ducts or rupture and bleed massively. In this chapter we discuss the pathophysiology of this small but interesting group of conditions that involve the arterial blood supply and venous drainage of the liver.

Normal Hepatic Artery/Portal Vein Hemodynamics

Under normal circumstances, the hepatic artery supplies approximately one-third of the blood flow and one-half of the oxygen used by the liver (1). The remainder of the liver's nutrition is derived from portal venous flow. The complex interrelationship between the liver's dual blood supply depends on a unique and complicated pattern of hemodynamics. Total hepatic blood flow tends to remain constant despite dramatic flow reduction in either system. A decrease in hepatic arterial or portal venous flow is rapidly followed by a compensatory increase of flow in the other system. The homeostatic mechanism which maintains this relationship is so effective that arterial blood flow cannot be kept reduced even if the hepatic artery is directly infused with a potent vasoconstrictor such as vasopressin. The local effect of the vasopressin escapes when systematic levels of the vasoconstrictor cause portal vein flow to diminish (2). Conversely, mechanical obstruction of flow in the hepatic artery is followed by a rapid increase in flow through the portal vein. The inverse relationship between arterial and venous flow to the liver is of considerable clinical importance since it tends to diminish the impact on hepatic function after obstruction of flow through either system.

Pathologic Conditions Related to the Hepatic Artery

Hepatic Artery Occlusion

Occlusion of the hepatic arterial blood supply in the dog routinely leads to infarction, infection, and death (3). On the other hand, in humans, therapeutic ligation and embolic occlusion of the hepatic artery are being used therapeutically with increasing frequency and are well tolerated in most cases. This species difference has been attributed to the fact that the canine portal vein contains bacteria, whereas human portal venous blood is normally sterile.

Occlusion of the hepatic artery proximal to the gastroduodenal artery is followed very rapidly by replacement of flow through pancreatic branches from the superior mesenteric artery. The efficiency of these collateral pathways is well known to most angiographers, who have seen excellent flow return to the distal hepatic artery branches within minutes after causing spasm or dissection of the common hepatic artery. Nor does liver infarction usually follow on occlusion that is distal to the gastroduodenal artery because of collateral pathways through the arteries around the common bile duct (Fig. 1). Chuang and Wallace (4) have intentionally obstructed flow in hepatic arterial branches and have shown that intrahepatic arterial communications exist which can restore segmental blood flow. They have used transarterial embolic therapy for a variety of pathologic conditions and claim that occlusion of segmental hepatic artery branches is well tolerated as long as flow in the portal vein is hepatopetal. Doppman confirmed that there are few significant sequelae to embolization of large intrahepatic branches, but showed that embolic obliteration at the arteriolar level leads to bile cysts similar to those seen in Caroli's disease (5).

Etiology of Hepatic Artery Occlusion

Occlusion of the hepatic artery and its branches is most commonly caused by *atherosclerotic disease*. It is therefore generally seen in elderly patients and is often discovered as an incidental finding during an arteriographic examination performed for

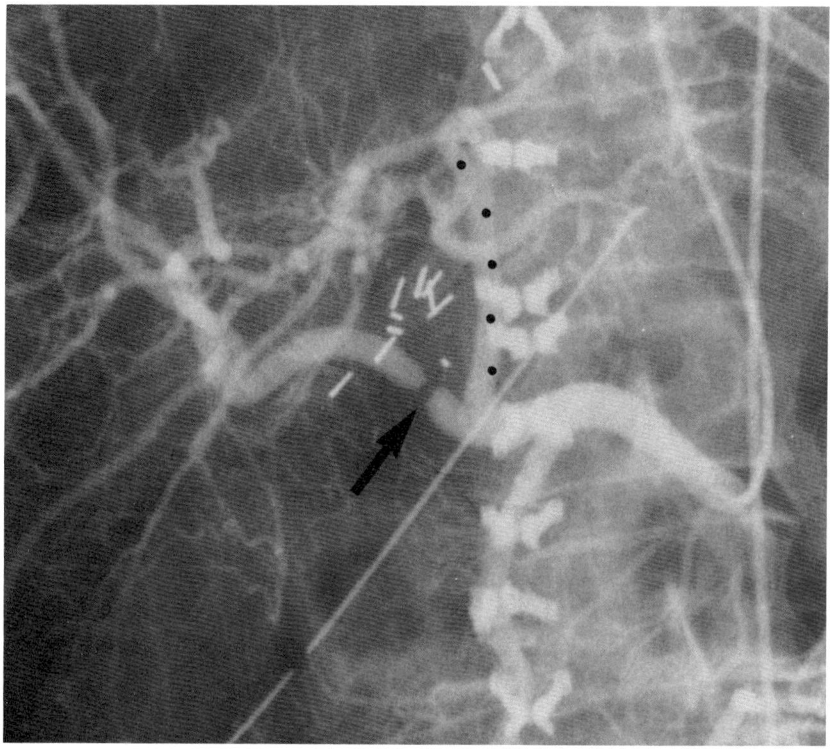

Figure 1 Return of intrahepatic arterial flow after surgical ligation of the right hepatic artery. A hepatic arteriogram demonstrates the efficiency of collateral arterial branches, here from the left hepatic artery (dots), in reconstituting flow immediately distal to a surgically placed ligature (arrow).

other reasons. Most atherosclerotic occlusions occur at the level of the celiac axis or common hepatic artery, but they can occasionally develop in any hepatic arterial branch. Fibromuscular hyperplasia and large vessel arteritis rarely involve the branches of the celiac axis or superior mesenteric artery, but can also result in occlusion of the hepatic artery or its branches.

Extrinsic compression from extension of malignant disease into the porta hepatis or along the course of the hepatic artery is another cause of hepatic artery occlusion. Pancreatic carcinoma commonly invades the portal vein and its tributaries, but its effect on the hepatic artery is usually that of encasement rather than occlusion. Cholangiocarcinoma occasionally causes sufficient encasement of hepatic artery branches that occlusion ultimately results.

Surgery and other iatrogenic trauma can precipitate hepatic artery thrombosis or occlusion. Intentional hepatic artery ligation has been used in the management of hemobilia and other causes of arterial bleeding from the liver, such as trauma. It is also being used for palliation of hypervascular liver tumors. Inadvertent dissection of the hepatic artery during an angiographic catheterization is an infrequent cause of acute occlusion and is fortunately only rarely followed by any significant complications.

Occlusion of multiple, small, intrahepatic branches may be seen in such diseases as *polyarteritis nodosa* or *subacute bacterial endocarditis*. Since these diseases are usually associated with superimposed infection, they lead to a much higher incidence of hepatic infarction or abscess than do sterile causes of occlusion.

Hepatic Artery Aneurysms

With the widespread use of angiography, hepatic artery aneurysms have been discovered with increasing frequency. Approximately 500 cases of localized hepatic artery aneurysms have already been described and this entity is no longer considered rare (6). The aneurysms are usually saccular and can vary in diameter from 2 to 10 cm (7). An aneurysm may exist for many years without causing symptoms, but when sufficiently large can obstruct the adjacent bile duct and lead to jaundice (7). Rupture leads to a clinical syndrome consisting of pain, gastrointestinal bleeding, and shock. The incidence

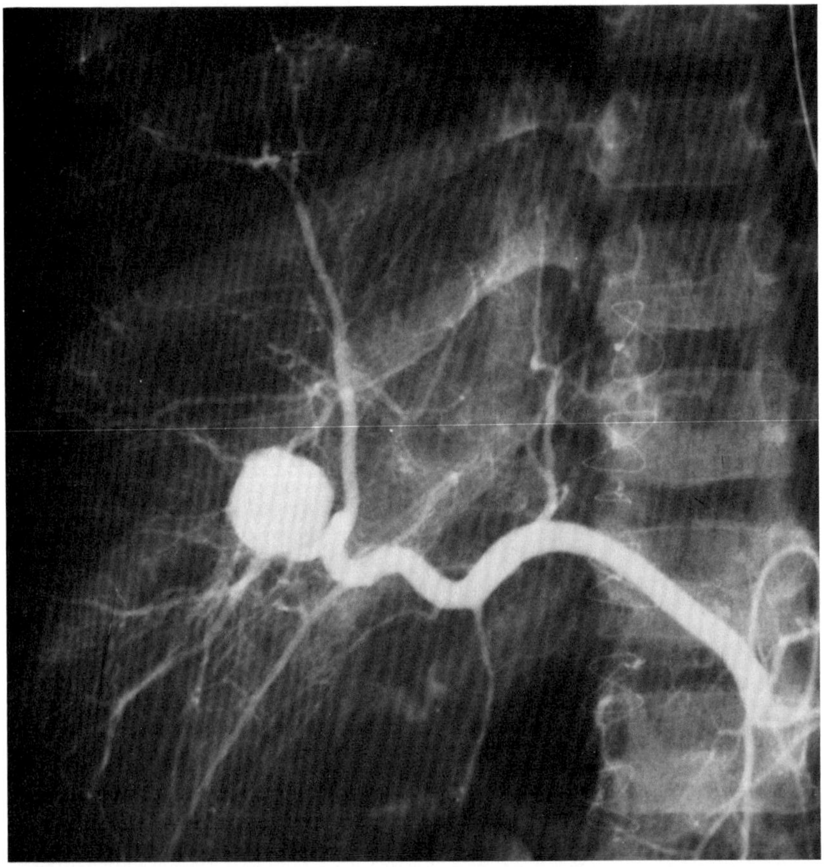

Figure 2A Selective embolization to control bleeding from a traumatic aneurysm of the right hepatic artery. A selective hepatic arteriogram demonstrates a 2-cm false aneurysm.

of rupture in untreated aneurysms is not definitely known, but it has been suggested that as many as 75–80% of untreated aneurysms will eventually rupture (6). Sixty percent of those that do rupture present with hemobilia; the remainder rupture into the free peritoneal cavity (8). The mortality rate after rupture of an hepatic artery aneurysm is extremely high.

Although the correct *diagnosis of hepatic artery aneurysm* can occasionally be suspected on the basis of plain radiographs, by filling defects shown on radioisotope liver scans, or a very large vascular structure seen on CT scanning, angiography is the only reliable way to make the diagnosis and determine the exact extent for surgical therapy. Therapy for hepatic artery aneurysms has traditionally been direct ligation of the common hepatic artery. More recently, transarterial catheter techniques have also been used to occlude the branch vessel leading to the aneurysm and avoid surgery (Fig. 2).

Etiology of Hepatic Artery Aneurysms

Although hepatic artery aneurysm may be associated with generalized *atherosclerosis*, they are not infrequently *mycotic*, caused by infections following intravascular drug

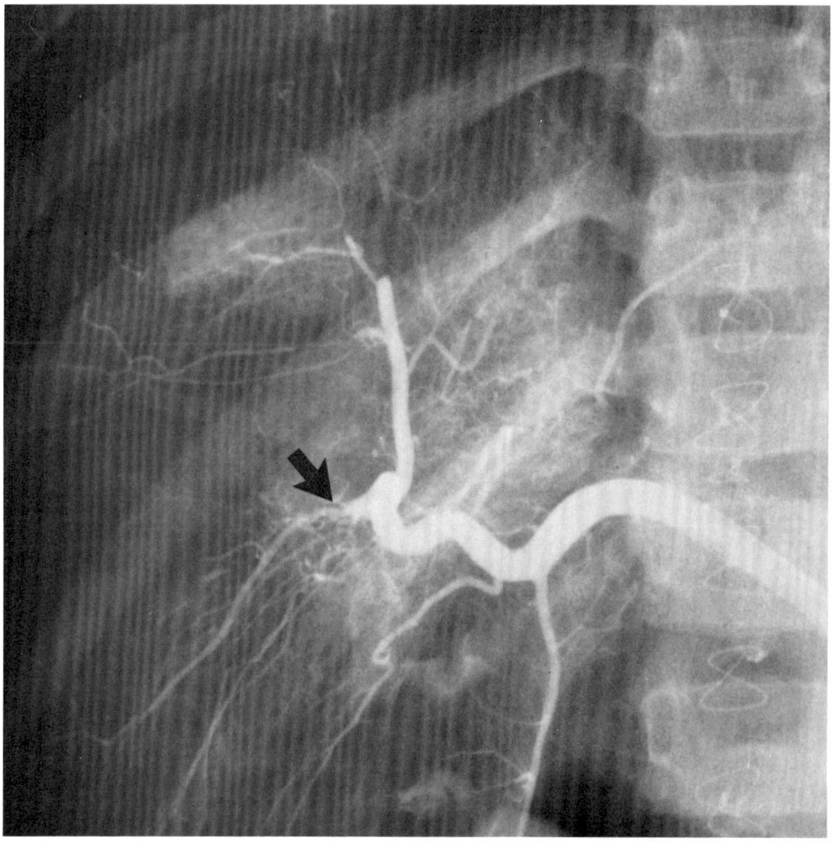

Figure 2B The branch vessel leading to the aneurysm was subselectively catheterized and embolized with Gelfoam. A repeat arteriogram after the embolization shows occlusion of the aneurysm and of its feeding branch (arrow). Bleeding was controlled.

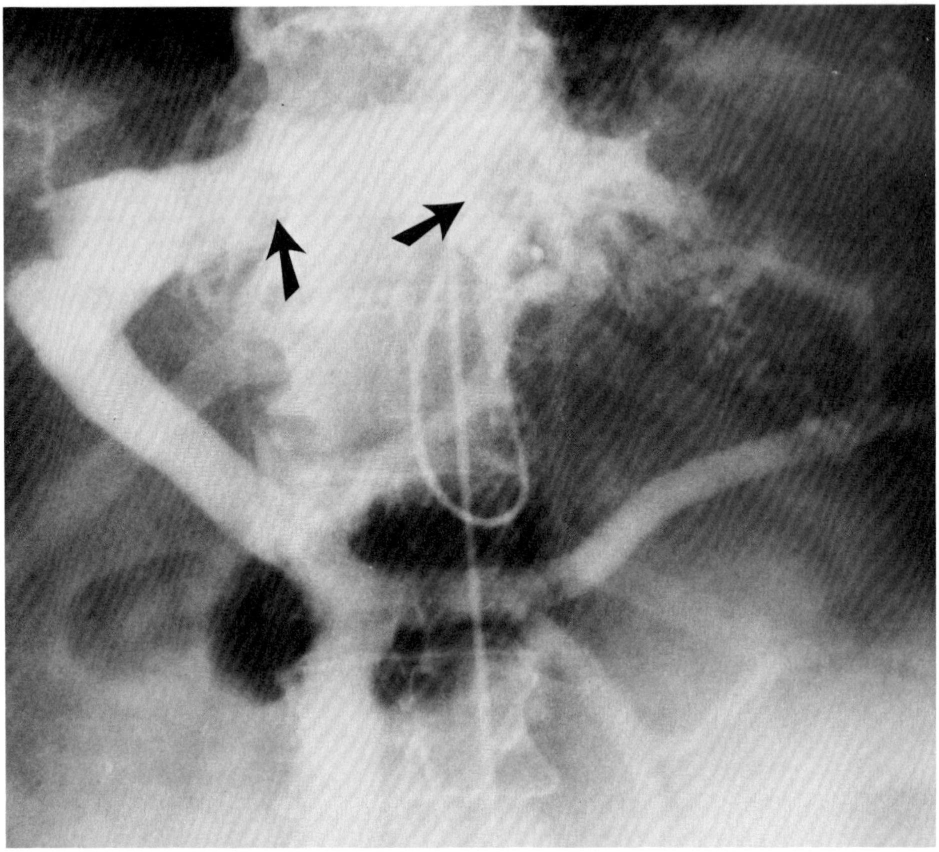

Figure 3A Hepatic arterioportal fistula secondary to a hepatoma embolized with a stainless steel coil. A selective left hepatic arteriogram performed on a patient actively bleeding from esophageal varices demonstrates rapid shunting direct into the left branch of the portal vein (arrows). Flow in the portal venous system is totally hepatofugal.

abuse. *False aneurysms* may follow surgery or trauma, usually during operations on the biliary tract. Collagen vascular diseases, such as polyarteritis nodosa, can produce a typical pattern of *miliary* aneurysms throughout the liver. Syphilis and tuberculosis have also been implicated as rare causes of mycotic hepatic aneurysms.

Hepatic Artery/Portal Vein Fistula

Arteriovenous fistulae commonly present clinically with abdominal pain and a bruit over the liver. They do not usually calcify and are therefore not recognizable either on routine radiography or any noninvasive imaging techniques. The angiographic diagnosis is readily established with the early opacification of the portal vein following injection of contrast material into the hepatic artery.

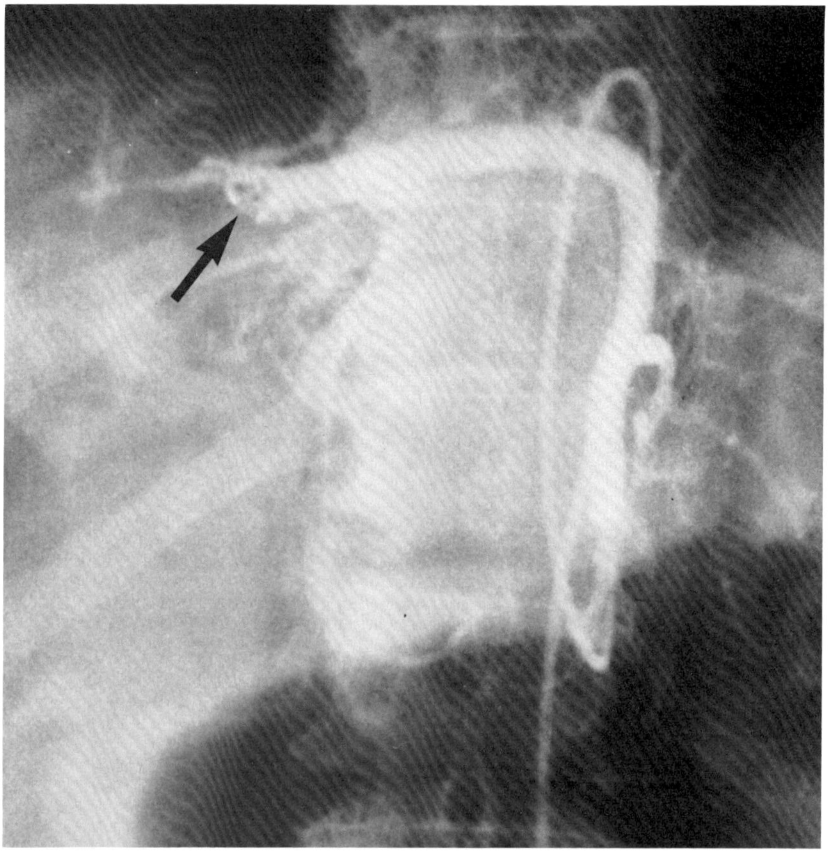

Figure 3B A stainless steel coil (arrow) was used to occlude the fistula and stop the hemorrhage.

Hepatic artery/portal vein fistulae do not affect the cardiovascular system to the same extent as arteriovenous fistulae elsewhere in the body. Increased flow through the portal venous system leads to an elevation of portal pressure which tends to reduce flow through the fistula. Single fistulae can be occluded with minimal risks using transcatheter techniques, provided that the angiographic catheter can be subselectively positioned (Fig. 3). Large and multiple fistulae cannot be remedied by any technique.

Etiology of Arterioportal Fistula

Abnormal arteriovenous communications are most commonly seen in association with *liver cirrhosis*. They may also occur with generalized vascular processes such as *Rendu-Osler-Weber disease* (Fig. 4). *Hepatomas* that invade the portal vein can create arterial portal shunting and are also frequently associated with portal thrombosis (Fig. 5). *Trauma* (surgical or otherwise) is another common cause of arterial venous fistulae in the liver. Abnormal communications between hepatic artery and portal vein branches have also been described with *schistosomiasis* (Fig. 6).

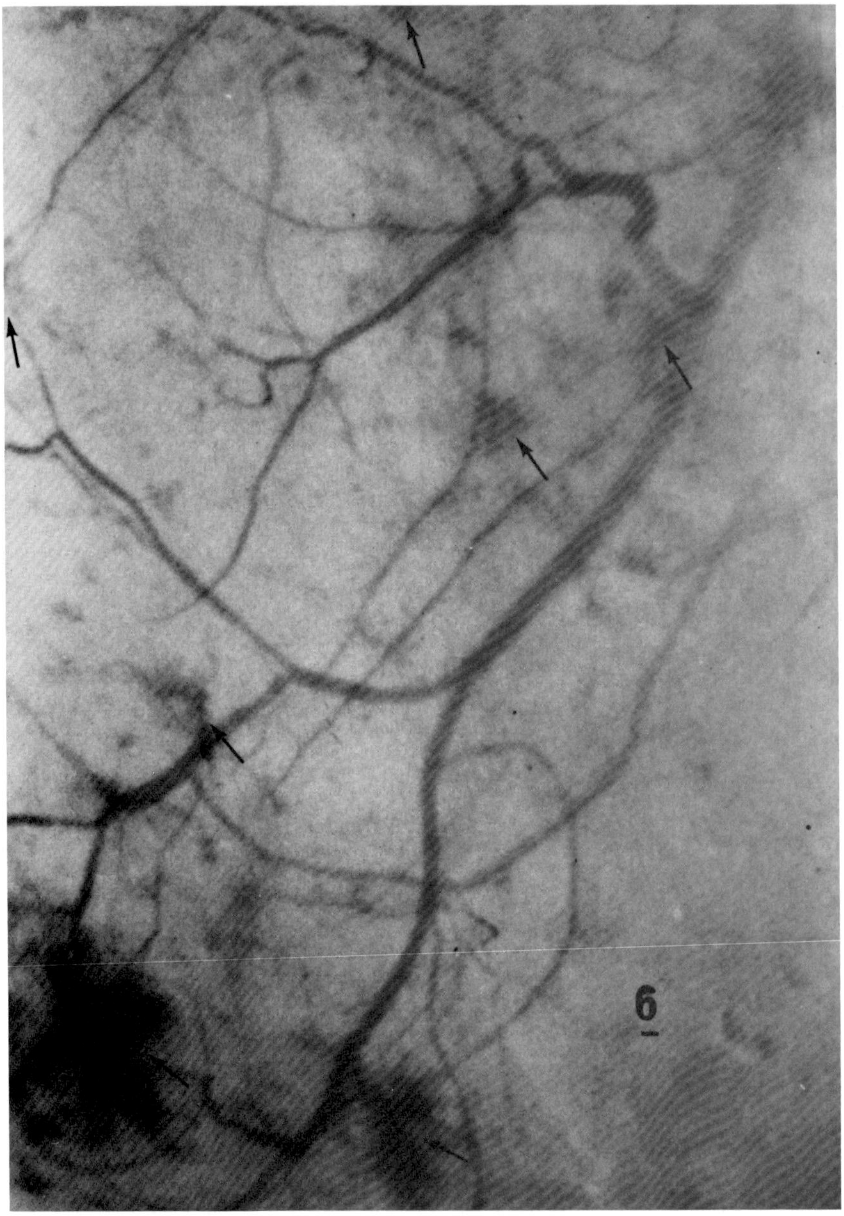

Figure 4 Multiple small hepatic arteriovenous fistulae (arrows) in a patient with Rendu-Osler-Weber disease.

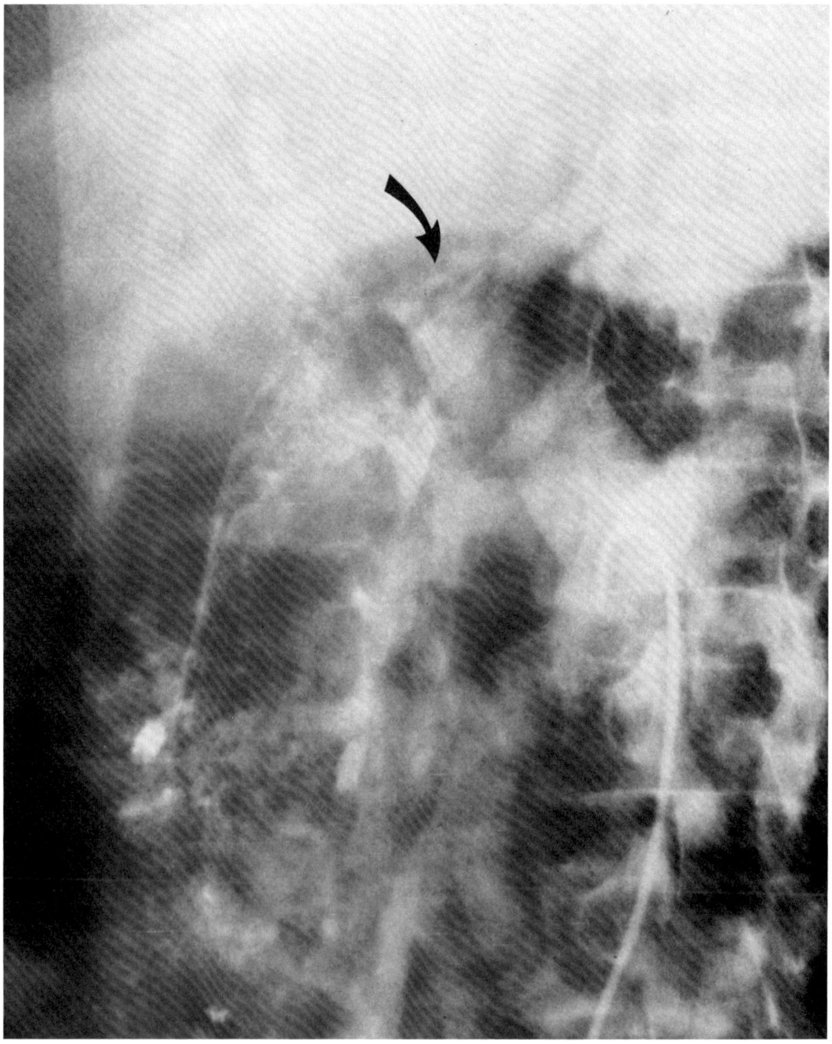

(A)

Figure 5 Hepatoma causing arterioportal communication and invasion of the portal vein. (A) The venous phase of a superior mesenteric arteriogram shows portal vein occlusion at the porta hepatis (arrow). (B) Hepatic arteriography reveals multiple tumor vessels (arrow). (C) During the late phase of the hepatic arteriogram the contrast outlines the right and left intrahepatic portal vein branches (arrows), which are almost completely filled with tumor thrombus.

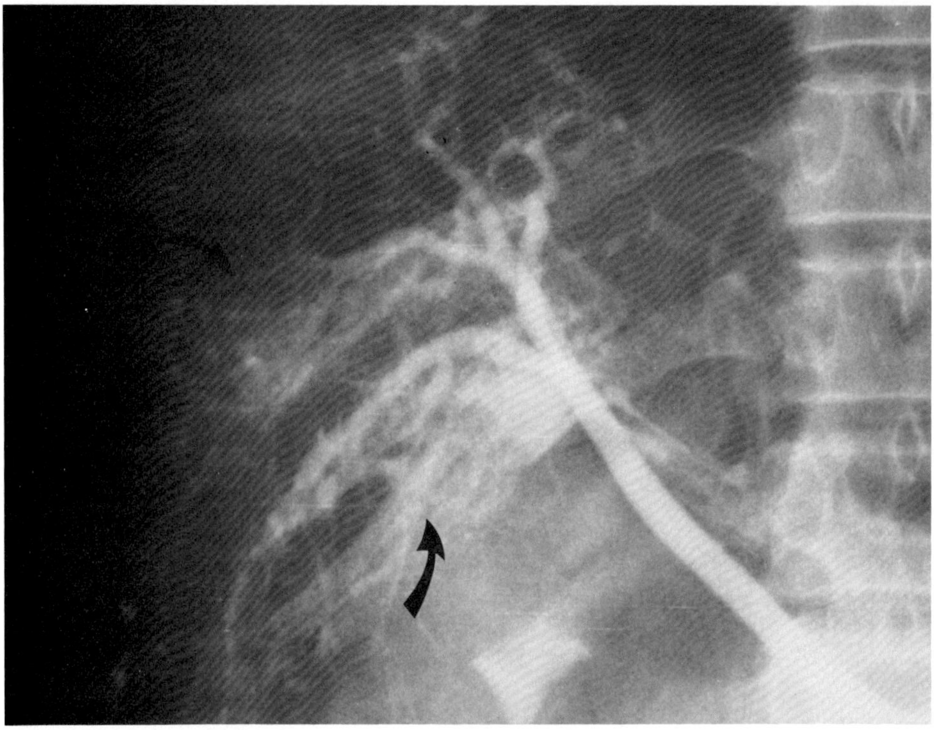

(B)

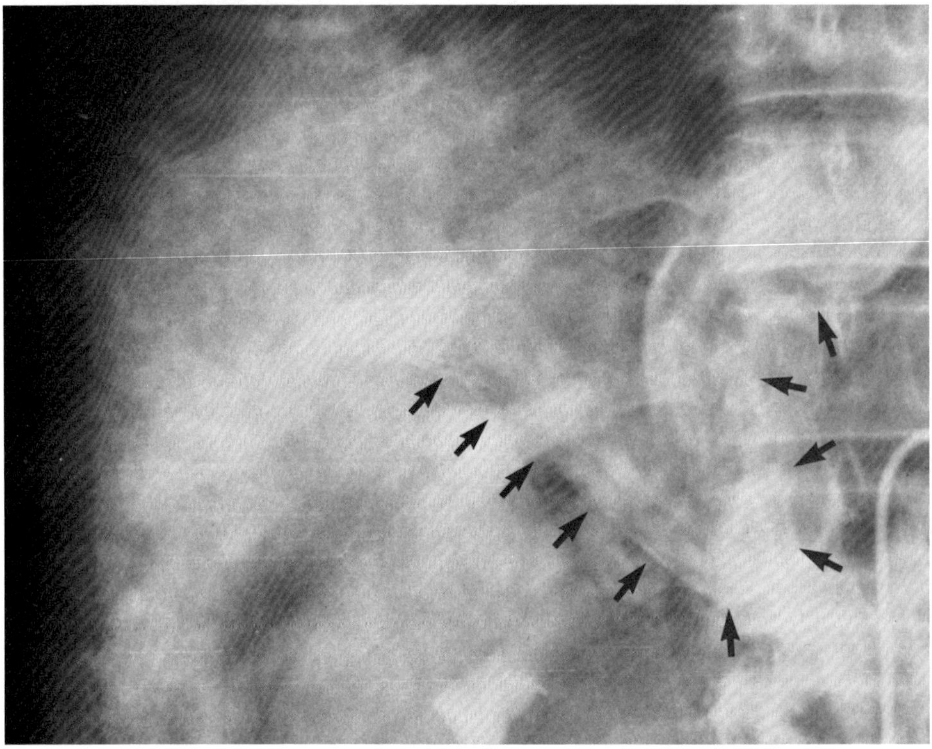

(C)

Figure 5 (continued)

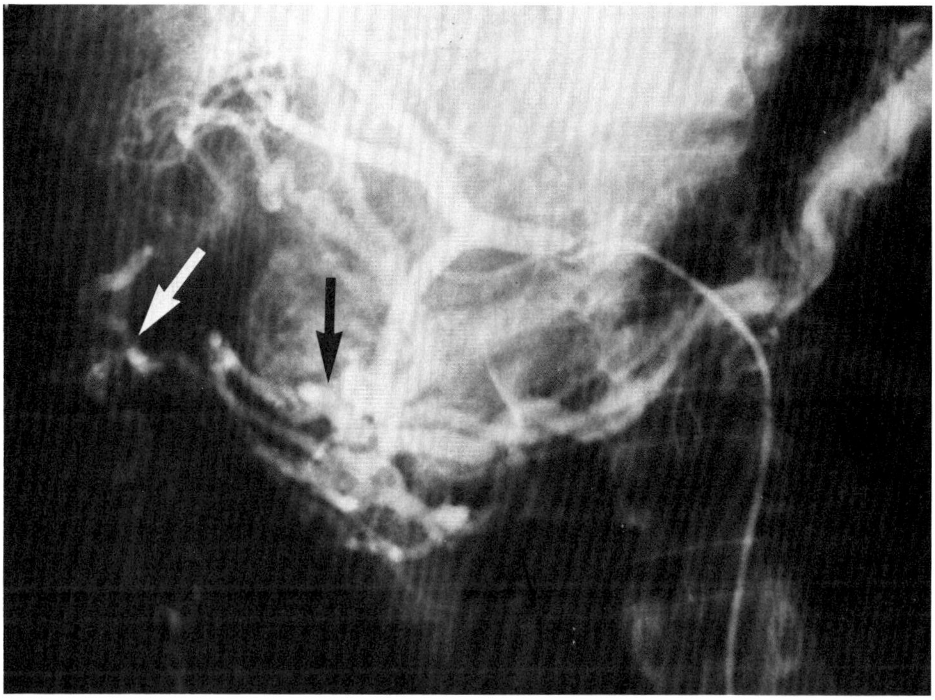

(A)

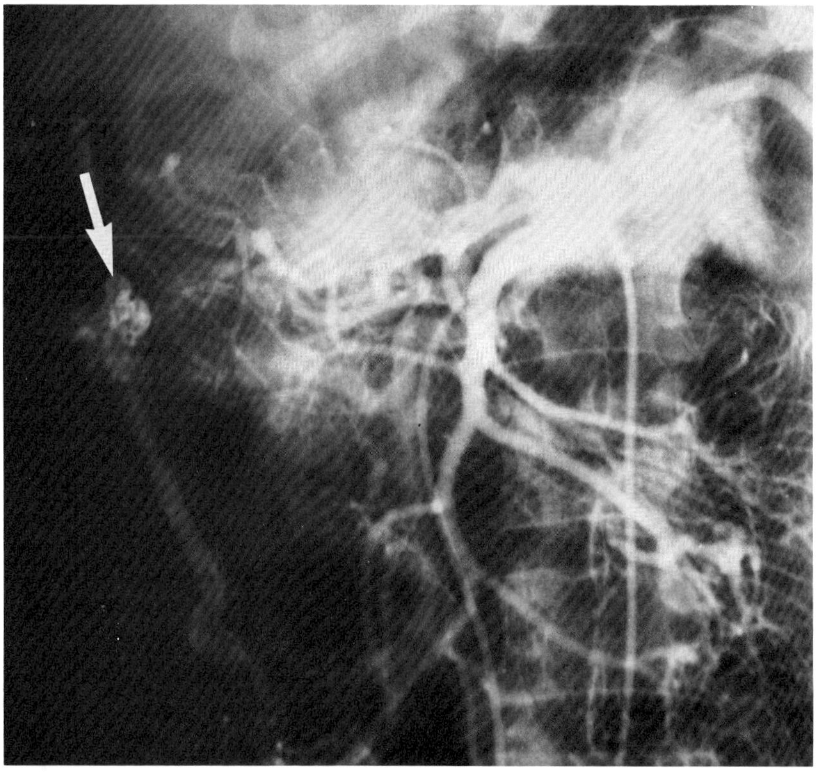

(B)

Figure 6

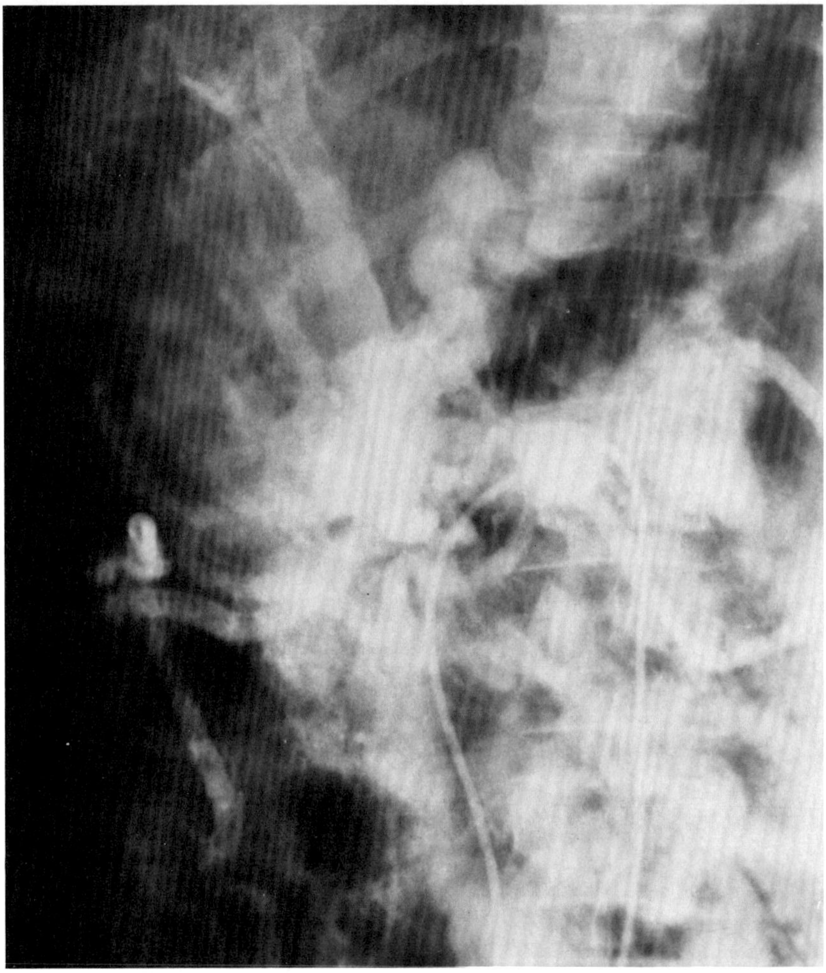

(C)

Figure 6 Multiple arterioportal fistulae in a patient with portal hypertension secondary to schistosomiasis. (A,B) Hepatic (A) and superior mesenteric (B) arteriography demonstrate multiple extrahepatic AV communications (arrows). (C) A late film in the superior mesenteric angiographic series shows massive shunting into the portal venous system.

Hemangiomas of the Liver

Hemangiomas of the liver are benign vascular tumors consisting of gross enlargement of the capillary spaces. Clinically significant hemangiomas are found mainly in children, where they may lead to a palpable mass or high-cardiac-output congestive heart failure. The diagnosis may be suggested in a child undergoing high-dose intravenous urography when the liver lesions may be demonstrated during the total body opacification phase of the examination. Further examination requires angiography to differentiate hemangioma from other vascular liver tumors. Angiographically, these lesions appear as large pools of contrast material, usually without abnormal arteries or veins. There is commonly also a central lucency caused by hemorrhage into the lesion. The dense opacification of the lesion typically persists throughout the capillary and venous phases (Fig. 7).

In adults, these lesions usually present with right upper quadrant pain or are discovered incidentally during a radioisotope liver scan or angiogram performed for another purpose. On radioisotope examination they may show either increased or decreased activity, both on static and flow scans. Needle biopsy is contraindicated in hemangiomas since massive bleeding may ensue. The definitive diagnosis is established by the typical angiographic pattern.

Peliosis Hepatis

Peliosis is a term that describes an abnormality of the liver where small blood-filled cystic spaces are seen throughout the parenchyma. Although this entity has been well described in the pathology literature, it has only been rarely reported by radiologists (9). Liver

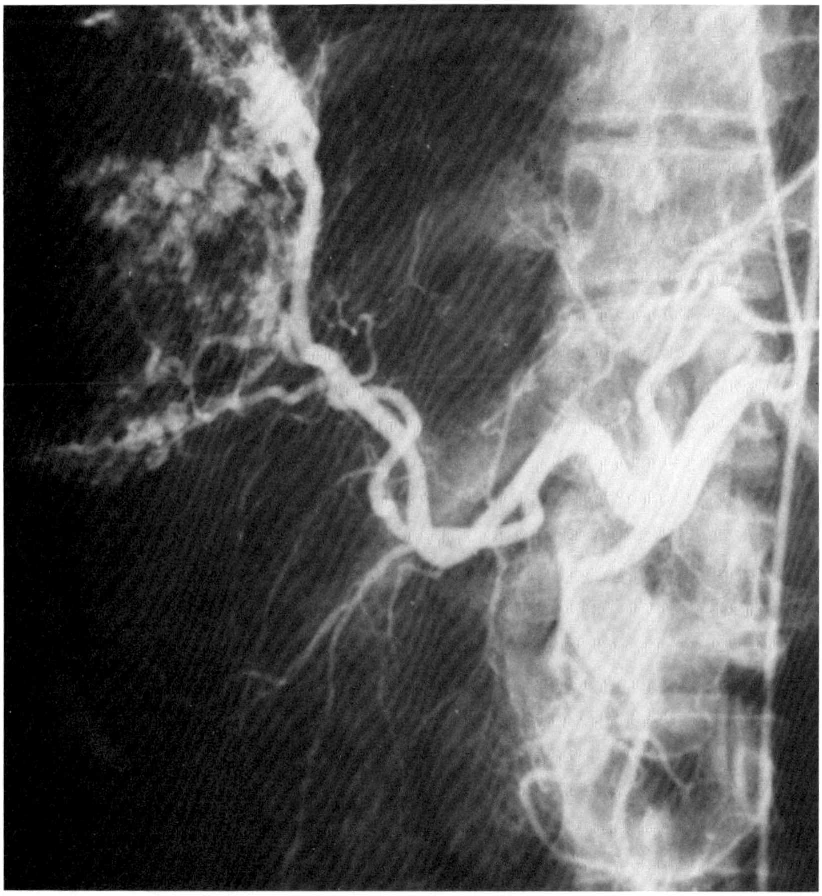

Figure 7A Cavernous hemangioma of the liver. During the arterial phase of a selective hepatic arteriogram, large pools of contrast material opacify a lesion in the right lobe of the liver.

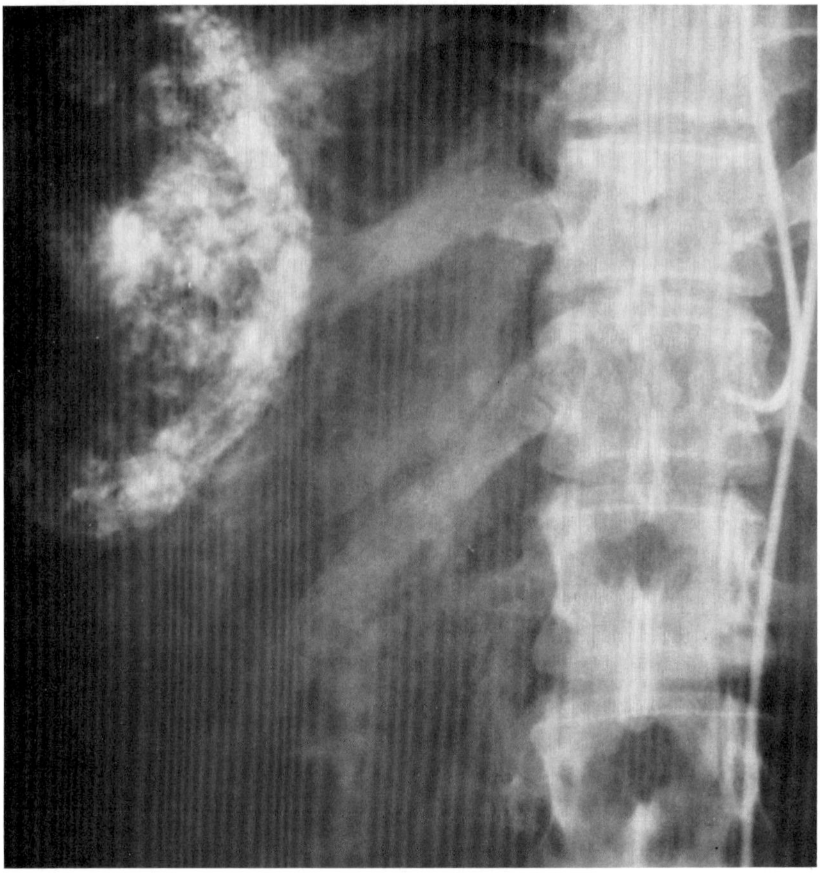

Figure 7B The dense opacification of the lesion typically persists beyond the capillary and venous phases.

function is not affected and the clinical significance is unclear. Some authors feel that these lesions are related to chronic hormone administration. Histologically, peliosis is characterized by blood-filled, endothelium-lined spaces that communicate with the hepatic sinusoids. The abnormalities are seen on hepatic arteriography during the parenchymal phase of the study. Small, opacifying nodules are seen diffusely throughout the otherwise normal liver parenchyma. The contrast staining does not persist as in hemangioma and there are no abnormal vessels to suggest tumors.

Abnormalities of the Portal Vein

Congenital Abnormalities

In the embryo, the portal venous system forms from the right and left vitelline veins, which empty into the primitive sinus venosus. Communicating anastomoses develop between these two veins ventrally, caudal to the common bile duct and near the porta hepatis, and dorsally, caudal to the dorsal pancreas. The normal adult portal vein depends on obliteration of the cranial segment of the left vitelline vein, the caudal segment of the right vitelline vein, and the ventral anastomoses. Congenital abnormalities of the portal vein occur from abnormal patterns of segmental obliteration. These include (1) ventral portal vein, (2) direct entry of the portal vein into the inferior vena cava, (3) duplication of the portal vein, (4) total anomalous pulmonary venous return into the portal vein, and (5) total portal vein atresia.

The *Cruveilhier-Baumgarten syndrome* describes the clinical findings of a venous hum and typical caput medusae of dilated veins about the umbilicus. Most commonly, it occurs in patients with portal hypertension who have a persistently patent umbilical vein or have recanalized the distal end of an obliterated umbilical vein (Fig. 8). As originally described (10), the condition was considered to be due to primary failure of closure of the umbilical vein, not associated with cirrhosis. This is now referred to as Cruveilhier-Baumgarten disease, an extremely rare entity if it exists at all.

Portal Vein Thrombosis

Thrombosis of the portal vein leads to different clinical syndromes depending on the rapidity of onset of the occlusion. Acute obstruction of flow in the portal vein is dramatic and usually fatal. Commonly, there is right upper quadrant pain with rapidly developing splenic enlargement, ascites, and bleeding esophageal varices. The acute congestion of the mesenteric vein can lead to bowel infarction. When portal vein occlusion develops more gradually, the clinical course is less dramatic and more closely parallels other causes of portal hypertension. In patients with preexisting severe portal hypertension and hepatofugal flow, the development of a superimposed thrombus in the portal vein may not be clinically evident and only found incidentally at angiography or autopsy (Fig. 9).

Etiology of Portal Vein Thrombosis

It has been estimated that up to 10% of patients with *cirrhosis* of the liver have associated thrombosis of the portal vein (11). Despite the high pressure in the portal venous system in these patients, flow can be relatively stagnant; this predisposes to thrombus formation. Other processes that cause portal vein stasis can similarly lead to thrombosis. These include hepatic venous occlusion (*Budd-Chiari syndrome*), chronic *congestive heart failure*, and *constrictive pericarditis*. *Coagulation abnormalities* such as those occurring in polycythemia rubra vera can cause portal thrombosis even in patients with normal portal pressure. *Tumors* such as pancreatic and gastric carcinoma may encase the portal vein or its tributaries and can lead to total occlusion.

Cavernous Transformation of the Portal Vein

Cavernous transformation forms a subgroup of portal vein thrombosis and is usually considered separately. Although the term can refer to any thrombosed portal vein which has partially recanalized, it is usually reserved to describe a process that occurs in children. Children with cavernous transformation have signs and symptoms of portal hypertension with relatively normal liver function. Angiographically, there is evidence of portal hypertension, hepatofugal flow, and esophageal varices. Depending on the degree of recanalization, the portal vein may be seen with multiple webs and contrast-filled

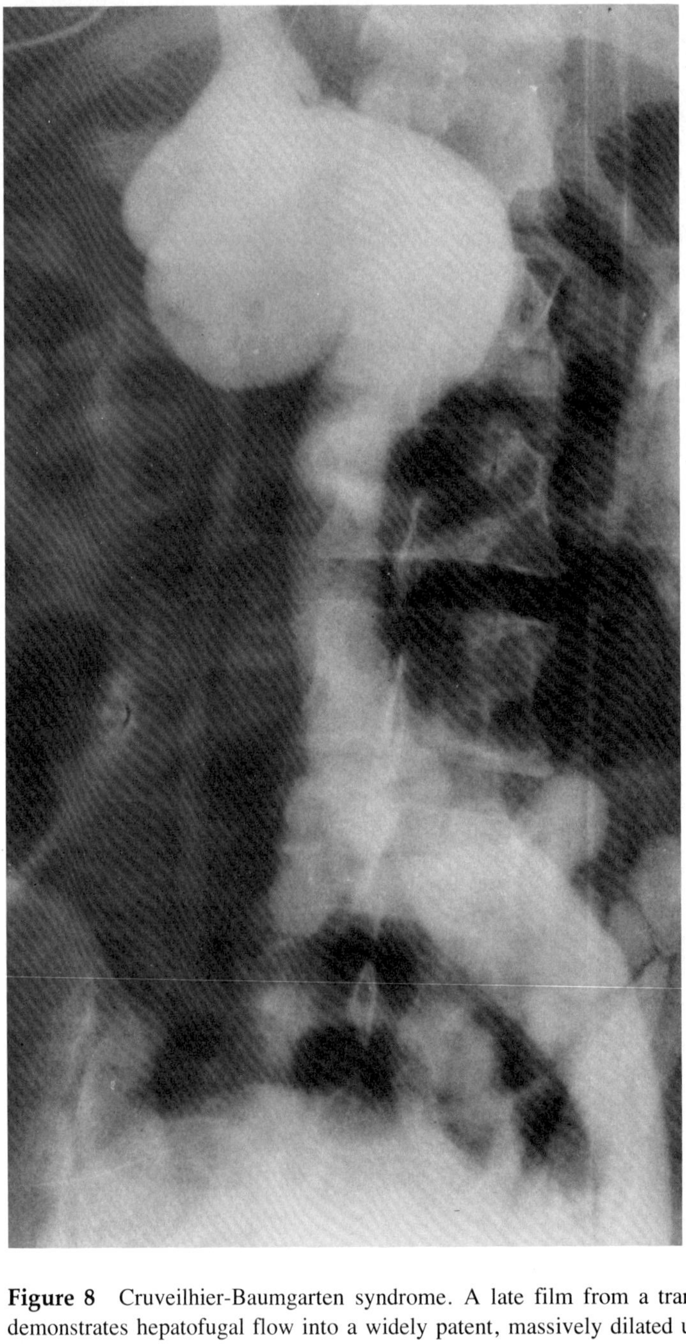

Figure 8 Cruveilhier-Baumgarten syndrome. A late film from a transhepatic portal venogram demonstrates hepatofugal flow into a widely patent, massively dilated umbilical vein.

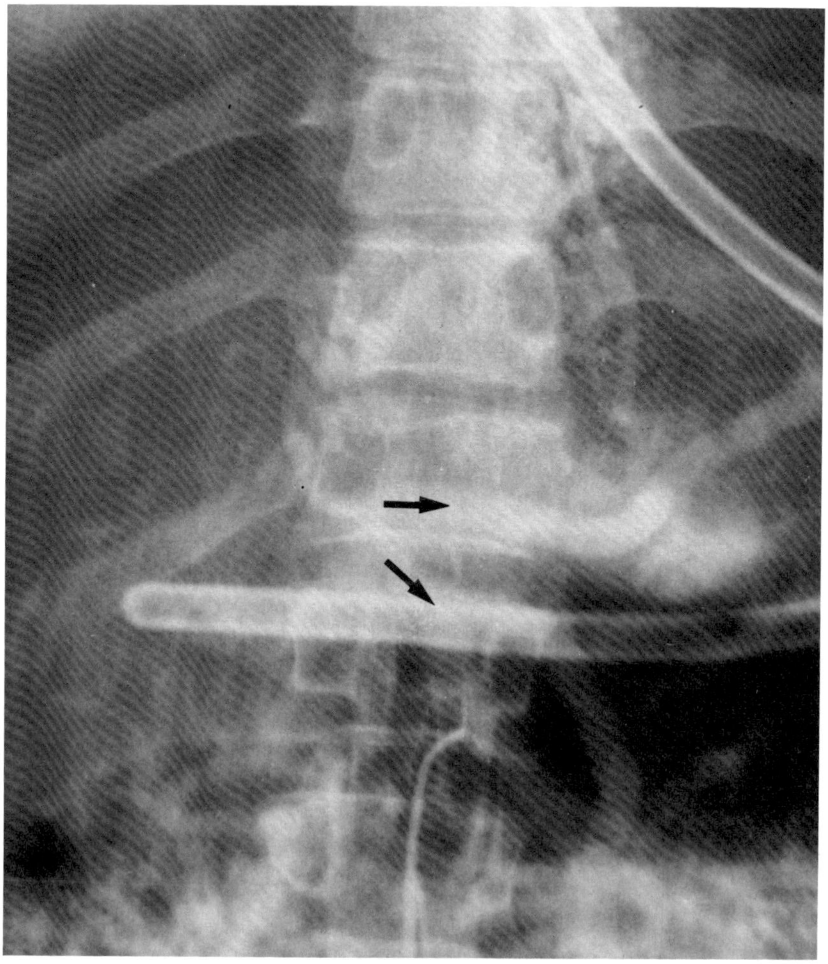

Figure 9A Portal vein thrombosis in a patient with micronodular cirrhosis. The venous phase of a superior mesenteric arteriogram fails to opacify the portal vein and shows hepatofugal flow (arrows) into major portal tributaries.

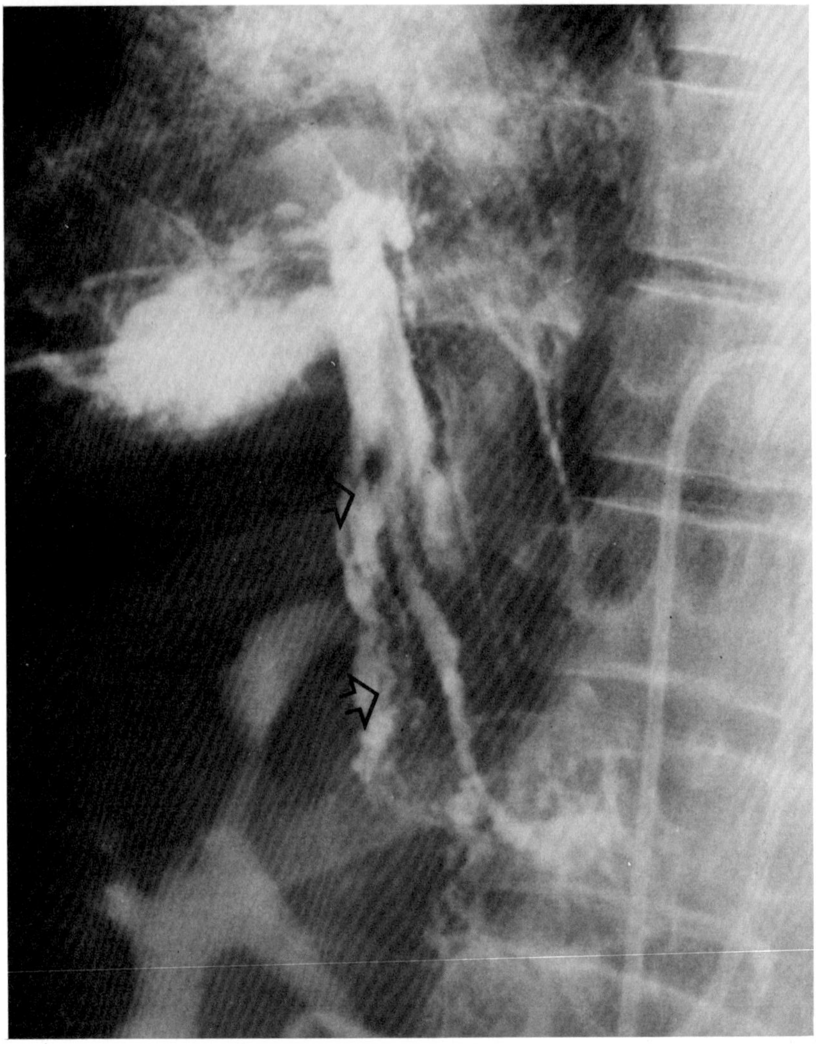

Figure 9B Attempts at directly catheterizing the portal vein through the liver were unsuccessful. An injection into a portal vein branch reveals multiple webs and partial recanalization of the portal vein mainstem (open arrows).

channels running through it, resembling an angiomatous malformation (Fig. 10). Multiple collateral veins are commonly seen around the portal structures which reconstitute flow to the intrahepatic branches of the portal vein. Although the precise etiology of cavernous transformation of the portal vein is not always known, there is often a history of neonatal sepsis and umbilical phlebitis.

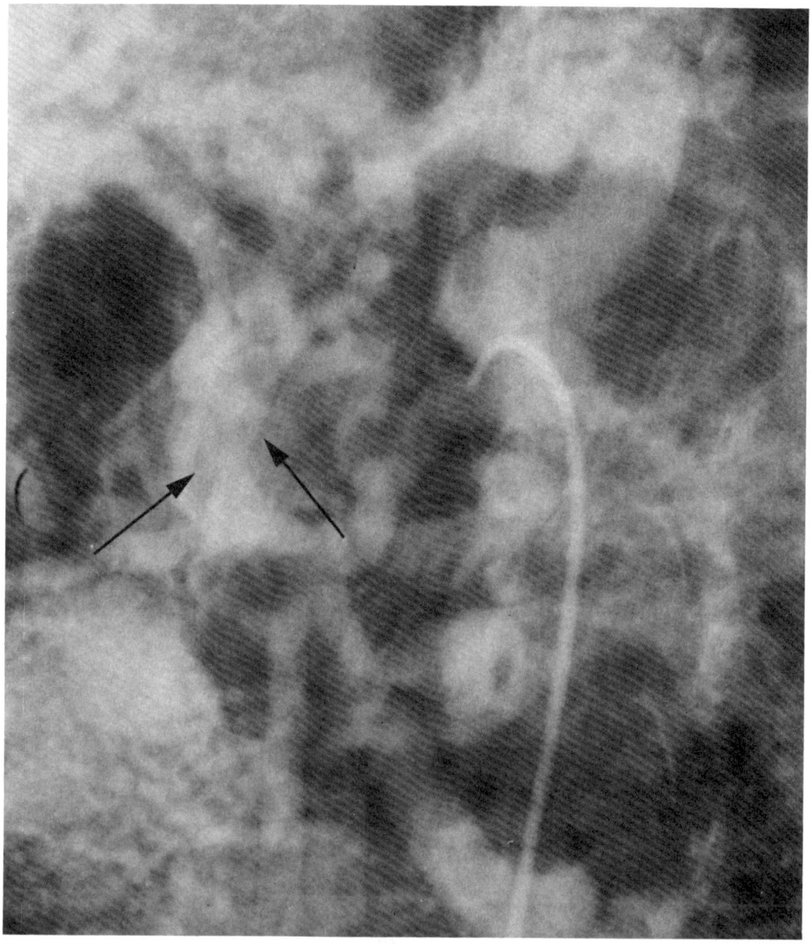

Figure 10 Cavernous transformation of the portal vein in a 9-year-old girl with bleeding esophageal varices. The venous phase of a superior mesenteric arteriogram shows linear webs in the portal vein (arrows). Multiple collateral venous channels in the porta hepatis reconstitute the intrahepatic portal branches.

Portal Vein Aneurysms

Portal vein aneurysms are extremely rare. In a few cases they can calcify and be suspected on plain radiographs (Fig. 11). Aneurysms of the portal vein have been diagnosed on computed tomography but are only apparent on isotope liver scans if extremely large. Arterial portography is usually required to make the diagnosis and is always necessary before any definitive therapy is performed. Portal vein aneurysms appear as localized saccular dilatations of the portal vein and occur almost exclusively in the presence of portal hypertension.

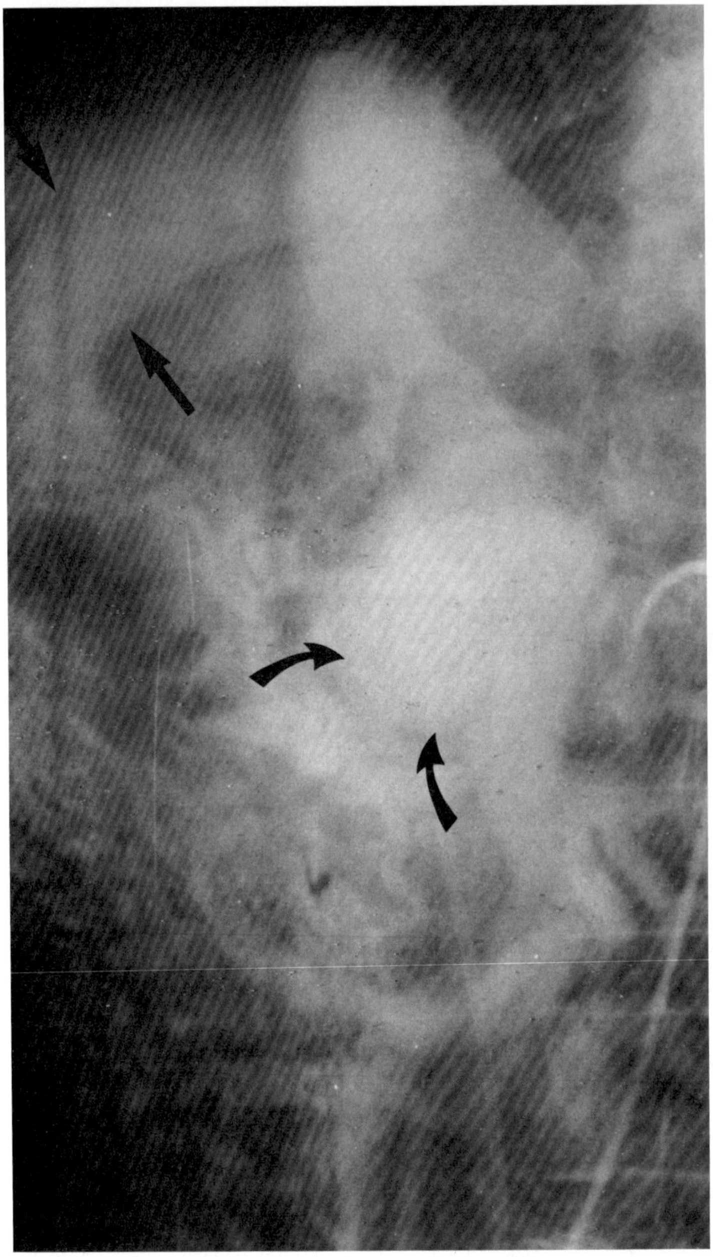

Figure 11 Portal vein aneurysm. Arterial portography demonstrates a saccular aneurysm of the portal vein (curved arrows) in a patient with underlying cirrhosis and portal hypertension. A wide umbilical vein is shown (arrows).

Diseases of the Hepatic Veins

Hepatic Vein Occlusion

The diseases associated with the occlusion of hepatic veins of whatever cause are described in Chapter 16. The diagnosis of Budd-Chiari syndrome is by angiography. The hepatic arteriographic findings are nonspecific and may demonstrate stretching of intrahepatic vessels by the congested, swollen parenchyma. Inferior vena cavography may reveal a site of obstruction adjacent to hepatic vein inflow. Selective catheterization of the hepatic veins is the only way to prove the diagnosis. If a selective angiographic catheter cannot be positioned into a hepatic vein, this implies complete thrombosis and usually confirms the diagnosis. In most cases, however, the catheter can be advanced through thrombus toward the origin of a hepatic vein and the upper end of the thrombus demonstrated by venography (Fig. 12). Since the vein draining the caudate lobe of the liver does not usually become involved in Budd-Chiari syndrome, it may be possible to catheterize this vessel selectively. Venography performed on such a collateral will also demonstrate a typical "spider's web" appearance of the intrahepatic venous structures.

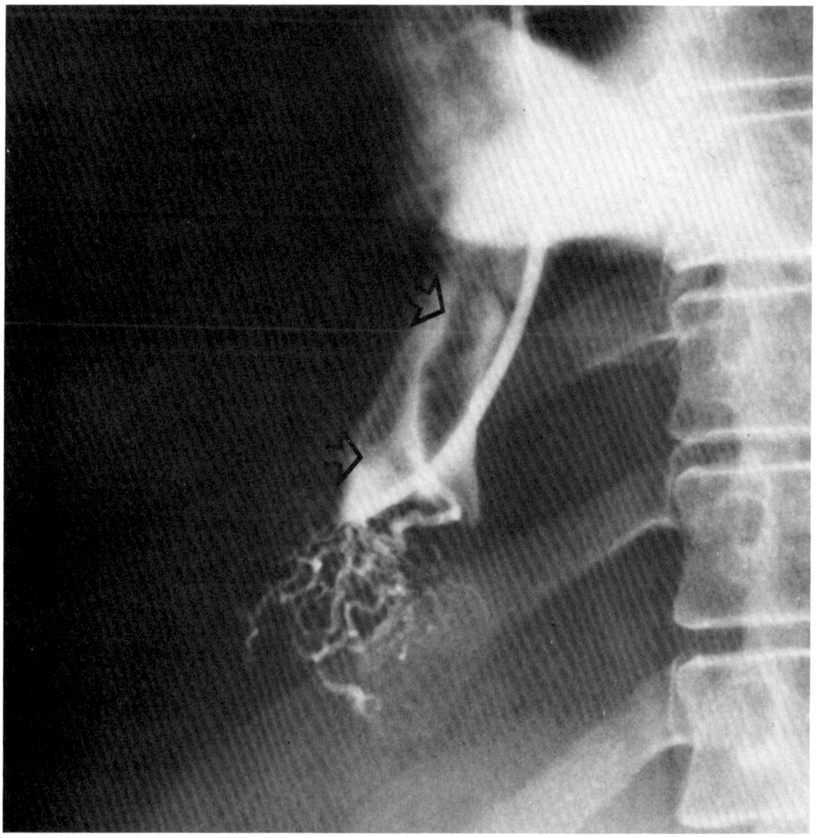

Figure 12 Hepatic vein thrombosis—Budd-Chiari syndrome. A selective hepatic venogram demonstrates thrombus (arrows) through which the catheter has passed. A spider's web pattern is also demonstrated.

References

1. Strandell B, Erwald R, Kulling KG: Simultaneous determination of portal vein and hepatic artery blood flow in awake man. *Acta Med Scand 191*:139, 1972.
2. Simmons JT, Ring EJ, Sheehan BA, Athanasoulis CA, Baum S: The effect of vasopressin on hepatic arterial blood flow. *Radiology 124*:637, 1977.
3. Propper HL, Jefferson NC, Necheles H: Survival of dogs after partial or total devascularization of the liver. *Ann Surg 140*:93, 1954.
4. Chuang VP, and Wallace S: Hepatic artery redistribution for intraarterial infusion of hepatic artery neoplasms. *Radiology 135*:295, 1980.
5. Doppman JL, Girton M, Kahn ER: Proximal versus peripheral hepatic artery embolization. Experimental study in monkeys. *Radiology 128*:577, 1978.
6. Ryan RJ: Hepatic artery aneurysm. *JAMA 219*:1762, 1972.
7. Bristol R, Gonzales P, Chassin J: Aneurysms of the hepatic artery. *Am J Surg 120*:97, 1970.
8. Ashbury GI: Ruptured hepatic artery aneurysm. *Am J Surg 36*:631, 1970.
9. Phiskin M: Peliosis hepatis. *Radiology 114*:29, 1975.
10. Baumgarten P: Über vollständiges Offenbleiben der Vena umbilicalis: Zugleich ein Beitrag zur Frage des Morbus Bantii. *Arb. Geb. Pathol. Anat Inst Tuebingen (Leipzig) 6*:93, 1907.
11. Marks C: *The Portal Venous System*. Charles C Thomas, Springfield, Ill, 1973.

30

Congenital and Pediatric Liver Disease

Edmund A. Franken, Jr., Wilbur L. Smith
The University of Iowa Hospitals and Clinics
Iowa City, Iowa

Aslam R. Siddiqui
Indiana University School of Medicine
Indianapolis, Indiana

Introduction

Radiology of the liver in the pediatric age group shares the problems of other aspects of pediatric radiology, that of recognition of the concept that infant and child are not miniature adults. Because even normal hepatic anatomy and physiology are different, diseases are often unique to or have unusual manifestations in children, and different techniques must be utilized for optimum imaging. Several practical problems arise. Plain film radiography requires short exposure time or respiratory motion blur will occur; conversely, the smaller size of the patient frequently allows the use of a small focal spot x-ray tube. Other imaging modalities are considered in similar fashion—for example, compound ultrasound images are difficult to obtain in a moving child, and real-time ultrasonography is frequently more suitable. Also, higher-frequency ultrasound transducers can be used in infants' examinations.

As in the adult, the child's liver can be studied with multiple imaging techniques: plain film, nuclear medicine, ultrasound, computed tomography, and more invasive procedures. At this time the literature on the appropriate modality for each circumstance is conflicting and confusing enough for the adult and even more so for the pediatric patient. Obviously, one need not use every available modality in every patient with suspected liver disease. Our approach has been to perform the study most apt to give the desired information, and follow with additional studies until the problem under investigation is solved. The order in which one utilizes the various modalities depends on the age of the patient, the clinical problem, and the available expertise in each imaging technique.

Development

The liver is a key organ in fetal life, as it receives oxygenated blood from the placenta and blood from the gastrointestinal tract, thereby essentially "screening" all inflow blood. It forms from a bud in the fetal foregut at the end of the fourth week of fetal life. The caudal portion of the bud develops into the gallbladder and cystic duct, while the cranial portion becomes the hepatic glandular tissue (1). The liver grows rapidly and descends into the abdomen. By the ninth week of fetal life the liver is at its largest size relative to the total body weight (2). Formation of recognizable lobes of near adult proportion occurs by the third month of fetal life. Bile secretion is noted in the gut lumen by 5 months (1). In utero the liver is an important organ in blood formation, and although this function largely ceases at birth, its potential for extramedullary hematopoiesis persists.

The blood supply in utero is derived from the vitelline (yolk sac) veins, which later form the basis for the portal system and the umbilical veins (3). Flow is entirely toward the liver, with drainage via the hepatic veins and the sinus venosus. The sinus venosus is an embryological structure connecting the left portal vein branch with the inferior vena cava. In utero it is widely patent, but at birth it usually closes. The sinus venosus is the usual pathway employed for placement of umbilical venous catheters into the inferior vena cava.

Developmental Anomalies

Despite the complex embryogenesis, major anomalies of the hepatic parenchyma are rare. Absence of the left lobe of the liver has been reported in a few patients and is associated with gastric volvulus due to absence of the stomach's suspensory ligaments (4). Absence of the right lobe of the liver, although reported, is very rare (5). Accessory hepatic lobes are unusual and when present are mostly incidental findings at surgery or autopsy (6). Anomalies of the portal venous system include atresia, duplication, and anomalous preduodenal position of the portal vein. The latter presents with a characteristic duodenal imprint on gastrointestinal barium studies (7). There is some overlap between portal vein atresia and neonatal patients with cavernous transformation of the portal vein (see portal hypertension). Both present with signs of severe portal hypertension during the newborn period. A final portal vein anomaly of note is the occasional drainage of all or some of the pulmonary veins into the portal system, a condition often causing congestive heart failure in the newborn.

The biliary tree and gallbladder are the most common sites of anomalies of the liver; duplications, atresias, and anomalous biliary insertion are well documented (3).

The accessibility of the umbilical vessels in the newborn make them likely sources of iatrogenic trauma. The umbilical vein has been used in the past as a route for parenteral infusion and exchange transfusion. Ideally, the catheter should be placed beyond the liver via the ductus venosus into the inferior vena cava before any materials are infused; however, this cannot always be accomplished. Intestinal perforation, ascending portal vein phlebitis, hepatic necrosis, and hepatic abscess have been reported after umbilical venous catheterization (8,9) (Fig. 1). About 1% of patients who have an umbilical venous catheter show some complication (10).

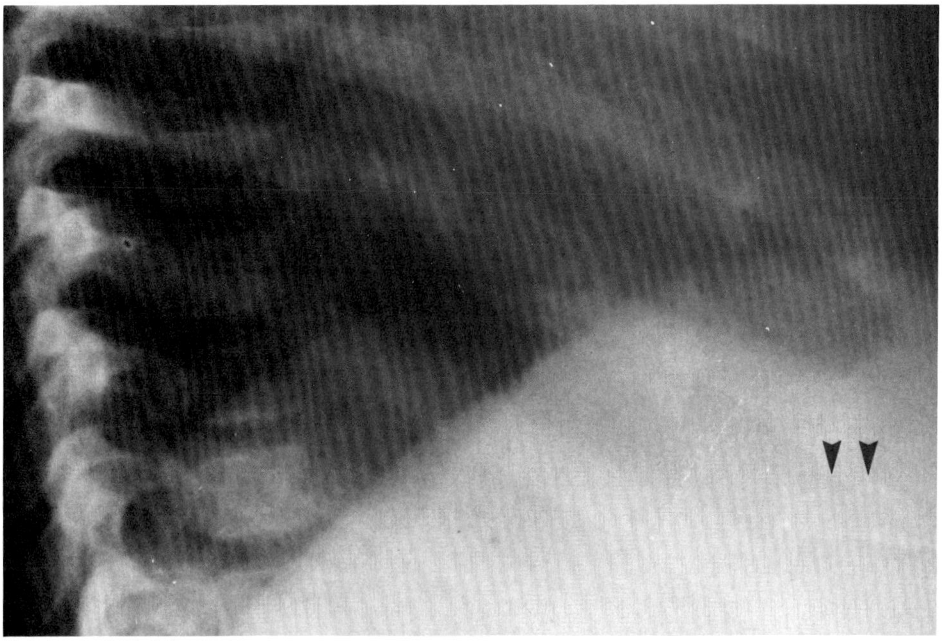

Figure 1 A child being evaluated for cardiac disease who has incidentally noted tubular calcification in the liver (arrows). Further history revealed that the child had an indwelling umbilical venous line in the newborn period. This is presumably a calcified portal vein thrombus.

Techniques and Uses of Examinations

Plain Film

The abdominal radiograph remains the base for hepatic evaluation, but other modalities are generally more rewarding in providing information. A massively enlarged liver is easily recognized on the plain film, but nuclear medicine studies are more exact in borderline situations.

Extensive hepatic calcification can be seen with routine radiography (Fig. 2); computed tomography identifies minimal deposits of calcium. Differential diagnosis of the common causes of hepatic calcifications in children is given in Table 1. A rare cause of hepatic calcification of infants is intrauterine portal vein thrombosis. In this condition single or multiple deposits are found beneath the liver capsule. These may have the appearance of phleboliths or show a branching arrangement (11).

The liver may be diffusely dense secondary to excessive iron storage. As with calcification, a gross increase in hepatic iron will be visible on plain films (Fig. 3), and a lesser degree of abnormality identified with computerized tomography (12). Idiopathic hemochromatosis is almost exclusively a disease of adults. In children increased iron storage occurs with accelerated gut absorption in a variety of diseases, or with multiple blood transfusions.

The normal child's liver contains less than 5% fat by weight. Any disease process in which the fat content increases may produce a reduction of radiographic density of the liver, and therefore allow its visibility as a lucent structure on the plain film (13). Reported

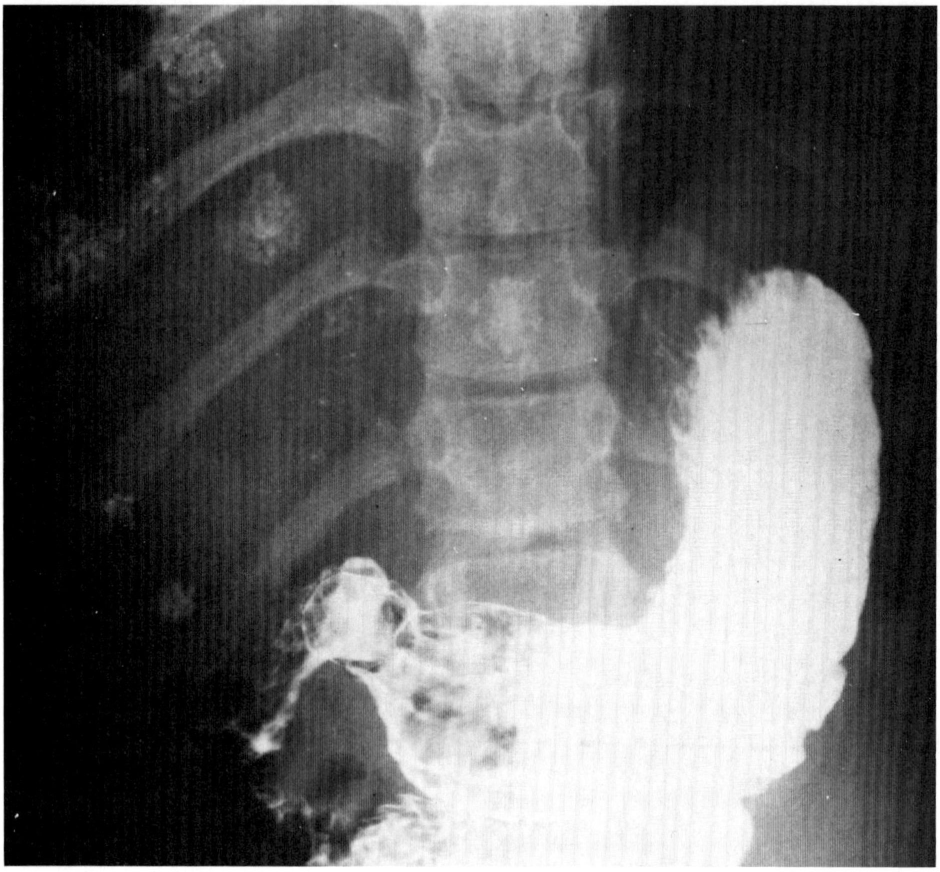

Figure 2 Multiple calcified liver abscesses in a patient with chronic granulomatous disease of childhood.

Table 1 Liver and Biliary Calcifications in Infants and Children

1.	Tumor: hepatoblastoma, hepatoma, hemangioma, hamartoma, metastasis (neuroblastoma), cyst
2.	Infection: intrauterine infection (cytomegalic inclusion disease, toxoplasmosis), tuberculosis, abscess, other granulomatous infections, parasites, chronic granulomatous disease of childhood
3.	Intraductal: intrahepatic calculi (especially Caroli's disease)
4.	Vascular: portal vein, hepatic artery thrombi
5.	Miscellaneous: capsular calcification of hypercalcemia or meconium peritonitis; sequel of umbilical venous catheterization

Source: Adapted from Ref. 11.

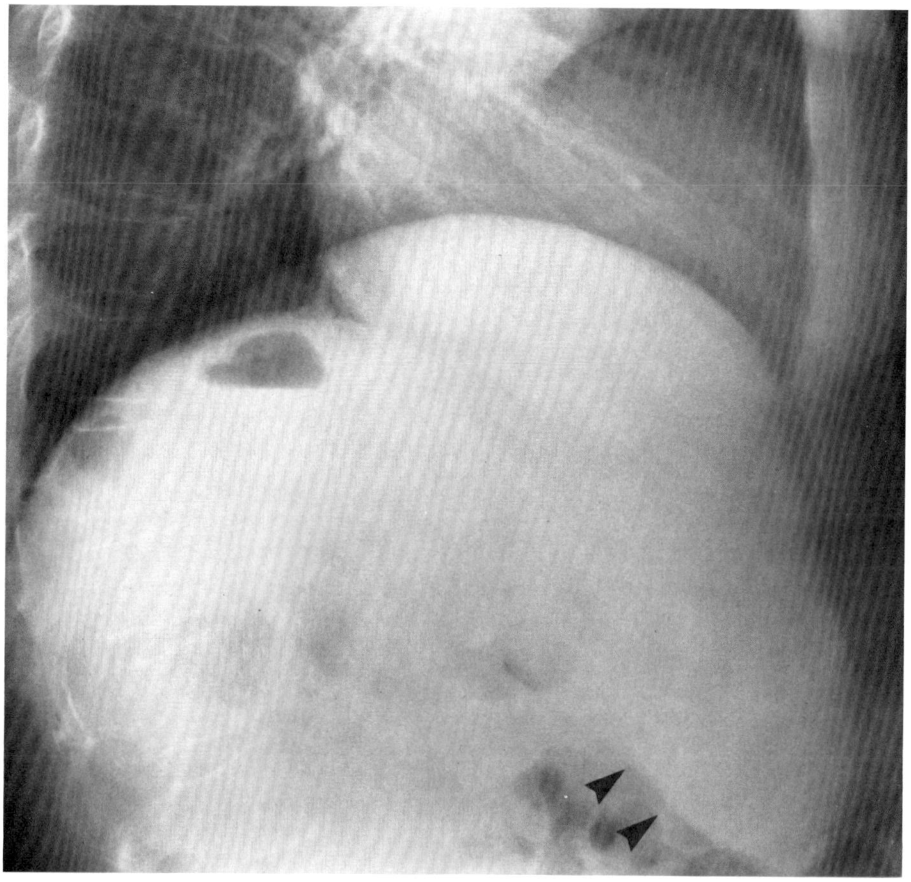

Figure 3 A teenager with primary aplastic anemia and a radiodense liver (arrowheads) on a lateral chest radiograph.

causes include cystic fibrosis, Reye's syndrome, acute and chronic starvation, malabsorption, steroid therapy, glycogen storage diseases, and hepatitis (14). The lucent liver is identified against surrounding muscle or other unit density (Fig. 4). Minimal fat infiltration may produce merely blurring of the medial margin of the right properitoneal flank stripe.

Total body opacification (TBO) is a technique first used in genitourinary radiology of infants and is sometimes useful for outlining liver or biliary tract masses. The TBO effect is based on the wide and immediate intravascular dispersion of intravenous contrast material throughout the body, thus increasing the radiographic density of normally perfused tissues. TBO is particularly effective in infants because of the lower kilovolt peak radiographic techniques used and the relatively large amounts of contrast material

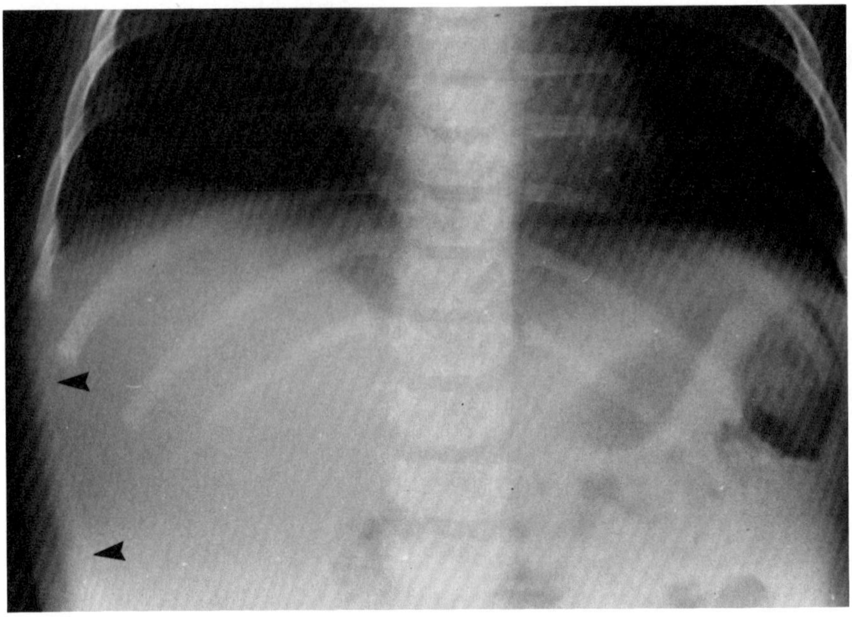

Figure 4 Visibly fatty liver outlined against the right flank stripe (arrowheads). CT is also an excellent method for delineating this abnormality. (From Ref. 14.)

administered. Hypovascular abdominal masses appear as lucencies on early films after injection (Fig. 5). In the liver, cyst, abscess, tumor, and areas of necrosis have been outlined (15).

Nuclear Medicine

Nuclear medicine procedures can study the anatomic and physiologic status of the liver in four different ways. These are the evaluation of the Kupffer's cells, hepatocytes, biliary system, and the vascular network of the liver.

The most widely used imaging agent is ^{99m}technetium sulfur colloid, which utilizes radiolabeled particles less than 1 μm in size. These particles are phagocytozed by the Kupffer's cells of the hepatic reticuloendothelial system. The sulfur colloid liver scan is valuable in documenting size, shape, and position of liver. From the scans information is also obtained regarding focal areas of abnormal function, diffuse liver disease, radiation injury, and liver regeneration.

For evaluation of the hepatocyte function and biliary system anatomy, the radiotracers available are ^{131}iodine labeled rose bengal and ^{99m}technetium labeled iminodiacetic acid (IDA) derivatives. Using these agents, one may visualize the biliary tree and its anatomy. Because these agents also rely on liver function, it is not always possible to use them to differentiate between biliary atresia and neonatal hepatitis. In some patients they are the definitive study.

The vascularity of the liver and liver lesions can be determined by rapid imaging over the right upper quadrant of the abdomen after the intravenous injection of various radiotracers. Usually, this is done at the time of the initial injection of ^{99m}technetium sulfur colloid for routine imaging. In certain lesions, such as cavernous hemangioma, the sulfur colloid perfusion study may give an impression that the lesion is avascular because of the very sluggish blood flow in it. A more definitive assessment of blood flow is obtained by using ^{99m}technetium labeled autologous red blood cells. Routine use of hepatic perfusion study is valuable not only in the characterization of liver lesions, but occasionally it also reveals extrahepatic vascular abnormalities.

Dosages for pediatric liver imaging procedures can be calculated from the formula described by Webster et al. (16). The formula is an age/mass approximation:

$$\text{Pediatric dose} = \frac{\text{age (yr)} + 1}{\text{age (yr)} + 7} \times \text{adult dose}$$

This formula can be further approximated in this way: for age 5 years or less, 25% of the adult dose; for ages 5–10 years, 50% of the adult dose; for ages 10–15 years, 75% of the adult dose; for ages 15 years or more, the adult dose.

Ultrasound and Computerized Tomography (CT)

Although ultrasound and CT are totally different imaging modalities, the information obtained by them relative to the liver is frequently complementary if not redundant. Indications for CT and ultrasound are approximately the same, and resemble those for adults (17,18) (Table 2). The choice of modality depends not only on the disease suspected, but also on the equipment and expertise available. Generally, the same techniques used for imaging in the adult can be used in children. Because of respiratory

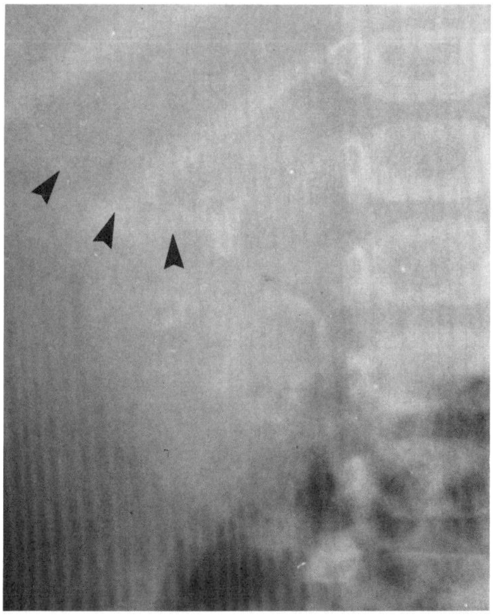

Figure 5 Total body opacification film after bolus injection of 2 cc/kg contrast outlines a faint lucency in the right upper quadrant (arrows). This is a hepatic cyst.

Table 2 Indications for CT and Ultrasound in Children

Cystic disease
Primary and metastatic tumors
Differential diagnosis of jaundice
Biopsy localization
Intrahepatic and perihepatic abscess
Portal hypertension (ultrasound only)

motion of the liver, the detection of hepatic masses and dilated intrahepatic ducts is significantly inhibited by CT (19); we occasionally use sedation in younger children, and have rarely used general anesthesia. In our own patients, access to a new generation CT unit with 1- to 2-sec scan times has been invaluable.

At one time CT was reserved for problem solving of cases with abnormal nuclear medicine or ultrasound studies (20). That is no longer the case, and some patients now have CT as the only definitive examination (e.g., demonstration of liver metastases).

Ultrasound has the ability to visualize the biliary tract independent of the secretory ability of the liver. With current equipment the normal common bile duct as well as the junction of right and left hepatic ducts can be identified even in infants (Fig. 6). Portal venous anatomy and its pathologic alternatives can be imaged to a degree heretofore impossible (see below). However, localized masses (tumors) are usually not as well demonstrated as with CT. Criteria for the ultrasonic diagnosis of diffuse liver disease remain imprecise.

CT seems most valuable in the unequivocal recognition of intrahepatic masses. For most other indications, CT and ultrasound are equally competitive. Although the portal vein can usually be identified on CT, our personal preference for study of portal venous aberrations is ultrasound.

Angiography

The necessity for angiography in the investigation of pediatric liver disease has diminished with the advent of ultrasound and CT; these modalities have made us aware of the limitations of angiographic accuracy (21). We now consider angiography essential only in two situations: the preoperative mapping of liver tumors prior to resection and the definitive study of portal hypertension. In the occasional neonate in whom abdominal arteriography is necessary, a flush aortogram via the umbilical artery usually provides adequate diagnostic information and avoids the dangers of femoral artery catheterization. After the first few days of life the umbilical route is no longer available and a femoral artery route is necessary. In this situation arteriography should be considered with caution, as the risk of femoral artery occlusion in the infant is substantial (22). Selective angiography of the abdominal arteries in the older child is performed as in the adult.

The angiographic methods of study of the liver in portal hypertension are now almost limitless, with several new techniques being described each year. As extrahepatic portal hypertension is most frequent in children, most of the newer methods are not appropriate or needed. The specific angiographic workup of portal hypertension is discussed below.

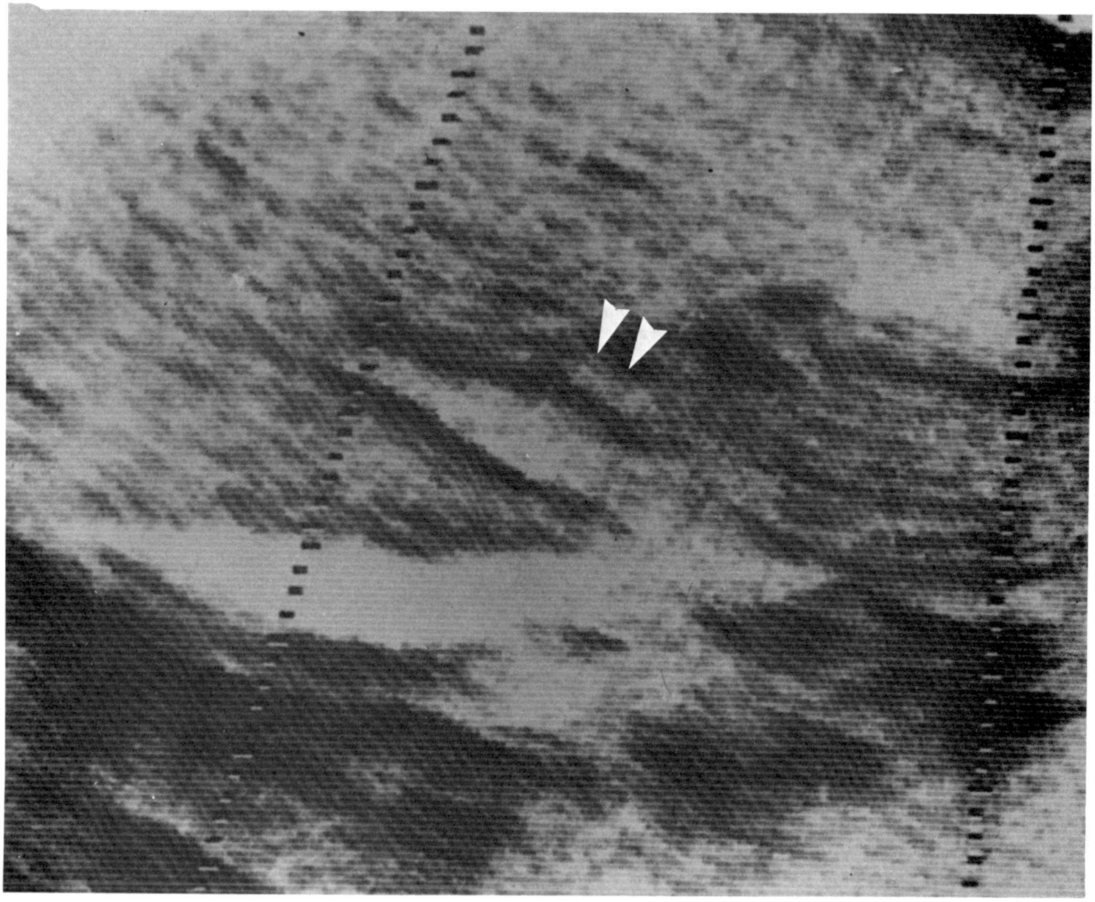

Figure 6 Common duct (arrows), of normal diameter, lying anterior to the portal vein in a 6-month-old child.

Other Investigative Methods

The intravenous cholangiogram is seldom used in the current practice of pediatric radiology, having been replaced by ultrasound and CT. Percutaneous cholangiography is feasible, even in the neonate with normal-size bile ducts (23). The technique involves the use of the Chiba needle; the only modification for infants is that general anesthesia is necessary.

Specific Liver and Biliary Tract Disease

This section includes those diseases which are unique to, or predominantly involve, or have differing manifestations in the pediatric age group. Pathologic entities that affect children on an occasional basis but have not specific pediatric features (e.g., hepatic trauma) are not covered.

Biliary Atresia and Neonatal Hepatitis

Jaundice in the first week of life has a variety of causes and infrequently needs radiographic investigation. Jaundice which is of cholestatic nature by laboratory studies and which persists beyond the first month of life is most often due to neonatal hepatitis or biliary atresia. Differentiation of these entities requires clinical, biochemical, nuclear medicine, and often radiological investigation. It must be stated that the subject of biliary atresia versus neonatal hepatitis is a complex and controversial area; what follows is the authors' interpretation of current literature.

Neonatal hepatitis is a clinical entity occurring in otherwise healthy babies between 1 and 4 weeks of age, with persistent jaundice accompanied by hepatomegaly. At one time "giant cell hepatitis" was the term used for this syndrome. It seems best to avoid this name, as giant cells are found in many liver diseases (24). It is now thought that the syndrome of neonatal hepatitis results from a variety of perinatal insults or metabolic deficits, rather than a single etiology. Possible infectious agents include viruses (cytomegalovirus, rubella, viral hepatitis), protozoa (toxoplasmosis), and spirochetes (syphilis). Metabolic causes include alpha$_1$-antitrypsin deficiency, familial recurrent cholestasis, cystic fibrosis, and others. Pathologic findings are somewhat variable, but in general there is parenchymal disruption, giant cells are present, and the biliary canaliculi are bile-free. Although some patients recover, cirrhosis subsequently develops in many.

There is a small group of patients with an intermediate entity between biliary atresia and neonatal hepatitis, that is, with disease limited predominantly to the bile ducts and a minimum of parenchymal inflammation. In this state the biliary tree is quite small, particularly its intrahepatic components. In the past these infants' condition has been labeled "intrahepatic biliary atresia" or "biliary hypoplasia." It is uncertain whether this is due to reduced bile flow secondary to cholestatic hepatitis (25) or is a separate disease entity associated with abnormal bile acids (24).

Biliary atresia has clinical manifestations identical to neonatal hepatitis, with persisting jaundice and hepatomegaly beyond 1–2 weeks of age. The etiology of biliary atresia is undetermined. Although previously assumed to occur during intrauterine life, several cases have now been described with patent bile ducts at birth progressing to occlusion within a few weeks (26). It may be associated with developmental defects such as polysplenia and abdominal vascular anomalies, as well as other syndromes (25). The extent of atresia is variable—any portion or all of the biliary tree may be without lumen. Only 10–15% of cases are potentially correctable (i.e., by anastomosing intrahepatic ducts with the gut). The bile ducts proximal to the point of atresia are usually not dilated; the nature of these proximal ducts determines the potential for successful surgical drainage (27). In biliary atresia the liver characteristically shows periportal fibrosis and bile duct proliferation.

As more infants with biliary atresia or neonatal hepatitis are investigated, the distinction between the two entities becomes more difficult. The concept is now advanced that biliary atresia and neonatal hepatitis may be variants of the same process, the cases of atresia having a component of sclerosing cholangitis of the extrahepatic ducts (28) (Fig. 7). This theory explains the indeterminate cases and accounts for the progressive development of bile occlusion.

Clinical distinction between biliary atresia and neonatal hepatitis is impossible. Biochemical studies, liver biopsy, and nuclear medicine investigations should allow differentiation in most patients (29).

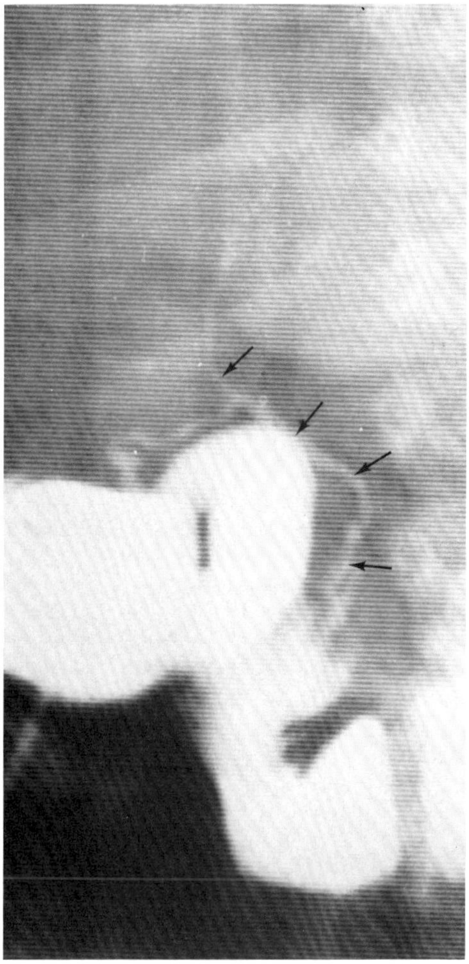

Figure 7 Intraoperative cholangiogram in a jaundiced child. A tiny common bile duct and intrahepatic ducts are present (arrows). Biopsy revealed a sclerosing cholangitis.

Nuclear medicine investigation of neonatal jaundice relies on ^{99m}Tc-iminodiacetic acid (IDA) compounds, particularly PIPIDA. In a normal infant after intravenous injection the gallbladder and gastrointestinal tract are visualized within 1 hr. There is a minimum of soft tissue background and virtually no renal excretion. In jaundiced patients there may be delayed clearance of the blood pool, increased soft tissue background, and increased renal excretion. The ^{99m}Tc-IDA compound study can be carried on for up to 24 hr. If at any time gastrointestinal excretion of the radiotracer is noted, the diagnosis of biliary atresia is virtually excluded. Prior treatment with phenobarbital for 3–7 days increases the accuracy of the exclusion result of the test (30). However, as the physical half-life of ^{99m}Tc is only 6 hr, compounds labeled with it are not suitable for long-term studies. If there is strong clinical doubt over the interpretation of an equivocal or negative ^{99m}Tc-PIPIDA scan, the next step may be rose bengal labelled with ^{131}Iodine. The long half-life of this radiotracer (8 days) is suitable for a long-term evaluation of excretion; however, the radiation dose to the patient is higher than with ^{99m}Tc. Therefore, only very small quantities (20–30 μCi) are used. Lugol's solution must be given to the patient for several days before to block the thyroid gland. As it is difficult to image liver and gastrointestinal tract with such a small amount of tracer, the procedure consists mainly of fecal and urinary monitoring. Urine and feces are collected every day for 5–7 days and excretion of ^{131}Iodine is measured in representative samples from each day. The kidneys are an alternate route of rose bengal excretion in the presence of severe hepatocellular disease, which makes it important that urine and feces are collected separately. Fecal excretion of less than 5% of the radioactivity over the study period is consistent with biliary atresia (31). Although a diagnosis can be made in most patients with neonatal jaundice by these techniques, there will still be a few patients with neonatal hepatitis who show a very poor and delayed excretion of ^{131}Iodine rose bengal.

One would expect ultrasound and/or computerized tomography to be of value in separating neonatal hepatitis from biliary atresia by demonstrating an intact biliary tree, but at this time results are poor. Percutaneous cholangiography has been moderately successful in demonstrating an intact biliary system in infants with neonatal hepatitis (23) (Fig. 8). In some instances laparotomy with operative cholangiography is necessary to confirm biliary atresia and its extent. At one time there was concern over referring

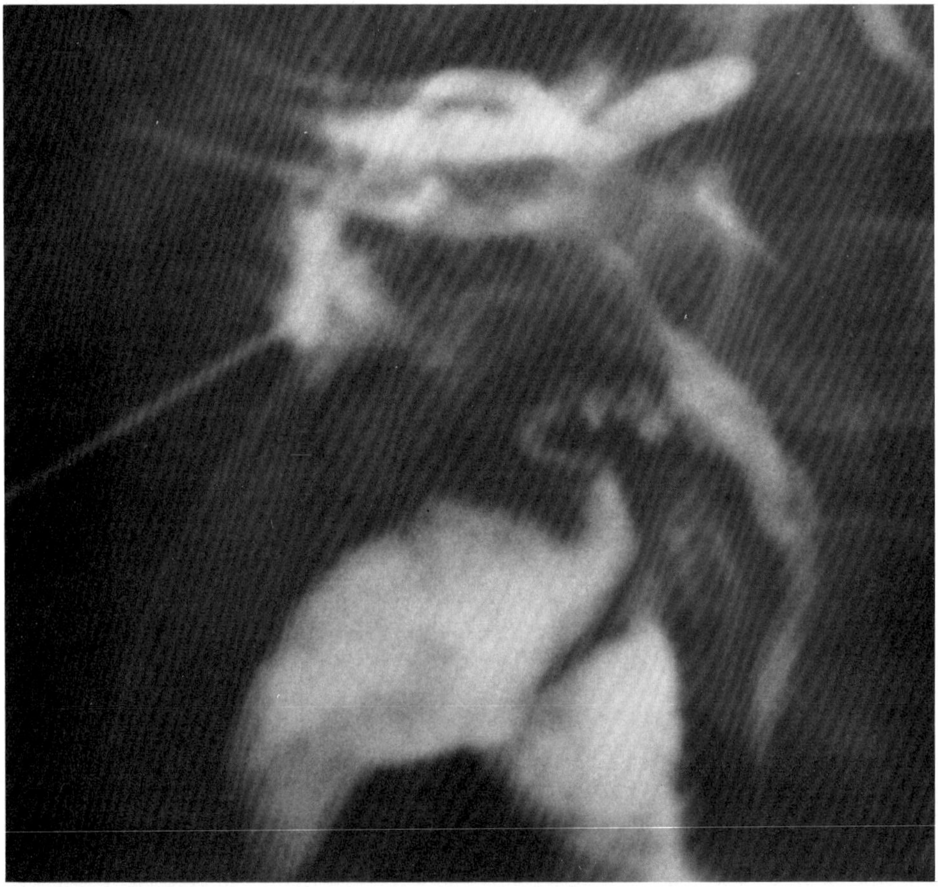

Figure 8 Transhepatic cholangiogram in a 2-month-old jaundiced child. Biopsy proven neonatal hepatitis.

jaundiced babies for laparotomy because of anesthetic risk; with contemporary surgery and anesthesia this is no longer the case (32).

There is a current wave of popularity for the Kasai procedure (portoenterostomy) in patients with uncorrectable biliary atresia. Surgery consists in excision of the atretic bile ducts, followed by anastomosis of an intestinal loop to the dissected porta hepatis. Results are variable—some groups are enthusiastic, others discouraging (25); surgery performed before 10 weeks of age seems to produce a better result (30). For evaluation of any surgical procedure to correct biliary atresia, ^{99m}Tc-IDA compounds are employed. With successful surgery, the radiotracer will be rapidly excreted into the gastrointestinal tract (Fig. 9).

The end stage of biliary atresia and neonatal hepatitis is cirrhosis; this develops in some hepatitis patients and almost all atresia patients with delayed surgery. Accompanying the chronic liver disease are bony changes of expansion of the marrow cavity and reduction in cortical depth. Cholangiocarcinoma has been reported as a late complication of the liver disease (33).

Choledochal Cyst

Choledochal cyst refers to a localized dilatation of the extrahepatic bile duct. The cyst may present at any age and is particularly common in Japanese patients.

The etiology of the choledochal cyst is not clear. A recent paper by Barlow et al. (34) proposes division of the cysts into two categories. The first group presents as jaundice in the neonate, is accompanied by atresia or stenosis of portions of the biliary tree, and is frequently complicated by portal hypertension and cirrhosis. Others (35) have related this group of patients to similar types of cystic disease of the liver. The second group of patients presents later in life, often has associated pancreatitis or choledocholithiasis, and is less apt to develop cirrhosis. In several patients Babbitt et al. (36) noted anomalous insertion of the common bile duct into the distal pancreatic duct; he proposed that the cyst develops from reflux of pancreatic secretions into the common bile duct, producing inflammation and subsequent cyst formation. Thus a current concept of the nature of choledochal cyst would include one group with bile duct cysts of congenital nature and related to other cystic disease of the liver, and another group with acquired cyst formation due to anomalous bile duct/pancreatic duct anastomosis.

The pattern of common duct dilatation can be one of three types (37): the more usual appearance of common duct widening and the much rarer common duct diverticulum or the choledochocele (Fig. 10).

The classic symptomatology of choledochal cyst is the triad of recurrent pain and jaundice with a palpable abdominal mass, but this is infrequent in the pediatric age group. In the neonate prolonged jaundice with or without a mass is usual; older children may present with the classic symptoms or with manifestations of cirrhosis and portal hypertension.

Radiographic diagnosis of choledochal cyst is possible with many imaging modalities. In the neonate the cystic mass may be relatively lucent with total body opacification. In the anicteric patient the cyst can be opacified with oral cholecystography or intravenous cholangiography; the latter study is seldom needed if other modalities are available.

Technetium-99m-labeled IDA compounds are often useful in the demonstration of a choledochal cyst. Upper gastrointestinal studies usually show the nonspecific but suggestive signs of anterior and medial displacement of the descending portion of the duodenum. Angiographic demonstration of choledochal cyst has been reported (38). The

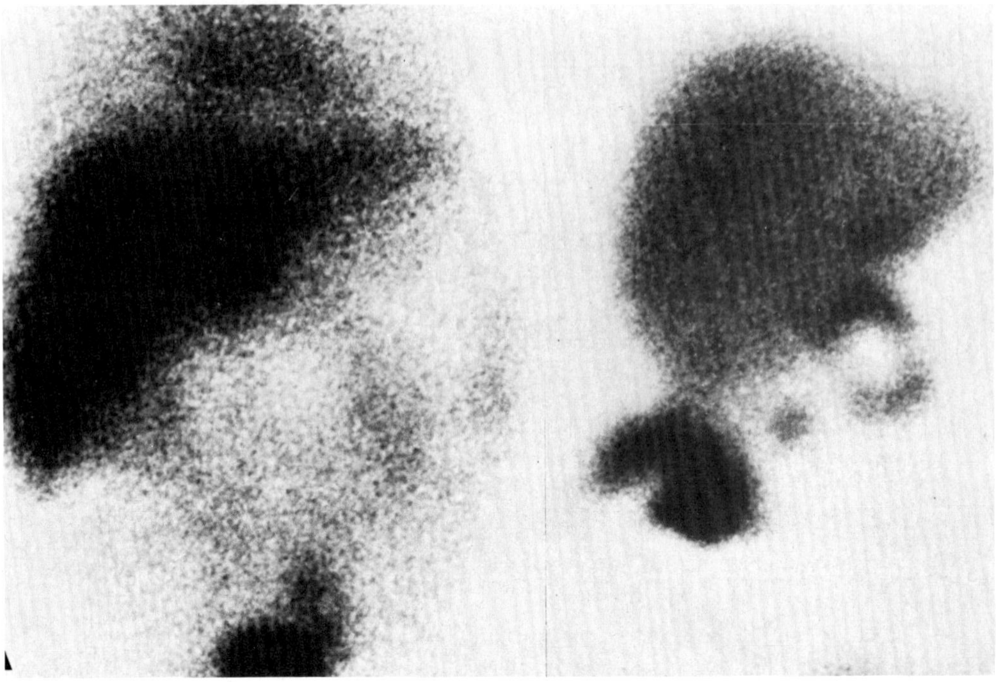

(A) **(B)**

Figure 9 Child with extrahepatic biliary atresia. (A) Initial technetium-IDA study shows no activity in bowel. (B) Study after Kasai procedure demonstrates radiotracer within the isolated bowel loop. Good operative result.

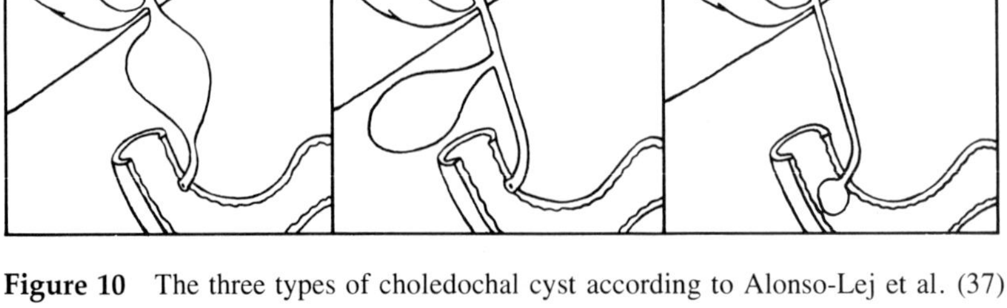

Figure 10 The three types of choledochal cyst according to Alonso-Lej et al. (37).

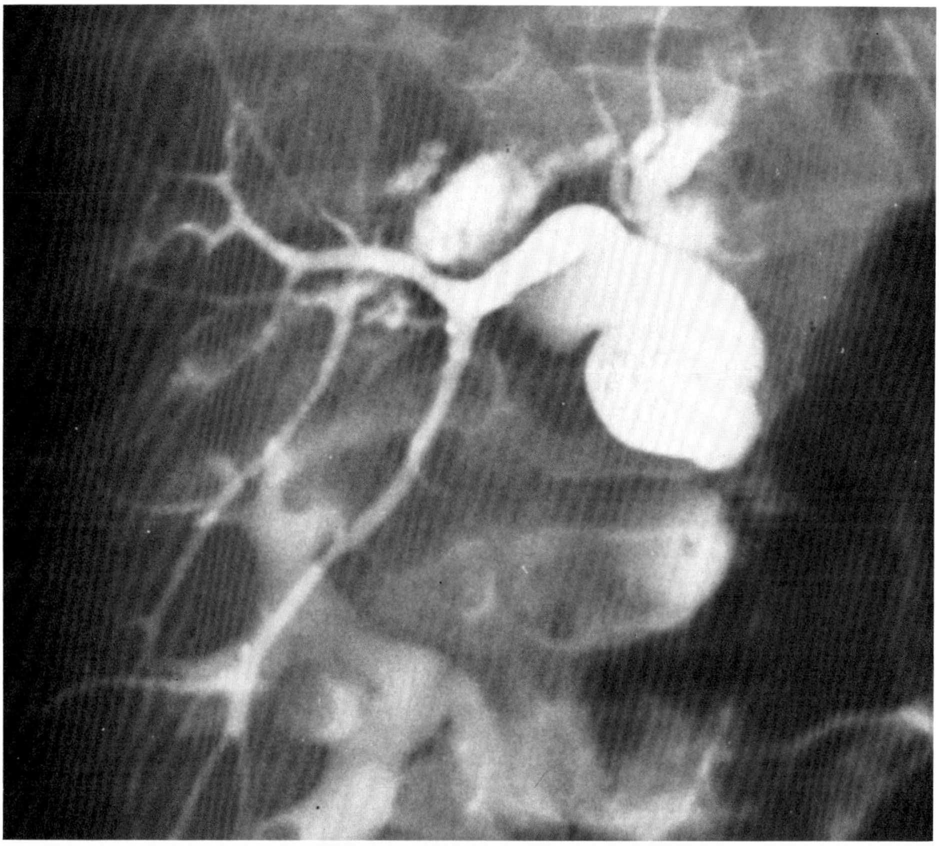

Figure 11 Percutaneous transhepatic cholangiogram demonstrates a choledochal cyst.

cyst is easily visualized by ultrasound (39) or computerized tomography. At this time we prefer percutaneous cholangiography for exact diagnosis and as a mapping procedure for the surgeon (23) (Fig. 11).

Treatment of a choledochal cyst usually involves some drainage procedure with anastomosis to the gastrointestinal tract. In some instances excision of the cyst may be feasible. A delayed complication of choledochal cyst is the development of biliary carcinoma. The increased risk in these patients for carcinoma is thought to be related to excessive exposure of the ductal epithelium to stagnant bile (40).

Congenital Hepatic Fibrosis

Congenital hepatic fibrosis is a disorder that usually manifests itself during childhood with hepatomegaly and portal hypertension. It is not unusual for these children to be initially hospitalized with acute gastrointestinal bleeding due to esophageal varices. The disease has a strong familial tendency and is probably inherited, although sporadic cases have been reported (41,42).

Pathologic evaluation of the liver demonstrates broad bands of fibrous tissue which in severe cases form a complete fibrous network encasing the functioning liver cell masses. Within these fibrous bands are multiple bile ducts of varying size, some even considerably dilated. In contradistinction to polycystic liver disease, no true cysts are present (43).

Radiography of the abdomen often shows hepatosplenomegaly. Calcifications due to nephrocalcinosis may also be present in a few cases. Barium studies are useful to confirm the presence of varices. Rosenfeld et al. have reported that ultrasound can show a distorted echo pattern within the liver without true cysts (44). Renal ultrasound or intravenous pyelography should be performed, as up to 80% of these patients will demonstrate some degree of renal tubular ectasia, often with nephromegaly (45). Studies of the biliary tree often show areas of ectasia closely resembling congenital dilatation of the intrahepatic ducts (Caroli's syndrome) (46).

Much of the mortality from congenital hepatic fibrosis relates to gastrointestinal hemorrhage from varices. Because of this fact and the reported high incidence of anomalies of the portal system in these patients, evaluation of the portal system by angiography is necessary (47). Our method of choice is a long, slow injection into the superior mesenteric artery with visualization of the portal system on late films. A splenic arteriogram often gives complementary information.

Cystic Disease of the Liver

Congenital cystic disease of the liver is considered in two categories: the solitary cyst and polycystic disease of the liver.

Solitary cysts occur in childhood but are more commonly found in adults as incidental findings at surgery or autopsy. There is a strong female predominance. The cysts are thought to arise from bile duct remnants. When symptomatic they usually present as hepatomegaly or a localized hepatic mass. Ultrasound and CT are definitive studies for cases that require investigation (48) (Fig. 12).

Polycystic disease of the liver represents a less clearly defined spectrum of disorders. About half of the patients have associated renal cystic disease. There is also an association between polycystic liver disease and cysts in the pancreas and spleen. Several instances of polycystic liver disease associated with intracranial aneurysms have been recorded and familial occurrence of this combination is documented (49).

Among the patients with polycystic disease of the liver and kidneys at least two well-defined genetically determined patterns are apparent. *Infantile polycystic disease* of the kidney and liver is an autosomal recessive disorder in which the renal component predominates. These infants usually die from renal failure during the newborn period and invariably have multiple cysts of the liver. *Adult-type polycystic disease* of the kidneys is inherited as an autosomal dominant disorder and in about one-third of these patients polycystic disease of the liver is found (50). Between these two disorders there is a whole spectrum of cystic disease of the liver and kidneys. Some authors have suggested an inverse relationship in severity between the renal and hepatic lesions (i.e., liver disease more severe, renal component less). The fact that the cysts of polycystic disease are derived from biliary structures and that Caroli's disease is seen in some cases of congenital hepatic fibrosis has led to speculation that there may be a link between these disorders. At present the histology of the renal lesions and hepatic lesions is not sufficiently well established to confirm this theory (51). At this time it seems prudent to recognize polycystic disease of the liver as an entity seen in several well-defined genetic disorders which comprise cystic disease of the kidneys and several other less clearly defined

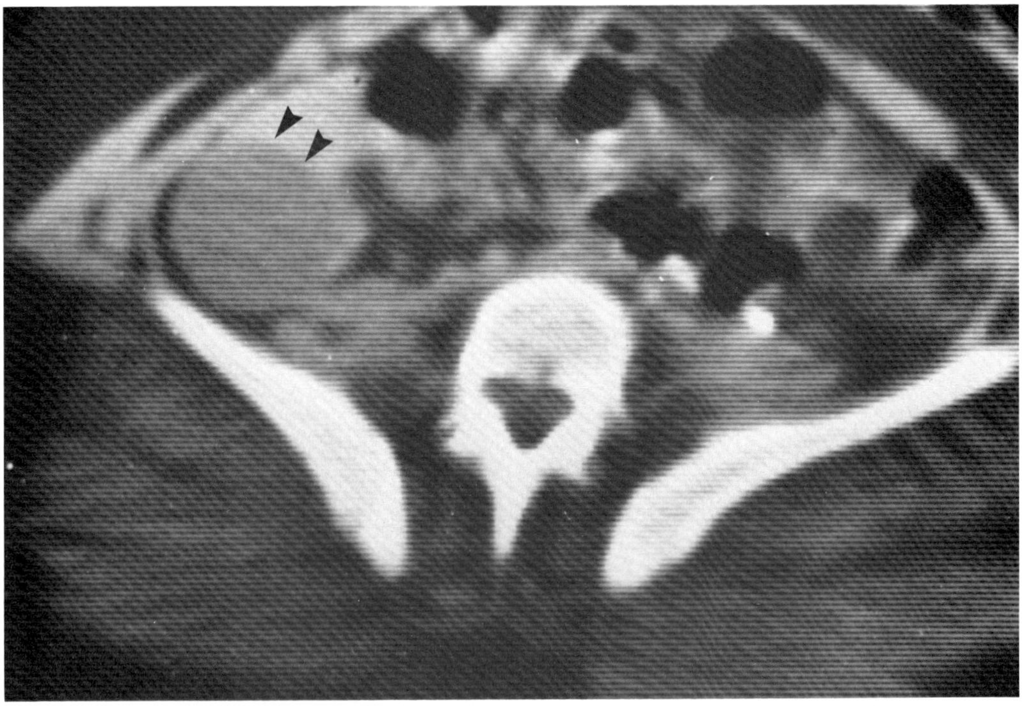

Figure 12 Simple hepatic cyst found incidentally in Riedel's lobe on the CT scan of a 12-year-old female (arrows). No treatment was undertaken.

conditions. In most of these lesions the hepatic disease is not life threatening, although occasionally patients do develop portal hypertension (43).

Radiographic evaluation of these children can be done with nuclear medicine, ultrasound, or CT. Intravenous pyelography is helpful in defining associated renal lesions but is often unnecessary with the information provided by CT or ultrasound. In unusual patients with obstruction of the biliary tract, transhepatic cholangiography is indicated. Angiography occasionally helps in difficult cases, but we have found noninvasive methods adequate in most instances (52).

Tumors

Tumors of the liver are unusual in children; however, several tumors are unique to children or differ enough from their counterparts in the adult to merit discussion in this section.

Benign tumors of epithelial origin include *hepatic adenomas* and *focal nodular hyperplasia*. The former are difficult to diagnose histologically and may become evident as a mass or as an incidental finding at surgery. Focal nodular hyperplasia has been reported in the pediatric age group and usually presents as a mass lesion (53) (Fig. 13).

Mesenchymal tumors of the liver are more characteristic in their presentation. The *hemangioendothelioma* is a unique lesion that often becomes evident through its

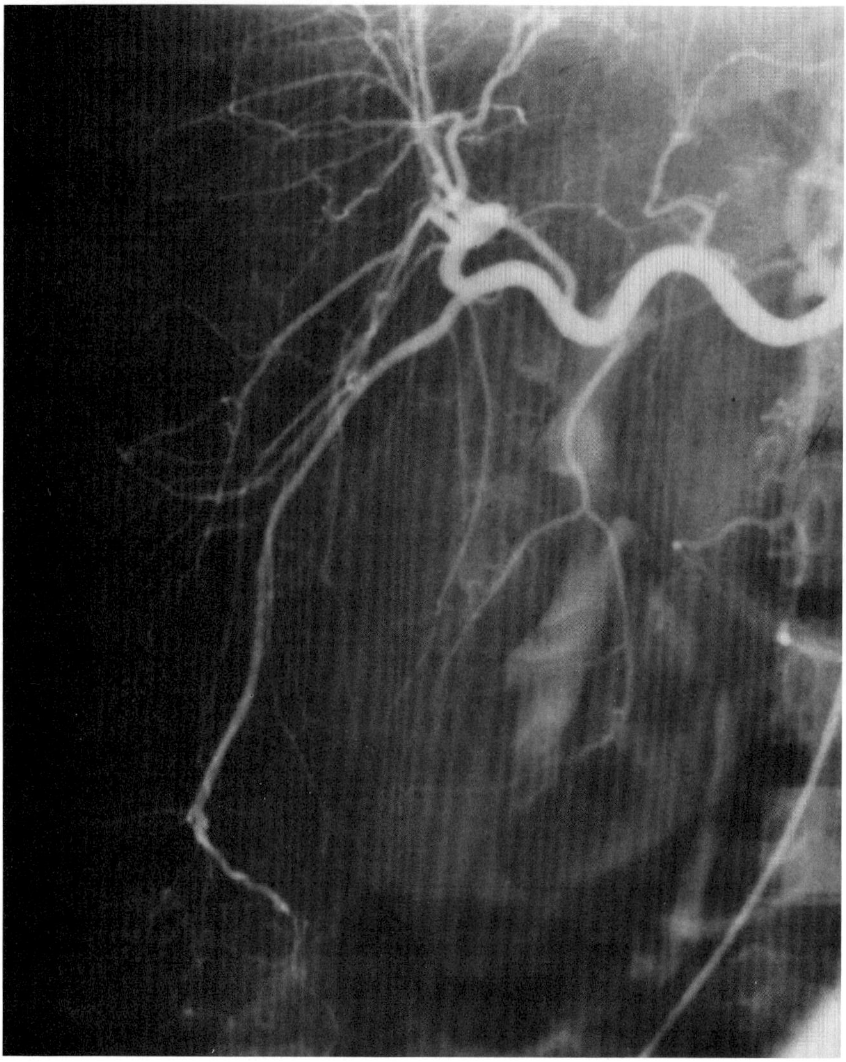

(A)

Figure 13

circulatory effects. These lesions have tremendous arteriovenous shunting, and the usual initial clinical findings are hepatomegaly and congestive heart failure. Physical examination reveals a bruit over the liver and may show evidence of cutaneous hemangiomas. Plain radiographs of the abdomen show hepatomegaly and may show either diffuse or focal areas of calcification (Fig. 14). Chest radiographs indicate cardiomegaly and varying degrees of congestive failure. Liver scan, CT, and ultrasound are helpful in demonstrating the number and size of defects, as these tumors are often multiple. Ultrasound offers the simplest method of demonstrating the extent of the lesion (Fig. 15). Arteriography has an important role if surgical excision or palliation are being considered (Fig. 16). Because these tumors are often multiple, careful preoperative

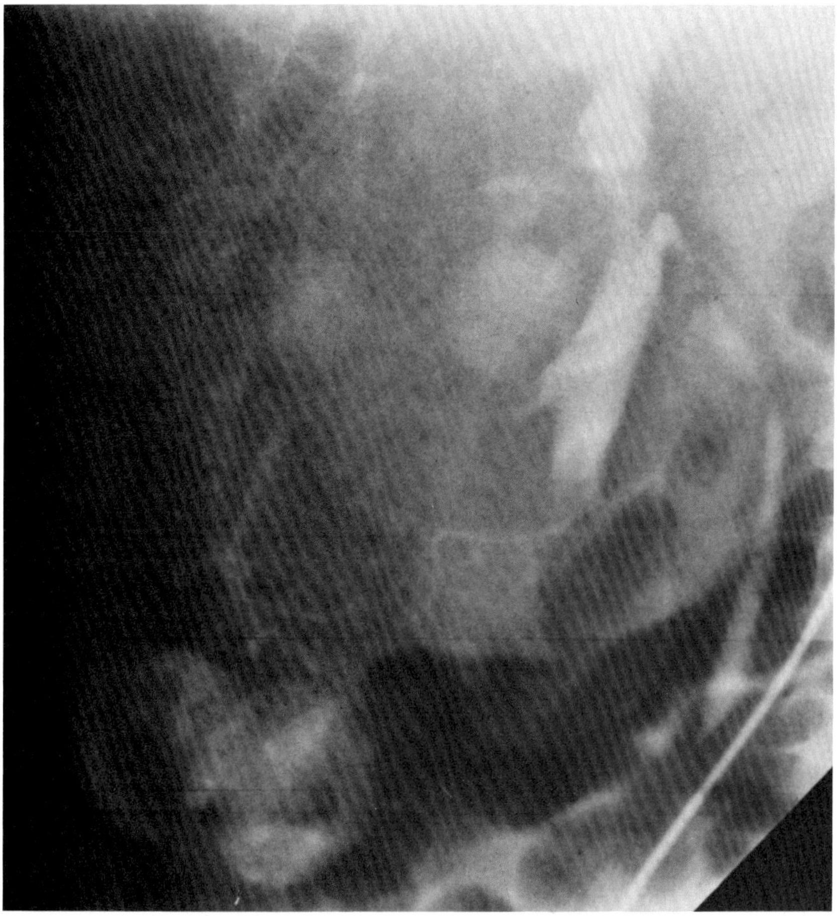

(B)

Figure 13 Focal nodular hyperplasia in von Gierke's disease. The arterial (A) and capillary (B) phases of a common hepatic arteriogram reveal multiple, homogeneous, well-circumscribed nodules.

selective angiography is needed. Embolization of the tumors, although theoretically possible, may be complicated by the size of the arteriovenous shunts. Medical treatment with corticosteroids is sometimes helpful in reducing the blood shunting and may cause regression of the tumors (54,55).

Other benign mesenchymal tumors occur much less commonly. *Cavernous hemangiomas* (Fig. 17) usually come to attention as an abdominal mass, although rarely they can trap platelets and present as bleeding disorder. *Lymphangiomas* cause diffuse hepatomegaly, although on occasion they can form a localized mass. The mesenchymal *hamartoma* (Fig. 18) represents an interface tumor between the hemangioma and a pure mesenchymal tumor. These rare tumors contain elements of all mesenchymal cells and usually present as a huge abdominal mass. Rarely, the angiomatous component predominates and produces congestive failure much as a hemangioendothelioma (56).

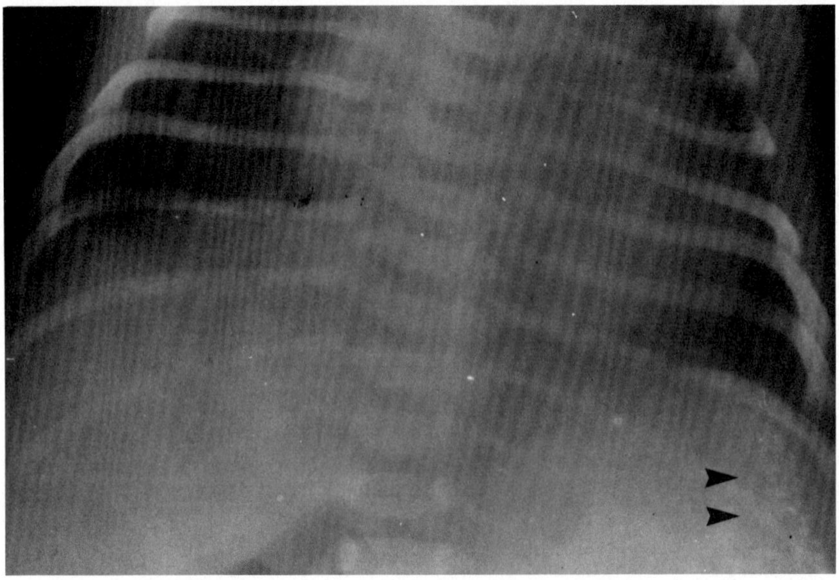

Figure 14 A newborn infant who presented in congestive heart failure. Calcifications (arrows) are seen within the left lobe of the enlarged liver on the chest radiograph. This combination of findings indicates the diagnosis of hemangioendothelioma of the liver.

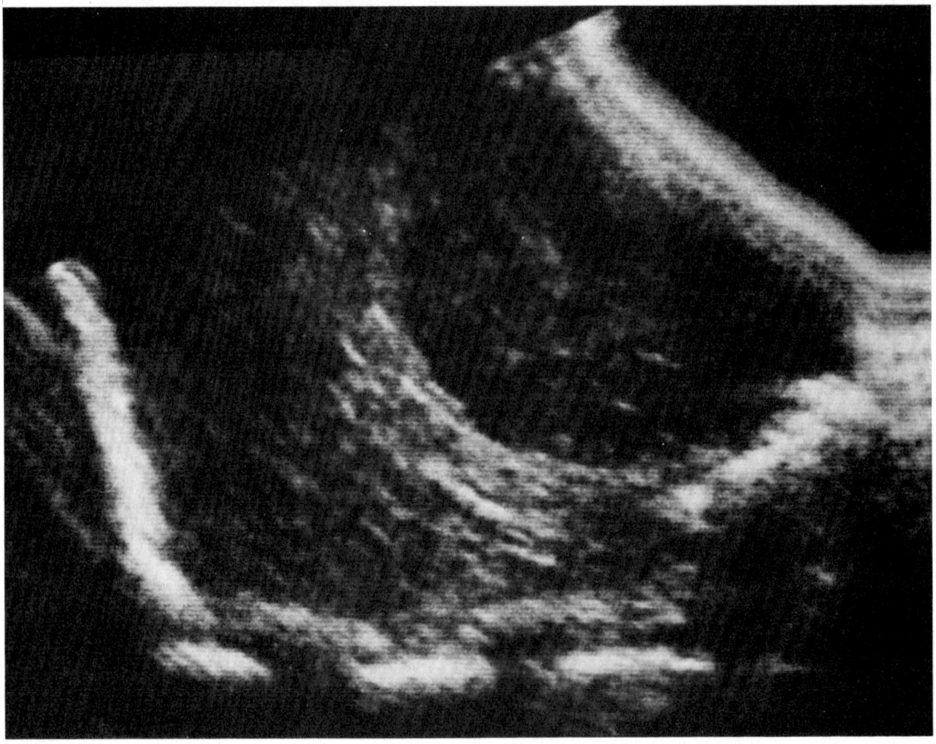

Figure 15 Hemangioendothelioma. Ultrasound of the liver demonstrates multiple irregular echoes within a generally less echogenic mass in the right lobe of the liver. Areas of cystic appearing venous lakes are present. The tumor was resected. (Courtesy of Dr. Charles Mulhern, Hospital of the University of Pennsylvania, Philadelphia.)

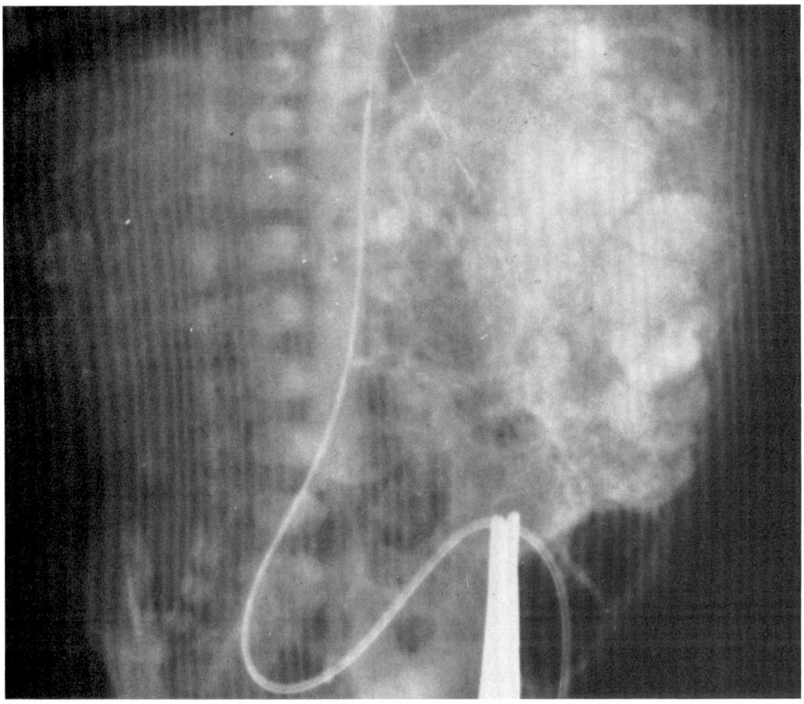

Figure 16 Hemangioendothelioma. Umbilical arteriogram demonstrating hypervascularity of the bulky tumor within the left lobe of the liver.

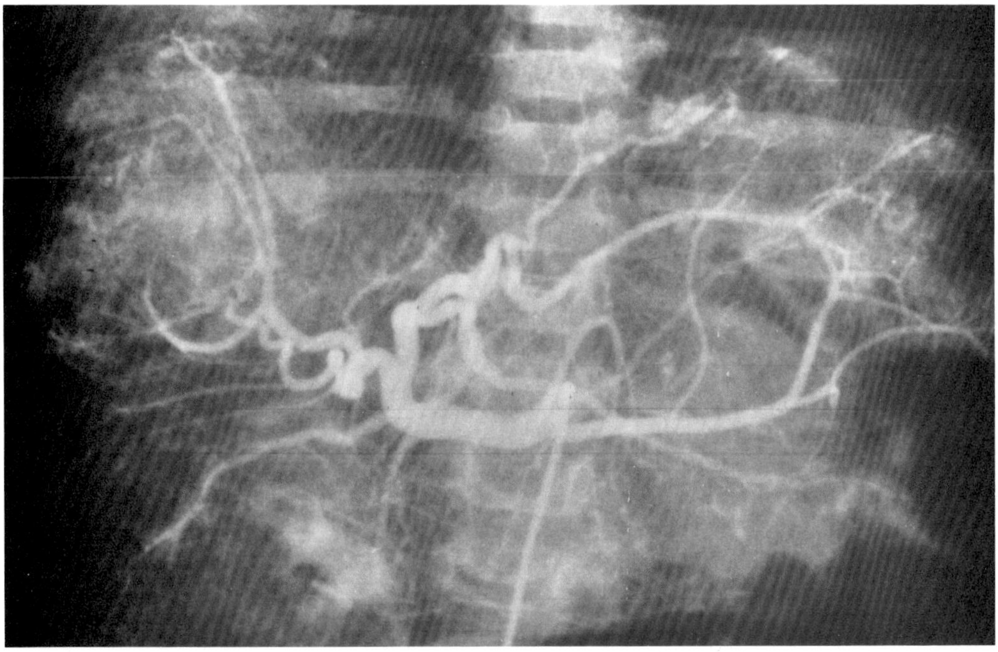

Figure 17A Cavernous hemangioma of the liver. Celiac arteriogram reveals multiple hypervascular masses in both lobes of the liver. Hepatic arteries taper normally and opacify large areas which remain opacified into the venous phase.

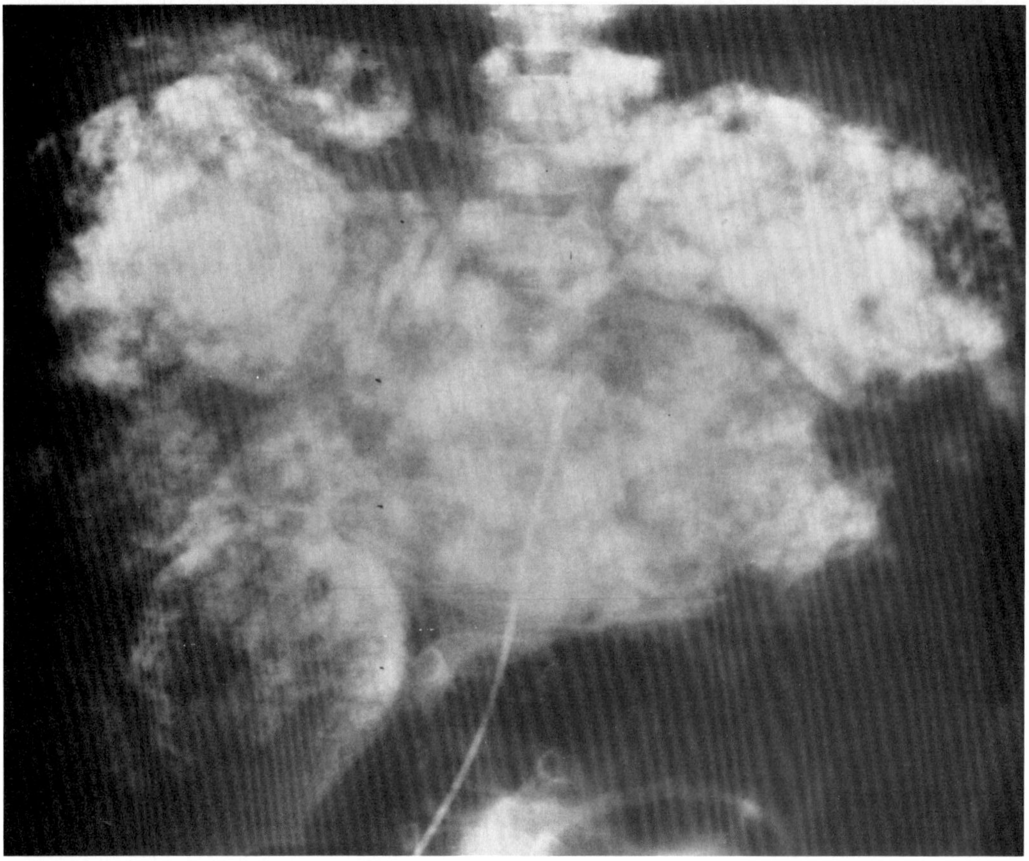

Figure 17B Intense opacification of several masses shown in the parenchymal phase.

Malignant tumors of the liver are fortunately rare. Most are epithelial in origin and have been classified on basis of their histology as *hepatocellular carcinoma* (more mature) and *hepatoblastoma* (less well differentiated). The distinction between the tumors is somewhat subjective. Hepatoblastoma tends to occur in children under the age of 3. Correlation between histological type and prognosis is not clear at the present time (57). The relationship between cirrhosis and hepatocellular carcinoma is not as definite in children as it is in adults. An association exists between childhood hepatocellular carcinoma and congenital anomalies, precocious puberty, and therapy with certain drugs, especially the anabolic steroids (58).

Abdominal radiographs often reveal only hepatomegaly, although about 20% of the tumors will have visible calcifications. The ^{99m}Tc sulfur colloid liver scan shows a cold defect (Fig. 19). Ultrasound can demonstrate diffuse distortion of the liver architecture or may show multicentricity, found in 15% of the tumors (Fig. 20). Computerized tomography is probably the definitive study to determine tumor extent (Fig. 21).

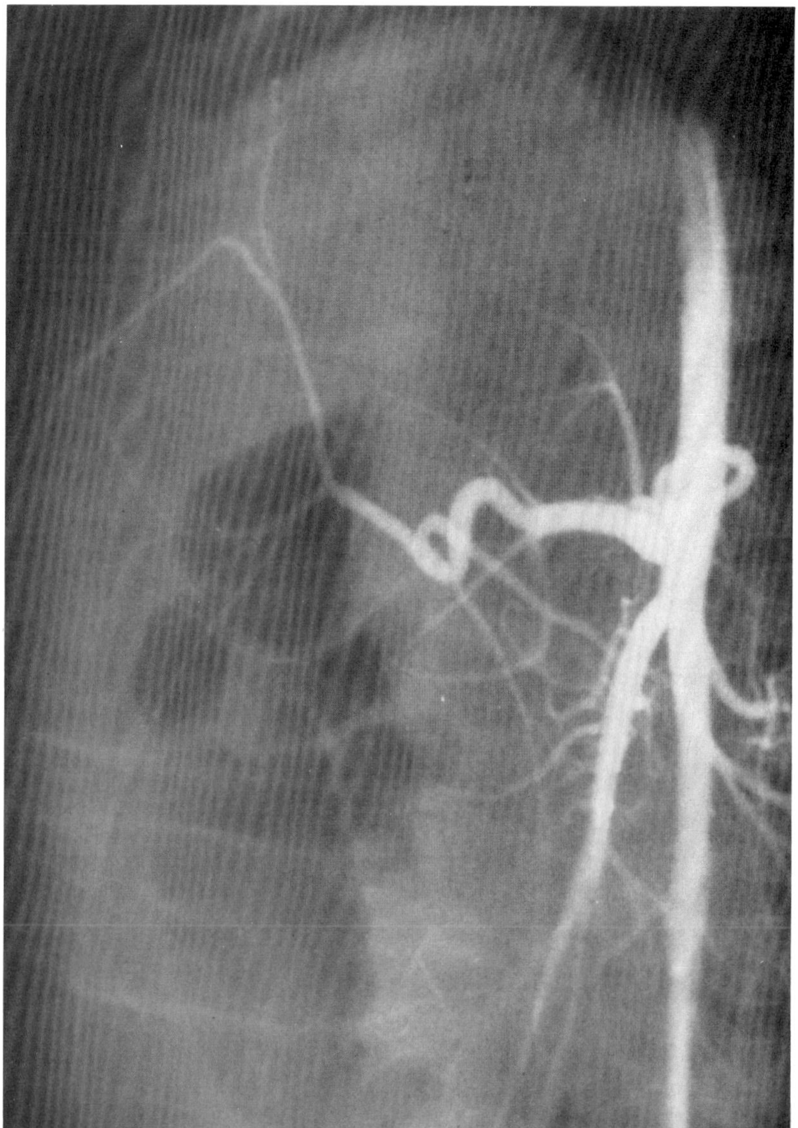

Figure 18A Cystic mesenchymal hamartoma. Aortogram. Marked displacement of branches of the hepatic artery by the multicystic tumor.

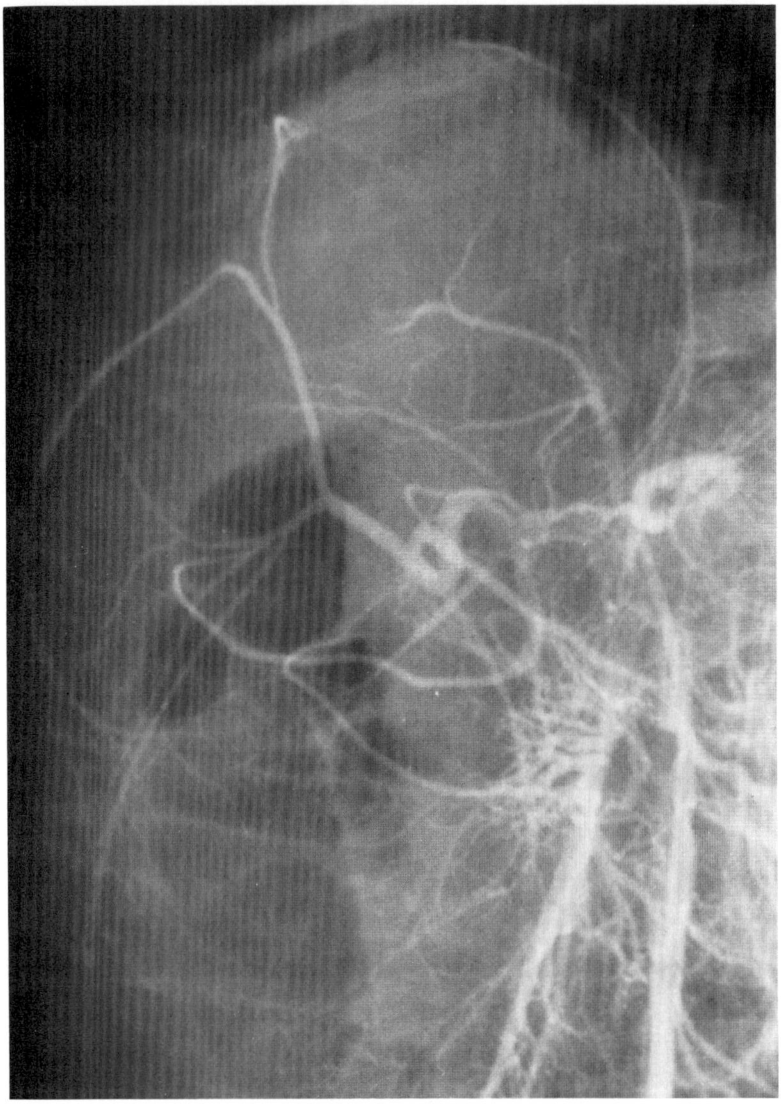

Figure 18B Late arterial phase. (Courtesy of Dr. Marie Capitano, St. Christopher's Hospital, Philadelphia.)

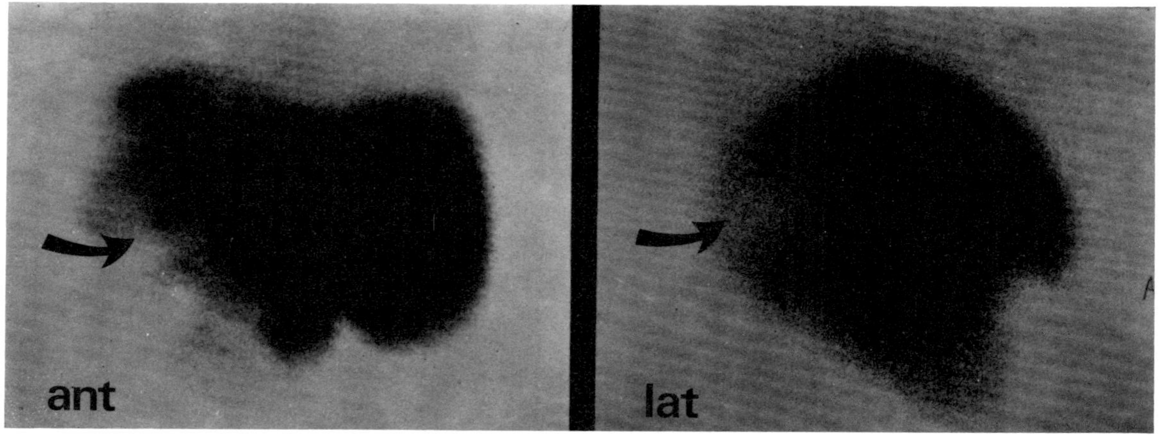

(A) (B)

Figure 19 Technetium-99m sulfur colloid scan of a patient with hepatocellular carcinoma. The tumor is multicentric and involves at least the entire right lobe of the liver. (A) Frontal view. (B) Lateral view.

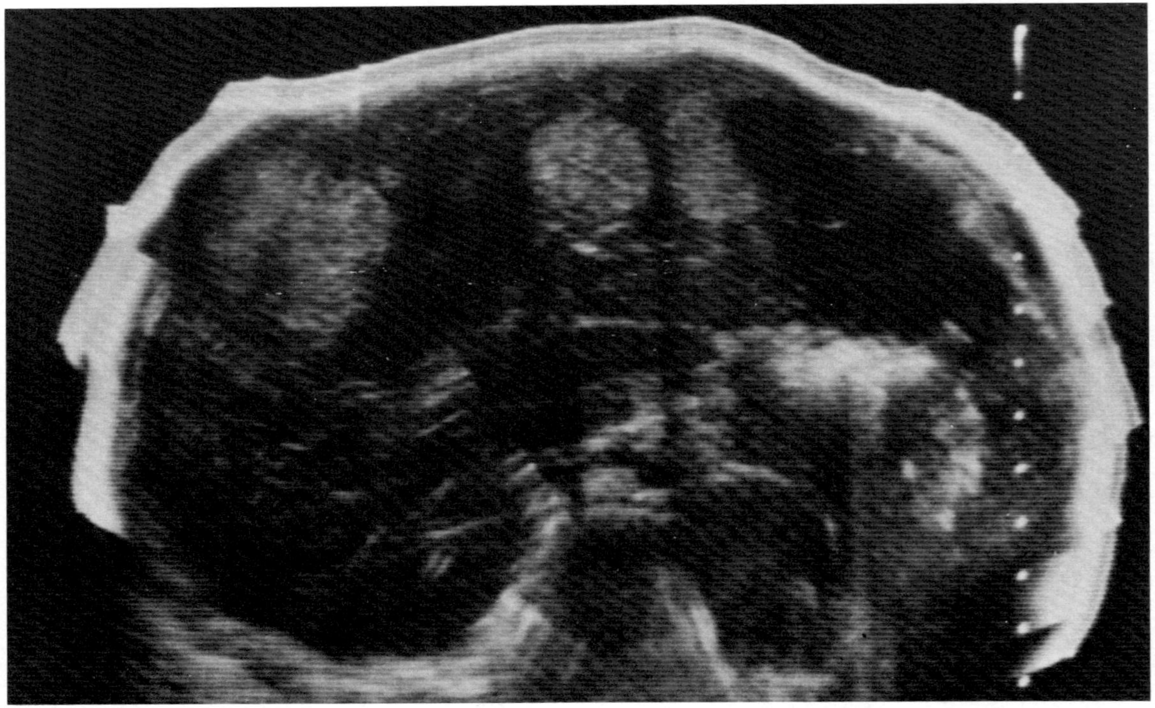

Figure 20 Ultrasound of a 2-year-old patient with hepatoblastoma. The tumor is multifocal, strongly echogenic in parts, almost transonic in others. It occupies most of the liver, sparing the posterior portion of the right lobe. (Courtesy of Dr. Charles Mulhern, Hospital of the University of Pennsylvania, Philadelphia.)

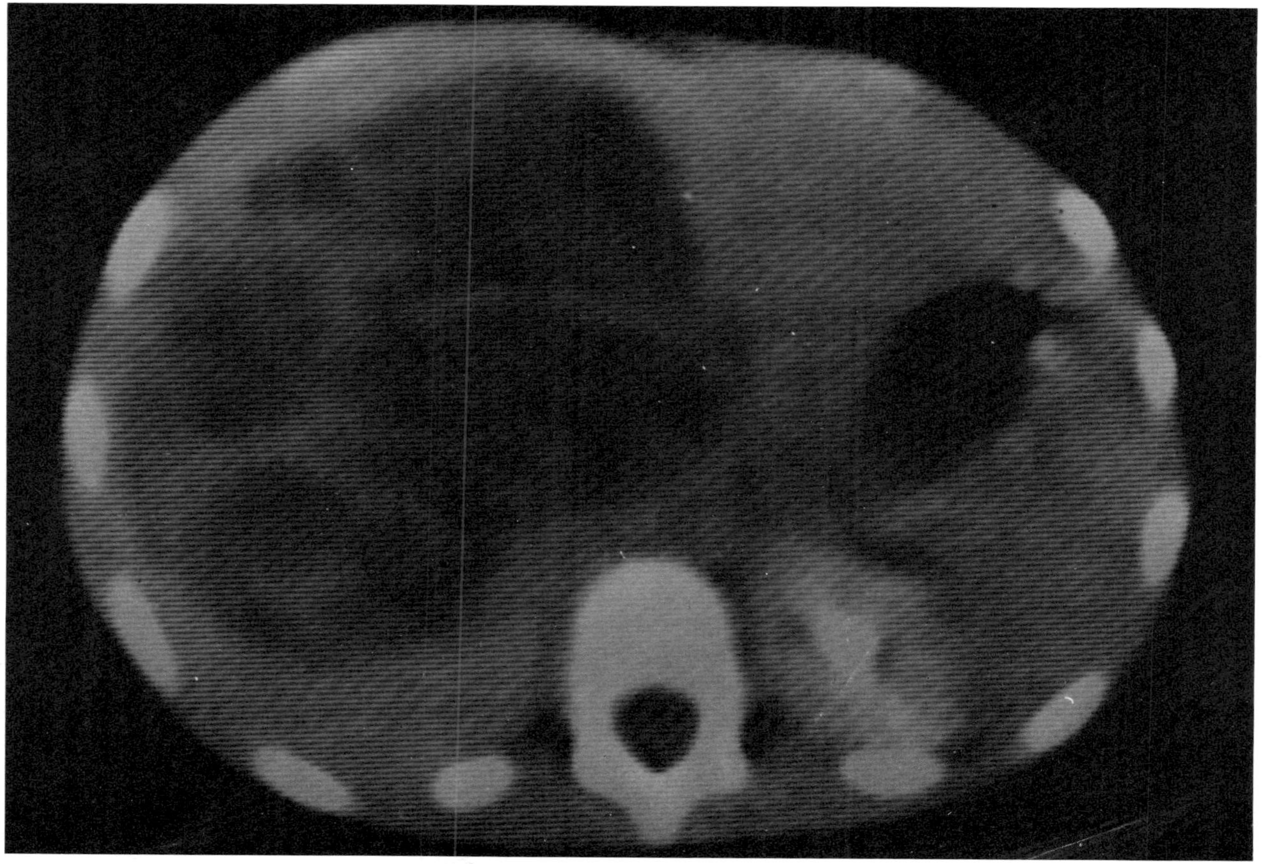

Figure 21 CT of the abdomen in a 13-year-old child with a large hepatocellular carcinoma of the liver. The CT was the definitive study for evaluating the extent of the tumor within the liver.

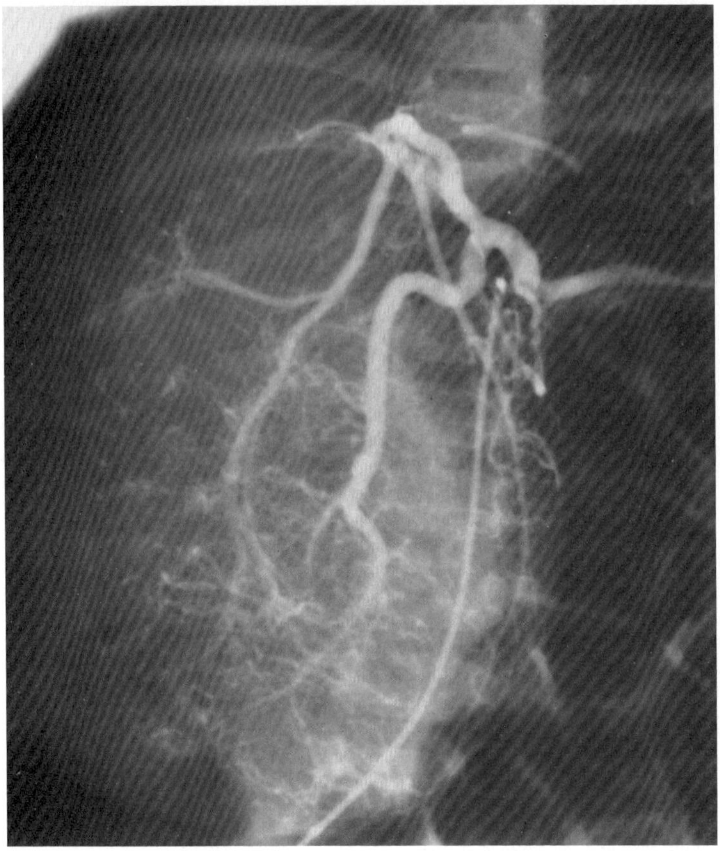

(A)

Figure 22 Hepatocellular carcinoma. (A) Celiac arteriography defines the medial aspect of the hypervascular mass. (B) Hepatogram phase, arterioportal communication, portal vein distortion (dots) by the tumor.

Angiography is invaluable in defining the vascular supply and lobar anatomy before surgical resection. The tumors are usually highly vascular (Figs. 22, 23). Venous phase films are necessary, as the tumors may cause portal vein occlusion or may extend into the portal vein (59). Since local invasion and pulmonary metastasis are the most common routes of spread, these areas should be studied closely at the time of evaluation.

Sarcomas of the liver are very rare in children and usually present as masses. Mesenchymal sarcoma, rhabdomyosarcoma, and angiosarcoma are the least rare liver sarcomas of childhood (57).

Metastases to the liver in the child are very similar to those in adults, with the exception of the stage IV-S neuroblastoma (Fig. 24). In this disease there is diffuse infiltration of the liver parenchyma by tumor cells, in addition to possible involvement of skin and bone marrow. The tumor may regress spontaneously and prognosis is good.

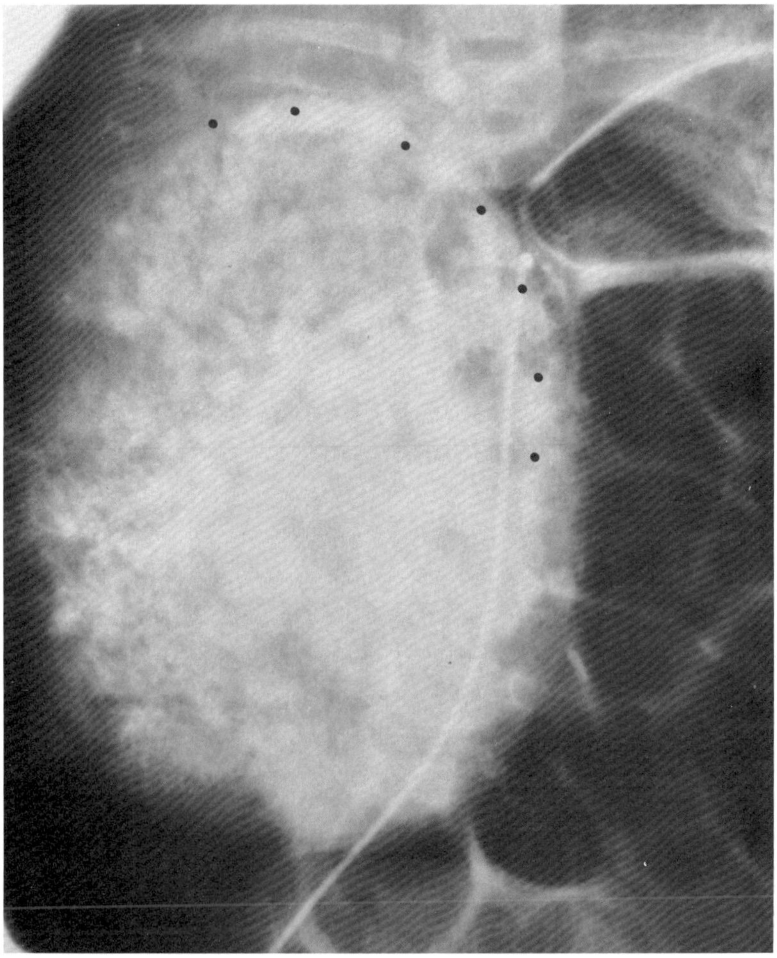

(B)

Figure 22 (continued)

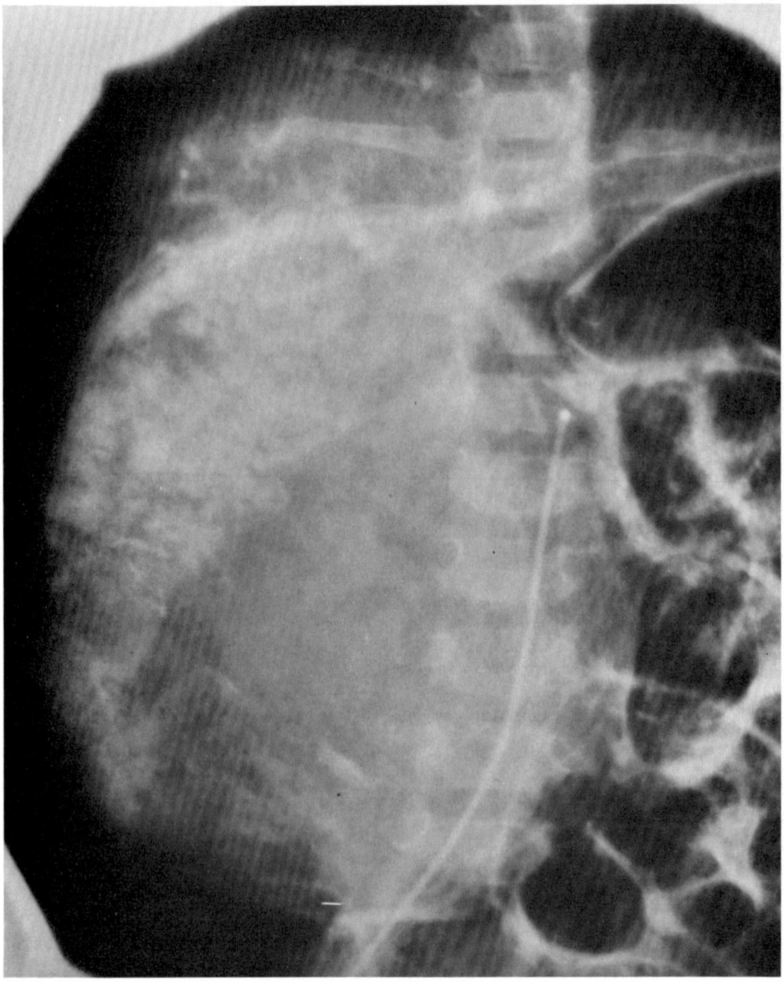

(C)

Figure 22 (continued)

(C) The lateral aspect of the mass was supplied by a right hepatic artery from the superior mesenteric. Portal venous communication. (D) The IVC is compressed by the tumor.

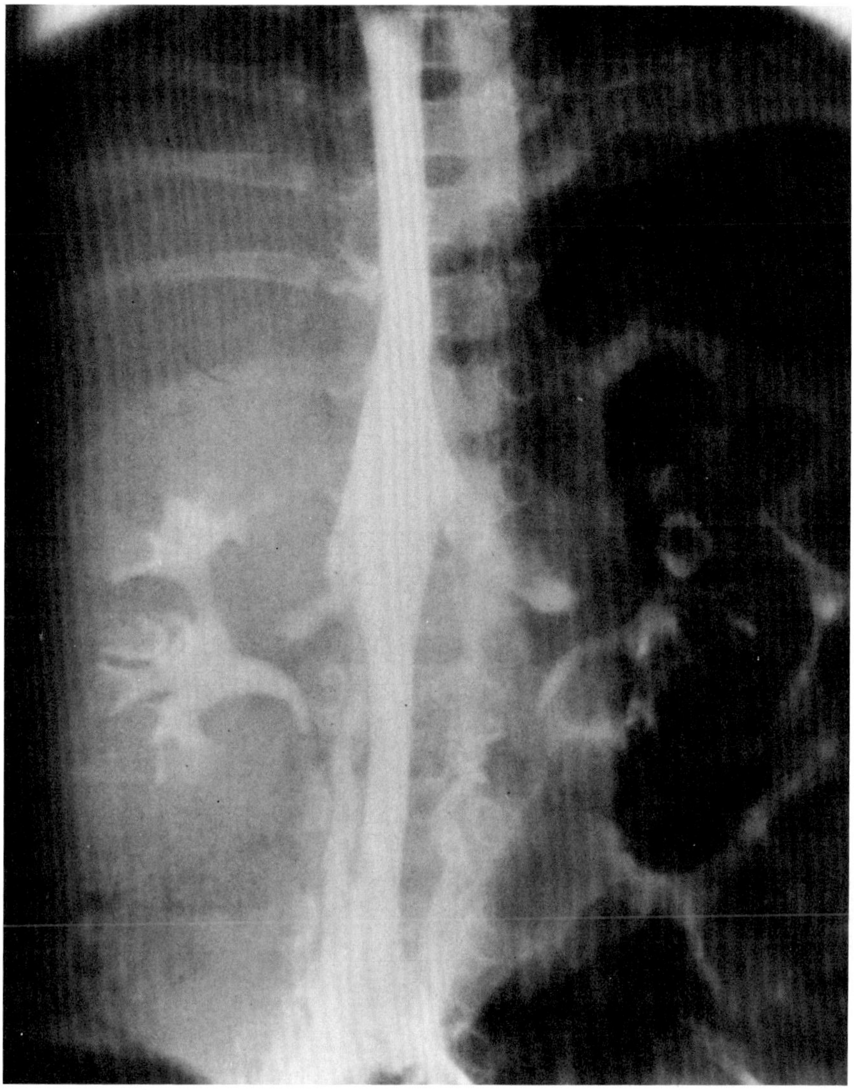

(D)

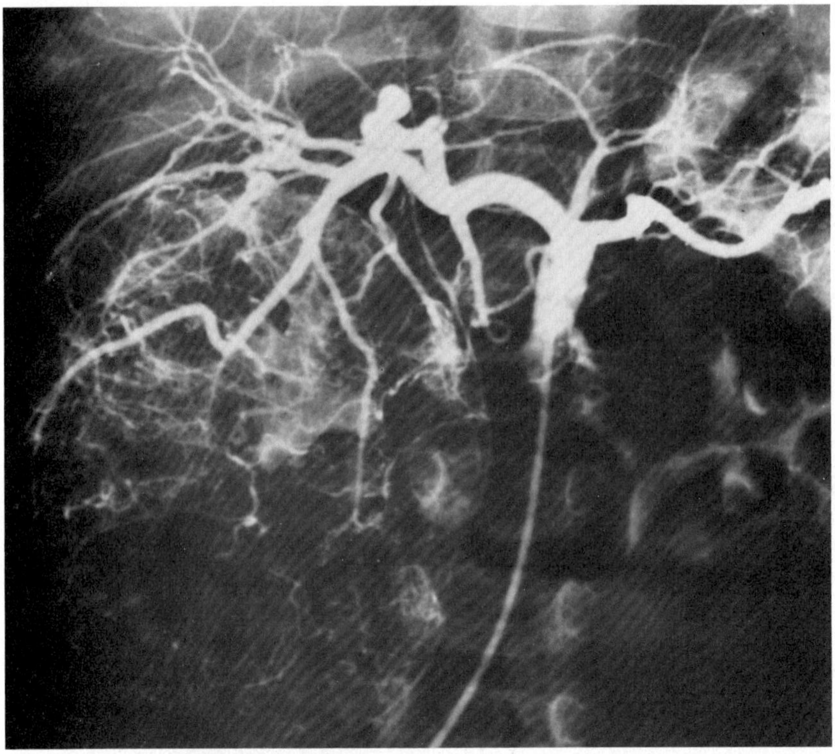

(A)

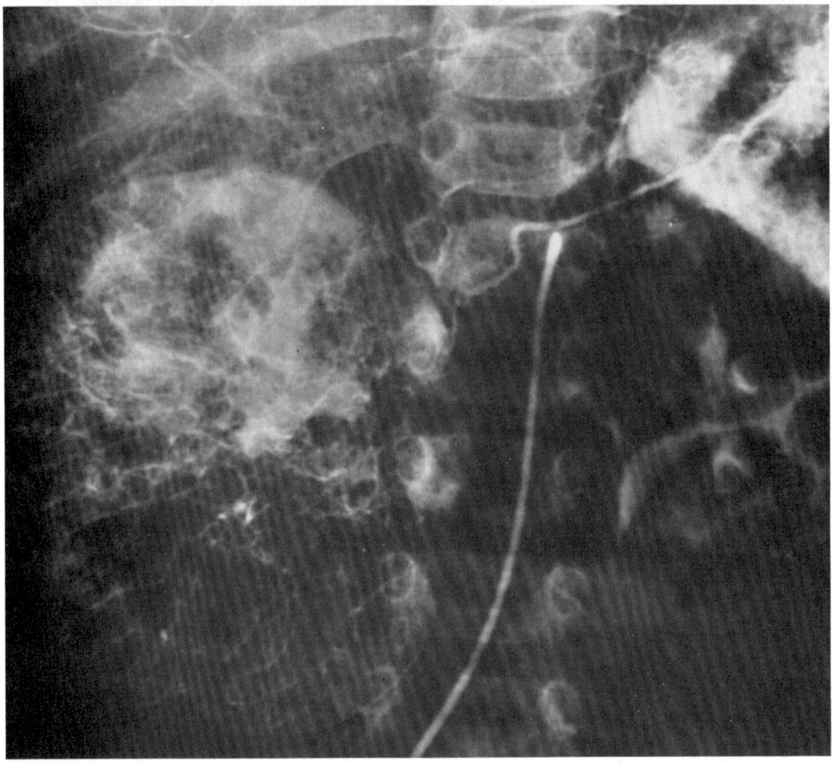

(B)

Figure 23

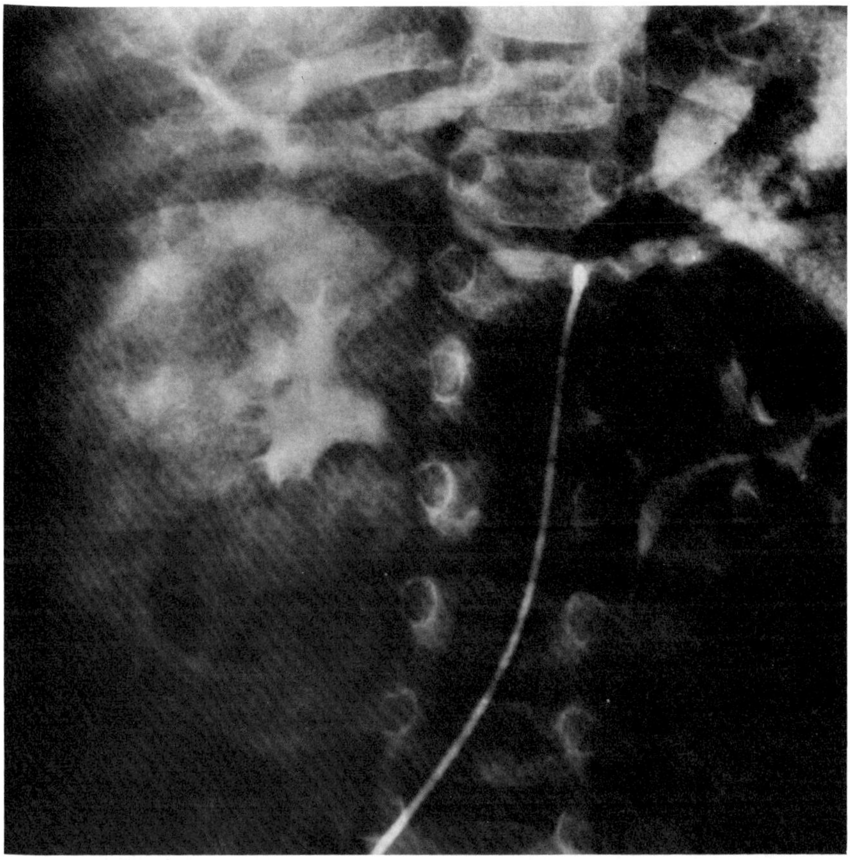

(C)

Figure 23 Hepatoblastoma in a 1-year-old child. (A) Celiac arteriography demonstrates a well-circumscribed hypervascular mass involving the inferior segments of the right lobe, extending into the medial segment of the left lobe. (B) Capillary phase. (C) Portal phase. (Courtesy of Dr. Paul Gerson, Texas Children's Hospital, Houston, Texas.)

Radiographic findings are those of hepatomegaly and a diffuse disturbance of the liver parenchyma as shown by radioisotope study or ultrasound.

Liver Abscess

Liver abscesses in children are most commonly associated with sepsis. This is in contradistinction to adults, where a liver abscess usually results from the ascent of bacteria out of an inflamed and obstructed biliary tract.

The majority of children who develop liver abscess are under 5 years old. The most common causative organism is *Staphylococcus aureus* (60). There is among these patients a high incidence of leukemia or other illnesses that alter host responsiveness. The abscesses are often multiple (61). A few infants develop a hepatic abscess after umbilical venous catheterization, presumably by direct innoculation of bacteria through the catheter tip (9).

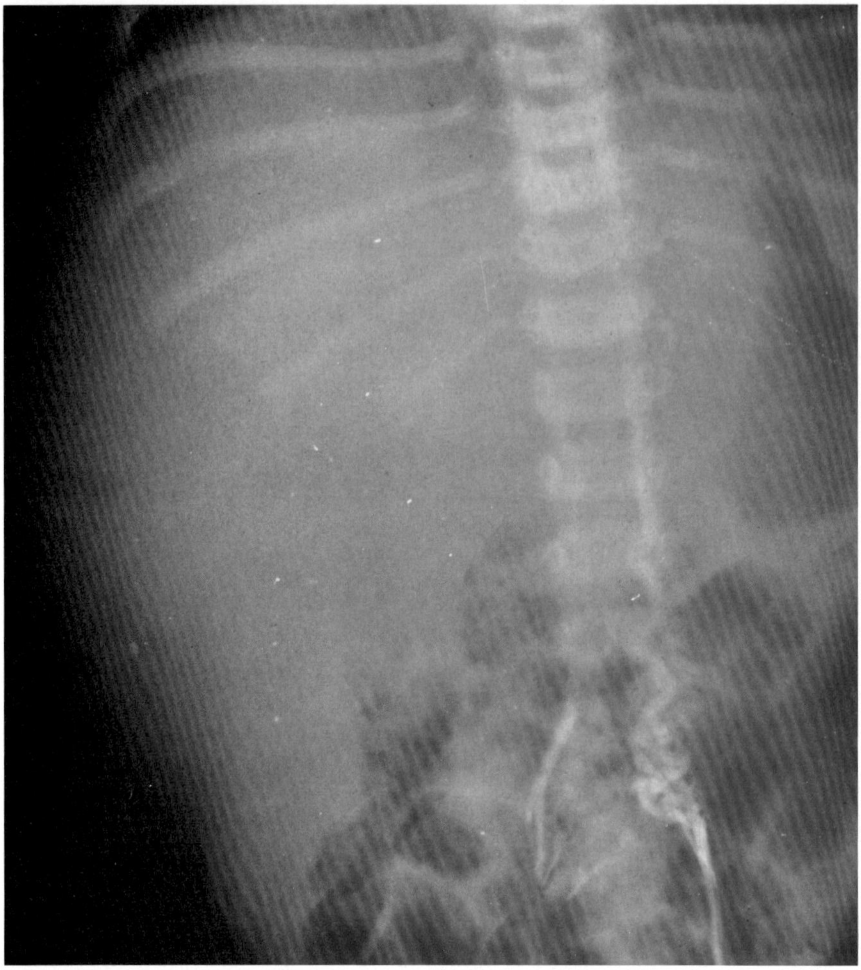

Figure 24 Abdominal radiograph of a child with hepatomegaly and cutaneous nodules. This is a classic presentation for stage IV's neuroblastoma (compressed inferior vena cava).

Radiographic evaluation is initially performed with a ^{99m}Tc sulfur colloid liver/spleen scan, although ultrasound and computerized tomography are also adequate. Uptake of the tracer by the lesion at a gallium scan suggests that an abscess exists (Fig. 25). Ultrasound and CT offer some advantage over nuclear medicine, as they can demonstrate the central center component of the abscess. Arteriography is needed only occasionally (Fig. 26). Percutaneous ultrasound or CT guided biopsy and drainage of the lesions are feasible.

Portal Hypertension

Elevated portal venous pressure produces the same deranged physiology in the child as in the adult. However, the causes, clinical and radiographic manifestations, and

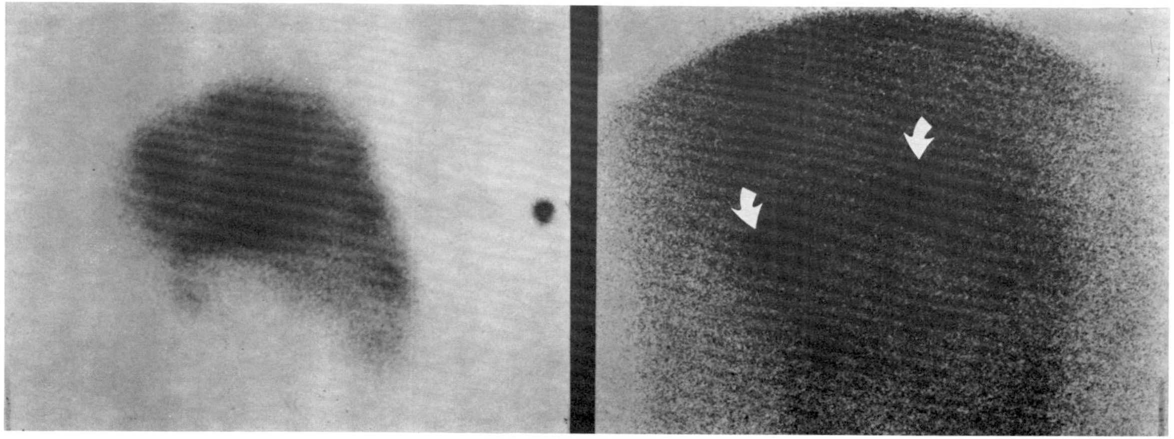

(A) (B)

Figure 25 Liver abscesses. (A) Technetium sulfur colloid scan shows several cold defects within the liver. (B) A gallium scan shows increased activity in areas previously presented as cold defects (arrows).

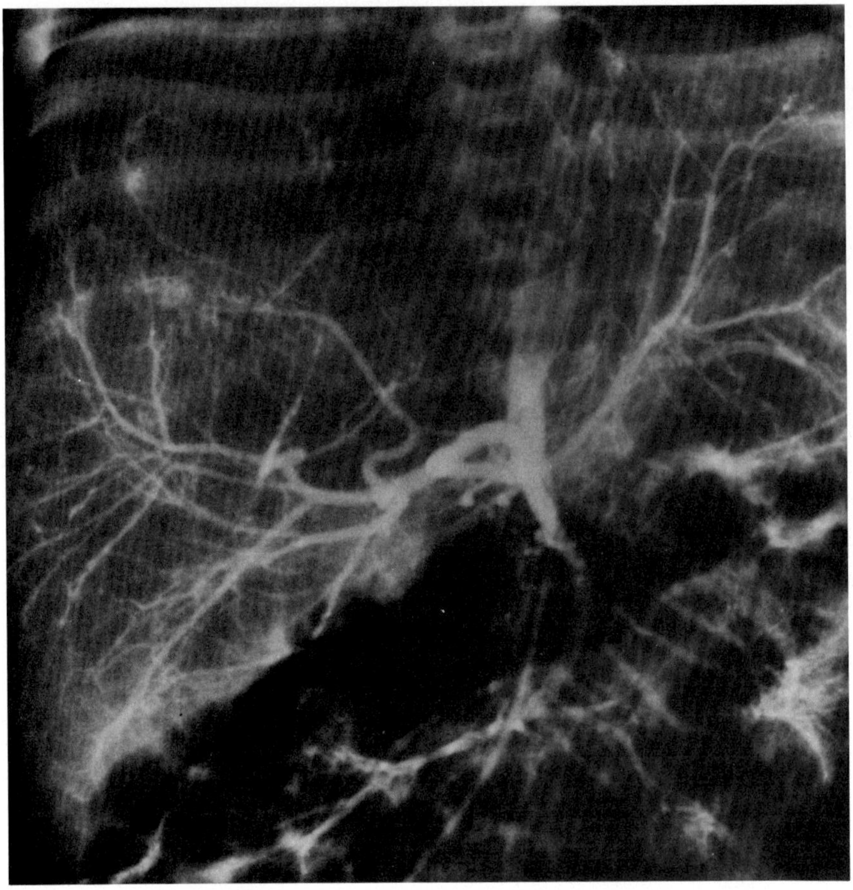

(A)

Figure 26 Bacterial abscess. (A) Huge mass in the central portion of the liver, displacing right and left hepatic arteries. Arterial phase of hepatic arteriogram.

management differ considerably in the pediatric patient. In this section we outline the peculiarities of portal hypertension in this younger age group.

The mechanics of elevated portal venous pressure are similar in all patients. In a few patients portal hypertension results from an increased flow through the portal system, usually as a result of arteriovenous fistulas in the spleen or bowel. The remaining cases have obstruction to portal vein drainage at some site: extrahepatic (portal vein or its precursors), intrahepatic, or suprahepatic (involving the hepatic veins). In pediatric practice the majority of cases are of the extrahepatic variety.

Intrahepatic Portal Hypertension

This condition is usually associated with cirrhosis; noncirrhotic causes include congenital hepatic fibrosis (see earlier) and Osler-Weber-Rendu disease. The causes of cirrhosis in children are multiple (62); a partial listing is seen in Table 3.

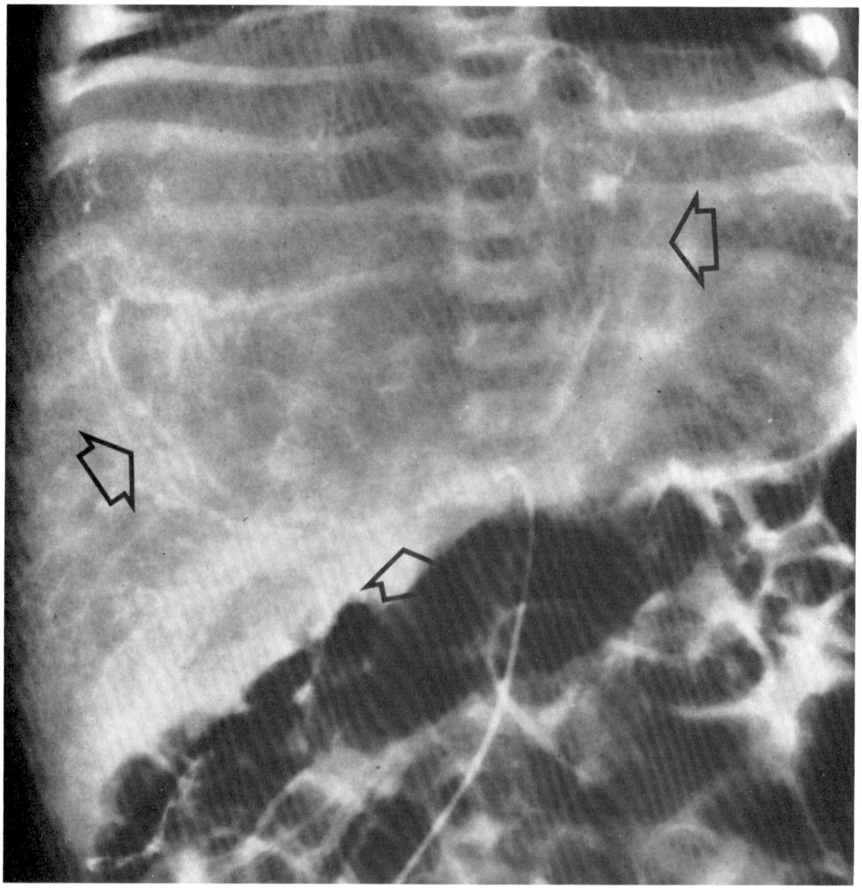

(B)

Figure 26 (continued)
(B) Hepatogram phase demonstrates the relatively hypovascular mass with increased density of the margins (arrows). (Courtesy of Dr. Joseph Rösch, University of Oregon, Portland, Oregon.)

In most children with liver disease and portal hypertension there are clinical indications of liver disease prior to the symptoms of portal hypertension. Wilson's disease and alpha$_1$ antitrypsin deficiency can be exceptions to this. Appropriate investigation and diagnosis of the type of liver disease is primarily biochemical and the province of the clinician, but occasionally there are radiologic manifestations which indicate the diagnosis (e.g., cystic fibrosis, mucopolysaccharidoses). Some children with chronic liver disease demonstrate osteopenia, perhaps related to protein deficit.

Extrahepatic Portal Hypertension

In this condition the portal vein is occluded, and multiple bridging collateral veins enter the liver hilus. "Cavernous transformation" is an appropriate descriptive term for the gross appearance. The etiology of portal venous occlusion in children is usually unclear. A few cases have been related to omphalitis at birth or indwelling umbilical venous

Table 3 Cirrhosis in Children

1. Post hepatic
   a. Post infectious hepatitis (A and B, non-AB)
   b. Neonatal hepatitis
2. Chronic active hepatitis
3. Genetic and metabolic
   a. Wilson's disease
   b. alpha$_1$-antitrypsin deficiency
   c. Histiocytosis X
   d. Hemoglobinopathies: sickle cell disease, thalassemia
   e. Other: mucopolysaccharidosis, glycogen storage disease, galactosemia, Gaucher's disease, porphyria
4. Indian, Egyptian, South African childhood cirrhosis
5. Kwashiorkor
6. Drugs, poisons, other toxins
7. Inflammatory bowel disease
8. Biliary cirrhosis
   a. Biliary atresia
   b. Choledochal cyst
   c. Cystic fibrosis
   d. Familial intrahepatic cholestasis
9. Passive venous congestion: pericarditis, congenital heart disease, Budd-Chiari syndrome

Source: Adapted from Ref. 62.

catheters (63), but in most children a precipitating event is not identified. Odievre et al. (64) report an increased incidence of congenital anomalies in patients with extrahepatic portal hypertension, suggesting that some cases are of congenital origin.

As liver function is normal with extrahepatic portal hypertension, the disease is usually clinically silent until the child develops sudden and unexpected hematemesis, most often between 3 and 5 years of age. Occasional patients will be discovered before bleeding because of asymptomatic splenomegaly. In a few patients the disease first becomes evident with the rather sudden appearance of ascites in late infancy; it is postulated that this may be the time when portal vein occlusion has taken place.

Radiology of portal hypertension Plain film studies may be abnormal in the child with portal hypertension. As collateral blood flow through the para-esophageal and mediastinal veins increases, such veins may be perceived as a posterior mediastinal mass, and the azygos vein may become visibly enlarged on the chest radiograph. Ascites is sometimes evident on abdominal films, particularly in a child with hypoproteinemia due to chronic liver disease.

Barium studies are valuable in the detection of varices. Although most often noted in the esophagus, they can occur at any point where there is communication between portal and systemic veins: distal esophagus and gastric fundus, pancreaticoduodenal area, base of mesentery, retroperitoneum, rectum, umbilicus, and at intestinal adhesions (65). Varices are most easily demonstrated in the distal esophagus. If the child is cooperative, the examination using barium suspension is similar to that of an adult. In equivocal cases, we use the method of Cockerill et al. (66), with a preliminary administration of probanthine. In the uncooperative child with suspected varices, a tube is inserted into the upper esophagus and contrast is administered under fluoroscopic control. The varices are often best visualized during the relaxation immediately following a crying episode (Fig. 27).

Although ultrasound may indicate multiple bridging collateral veins in the region of the occluded portal vein (67), a definitive diagnosis of the pathologic anatomy in portal hypertension requires angiography. Most of the new techniques for angiographic investigation are intended for the patient with intrahepatic disease; therefore, they are less applicable for the child. Our current policy for diagnostic evaluation is to use arterioportography with selective contrast injection into the celiac and superior mesenteric arteries to produce subsequent venous opacification. If approximately 1 cc/kg of contrast

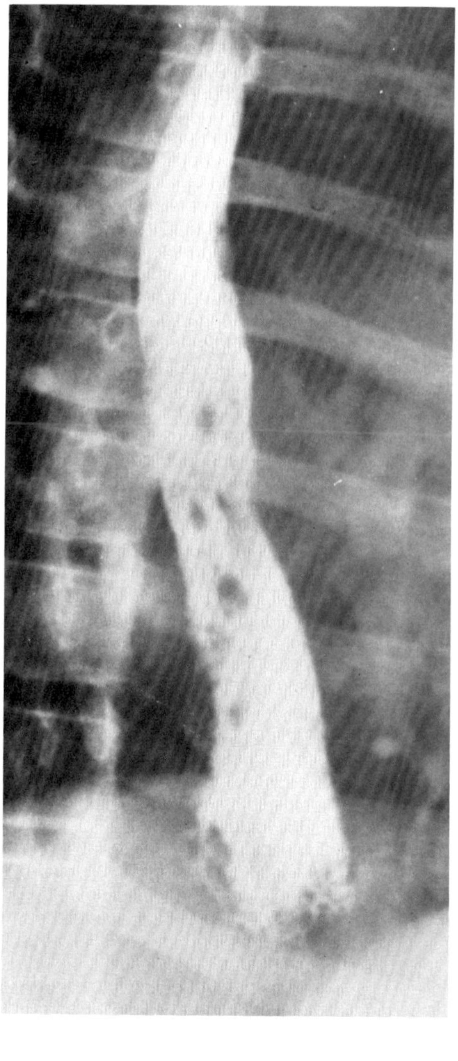

Figure 27 Esophageal varices in a 6-year-old child.

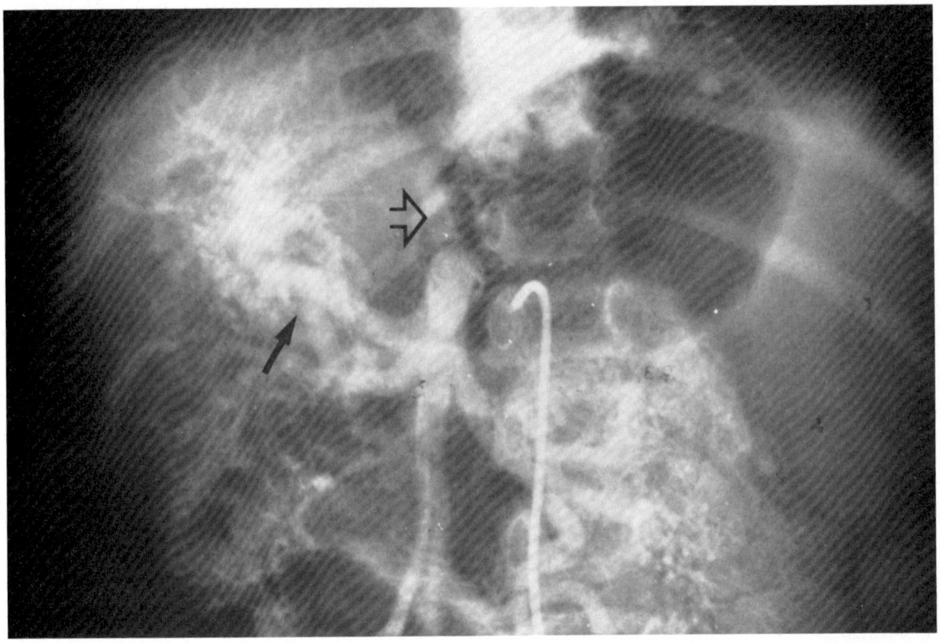

Figure 28 Portal venous phase after superior mesenteric artery injection shows a coronary vein opacifying esophageal varices (open arrow). A typical racemose pattern of venous collaterals (arrow) represent cavernous transformation of the portal vein.

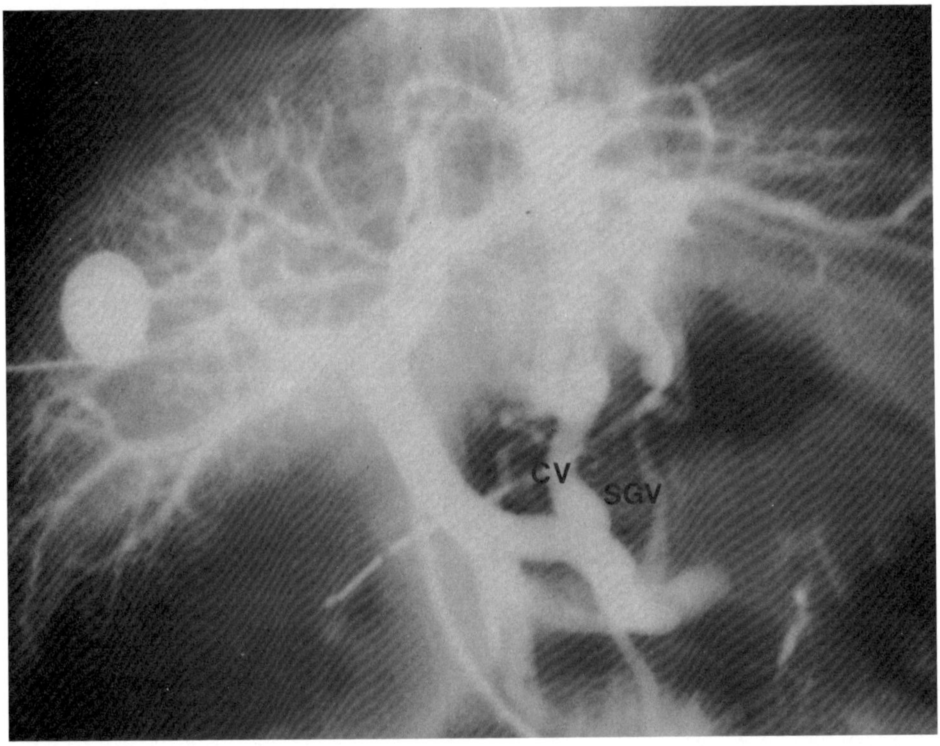

Figure 29 Umbilical venogram in a child with intrahepatic portal hypertension due to cirrhosis. A coronary vein (CV) and short gastric vein (SGV) carry hepatofugal flow. The portal vein is patent.

is used, visualization of the portal abnormality is generally sufficient for diagnosis (Fig. 28).

When surgery is indicated, some centers still perform a percutaneous splenoportogram, to measure splenic pulp pressure and obtain an improved visualization of the splenic and portal vein as well as collateral vessels (68). As there is a small but definite risk of splenic hemorrhage, we customarily defer the examination until the day of surgery. Characteristic examples of the radiographic anatomy in intrahepatic and extrahepatic portal hypertension are shown in Figures 28 and 29.

A variety of surgical procedures are performed in children with portal hypertension (69). The indications and techniques for their use are beyond the scope of this discussion. The child bleeding due to extrahepatic portal hypertension has a better prognosis than the adult with bleeding varices, because liver function is normal.

References

1. Arey LB: *Developmental Anatomy*. W. B. Saunders, Philadelphia, 1974, p 255.
2. Popper H and Schaffner F: *Liver, Structure and Function*. McGraw-Hill, New York, 1957, p 167.
3. Bremer JL: *Congenital Anomalies of the Viscera: Their Embryological Basis*. Harvard University Press, Cambridge, Mass, 1957, pp 73–75.
4. Leorente J and Dardick H: Symptomatic accessory lobe of the liver associated with absence of the left lobe. *Arch Surg 102*:221–223, 1971.
5. Morgenstein L and Mozer M: Hypoplasia of the right hepatic lobe. *Am J Surg 98*:629, 1959.
6. Pujari BD and Deodhare SG: Symptomatic accessory lobe of the liver. *Postgrad Med J 52*:234, 1976.
7. Johnson GF: Congenital preduodenal portal vein. *Am J Roentgenol 112*:93, 1971.
8. Taber P, Lackey DA, Mikity V: Roentgenographic findings of complications with neonatal umbilical vascular catheterization. *Am J Roentgenol 118*:49, 1973.
9. Brans YW, Deballos R, Cassady G: Umbilical catheters and hepatic abscesses. *Pediatrics 53*:264, 1974.
10. Johns AW, Kitchen WH, Leslie DW: Complication of umbilical vessel catheters. *Med J Aust 2*:810, 1972.
11. McNulty JG: *Radiology of the Liver*. W. B. Saunders, Philadelphia, 1977.
12. Mills SR, Doppman JL, Nienhuis AW: Computed tomography in the diagnosis of disorders of excessive iron storage of the liver. *J Compt Assist Tomogr 1*:101, 1977.
13. Griscom NT, Capitanio MA, Wagoner ML, Culham G, Morris L: The visible fatty liver. *Radiology 117*:385, 1975.
14. Yousefzadeh DK, Lupetin AR, Jackson JH Jr: The radiographic signs of fatty liver. *Radiology 131*:351, 1979.
15. Martin DJ, Griscom NT, Neuhauser EBD: A further look at the total body opacification effect. *Br J Radiol 45*:185, 1972.
16. Webster EW, Alper NM, Brownell GL: Radiation doses in pediatric nuclear medicine and diagnostic x-ray procedures. In *Pediatric Nuclear Medicine*, James AE, Wagner HN, Cooke RF (Eds). W. B. Saunders, Philadelphia, 1974, pp 34–58.
17. Haaga J and Reich NE: *Computed Tomography of Abdominal Abnormalities*. C. V. Mosby, St. Louis, 1978.
18. Goldberg BB and Pollack HM: Aspiration—biopsy techniques. In *Abdominal Gray Scale Ultrasonography*, Goldberg BB (Ed). Wiley, New York, 1977, pp 341–363.
19. Alfidi RJ, MacIntyre WJ, Haaga JR: The effects of biological motion on CT resolution. *Am J Roentgenol 127*:11, 1976.

20. Stanley RJ, Sagel SS, Levitt RG: Computed tomography of the liver. *Radiol Clin North Am 15*:331, 1977.
21. Gutierrez OH and Rosch J: Limitations of angiographic differential diagnosis in major hepatic processes. *Fortschr Roentgenstr 127*:1, 1977.
22. Hurwitz RA, Franken EA Jr, Girod DA, Smith JA, Smith WL: Angiographic determination of arterial patency after percutaneous catheterization in infants and small children. *Circulation 56*:102, 1977.
23. Franken EA Jr, Smith WL, Smith JA, Fitzgerald JF: Percutaneous cholangiography in infants. *Am J Roentgenol 130*:1057, 1978.
24. Poley R: Differential diagnosis of persistent cholestatic jaundice in infancy. *South Med J 70*:91, 1977.
25. Howard ER and Mowat AP: Extrahepatic biliary atresia. Recent developments in management. *Arch Dis Child 52*:825, 1977.
26. Poley JR, Smith EI, Boon DJ, Bhatia M, Smith CW, Thompson JB: Lipoprotein-X and the double ^{131}-I-Rose Bengal test in the diagnosis of prolonged infantile jaundice. *J Pediatr Surg 7*:660, 1972.
27. Arima E, Kikuchi J, Sakoguchi Y, Akita K: Surgically correctable biliary atresia. A follow-up study. *Acta Med Univ Kagoshima 18*:39, 1976.
28. Bill AH, Brennom WS, Huseby TL: Biliary atresia. New concepts of pathology, diagnosis and management. *Arch Surg 109*:367, 1974.
29. Mowat AP, Psacharopoulos HL, Williams R: Extrahepatic biliary atresia versus neonatal hepatitis. Review of 137 prospectively investigated infants. *Arch Dis Child 51*:763, 1976.
30. Majd M, Reba RC, Altman RP: Hepatobiliary scintigraphy with ^{99m}Tc-PIPIDA in the evaluation of neonatal jaundice. *Pediatrics 67*:140, 1981.
31. Rosenthall L: Differentiation of intrahepatic disease and extrahepatic biliary atresia in infants. In *The Applications of Radioiodinated Rose Bengal and Colloid Radiogold in the Detection of Hepatobiliary Disease*, Rosenthall L (Ed). Warren H. Green, St. Louis, 1969, pp 79–86.
32. Gellis SS: Biliary atresia. *Pediatrics 55*:8, 1975.
33. Kulkarni PB and Beatty EC Jr: Cholangiocarcinoma associated with biliary cirrhosis due to congenital biliary atresia. *Am J Dis Child 131*:442, 1977.
34. Barlow B, Tabor E, Blanc WA, Santulli TV, Harris RC: Choledochal cyst: a review of 19 cases. *J Pediatr 89*:934, 1976.
35. Wechsler RL and Van Thiel D: Fibropolycystic disease of the hepatobiliary system and kidneys. *Am J Dig Dis 21*:1058, 1979.
36. Babbitt DP, Starshak RJ, Clenett AR: Choledochal cyst; a concept of etiology. *Am J Roentgenol 119*:57, 1973.
37. Alonso-Lej F, Rever WB Jr, Pessagno DJ: Congenital choledochal cyst with a report of 2 and an analysis of 94 cases. *Surg Gynecol Obstet (Int Abstr Surg) 108*:1, 1959.
38. Jacobs RP and Palubinskas AJ: Angiographic findings of cholecohal cyst. *Br J Radiol 48*:51, 1975.
39. Kobayashi A and Ohbe Y: Choledochal cyst in infancy and childhood. Analysis of 16 cases. *Arch Dis Child 52*:121, 1977.
40. Bloustein PA: Association of carcinoma with congenital cystic conditions of the liver and bile ducts. *Am J Gastroenterol 67*:40, 1977.
41. Kerr DNA, Harrison CV, Sherlock S, Walker RM: Congenital hepatic fibrosis. *Q J Med 30*:91, 1961.
42. Hodgson HJF, Davies DR, Thompson RPH: Congenital hepatic fibrosis. *J Clin Pathol 29*:11, 1976.
43. Adams CM, Danks DM, Campbell PE: Comments upon the classification of infantile polycystic diseases of the liver and kidney, based upon three-dimensional reconstruction of the liver. *J Med Genet 11*:234, 1974.

44. Rosenfield AT, Siegel NJ, Kappelman NB, Taylor KJW: Gray scale ultrasonography in medullary cystic disease of the kidney and congenital hepatic fibrosis with tubular ectasia: new observations. *Am J Roentgenol 129*:297, 1977.
45. Unite I, Maitem A, Bagnasco FM, Irwin GAL: Congenital hepatic fibrosis associated with renal tubular ectasia. *Radiology 109*:565, 1973.
46. Grossman H and Seed W: Congenital hepatic fibrosis, bile duct dilatation, and renal lesion resembling medullary sponge kidney. *Radiology 87*:46, 1966.
47. Odievre M, Chaumont P, Montagne J: Anomalies of the intrahepatic portal venous system in congenital hepatic fibrosis. *Radiology 122*:427, 1977.
48. Spiegel RM, King DL, Green WM: Ultrasonography of primary cysts of the liver. *Am J Roentgenol 131*:235, 1978.
49. Szuchmacher PH and Wilk P: Cystic diseases of the liver. *Mt Sinai J Med 43*:68, 1976.
50. Blyth H and Ockenden B: Polycystic disease of kidneys and liver presenting in childhood. *J Med Genet 8*:257, 1971.
51. Six R, Oliphant M, Grossman H: A spectrum of renal tubular ectasia and hepatic fibrosis. *Radiology 117*:117, 1975.
52. McLoughlin MJ, Mishkin M, Thompson CP: Congenital cystic disease of the liver; isotope scanning, ultrasonography and angiography. *J Can Assoc Radiol 28*:243, 1977.
53. McLoughlin MJ, Colapinto RF, Gilday DL, et al: Focal nodular hyperplasia of the liver. *Radiology 107*:257, 1973.
54. Rocchini AP, Rosenthal A, Issenberg HJ, Nadas AS: Hepatic hemangioendothelioma: hemodynamic observations and treatment. *Pediatrics 57*:131, 1976.
55. McLean RH, Moller JH, Warwick WJ, Satran L, Lucas RV Jr: Multinodular hemangiomatosis of the liver in infancy. *Pediatrics 49*:563, 1972.
56. Smith WL, Ballantine TVN, Gonzalez-Crussi F: Hepatic mesenchymal hamartoma causing heart failure in the neonate. *J Pediatr Surg 13*:183, 1978.
57. Exelby PR, Filler RM, Grosfeld JL: Liver tumors in children in the particular reference to hepatoblastoma and hepatocellular carcinoma: American Academy of Pediatrics Surgical Section Survey. *J Pediatr Surg 10*:329, 1975.
58. Fraumeni JF, Miller RW, Hill JA: Primary carcinoma of the liver in childhood: an epidemiologic study. *J Natl Cancer Inst 40*:1087, 1968.
59. Brunelle F, Garel L, Harry G, Chaumont P: Portal angiography in hepatic tumors in children. *Ann Radiol 22*:142, 1979.
60. Chusid MJ: Pyogenic hepatic abscess in infancy and childhood. *Pediatrics 62*:554, 1978.
61. Dehner LP and Kissane JM: Pyogenic hepatic abscess in infancy and childhood. *J Pediatr 74*:763, 1969.
62. Roy CC, Silverman A, Cozzetto FJ: *Pediatric Clinical Gastroenterology*, 2nd ed. C. V. Mosby, St. Louis, 1975.
63. Junker P, Egeblad M, Nielson O, Kamper J: Umbilical vein catheterization and portal hypertension. *Acta Paediatr Scand 65*:499, 1976.
64. Odievre M, Pige G, Alagille D: Congenital abnormalities associated with extrahepatic portal hypertension. *Arch Dis Child 52*:383, 1977.
65. Franken EA Jr: *Gastrointestinal Radiology in Pediatrics*. Harper & Row, New York, 1975.
66. Cockerill EM, Miller RE, Chernish SM, McLaughlin SC, Rodda BE: Optimal visualization of esophageal varices. *Am J Roentgenol 126*:512, 1976.
67. Weill FS: *Ultrasonography of Digestive Diseases*. C. V. Mosby, St. Louis, 1978.
68. Kogutt MS and Jander HP: Splenoportography—a valuable diagnostic technic, revisited. *South Med J 70*:1210, 1977.
69. Hermann RE: Shunt operations for portal hypertension. *Surg Clin North Am 55*:1073, 1975.

31

Liver Disease in the Tropics

W. Peter Cockshott
McMaster University
Hamilton, Ontario, Canada

Liver enlargement occurs in several tropical disorders. Often there are no specific radiographic features, as in *Leishmania* and *Histoplasma dubosii* infiltrations, or in the congestive changes of malaria and tropical splenomegaly syndromes, where radiology merely documents the hepatic enlargement as such. By contrast, there are a number of specific entities which lead to focal alterations of the liver parenchymal structures, perhaps affecting vascular or biliary pathways, so that imaging studies may provide more useful diagnostic and management information. This chapter considers the appearances that may be seen in certain specific parasitisms, infections, and clinical syndromes that manifest themselves predominantly in tropical communities.

It should be emphasized that although radiology can provide helpful information, the specific diagnosis often depends on laboratory parasitic, immunologic, cultural, or biopsy studies, as the radiological features are not pathognomic. In many parts of the tropics, radiologic facilities are not highly developed. Consequently, the full value of x-ray and other imaging modalities has not yet been fully exploited, so that much remains unknown in some of the clinical entities to be described.

Biliary Tract Infections

In certain tropical areas parasitic diseases assume importance as a factor causing obstructive jaundice and cholangitis. Parasites may normally pass a stage of their life cycle in the biliary passages, as in clonorchiasis, opisthorchiasis, and fascioliasis; or the biliary tree may be an ectopic parasitic location, as with ascariasis. Biliary parasites are well recognized in animals varying from small liver flukes in sheep to larger Cestodes such as *Stilesia* of sheep and the enormous 21-m-long *Multiductus physeteris* of sperm whales (1). In humans biliary parasites may cause few symptoms but can also be responsible for acute episodes and chronic ill health. Some chronic parasitic infections may predispose to cholangitic carcinoma.

Ascariasis

Ascariasis is the most frequent parasitism of the alimentary tract, with hundreds of millions of people affected. Its transmission is associated with poor sanitary facilities or habits, so that it is more common in children and in the rural areas of the humid tropics. Ova are excreted in the stool of humans and contaminate soil. Given suitable environmental circumstances a rhabtidiform larva develops within the chitinous envelope of a fertile egg. If a human swallows the egg with contaminated food or objects, the larva is released to enter the portal system or gut lymphatics and thence reaches the capillary bed of the lung, where further maturation molts occur. These may excite eosinophilic reaction and at times transient alveolar infiltrates. Ultimately, the parasite ascends the trachea and passes down the esophagus to reach the small bowel, where sexual maturity is attained.

Adult worms reside in the jejunum with a life span of about 1 year. The males are about 20 cm long by 3 mm, whereas females are larger, 30 cm by 4–6 mm wide. Worms keep their head directed against the peristaltic stream and maintain station or advance by active propulsive movements which intensify when they meet an obstruction (2). It is because of this habit that they can migrate through the sphincter of Oddi and enter the biliary passages. Initially, there may be one or more worms with the head through the papilla and part of the body in the duodenum. This forceful dilatation of the sphincter causes severe pain. A single worm is present in over 80% of clinical cases (3), but up to 48 have been recorded. Worms may pass beyond the common duct to lie in the gallbladder, cystic, or hepatic ducts. A single worm does not usually obstruct the duct, although multiple parasites can do so. Unfortunately, the passage of a bacterially contaminated intestinal parasite can lead to cholangitis. Often, the ascaris spontaneously returns to the bowel. When a female deposits ova in the biliary tract or the parasite dies, a marked reaction occurs within the liver to the foreign tissue, which can result in suppurative cholangitis and liver and subhepatic abscess formation. Parasitic biliary disease is not rare, with large series being reported from the Far East and Africa [600 cases in the series of Schmauss and Tung (4)].

Plain film signs can be suggestive. The entry of the worm through the papilla may allow gas into the biliary tree. If there is a heavy worm load, parasites may be seen outlined by gas in the small bowel. Visualization of the tail of worms protruding from the papilla into the barium-filled duodenum has been described (5). Sometimes, if the sphincter is incompetent, barium can reflux into the common duct and reveal an ascaris there.

More specific information on biliary ascariasis is provided by intravenous cholangiography, which usually demonstrates a linear filling defect within the opacified duct. Tomography (6) is of particular assistance in this regard (Figs. 1–3B). Conservative management is usual, but if a repeat study in 10 days or so shows a persistent worm,

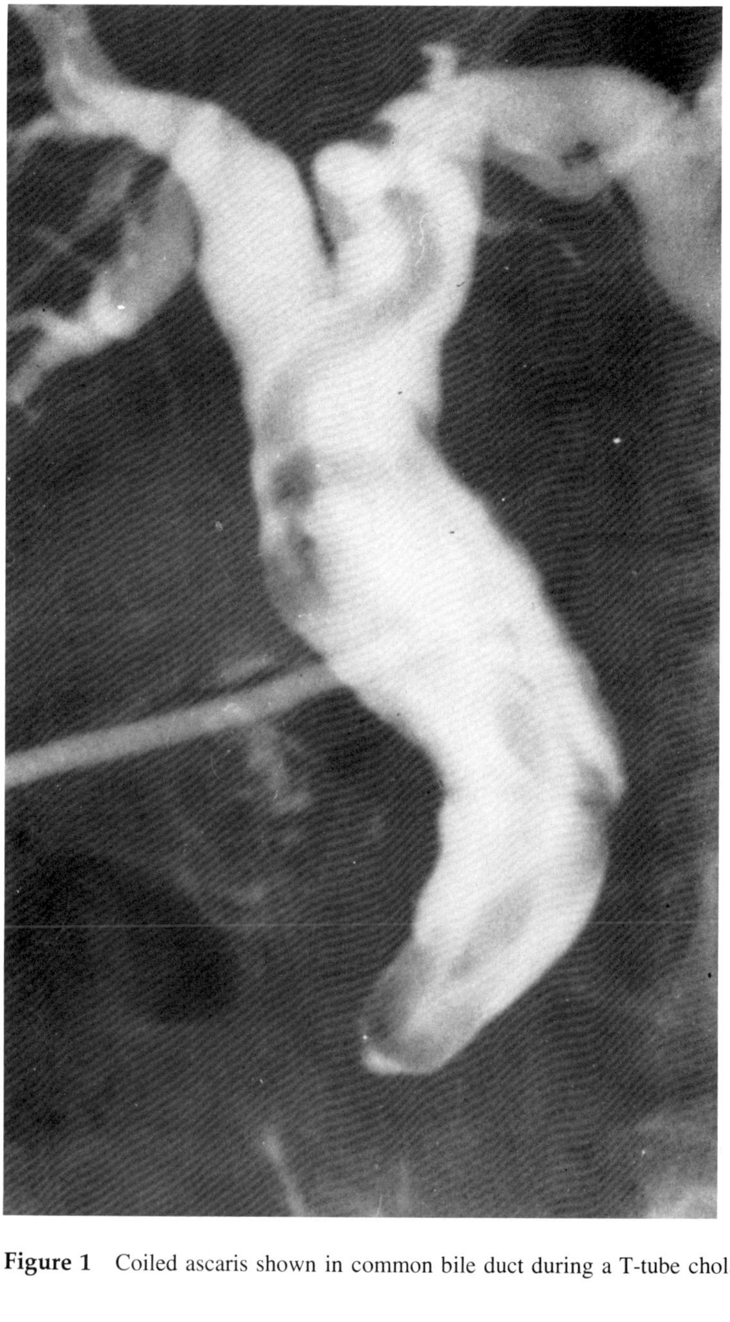

Figure 1 Coiled ascaris shown in common bile duct during a T-tube cholangiogram.

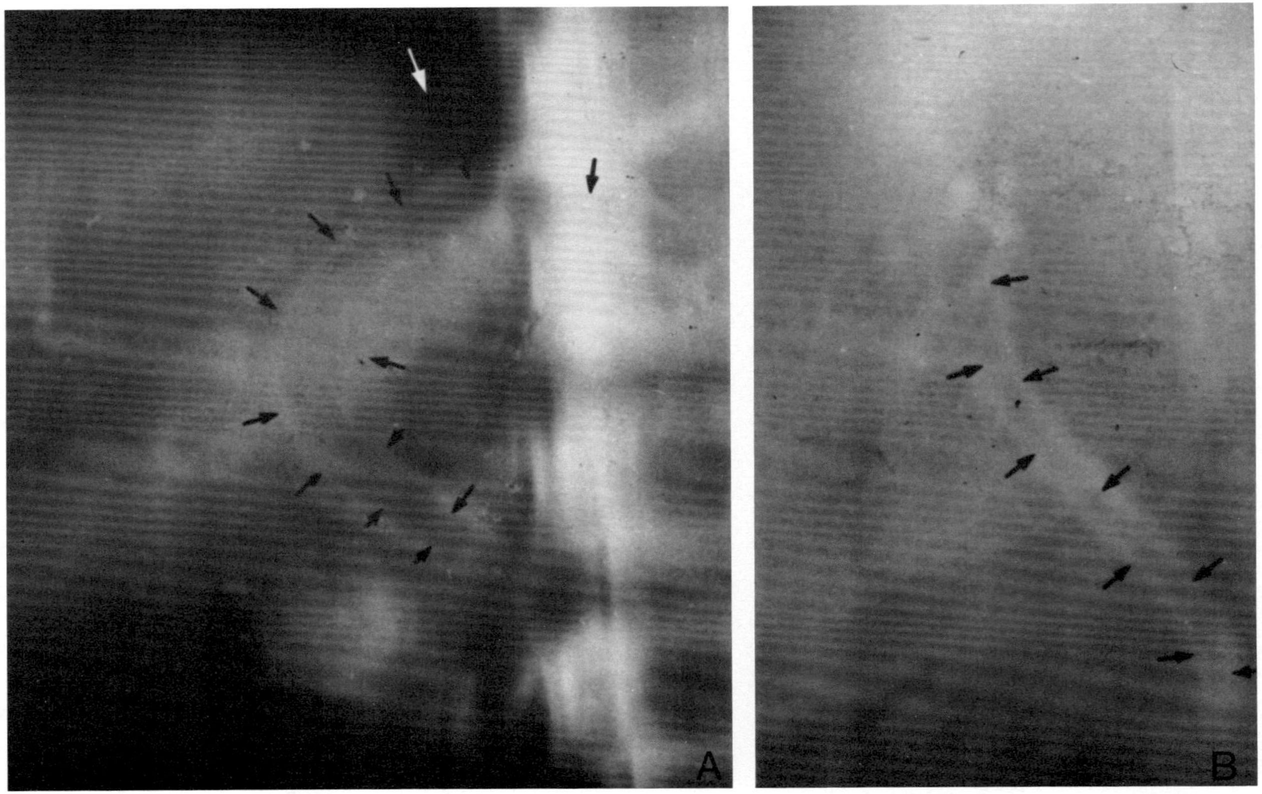

Figure 2 Cholangiograms revealing an ascaris worm (arrows) in the common bile duct of two South African children. (Courtesy of Krige and B. J. Cremin; from Ref. 22.)

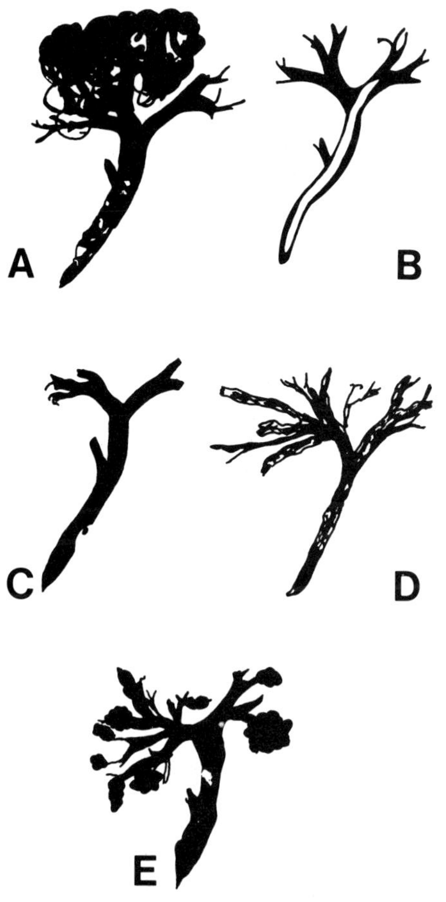

Figure 3 Schematic features of various parasites demonstrated during cholangiography. (A) Hydatid liver cyst with rupture of daughter cysts into biliary passages. (B) Ascaris in common bile duct. (C) *Fasciola hepatica* in common bile duct with contrast medium in the region of its ventral sucker. (D) Clonorchiasis or opisthorchiasis with distortion of normal biliary duct architecture and numerous small parasitic filling defects. (E) Pyogenic cholangitis of Southeast Asia.

surgical measures are indicated, as the death of an ectopic worm can lead to severe complications.

Needless to say, stool examination for the characteristic ova or evacuated adult worms is a necessary part of the workup of these patients.

Liver Flukes

Various species of flat, leaflike hermaphrodites can parasitize the biliary passages of humans. *Fasciola hepatica* though widespread in global terms has a patchy geographical distribution that includes France, North Africa, parts of the USSR and Eastern Europe, Peru, China, and some Caribbean foci. *Fasciola gigantica* has a predominantly tropical endemicity, being found in Southeast Asia, the Middle East, Hawaii, and parts of Africa.

The normal hosts are sheep and cattle, who pass the eggs in their droppings. In water, eggs produce miracidium forms that develop further in the liver of certain water snails. Subsequently, metacercarial forms are produced which become attached to water vegetation such as watercress and there encyst. Consumption of such contaminated vegetation by cattle or humans leads to release of larvae from the cysts when these reach the small bowel. The larvae penetrate the bowel wall and via the peritoneal cavity seek the surface of the liver. The successful parasites burrow through the liver to attain the biliary passages, where they reach sexual maturity and begin laying eggs. As adults they vary in length from 15 to 25 mm.

During their transperitoneal migration a patient may develop nonspecific fever, urticarial symptoms, and eosinophilia; obstructive jaundice of an intermittent type may ultimately occur. The diagnosis is not usually suspected. As the parasite can be visualized at cholangiography, the appearances need to be known (7,8). There is usually a narrowed area of the common duct associated with a filling defect due to the leaflike adult fluke. A small collection of contrast medium with a ring-shaped filling defect has been described (9) and attributed to the sucker of the parasite (Fig. 3C).

Stool inspection for ova confirms the species diagnosis.

The size of the parasite, their paucity, their distal location, and the normal appearance of the hepatic biliary tree distinguish biliary liver flukes from the distomata infections of the Far East: clonorchiasis and opisthorchiasis.

Clonorchiasis and Opisthorchiasis

Both these parasitisms exist in the Far East and exhibit similarities in their life cycles. *Clonorchis sinensis* is seen in southern China, Korea, Taiwan, and Japan but, owing to control measures and industrial pollution affecting the snail intermediate hosts, the disease is now on the wane. *Opisthorca felineus* and *O. viverini* are endemic in some of the clonorchiasis areas but also occur in western Malaysia, Thailand, Laos, and the Philippines.

The parasite may persist in a symptomless fashion for up to 50 years. Thus 26% of Kwantung Province immigrants to New York City still harbored parasites 20 years after their arrival in the United States (10).

These parasites both require a first snail intermediate vector and then a fish, usually a carp, as second-stage host. The snails become contaminated from human soil containing eggs with miracidia. Humans are involved by eating raw fish containing encysted forms. These excyst in the duodenum and the flukes ascend the common bile duct and hepatic radicles until they can progress no further. They start laying eggs and settle down to a long hepatic career. Patients with light parasitic burdens may have no symptoms, but ultimately the prolonged presence of the parasites causes problems to the human host (11).

The presence of the biliary parasites leads to a proliferative change in the epithelium of the ducts and fibrosis of the walls. In addition to the flukes, which measure about 1 to 1.5 cm in length and just over 1 mm in thickness, desquamated epithelial sludge may be present in the ducts. As these obstructive events are multifocal, many fusiform dilatations develop in the proximal biliary tree. If stenosis is severe, large ductal sacculations may form.

These alterations can be studied by interoperative, percutaneous transhepatic, or endoscopic retrograde cholangiography (11–13). These contrast studies reveal the caliber changes of the hepatic ducts, the presence of sludge, and multiple small tea-leaf-like filling defects due to the parasites (Figs. 3D, 4, 5). Ductal biliary concretions may be evident in clonorchiasis but are exceptional in opisthorchiasis (14). Gallstones may be present.

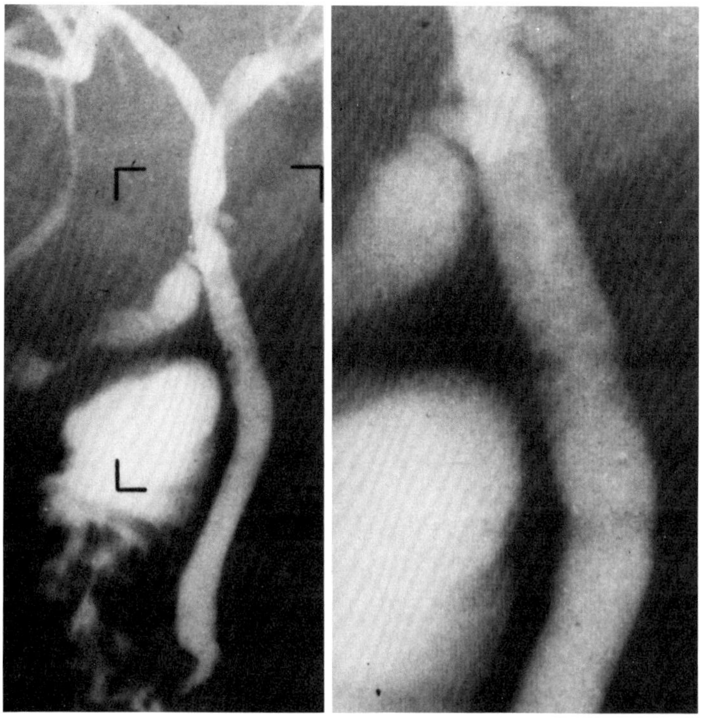

Figure 4 Clonorchis sinensis parasites in common bile duct. (Courtesy of Professor K. Okuda; from Ref. 22.)

Suppurative cholangitis is a recognized complication. Liver infection can lead to subphrenic collections and even pulmonary biliary fistulae (15). A chronic typhoid carrier state has been associated with clonorchiasis (16).

Cholangiocarcinoma is a recognized late complication of opisthorchiasis (Fig. 6) and carcinoma of the cystic duct has also been associated (17). Although a specific diagnosis depends on the isolation of ova in the stool, radiologists examining a patient from an endemic area should think of this form of parasitism in patients who have cholangitis and who at cholangiography show a distorted ductal architecture, have debris in the ducts, and possible small filling defects due to parasitic elements.

Echinococcosis

In some patients with hydatid disease liver cysts may establish communication with the biliary tree and discharge fluid, daughter cysts, and membranes. This development is discussed later in the chapter.

Far Eastern Pyogenic Cholangitis

Chronic suppurative cholangitis is a well-recognized clinical entity on the Malaysian peninsula and Singapore, in Hong Kong, and adjacent areas. By the time patients present,

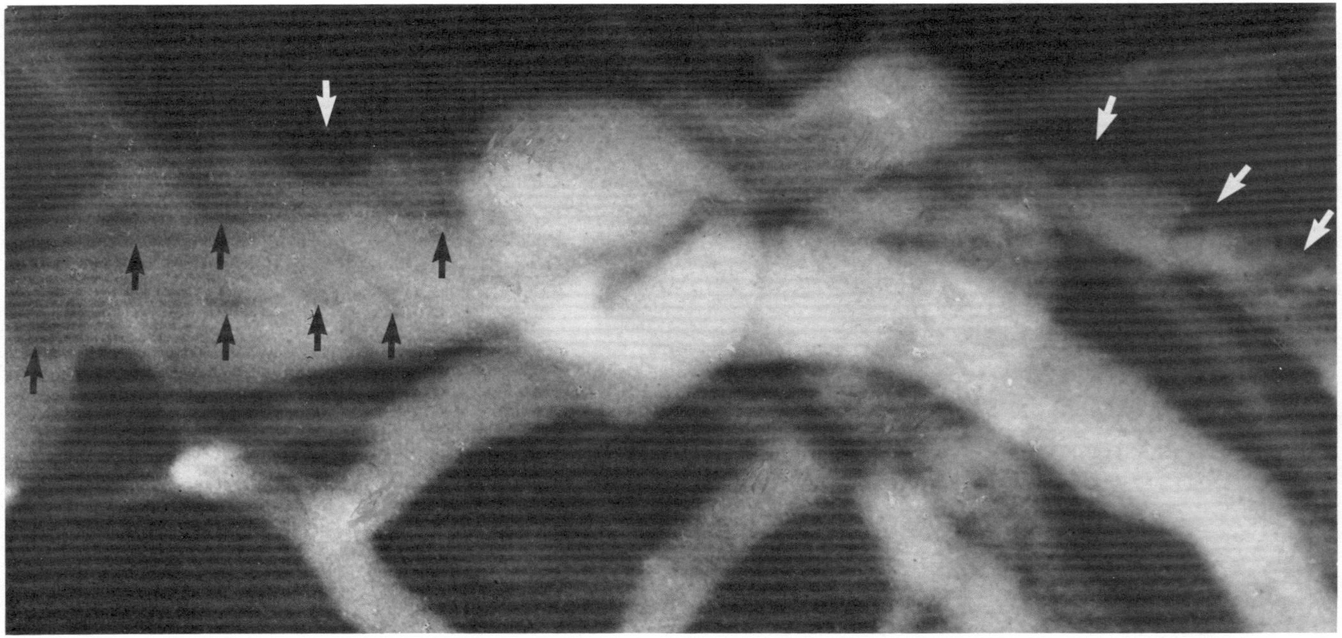

Figure 5 Transhepatic cholangiogram. Opacified intrahepatic ducts show filling defects due to *Clonorchis sinensis* (arrows). (Courtesy of Professor J. Ho.)

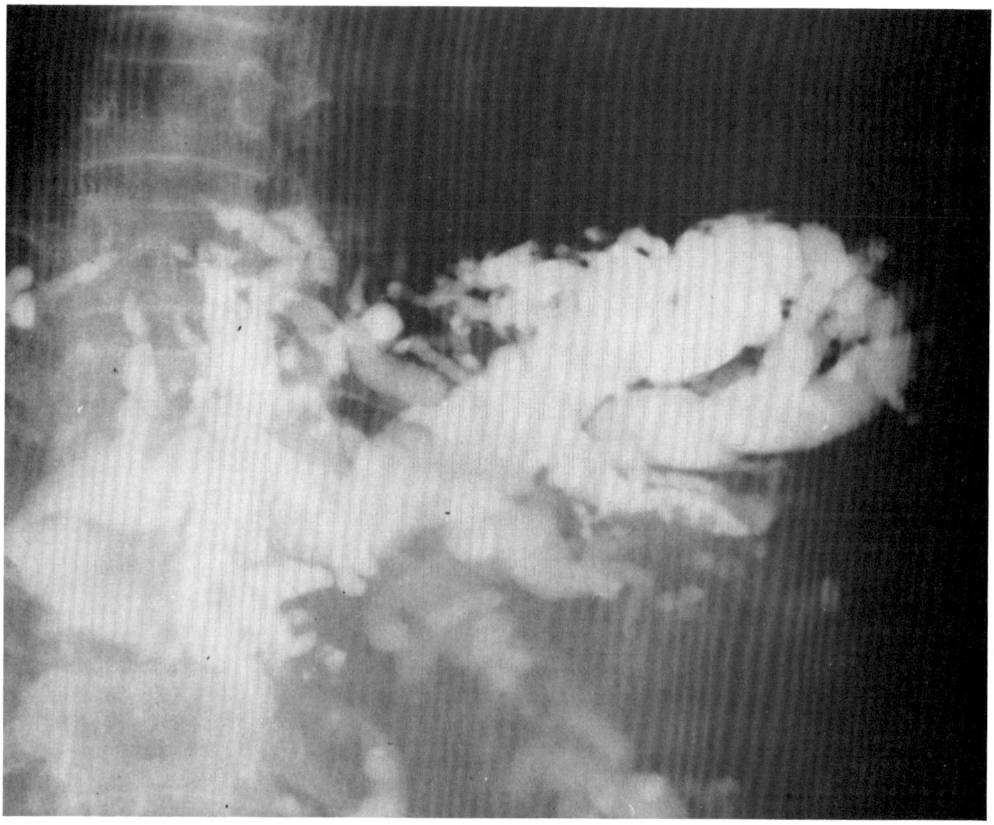

Figure 6 Opacified dilated hepatic ducts above an obstruction due to cholangiocarcinoma secondary to opisthorchiasis.

the underlying etiology is often obscure and it is uncertain whether distomata or ascaris or another as yet undefined cause is responsible (18,19). Parasites may well have disappeared in the hostile and infected intrabiliary environment. The septic process is associated with sludge and debris casts within the ducts, and this may become visible on cholangiography. Gallstone or hepatic duct concretions may be present. Ducts may show small irregular connecting abscess cavities or ductal outpouchings (Figs. 3E,7). Yu et al. (20) have emphasized that in chronic cholangitis the ducts do not readily dilate because of intramural fibrosis, whereas in most other types of obstructive jaundice, generalized dilatation and tortuosity tend to develop. This can be a useful differential cholangiographic feature.

Biliary Calculi

The incidence of gallstones is subject to considerable ethnic and geographic variations. In much of equatorial Africa and in the Far East, Indonesia, and Thailand, gallstones are rare at autopsy. Thus compared to a 20% autopsy frequency in the United Kingdom, gallstones

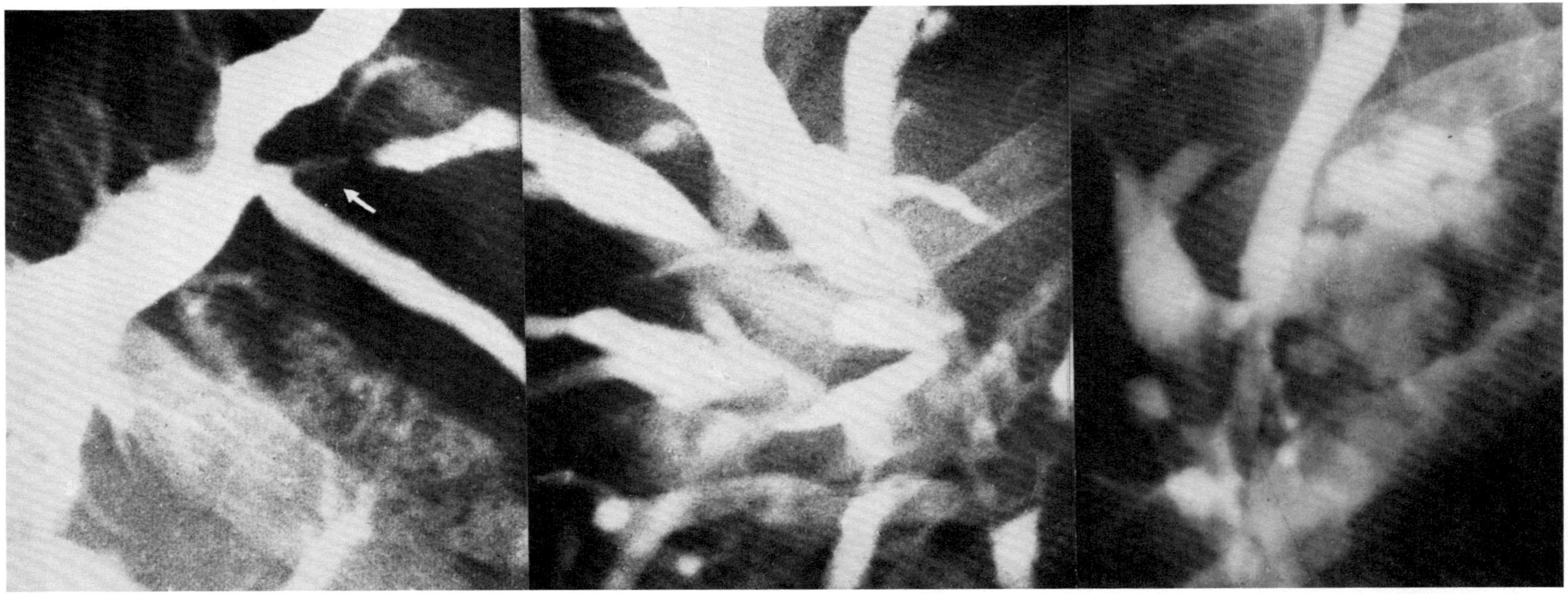

Figure 7 Distorted duct architecture with dilatation, stenosis, and communicating cavities in patients with Southeast Asian cholangitis. (From Ref. 22.)

were found in only 0.1% in Kenya, 0.87% in Uganda, 1.4% in Thailand, and 2.3% in China (21). Clinical experience from Nigeria, Ghana, Uganda, and Zaire similarly attests to the paucity of cases (22–24). In some parts of the Far East, intrahepatic ductal stones are much more frequent than gallbladder stones. This relative frequency inversion is probably related to the parasitic disorders described in the preceding portion of this chapter.

It is also strange to note how much more often cholelithiasis is detected at cholecystography in the American Negro with sickle cell disease than in West Africans with the homozygous disease process.

Mass Lesions of the Liver

Hepatic Amebiasis

By the use of radiographic, isotopic, ultrasound, and CT imaging techniques the radiologist can assist in the diagnosis and management of hepatic amebiasis by detecting hepatomegaly, the presence of an abscess, and whether the abscess has extended beyond the confines of the liver.

The problem of liver amebiasis is that of the liver abscess. Although amebic hepatitis has been postulated as a specific entity separate from abscess formation, no sound pathological histological basis has been produced for it (25).

The frequency of liver abscess complicating colonic amebiases cannot be accurately judged from autopsy series or even clinical experience, as the selection of patients renders rate assessment unreliable. Since antiamebic therapy for colonic disease may abort a developing amebic abscess, the present frequency of the complication is difficult to gauge. It probably occurs in fewer than 5% of patients.

Abscesses are most frequent in the right lobe (80%). This has been attributed to the larger size of the right lobe, the streaming of ascending colon portal flow to the right side, and to the heavier infection density of the right colon. The surprising feature is how rarely there are multiple abscesses despite venous dissemination. Over 75% of abscesses are solitary (26,27).

The condition is seen most frequently in males between 20 and 40 years of age. Classically, a tender enlarged liver associated with fever and leukocytosis and accompanied by impaired liver function suggests the diagnosis. A previous history of diarrhea or dysentery is absent in over half the patients. The presence of *Entamoeba histolytica* trophozoites in the stools or rectal exudate is inconstant, but serological tests are positive. This immunological index of invasive amebiasis is particularly useful for diagnosis in nonendemic areas.

An abnormal chest or abdominal film is found in most cases, but as the changes detected are not specific, additional considerations are necessary for the diagnosis. A radiographically normal liver is often noted in those with a left lobe abscess or an abscess near the inferior surface of the liver. These "silent" lesions may perforate into the pericardium or free peritoneal cavity when still small.

The chest abnormalities, such as diaphragmatic elevation, basal atelectasis, relative immobility of a leaf of diaphragm, extension into the fissues, effusions, and so on, are well known and described in standard texts (22,28,29). Some workers have used pneumoperitoneum to aid in the diagnosis of a liver focus, but the indications for such a study are now exceptional. Rarely, an amebic abscess may calcify on resolution (30) and its site become visible on plain film (Fig. 8).

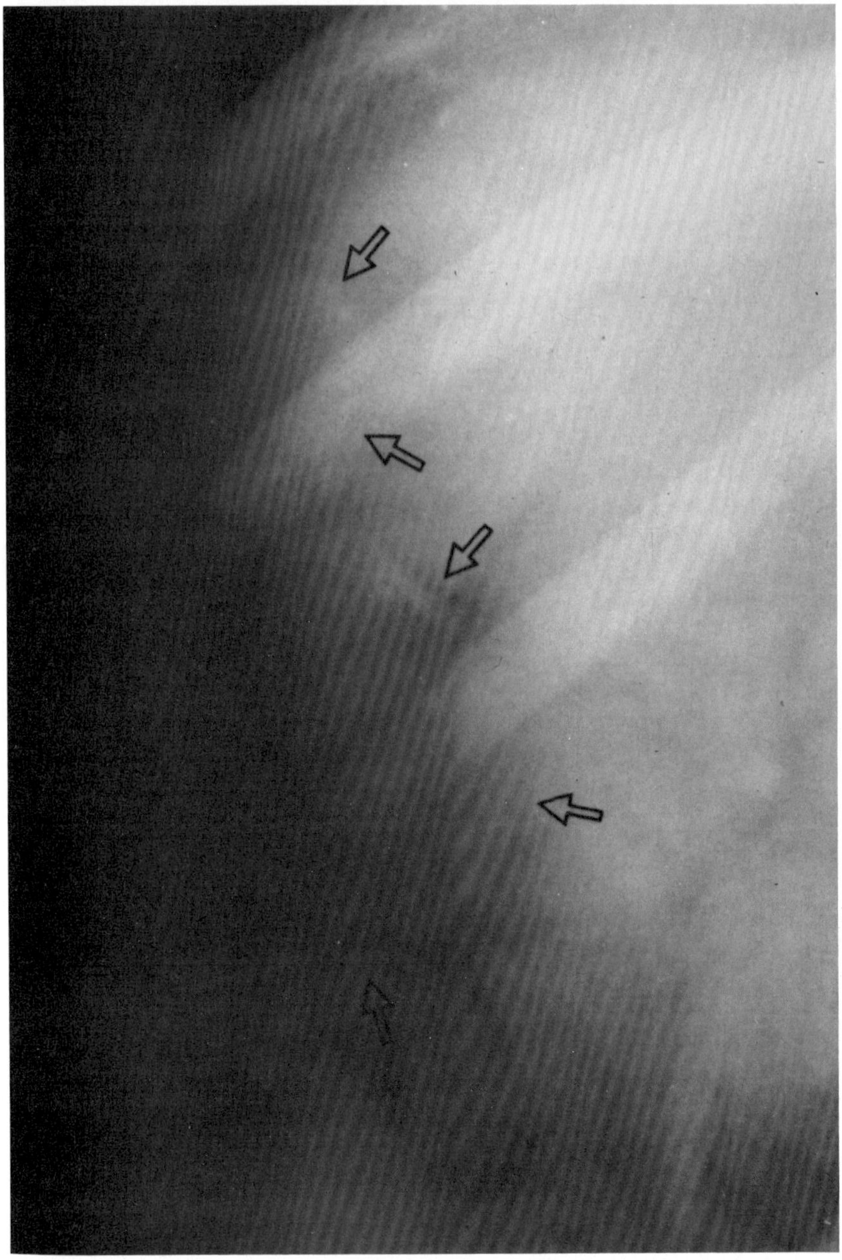

Figure 8 Calcified walls of hepatic amebic abscesses—an exceptional finding. (Courtesy of Dr. Rogers.)

Since the core of the clinical problem is the detection of an abscess, methods that will delineate an intrahepatic mass lesion are helpful. The choice depends on availability and cost.

The simplest radiographic method is to inject a large bolus of contrast medium (2 ml/kg body weight) and carry out hepatotomography (31,32). The lack of circulation within a liver abscess causes the cavity to appear as a radiolucent defect relative to the perfused and opacified liver parenchyma (Fig. 9A). This is easy to carry out, helpful, and inexpensive.

Ultrasonography of the liver is a valuable procedure that locates an abscess and demonstrates its size. The contents are less echogenic than normal liver tissue and there may be distal sonic enhancement (33). The walls are slightly irregular, in contrast to the smooth edges of a hydatid cyst (Fig. 9B).

Isotope liver investigation can readily demonstrate the liver mass but will not differentiate among abscess, cyst, and solid tumor (Fig. 9C). If computed tomography (CT) is available, this modality will give a good demonstration of the size and position of the mass, will show whether it is cystic or solid, and whether its outline is smooth or irregular. Intravenous contrast enhancement can increase this information. An abscess wall may not be seen at an early stage when contents are nearly isodense with normal liver tissue (Fig. 9D), but as the abscess matures the wall becomes distinct (Fig. 10).

At times liver abscesses have been radiographically demonstrated after aspiration by injecting air, iodine contrast material (Fig. 11), or sterile particulate barium. Barium particles become ingested by phagocytes in the abscess wall, permitting serial assessment of resolution with therapy (34). As such procedures are not without risk and since aspiration is rarely necessary with effective chemotherapy, these forms of studies are now exceptional.

Angiography, including splenoportal phlebography, has been used to show abscesses. Since these procedures add nothing to the simpler infusion studies, they are best reserved for patients where hepatoma is suspected in the differential diagnosis.

To conclude, both ultrasound and CT scanning can clearly identify the site and size of a liver abscess and follow its resolution during therapy. When available these techniques are preferable to other radiographic and isotopic imaging methods. Chest radiography should invariably precede other studies.

Hydatid Disease

Echinococcosis is more prevalent in temperate climes than in the tropics. The disease is seen in central and northern parts of South America due to *Echinococcus oligarthus* with a feline rodent cycle; in the Middle East, North Africa, South America, and Australia, from *E. granulosus*, where a canine-ungulate cycle occurs; and in Australia, where a dog-sheep and a dog-kangaroo cycle have been observed. *E. multilocularis* does not occur in the tropics and will not be considered here.

E. granulosus can be considered the representative parasite. The sexually mature small tapeworm in the intestinal tract of dogs releases a terminal segment containing eggs.

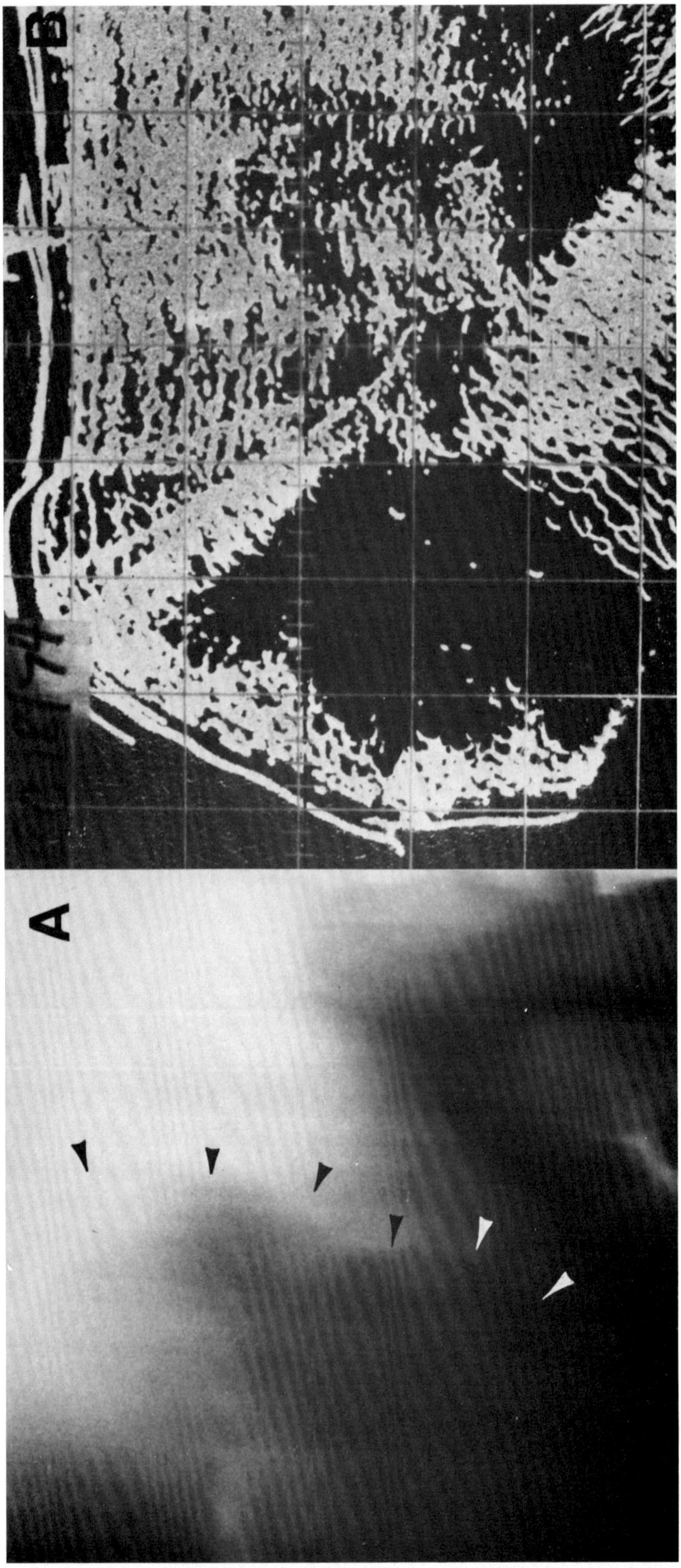
B
A

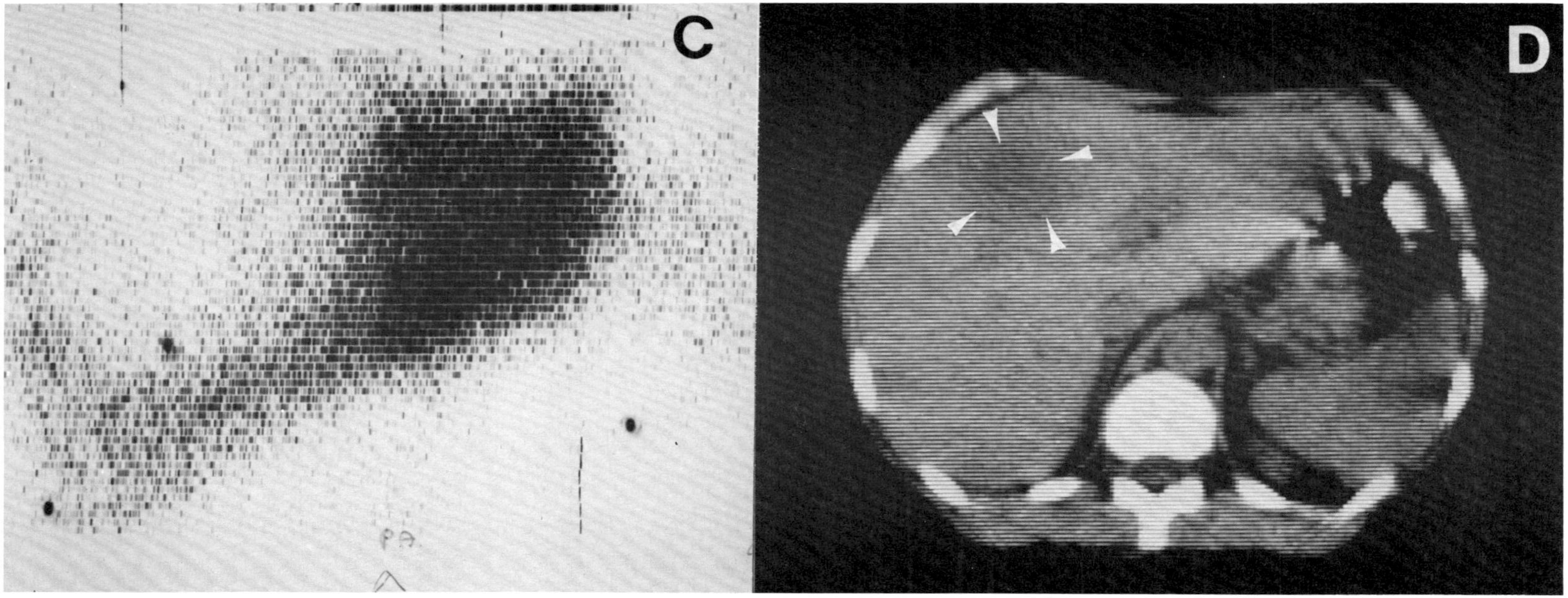

Figure 9 Hepatic amebic liver abscesses. (A) Lucent nonperfused area of abscess (arrowheads) demonstrated by hepatotomography following bolus injection of contrast material. (B) Bistable ultrasonography demonstrates a large sonolucent abscess cavity in the right lobe. (C) Massive amebic abscess demonstrated by isotope scan. (D) Ill-defined low-attenuation area of an early amebic liver abscess (arrowheads) demonstrated by CT. (From Ref. 22.)

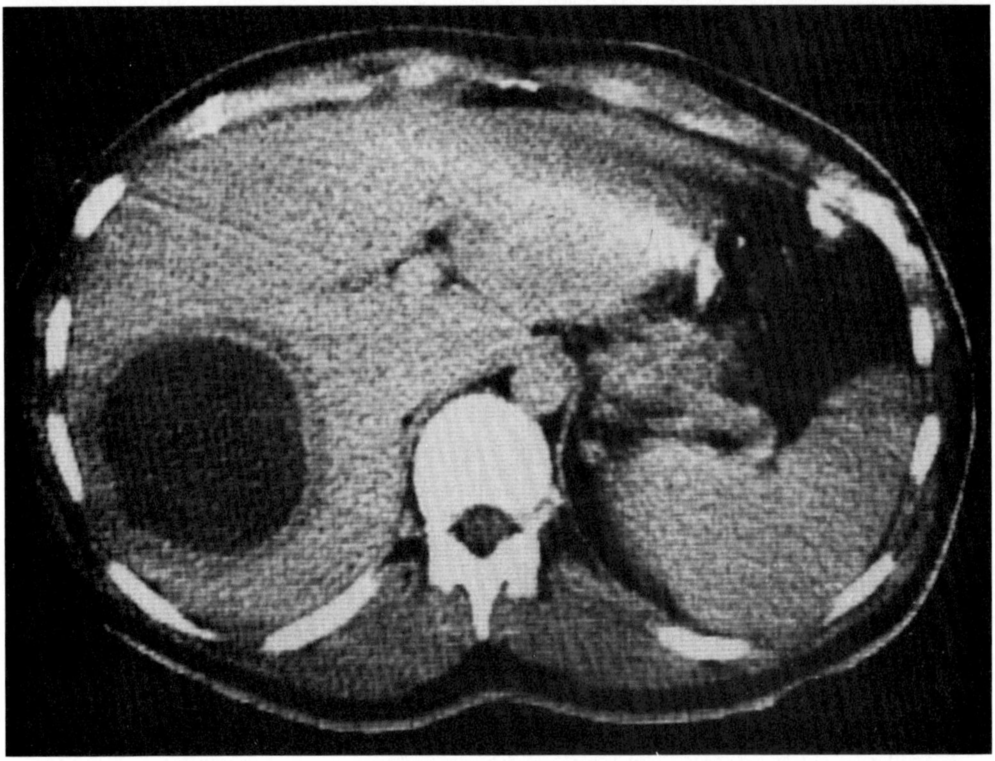

Figure 10 Well-defined area of low attenuation with an investing ring of low attenuation in amebic liver abscess. (CT scan courtesy of Dr. R. E. Koehler.)

The intermediate host becomes infected by consuming contaminated food in a pasture. In the duodenum the embryo is liberated, burrows through the mucosa to enter the circulation, and embolizes. There a cyst forms with an outer adventitial host layer, an ectocyst laminated capsule, and an internal germinal layer. Cysts are usually unilocular but can become multiseptate when daughter cysts develop from the germinal layer.

Embolization occurs in the liver in about 50% of infected individuals. The remaining oncospheres arrest in the pulmonary circulation and a few pass on to even more distal sites. Multiple cysts are frequent, so that 25% with liver cysts have lung lesions and 40% of those with pulmonary foci also have hepatic hydatids (35). About 80% of cysts lie in the right lobe of the liver. Hydatid cysts grow about 1 mm a month, so there is usually a long silent period before clinical symptoms appear. At the time of presentation, half to two-thirds of cases show some calcification in the cyst wall formed by the host (35,36).

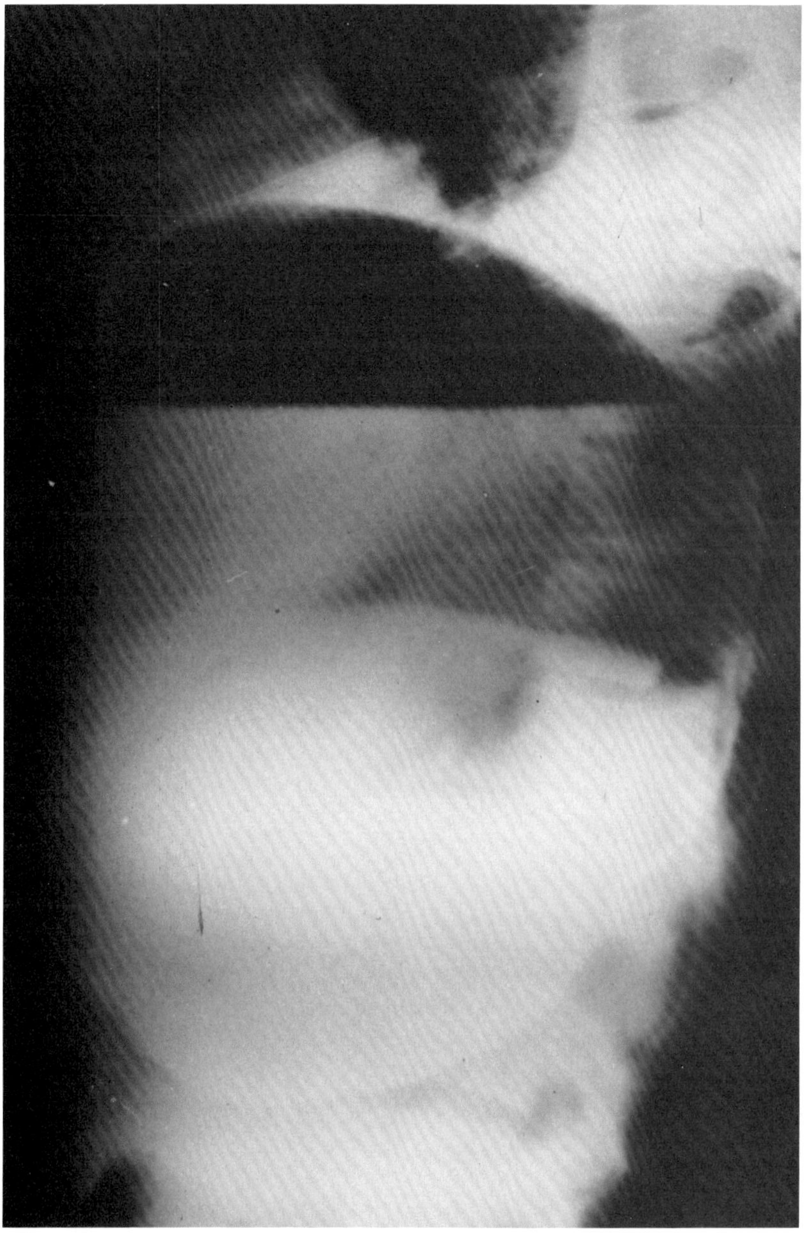

Figure 11 Large liver abscess that has been partially drained and air and contrast injected. (Courtesy of Dr. Cave, Dakar.)

Calcification may be circular due to total spherical mineral deposition, but a partial curvilinear appearance is more frequent (Fig. 12). Dense flocular amorphous calcification is a feature of the invasive *E. multilocularis* of central Europe, Siberia, Alaska, and the Canadian Arctic (37). Patchy calcification of the rim of the host tissue is not necessarily indicative of death of the inner germinal layer, but massive calcification of the wall implies death of the germinal layer. A lucent rounded defect in the liver detectable by plain films has been reported, but this appearance is exceptional (38).

Hydatid cysts can be demonstrated as space-occupying masses by many imaging methods. As with amebic abscess, large dose infusion or bolus injection hepatotomography is a simple, cheap, and sensitive but not absolutely specific technique. The lucent area usually has a much better defined wall than in amebic liver abscess, and often there is a more dense, hypervascular rim due to the vascular pericyst.

Isotopic scintigrams reveal a well-defined cold area. The procedure has a high sensitivity but lacks specificity.

Ultrasound and CT studies possess sensitivity and specificity of a high order (Figs. 13,14). Both investigations clearly show the well-defined capsule and detect the multilocular features of daughter cysts of *E. granulosus*. By contrast the infiltrative features of the nontropical *E. alveolaris* are less clear cut and can be confused with malignant processes (39). In the CT scans the images show a well-defined water density within the cyst. Multilocularity may be due to septa of daughter cysts or the coalition of two adjacent cysts. With intravenous contrast enhancement the vascular pericyst tissue displays a well-defined rim of high attenuation. This will assist in the differentiation between lymphatic hepatic cysts and echinococcosis.

Some hydatid cysts rupture into biliary passages, causing acute symptoms of fever, obstructive jaundice that may be intermittent, and sometimes urticaria. This complication may occur in 16% of patients (40). Methods already discussed to detect hepatic cysts would aid in the diagnosis. Preoperative transhepatic cholangiography can outline communications between cysts and bile ducts and may show membranes or daughter cysts in the main biliary passages (Figs. 3A, 15). However, because of the danger of "blind" needle puncture, interoperative contrast studies are probably to be preferred. Retrograde endoscopic cholangiography would be useful in such a situation.

Until recently surgery was the only therapeutic approach available, but since mebendazole has been shown to be effective in some patients with liver hydatidosis, the value of ultrasound or CT follow-up has increased, as IgE, specific antibody, and circulating immune complex immunological studies can then be difficult to interpret (41,42).

Malignant Hepatoma

Primary hepatoma is a frequent malignancy in tropical Africa, New Guinea, Taiwan, and Singapore. In those parts of the Far East, where clonorchiasis and opisthorchiasis are prevalent, cholangiocarcinoma rates are elevated.

In Mozambique, 55% of all malignancies are attributed to hepatoma, 19% in Nigeria, and 15% in Taiwan. In Mozambique the tumor has been recorded as 500 times more frequent in males between 25 and 36 years of age than in the United States.

The diagnostic problems posed in the tropics differ from those seen in the temperate world mainly because of the advanced stage of presentation combined with the paucity of well-equipped investigative centers.

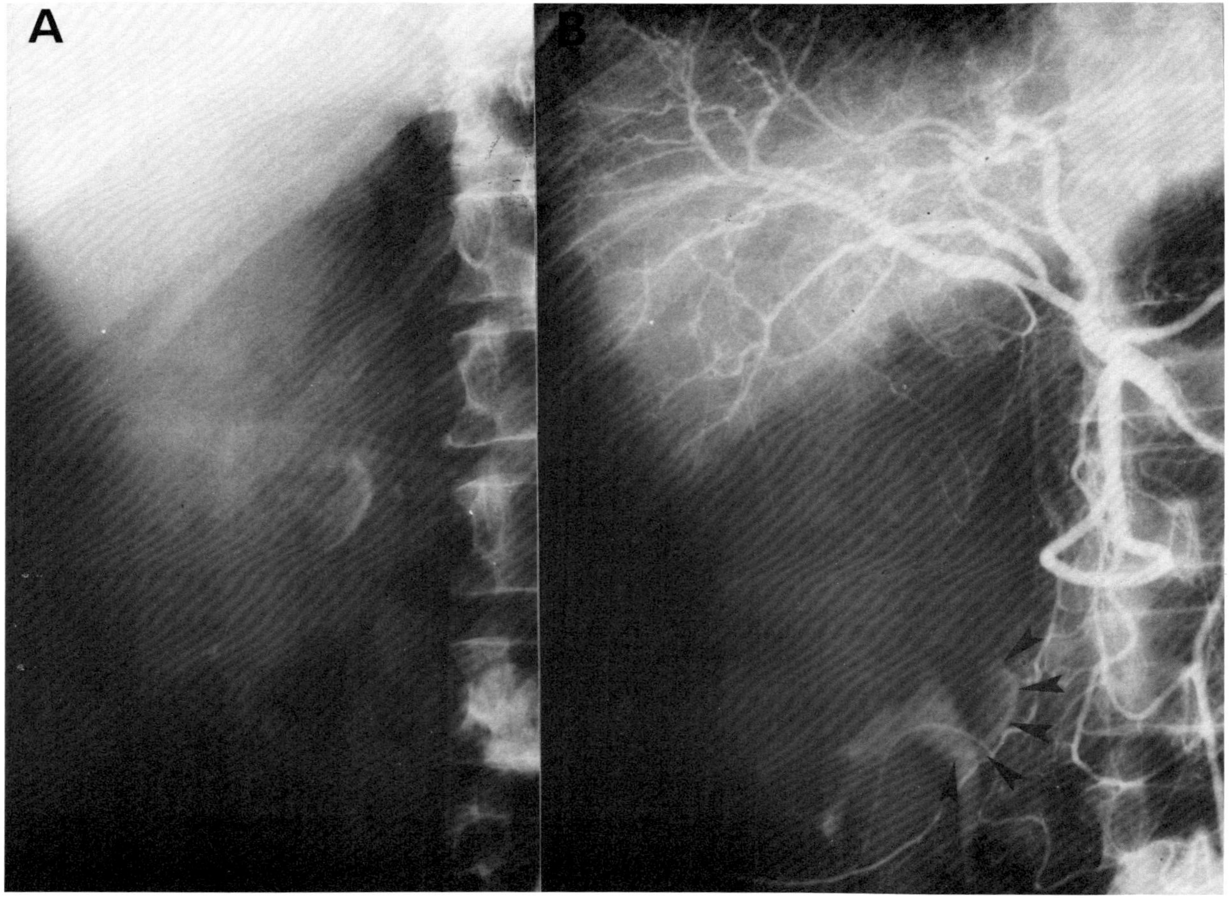

Figure 12 (A) Curvilinear calcification in a segment of the wall of a hydatid liver cyst. (B) A celiac angiogram shows displaced stretched vessels, indicating that the cyst is considerably larger than suggested by the segment of calcified wall (arrows). (Courtesy of Dr. Prem Kapur.)

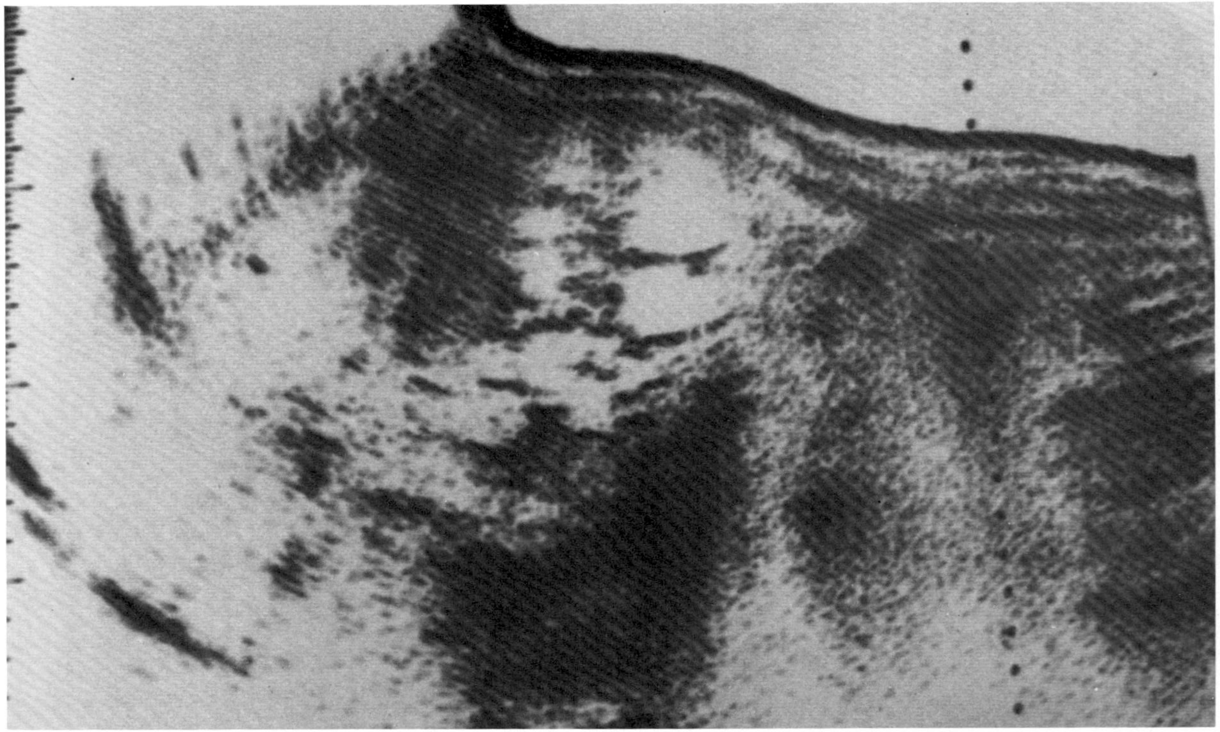

Figure 13 Ultrasound study revealing multiple sonolucent areas near the inferior border of the right lobe of the liver due to hydatid cysts.

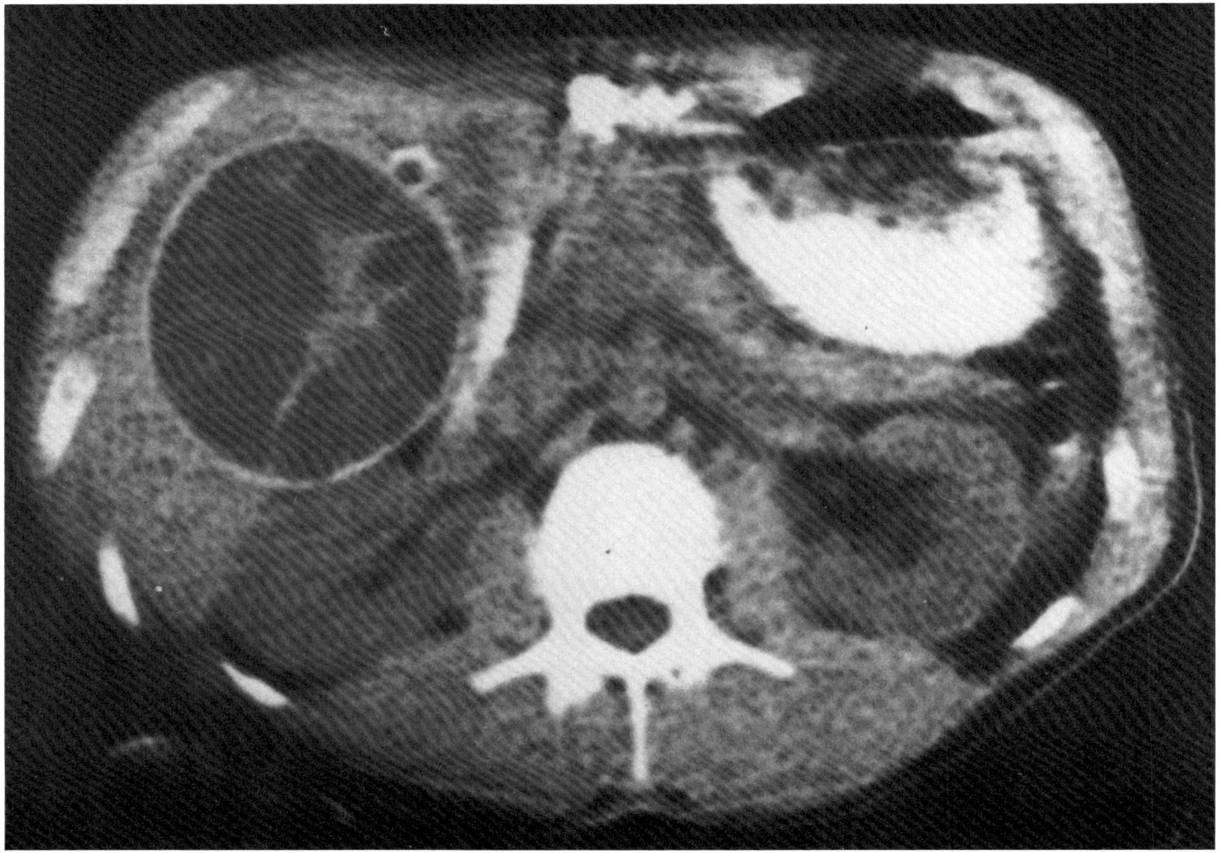

Figure 14 CT scan of large hydatid in the right lobe of the liver showing a well-defined wall and multilocular septa. Some calcium is present within the wall.

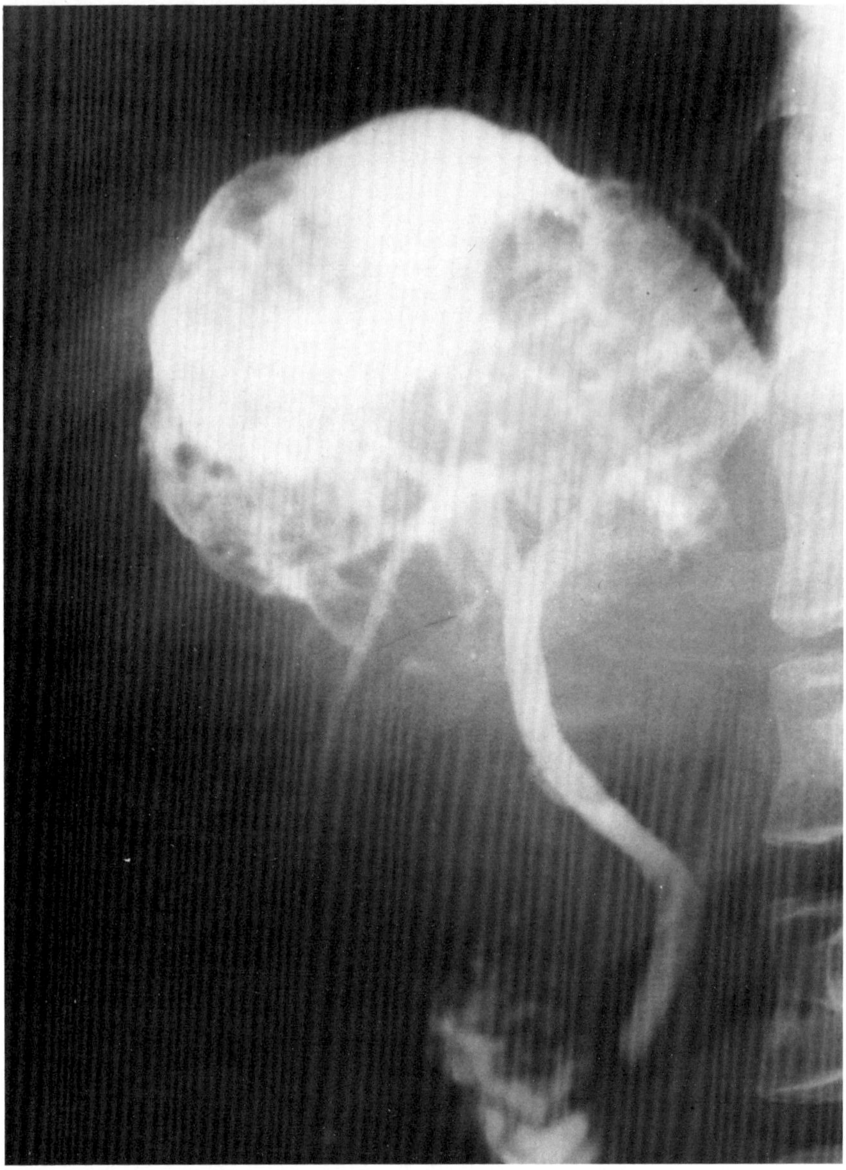

Figure 15 Percutaneous transhepatic cholangiogram in a patient with obstructive jaundice. Unexpected opacification of liver hydatid cyst in communication with the biliary tree. Rounded filling defects due to daughter cysts. (Courtesy of Dr. R. Tuttle.)

Portal Hypertension

In addition to conventional etiologies, portal hypertension in the tropics may result from such causes as *umbilical sepsis*, causing portal obliterative processes (22); *veno-occlusive hepatic disease* of Jamaica (43); as a sequel to *cholangitis* of the Far East; and most particularly as a complication of schistosomal infections.

Schistosomiasis

Ova of schistosomes embolize into the portal system and produce an obliterative portal fibrosis with considerable thickening of vessel walls. Paired schistosomes live in permanent copulation in veins. *Schistosoma haematobium* inhabit initially and predominantly the vesical plexus of veins; *S. mansoni* are in the ileocolic, colic, and sigmoidal veins; *S. intercalatum* in the rectal and sigmoidal veins; and *S. japonicum* in the mesenteric veins. The flukes produce ova which initially enter the bowel lumen. However, as time goes on the ovideposition leads to local fibrosis and eggs begin to embolize to the liver. Some flukes may also embolize to the liver (22).

In endemic areas portal hypertension can be an important complication of *S. mansoni* and *S. japonicum* infections. For example, in Zambia, 70% of esophageal varices are attributed to schistosomiasis (44).

In eary disease fibrosis due to ovideposition is periportal and the cirrhosis is presinusoidal, with normal sinusoidal or wedged hepatic venous pressures. Later, hepatic fibrosis becomes generalized (45). The radiological investigation of schistosomal portal hypertension is by standard angiography. Elevated flow is seen in a dilated hepatic artery, and development of a hepatofugal collateral portal flow system occurs. There is no increase in the incidence of hepatoma in schistosomal cirrhosis (45).

Tropical Splenomegaly Syndrome

This syndrome occurs in malarial areas and is reported particularly from equatorial Africa, New Guinea, India, and in the Amazon valley (22). Although portal hypertension is a feature of the disorder, massive splenomegaly and hematological abnormalities due to hypersplenism dominate the clinical picture (46). There is no need to investigate the portal system radiologically.

References

1. Clarke MR: *Multiductus physeteris* gen. et sp. nov. —a new diphyllocothriid cestode from a sperm whale. *J Helminthol 36*:1, 1962.
2. Makidono J: Observations on Ascaris during fluoroscopy. *Am J Trop Med Hyg 5*:699, 1956.
3. Guang ND, Schnauss AK, Thu NX: Ascaridiasis der Gallenwege beim Kind. *Tropenmed Parasitol 13*:318, 1962.

4. Schnauss AK and Tung TT: Erfahrungen bei dem durch Parasitenbefall der tiefen Gallenwage ausgelösten akuten Pankreasoedem und der Pankreasnekrose nach Ulcusresektionen. *Langenbecks Arch Chir 292*:890, 1959.
5. Lein SH: Radiographic diagnosis of biliary ascariasis. *Chin Med J 78*:545, 1959.
6. Cremin BJ: Biliary parasites. *Br J Radiol 42*:506,1969.
7. Levrat M, Tissot A, Pasquier J: Distomatose hépato biliaire à forme d'ictère par retention guérie par le traitement médical. *Mal Appar Dig 52*:351, 1962.
8. Courbier R, Villani R, Faini M: Distomatose des voies biliaires. *Mars Chir 16*:638, 1966.
9. Vayre T and Robin B: Distomatose cholédocienne découverte par cholangiographie per-opératoire lors d'une cholécystite lithiasique. *J Chir 96*:553, 1968.
10. Kammerer WS, Van der Decker JA, Keith TB, Mott KE: Clonorchiasis in New York City Chinese.*Trop Doct 7*:105, 1977.
11. Evans H, Bourgeois CH, Comer D, Keschamras N: Biliary tract changes in opisthorchiasis. *Am J Trop Med Hyg 20*:667, 1971.
12. Ho HC: *Tropical Radiology*, Middlemiss H (Ed). Heinemann, London, 1961.
13. Okuda K, Emura T, Morokuma K, Kokima S, Yokagawa M: Clonorchiasis studies by percutaneous cholangiography: a therapeutic trial of toluene-2,4-diisothiocyanate. *Gastroenterology 65*:457, 1973.
14. Wilde H: Biliary calculus associated with opisthorchiasis. *Am J Trop Med Hyg 22*:819, 1973.
15. Prijyanonda, B and Tandhanand S: Opisthorchiasis with pulmonary involvement. *Ann Intern Med 54*:795, 1961.
16. McFadzean AJS and Ong GB: Intrahepatic typhoid carriers. *Br Med J 1*:1567, 1966.
17. Chainuvati T, Paosawadhi A, Sripranoth M, Mamasatith S, Viranuvatti V: Carcinoma of cystic duct associated with opisthorchiasis. *Am J Trop Med Hyg 27*:482, 1976.
18. Harrison-Levy A: The biliary obstruction syndrome of the Chinese. *Br J Surg 49*:674, 1962.
19. Ong GB: A study of recurrent pyogenic cholangitis. *Arch Surg 84*:199, 1962.
20. Yu SF, Oon CL, Kho KM: Local experience of percutaneous transhepatic cholangiography. *Singapore Med J 14*:13, 1978.
21. Stitnimankarn T: The necropsy incidence of gallstones in Thailand. *Am J Med Sci 240*:349, 1960.
22. Cockshott WP and Middlemiss H: *Clinical Radiology in the Tropics*. Churchill Livingstone, Edinburgh, 1979.
23. Ngala Kenda JF: Lithiase biliaire chez l'africain, une revue de 16 ans au Clinique Universitaire de Kinshasa. *Ann Soc Belg Med Trop 57*:61, 1977.
24. Akinyanju O and Ladapo F: Cholelithiasis and biliary tract disease in sickle-cell disease in Nigerians. *Postgrad Med J 55*:400, 1979.
25. Lamont NMcCE and Pooler NR: Hepatic amebiasis. *Q J Med 27*:389, 1958.
26. Pittman FE, Ee-Hashimi W, Pittman JC: Studies on human amebiasis. *Gastroenterology 65*:581, 1973.
27. Lamont AC and Wicks ACB: Amoebic liver abscess in Rhodesian Africans. *Trans R Soc Trop Med Hyg 70*:302, 1976.
28. Rowlands HAK: Radiological changes in amoebic liver abscess. *J Trop Med Hyg 66*:113, 1963.
29. Schmidt AG: Plain film roentgen diagnosis of amebic hepatic abscess. *Am J Roentgenol 107*:47, 1969.
30. d'Alexandro A, Laga J, Vera MA: Cystic calcification of liver in Columbia. Echinococcosis or calcified abscess. *Am J Trop Med Hyg 15*:908, 1966.
31. Palma LD, Bacarini L, Bazzochi M: The use of abdominal contrast tomography in liver disease. *Br J Rad 50*:483, 1977.
32. DeMorais JAD and Medina D: Essai sur la technique de visualisation des abscès amibiens hépatique par coupes tomographiques après perfusion de sels de l'acide triobenzoique. *Ann Soc Belg Med Trop 56*:449, 1976.

Chronic Hepatic Cell Failure

In chronic liver cell failure arterial "spiders" may be seen on the pleura, but these are too small to be shown radiologically. The functional significance of these small vessels is uncertain, but by acting as shunts between the pulmonary arterial and venous circulation, they may make a small contribution to the peripheral arterial oxygen desaturation frequently found in patients with advanced cirrhosis. Some arteriovenous shunting is suspected to be the main cause of desaturation (4). Multiple pulmonary arteriovenous aneurysms were shown in two patients with cirrhosis (14), although it was considered unlikely that such shunts could ever be large enough to produce significant arterial oxygen desaturation. Hutchison et al. (15) have been able to show by angiography multiple pulmonary arteriovenous anastomoses in patients with cirrhosis, cyanosis, and polycythemia. Arteriovenous shunting may also occur via the portopulmonary pathway (16), as for example, from the portal vein via periesophageal and mediastinal veins to the pulmonary veins.

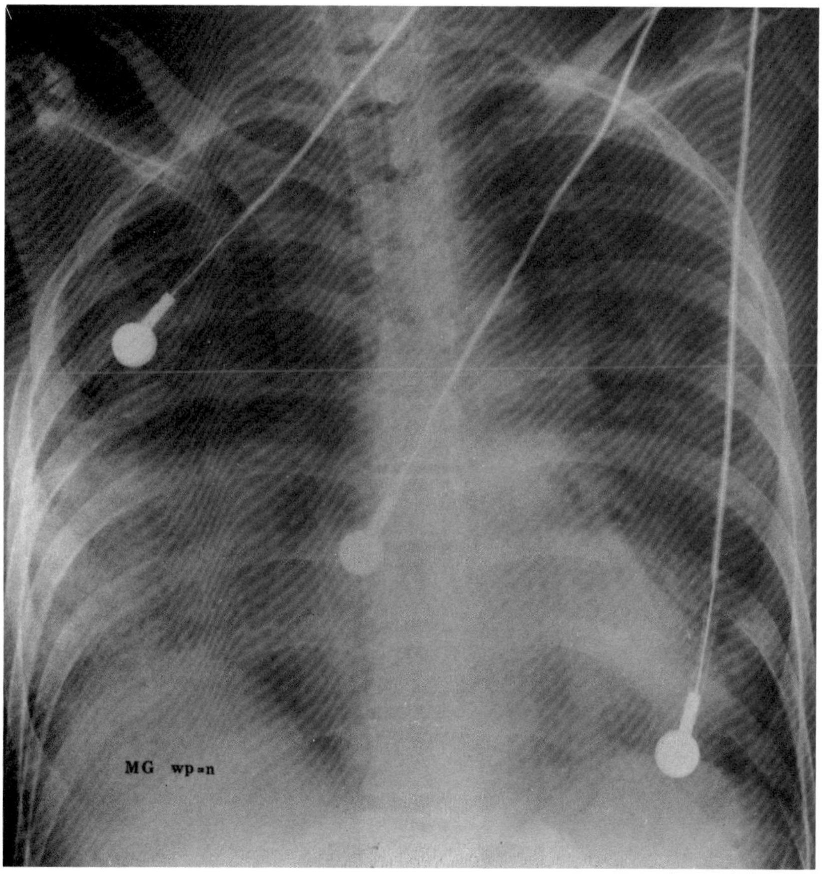

Figure 2 Female, 39 years. Acute fulminant hepatic failure. Bilateral pulmonary edema with normal pulmonary wedge pressure.

Changes Due to a Common Etiology

Granulomatous Disease

When granulomatous disease affects the lung and the liver, the pulmonary disease commonly predominates in the clinical picture. For example, in sarcoidosis and tuberculosis there may be widespread nodules throughout the lung with lymph node enlargement in the hilar and paratracheal regions, while biopsy of the liver may reveal only a few scattered granulomata.

Alpha$_1$-Antitrypsin Deficiency

Alpha$_1$-antitrypsin is a glycoprotein whose synthesis in the liver is controlled by a pair of autosomal codominant genes (17). Decreased serum levels of alpha$_1$-antitrypsin are associated with decreased activity of the *Pi***2** and *Pi***s** alleles, the lowest serum level being found with homozygous Z phenotype. Ten percent of homozygous Z adults develop cirrhosis of the liver, and this is typically a rapidly progressive process occurring after 50 years of age and leading to death from hepatic coma or bleeding. The cirrhosis may be macronodular, micronodular, or biliary in type. Of 14 homozygous cases studied by Berg and Eriksson (18), 5 had cirrhosis and 3 fibrosis of the liver. Two of the cirrhotics had highly differentiated hepatocellular carcinomata, and in another noncirrhotic liver a cholangiocarcinoma was found. In a review of 78 primary liver carcinomas from Lund (18), these workers also found pathological changes in the liver characteristic of alpha$_1$-antitrypsin deficiency in seven patients (9%). It therefore seems likely that alpha$_1$-antitrypsin deficiency predisposes to cirrhosis and hepatic carcinoma in adults (Fig. 3).

The pulmonary manifestations of alpha$_1$-antitrypsin deficiency are a severe and progressive shortness of breath occurring around the age of 40 due to the onset of panlobular emphysema. Cigarette smoking probably hastens the onset of emphysema. Radiologically, the emphysema is typically basal (17). Virtually all patients with cirrhosis of the liver due to alpha$_1$-antitrypsin deficiency also have pulmonary emphysema (Fig. 3).

In infancy 10–20% of homozygous alpha$_1$-antitrypsin-deficient children have a cholestatic type of neonatal hepatitis which leads to a progressive cirrhosis. Most such children die before reaching adult life (17).

Cirrhosis of Autoimmune and Alcoholic Origin

Pulmonary changes may be seen in patients with cirrhosis of both autoimmune and alcoholic etiology. The significance and method of production of these changes is less well understood than the conditions described above.

In active chronic hepatitis about 40% of patients have an abnormal chest radiograph (19). In addition to pleural effusions and segmental or subsegmental collapse, ill-defined rounded shadows are seen at the bases in 16% of this group. A similar appearance was found by Turner-Warwick (20) in six of eight patients with fibrosing alveolitis, chronic liver disease, and multiple autoantibodies. Five of the patients had chronic active hepatitis and three had active interlobular hepatitis, and in seven of the eight patients the course of the liver and lung disease was similar. Golding et al. (21) studied a series of 218 patients with chronic active hepatitis, primary biliary cirrhosis, and cryptogenic cirrhosis. Seventeen of 70 patients tested had a reduced gas transfer factor, and of these 9 had fibrosing alveolitis, based on radiological signs and lung function tests. Biopsy of 2 of these patients showed a mixture of the desquamative and mural types of fibrosing

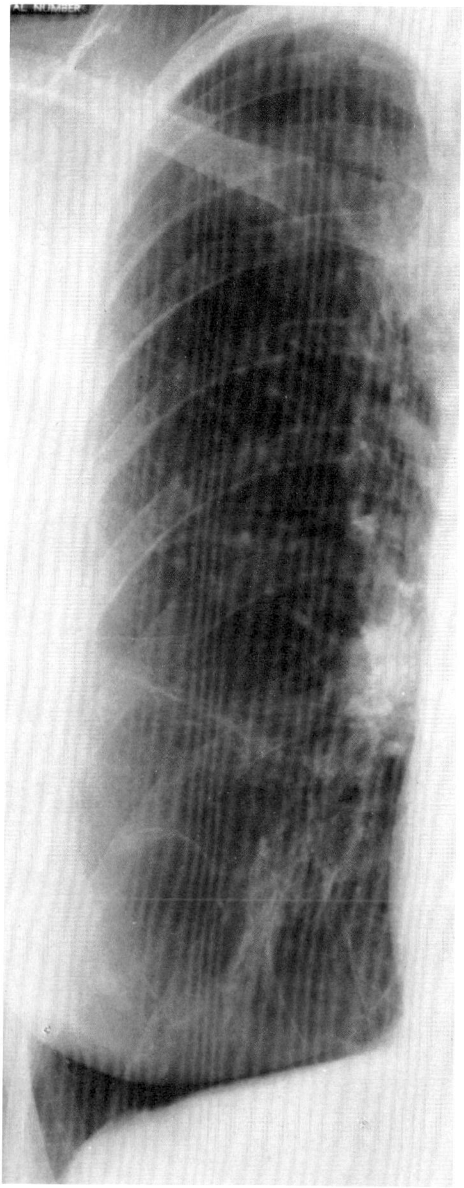

(A)

Figure 3 Female, 53 years. $Alpha_1$-antitrypsin deficiency. (A) Right lung showing lower zone emphysema. (B) Celiac axis angiogram showing cirrhosis with a hepatocellular carcinoma in the right lobe.

alveolitis. The remaining 8 patients with a reduced transfer factor were considered to have increased "vascular markings" best seen at the bases.

The anatomical basis for these basal shadows is uncertain and may vary in different patients. In some cirrhotic patients they are due to the changes of fibrosing alveolitis (20), but in alcoholic cirrhosis the shadows are probably due to the increased number of alveolar wall blood vessels (6) and to a dilatation of vessels up to 16 μm in diameter in both upper and lower lobes, as described earlier.

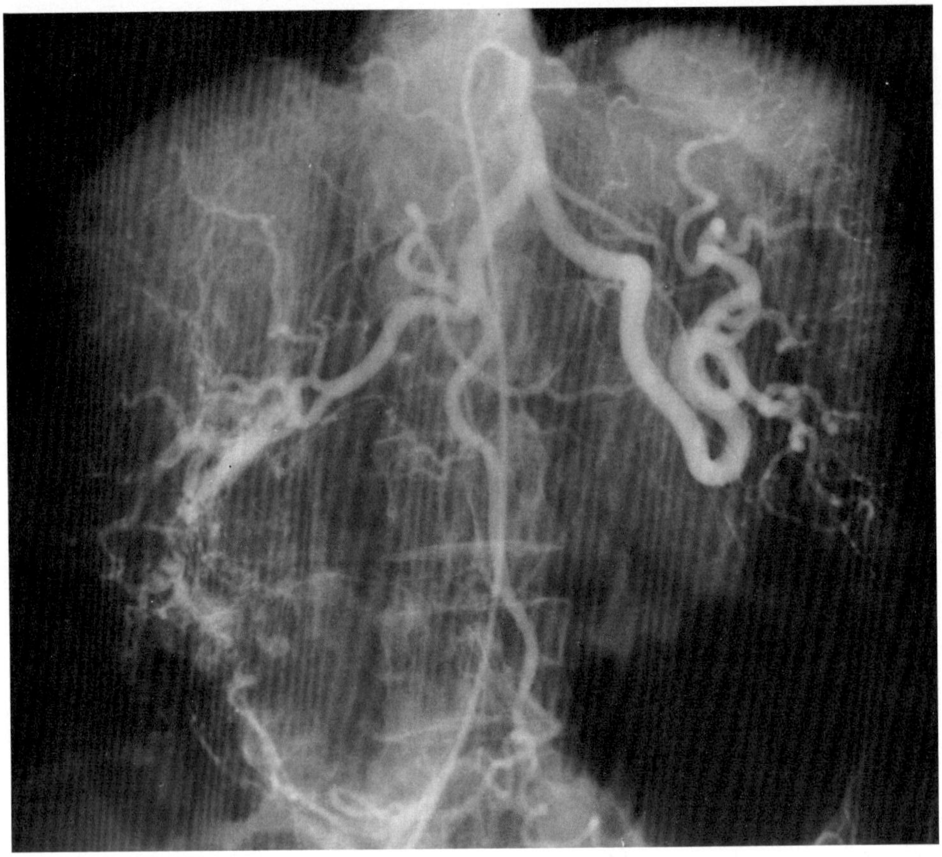

(B)

Figure 3 (continued)

Urinary System

Two aspects of renal disease occurring in patients with hepatic disease will be discussed: renal failure and cystic disease.

Renal Failure

Renal and hepatic failure both due to a common infection as may occur in Weil's disease or due to a common toxin will not be discussed. We wish to discuss the functional renal failure that may occur in association with acute fulminant hepatic failure or advanced cirrhosis and which is practically always fatal (22). Recovery of renal function occurs only in those patients with reversible liver disease. The term *hepatorenal syndrome* has been used to describe this clinical condition, but since the term is sometimes used to include any disease having both hepatic and renal manifestations, it is probably better to use the term *functional renal failure* to describe those patients who develop renal failure as a complication of hepatic cell failure.

The onset of renal failure in such patients is often gradual and spontaneous, although it may be precipitated by upper gastrointestinal hemorrhage. At first the blood urea is normal, but there is subclinical renal impairment. Later the blood urea starts to rise, and terminally there is severe polyuria, arterial hypotension, and coma leading to death.

Epstein et al. (23) performed selective renal angiography on patients with cirrhosis and functional renal failure. They found consistent angiographic abnormalities in the kidneys of their patients: beading and tortuosity of the interlobar and proximal arteries, in some cases like the microaneurysms described in polyarteritis nodosa. Filling of cortical vessels or a distinct cortical nephrogram were not seen and this is similar to the findings in oliguric renal failure or during immunological rejection of a renal transplant. It was considered that the decrease in the peripheral vascular bed gave rise to an increase in the renal vascular resistance, a theory supported by the reflux of contrast medium into the aorta with selective injections. The same works noted extreme hemodynamic instability in their patients, as shown by a variability and irregularity of the ^{133}xenon washout, suggesting that the decreased renal blood flow was secondary to active vasoconstriction rather than intrarenal edema or other mechanical factors.

There is little good evidence on the pathological changes that occur in the kidney. Bloodworth and Summers (24) have shown a variant of glomerulosclerosis, and immunofluorescent studies have demonstrated a gamma globulin in the glomerulus, which would suggest an autoimmune cause. Postmortem renal angiography (23) showed normal filling of the peripheral vessels with smooth arteries and no sign of the tortuosity and aneurysmal dilatations seen in life. This evidence that the vascular changes are potentially reversible is supported by the fact that kidneys removed from patients dying in functional renal failure due to cirrhosis perform normally when transplanted into a patient with normal hepatic function (25). The mechanism of this vasoconstriction, which causes a redistribution of blood flow away from the cortical nephrons to medullary and juxtamedullary nephrons, is unclear. Renin is the most likely agent since its level is raised in cirrhosis, but it would be necessary to show that the renin level is the cause and not the result of the decreased renal blood flow. If a specific vasoactive substance could be identified in patients with hepatic cell failure as responsible for the fall in renal perfusion either by its presence or absence, the prospect for therapy of this usually fatal complication of liver failure would be improved. In the early stages at least, drugs that increase renal blood flow may return renal function to normal (26).

Cystic Disease

There are two main forms of cystic disease of the liver associated with cysts in the kidneys. Cysts occurring in the parenchyma of the liver are functionally benign and are found in adults with polycystic disease of the kidneys. Cysts and ectasia of the bile ducts with hepatic fibrosis are an important cause of morbidity and are usually associated with infantile polycystic kidneys and medullary tubular ectasia.

Polycystic Disease of the Liver and Kidneys

The liver and spleen are enlarged (27) and the liver contains spherical unilocular cysts not more than a few centimeters in diameter (28) which contain mucus under pressure (29).

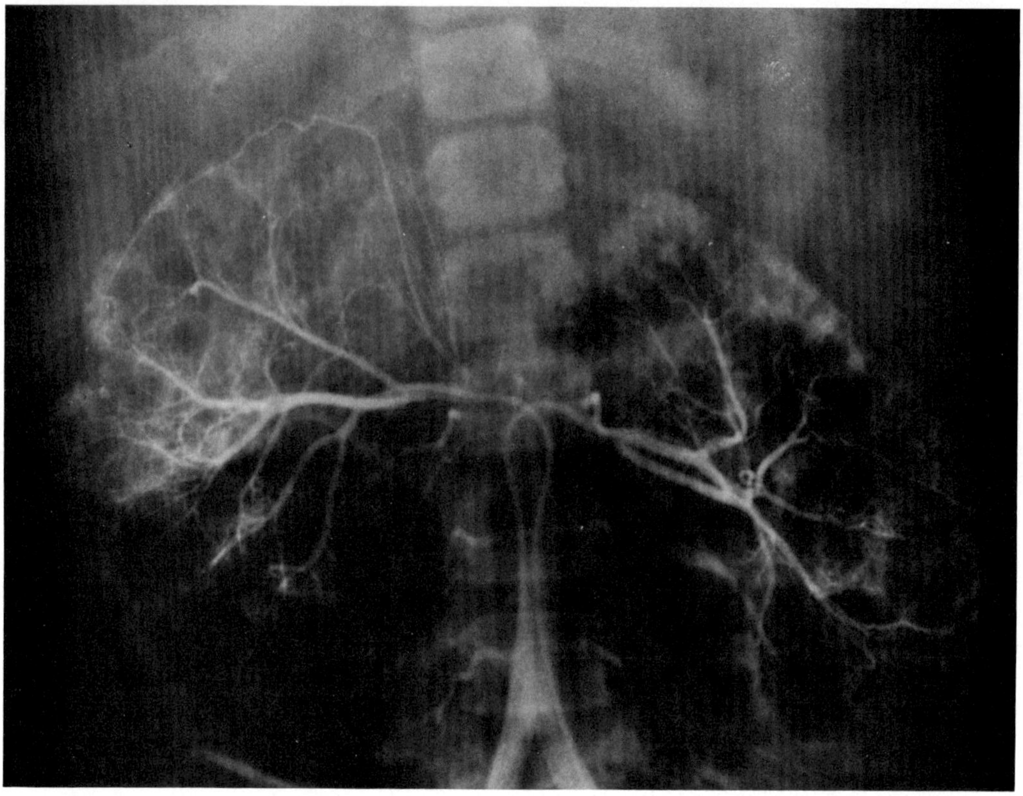

(A)

Figure 4 Female, 13 years. Infantile polycystic kidneys with hepatic fibrosis. (A) Bilateral selective renal angiograms showing multiple cysts throughout both kidneys. (B) Venous phase of arterioportogram showing enlarged spleen, with dilated portal vein, gastroesophageal collaterals, and diminished intrahepatic radicals of the portal vein.

Although the liver may be very large, the hepatic function is normal and the cysts are usually asymptomatic and are found by chance. The majority of the polycystic livers are not detected before autopsy (30). None of the 58 patients with polycystic disease of the kidneys studied by Hatfield and Pfister (30) had clinically significant liver disease. In one autopsy series (31) 53% of patients with hepatic cysts had polycystic disease of the kidneys, and conversly one-third of patients with polycystic kidneys had hepatic cysts. Probably the most important aspect of polycystic liver disease is in aiding the diagnosis of adult polycystic disease of the kidneys. Indeed, the presence of extrarenal cysts is the only way of distinguishing between patients with polycystic kidneys and normal renal function and patients with multiple simple cysts of the kidneys.

Congenital Biliary Ectasia and Renal Cystic Disease

Congenital ectasia or cystic disease of the biliary system may present in two forms, which could well represent variations of the same disease process. The simple form of congenital

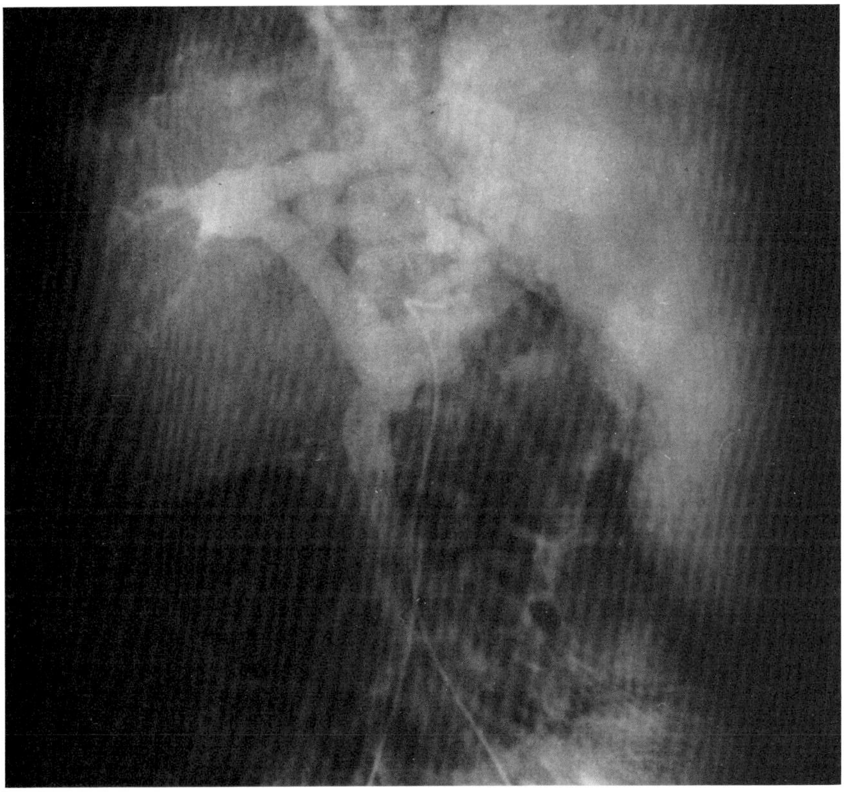

(B)

Figure 4 (continued)

bile duct dilatation was described by Caroli in 1958 (29) and is the rarer of the two, there being fewer than 10 cases in the literature up to 1973, although more have been described since. There is gross enlargement of the liver, which contains round or oval dilatations of the intrahepatic ducts, the invervening bile ducts being relatively normal. The hepatic parenchyma is normal, with no evidence of cirrhosis or periportal fibrosis. The extrahepatic ducts are always dilated, apparently not due to obstruction. The main complication of this disease is the formation of calculi within the cysts giving rise to infection and obstruction. Cirrhosis and portal hypertension do not occur.

The second form of congenital biliary dilatation is associated with portal fibrosis and was described by Crumach in 1954 (32). It is much more common than the simple form and is seen in children and young adults. The liver is grossly enlarged and the larger segmental biliary ducts are dilated. Recurrent cholangitis occurs as in the simple form, but there is also dilatation and hyperplasia of the smaller bile ducts in the portal triads, which become surrounded by an intense fibrous reaction. This gives rise to portal hypertension, giving these patients splenomegaly and hematemeses, which may be the cause of death before the first decade. Both of these forms of cystic disease of the bile ducts can be associated with infantile polycystic kidneys (Fig. 4).

Infantile polycystic disease has been classified in a number of ways depending on the age of presentation and the degree of renal impairment. Blyth and Ockendon (33) described groups I and II, with severe renal disease which gives rise to death before the hepatic lesions become significant. This corresponds to the newborn form of infantile polycystic disease (34). In groups III and IV renal disease is less severe but there is significant liver disease, which gives rise to portal hypertension. This corresponds to the childhood form of infantile polycystic kidney disease. In both forms the underlying pathological abnormality is dilatation of the nephrons, tubules, and the collecting ducts in the medulla and papillae. This is in contrast to medullary sponge kidney of the adult, in which the cystic changes are limited to the collecting tubules in the renal pyramids (35).

In the newborn form, both kidneys are enlarged. Death may occur in the first few days from respiratory problems such as pneumothorax, pneumomediastinum, and compression of the lungs by the high diaphragm. Hypertension is also a major problem at all ages. The intravenous urogram shows two massively enlarged kidneys. The nephrogram may persist from minutes to hours after injection of the contrast medium. The nephrogram may be homogeneous, but typically it shows streaks of contrast and radiolucent areas. The streaks represent contrast medium in the dilated ducts in the same way as the "brush border" seen in adult medullary sponge kidneys. Concentration may be so poor that the collecting systems are not seen at all or blunt calyces with foreshortened infundibula may be shown.

Survivors beyond the newborn period became more like the patients with the childhood form of infantile polycystic kidney disease. The kidneys are not as large as in the newborn form and the cysts are smaller, but the collecting ducts visible after contrast still present as a brush border and the calyces may be blunt or normal. The pattern of alternating radiolucency and streaks of contrast may be seen, or the appearance may be that of an adult polycystic kidney. These children may have no symptoms from their renal disease or show hypertension or uremia. However, the hepatic fibrosis progresses and produces portal hypertension and they tend to present with hematemesis in the first or second decade.

Skeletal System

Joint Disease

Hemochromatosis

It was Schumacher (36) who first suggested that the *arthropathy* found in two patients with idiopathic hemochromatosis might be a previously unrecognized complication of the diseases. Since then detailed descriptions of the joint changes have been recorded by other workers (37–39). The condition presents as a progressive degenerative arthropathy with a distribution similar to that found in rheumatoid arthritis. There are frequently episodes of acute crystal synovitis resembling gout when crystals of calcium pyrophosphate may be found in the synovial fluid.

Dymock et al. (39) analyzed the radiological appearances of the joint changes in 63 patients with hemochromatosis and related these to the clinical and biochemical features of the disease. Thirty-one of the 54 (57%) male patients in this series had an arthropathy. In 5 of these patients the arthropathy occurred before any other symptom of hemochromatosis and in a further 5 it was one of the initial symptoms of the condition.

The most frequent and characteristic radiological changes were found in the hands, in the second, third, and fourth metacarpophalangeal joints (Fig. 5); the interphalangeal joints were much less frequently affected, usually only mildly. The most common and

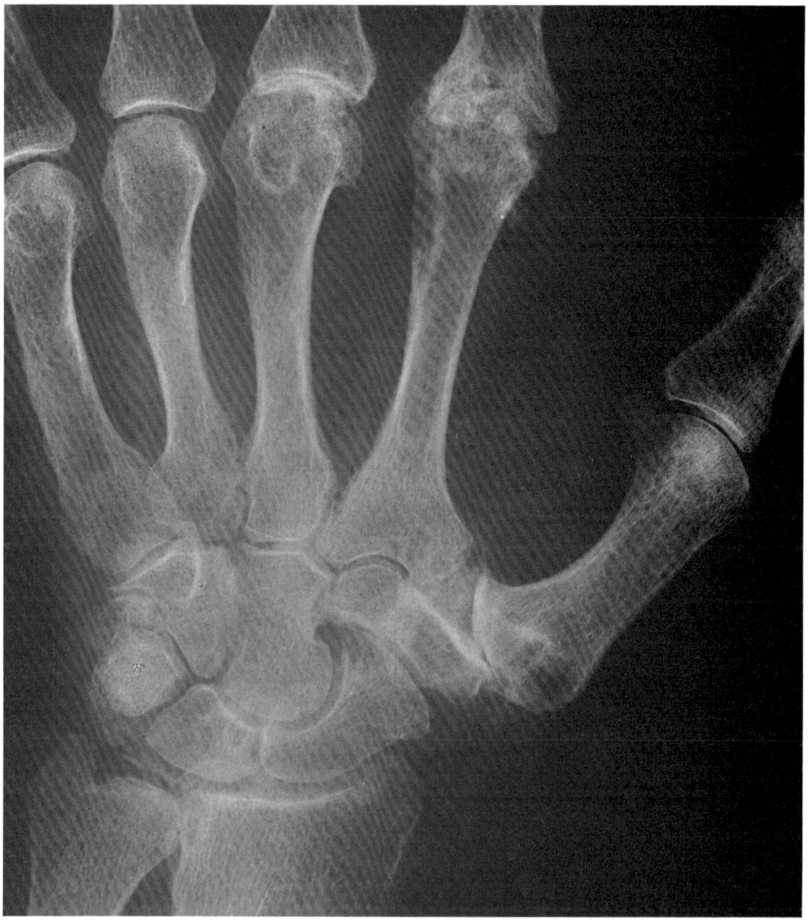

Figure 5 Male, 69 years. Hemochromatotic arthropathy for 13 years. Sclerosis, cysts, and loss of cartilage in second and third metacarpophalangeal joints and calcification in the triangular ligament.

probably the earliest feature was the development of small, 1- to 3-mm-diameter, well-defined cysts with sclerotic margins in the subarticular areas of the metacarpal heads and in the bases of the proximal phalanges. There was frequently some loss of cartilage but this was not an early feature. Juxtarticular porosis was not seen but there was frequently a reduction in the thickness of the cortex when compared with the normal range (40).

The wrists were also commonly affected. Cyst formation was found in the carpal bones in about half the patients with arthropathy and it was often associated with some loss of cartilage. Cyst formation in the lower end of the radius and ulna was common but the joint space was usually normal. The shoulders and elbows were affected in about one-fourth of the patients. The knees and hips were affected in over half the patients and differed from the changes found in the other joints in that cystic changes did not occur although loss of cartilage and lipping were common.

Chondrocalcinosis was found in over half the patients with arthropathy and in about one-fourth of those with no evidence of arthropathy. Calcification was seen in both fibrocartilage and hyaline articular cartilage. The commonest joints to be affected were the knee (36%), the wrist (20%), and the hip (10%). Calcification was also seen in the symphysis pubis, tendo Achillis, plantar fascia, and the triangular ligament of the wrist joint. In the spine, amorphous calcificiation was seen in the nucleus pulposus of the intervertebral disks as well as linear calcification in the annulus fibrosus (41). Calcification may occasionally be seen in fibrocartilage, such as the meniscus of the knee, in the absence of any underlying disease, particularly in the elderly. Calcification in hyaline articular cartilage usually indicates some underlying metabolic disorder, such as hemochromatosis, hyperparathyroidism, or hypophosphatasia.

The cause of the arthropathy in patients with hemochromatosis with iron overload is unknown. It has been suggested that it is due to the deposition of iron in the joint tissues. Certainly, hemosiderin deposits have been found in the articular cartilage and synovium of patients with hemochromatosis (42,43). The finding of a similar type of arthropathy in one patient with secondary iron overload provided supporting evidence that iron overload may be the initiating factor (39). Both the arthropathy and chondrocalcinosis found in association with hemochromatosis are progressive conditions. In a follow-up of 18 patients with hemochromatotic arthropathy over an average period of 9.6 years, Hamilton et al. (44) found that the joints affected by the arthropathy became worse due to further bone destruction and reduction in joint space and that joints previously normal became affected (Fig. 6). In no case did any improvement occur. Similarly, chondrocalcinosis increased in joints previously affected and appeared in joints previously demonstrated to be free (Fig. 7). In no case did the chondrocalcinosis improve. This deterioration was seen in spite of treatment of the hemochromatosis throughout the period of the survey.

Primary Biliary Cirrhosis

Patients with primary biliary cirrhosis may show either a destructive arthropathy of the large joints or an inflammatory polyarthritis. Clarke et al. (45), in a study of 83 patients with primary biliary cirrhosis, found 4 with an inflammatory polyarthritis closely resembling rheumatoid arthritis.

The destructive arthropathy was also seen in four of the author's patients. The radiographic appearances were those of an avascular necrosis of the subchrondral bone of the humerus and femur (Figs. 8, 9). In two patients submitted to surgery, the histological picture was of gross osteoarthritis, without any evidence of deposits of either foam cells or cholesterol. None of the patients had had local or systemic steroids to produce such a lesion, nor did they have any degree of hypercholesterolosis, a condition in which cystic bone disease has been described (46). It would seem, therefore, that primary biliary cirrhosis should be added to the list of causes of avascular necrosis of bone. The significance of the inflammatory polyarthritis found in four patients is uncertain. Since the group of patients with primary biliary cirrhosis was composed mainly of middle-aged females, an incidence of rheumatoid arthritis of approximately 5% might have been expected (47). Consequently, it was not claimed that a specific inflammatory arthritis related to primary biliary cirrhosis had been described (45). In the same group of 83 patients with primary biliary cirrhosis, 14 (17%) had clinical or radiological evidence of scleroderma, two with calcinosis circumscripta (45).

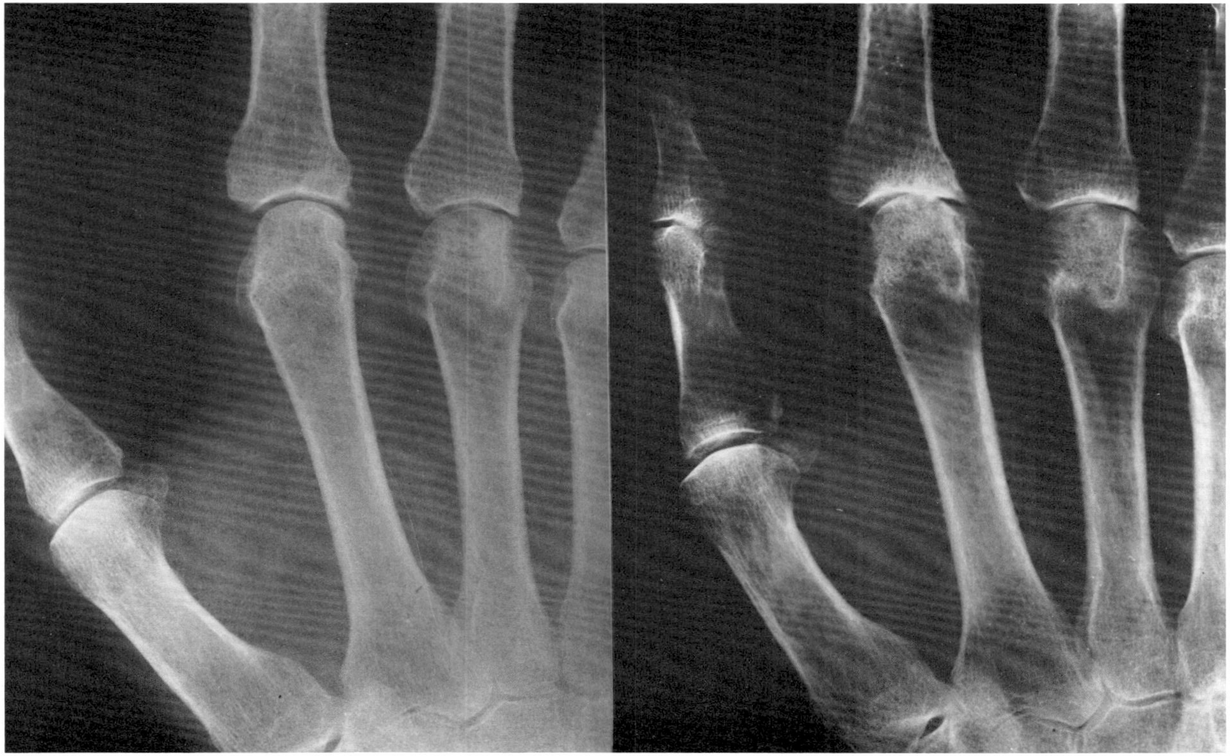

(A) (B)

Figure 6 Male, 53 years. Hemochromatotic arthropathy. (A) Small cysts in the heads of the second and third metacarpals with slight loss of cartilage in the third metacarpophalangeal joint. (B) Same patient 5 years later, showing progressive sclerosis, cyst formation, and further loss of cartilage.

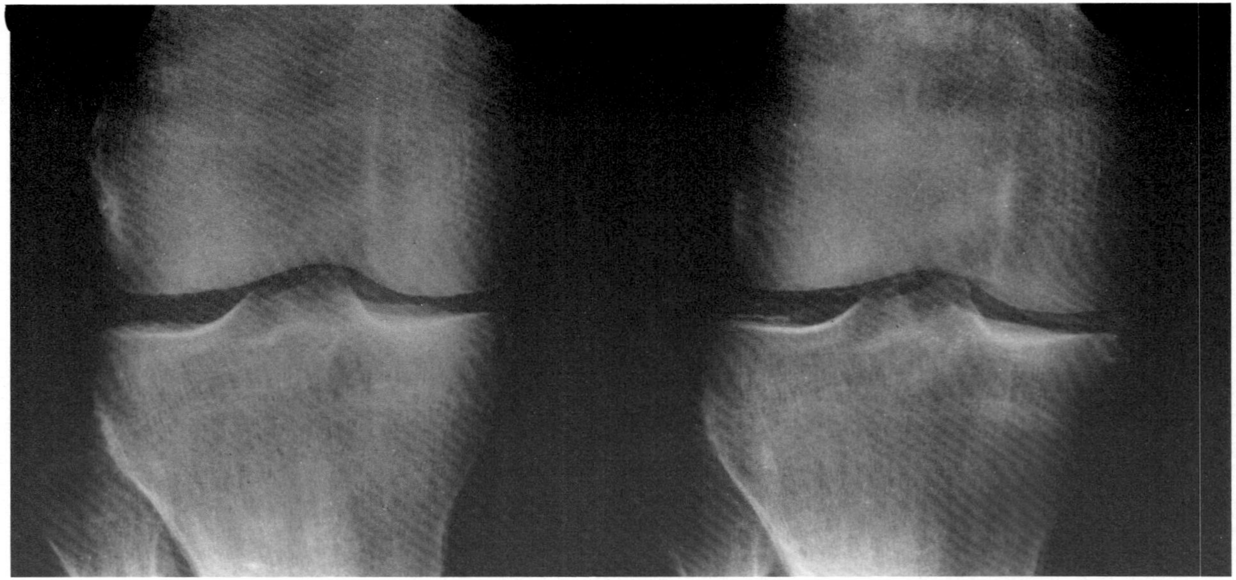

(A) (B)

Figure 7 Male, 45 years. Hemochromatotic arthropathy. (A) Right knee showing chondrocalcinosis in both hyaline and fibrocartilage. (B) Same patient 10 years later, showing marked increase in the amount of calcification, but no further loss of cartilage in the joint.

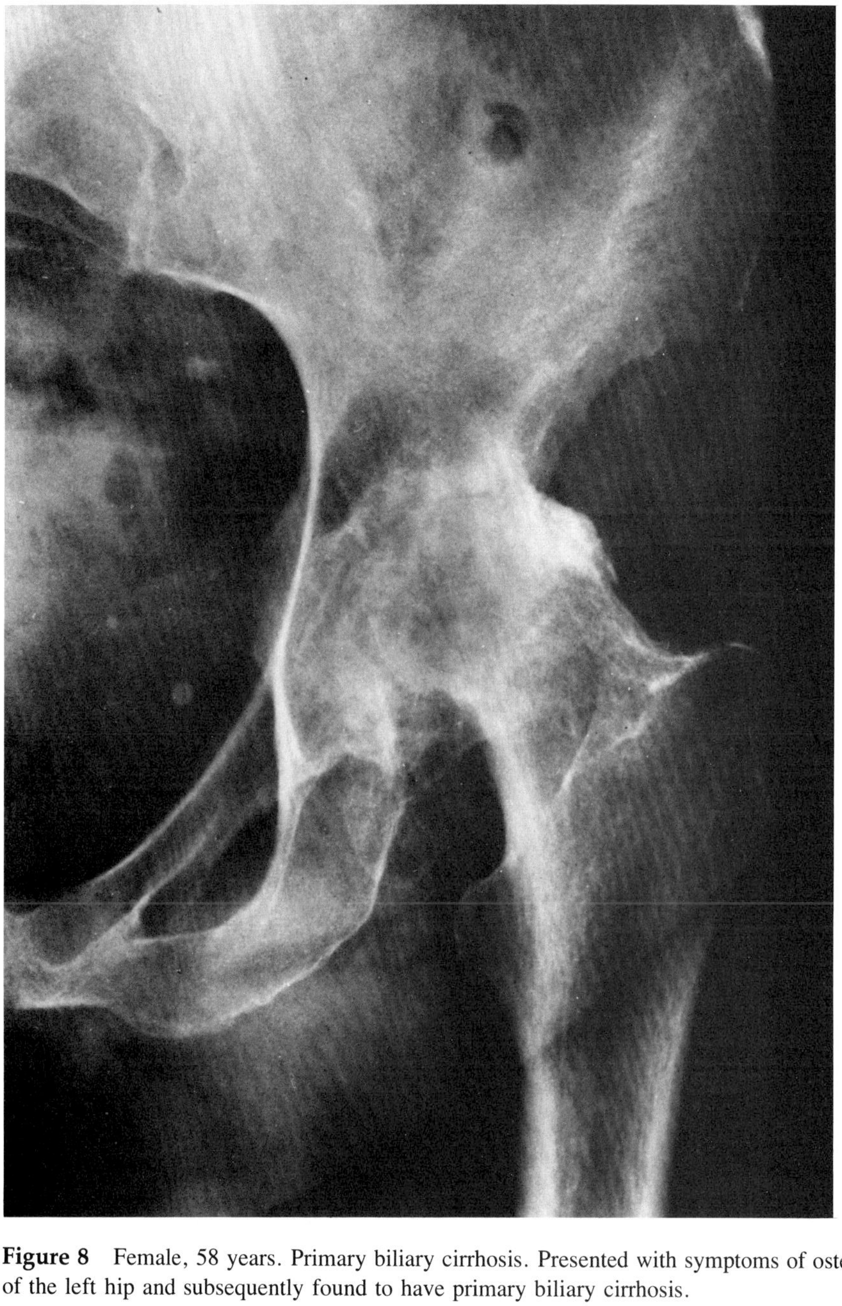

Figure 8 Female, 58 years. Primary biliary cirrhosis. Presented with symptoms of osteoarthritis of the left hip and subsequently found to have primary biliary cirrhosis.

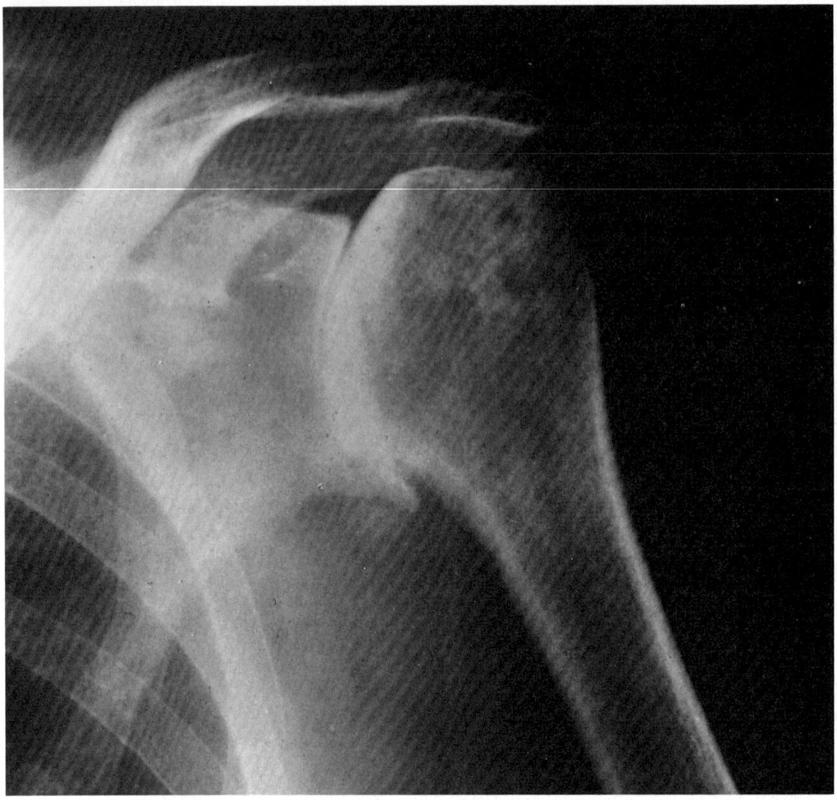

Figure 9 Female, 45 years. Primary biliary cirrhosis. Left shoulder joint showing severe arthropathy with complete loss of joint space. Sclerosis of the bones.

Metabolic Bone Disease

Osteomalacia

Renal tubular acidosis occurs in about half the patients with primary biliary cirrhosis, is less common in chronic active hepatitis and cryptogenic cirrhosis, and is rare in alcoholic cirrhosis (21). The defect usually causes no symptoms but in about 10% may cause polydypsia, polyuria, muscular weakness, nausea, and vomiting and may be the presenting feature of the disease. Severe bone pain due to osteomalacia may be present and respond to prolonged treatment with calcium and vitamin D. In some patients with primary biliary cirrhosis the osteoporosis (Fig. 10) and osteomalacia found may be due to the malabsorption associated with any obstructive jaundice (21).

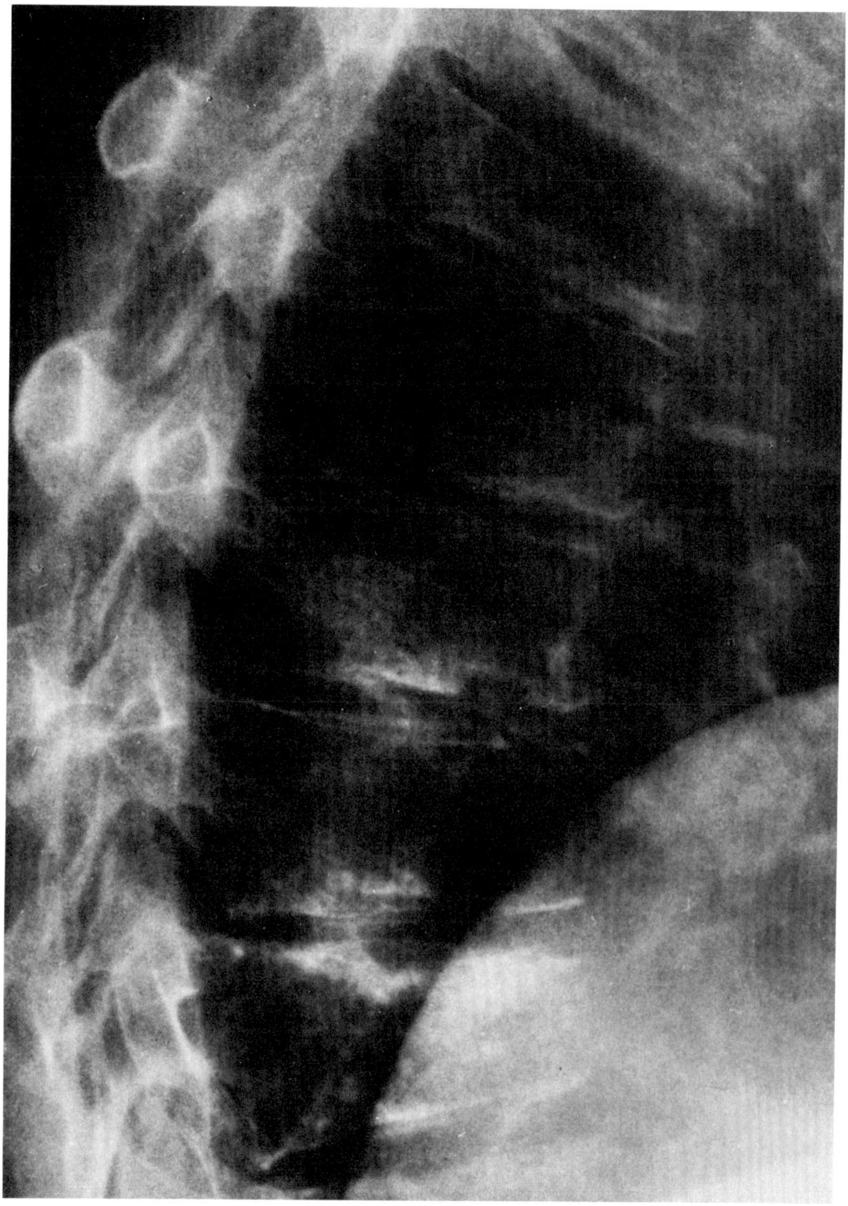

Figure 10 Male, 51 years. Primary biliary cirrhosis with severe bone pain due to osteoporosis. Lateral view of spine showing wedging of lower dorsal vertebral bodies with demineralization.

Storage Disease

Gaucher's disease, the inborn error of metabolism in which there is deficiency of the enzyme which catalyzes glucocerebroside, may present in adult life with unexplained hepatosplenomegaly. The spleen may be enormous and the liver moderately enlarged, smooth, and firm. Portal hypertension is rare.

The long bones, especially the lower end of the femora, are expanded, with failure of the normal tubulation. There may be collapse of vertebral bodies and fractures of long bones. Avascular necrosis of the subchondral bone in the large joints causes a severe arthropathy. Infection of necrotic bone may give rise to an intractable osteomyelitis which may eventually be responsible for amyloid disease and the death of the patient.

Rarely, nodular shadows may be seen in the lower zones of the lung. These have been demonstrated to be due to the presence of a large number of Gaucher's cells within the lung parenchyma (48).

Alimentary System

All parts of the alimentary system may be affected in patients with liver disease. For example, portal hypertension may produce varices affecting the esophagus, the stomach, proximal duodenum, and colon. In portal hypertension, particularly when complicated by thrombosis of the portal vein, there may be calcification within the portal vein or within the clot itself. This calcification and the subsequent ascites may be seen on the plain radiograph of the abdomen.

Cystic Fibrosis of the Pancreas

The extrahepatic manifestations of cystic fibrosis, affecting chiefly the lungs and small bowel, are generally more important than those affecting the liver. However, as the overall survival improves due to better treatment of the lung condition, the importance of the hepatic and biliary disease is likely to become greater.

Cystic fibrosis of the pancreas is transmitted as an autososomal recessive with an incidence of about 1 per 2400 Caucasians in the United Kingdom (49). The exact nature of the abnormality is not known, but in all patients there is an obstruction of the ducts from the exocrine glands of the pancreas associated with abnormal secretions containing a high electrolyte content and with impaired mucociliary transport mechanisms. In the liver there are eosinophilic concretions in the intrahepatic ducts, with focal biliary cirrhosis found in 20–25% of patients at autopsy. In the first 3 months of life, periportal changes including excess mucus in bile duct radicles or the lining epithelial cells are more common. Focal biliary cirrhosis occurs later. The combination of these lesions is pathognomonic (50).

Fatty change in the liver occurs in about 30% of patients in spite of vitamin supplements, adequate diet, and replacement of pancreatic enzymes, but cirrhosis develops in only about 4–6% of patients. Occasionally, however, cirrhosis may be the initial clinical manifestation of cystic fibrosis. The mechanism of its production is unknown and it may occur in the presence of normal hepatic enzyme levels, although cystic fibrosis patients tend to show increasing enzyme levels with advancing age. The liver may be small or large. Severe liver disease with hepatic cell failure is rare. Portal hypertension and bleeding varices occur in only 2–4% of the patients with fibrocystic disease. Patients with bleeding varices may improve dramatically with a portocaval shunt, which is the treatment of choice.

All patients with liver disease have symptoms from their pancreatic disease. Failure of pancreatic exocrine function leads to malabsorption and that of endocrine function to diabetes mellitus. Recurrent attacks of acute pancreatitis may occur when there is some residue of exocrine function. Pancreatic calcification is seen in less than 2% of the patients (50), and in our experience is similar to that seen in chronic pancreatitis. Its presence does not correlate with symptoms or signs referrable to the pancreas.

Apart from those babies dying with meconium ileus or its complications, more than 95% of deaths from cystic fibrosis are due to the respiratory complications of the disease. The clinical and radiological features of the respiratory and other alimentary abnormalities are well known and will not be further discussed.

Inflammatory Bowel Disease

There is an association, which is poorly understood, between certain liver and biliary disorders and inflammatory disease of the bowel, mainly ulcerative colitis and Crohn's disease. Toxins in the portal vein or bacteria absorbed through diseased bowel may cause liver disease or there may be an autoimmune attack on both bowel and liver, but at the moment there is inadequate evidence for both hypotheses.

Sclerosing cholangitis is an uncommon condition with a variable age of onset. It presents with signs of obstructive jaundice or recurrent cholangitis. Usually, both the intra- and extrahepatic bile ducts are affected by an irregular narrowing with intervening lengths of focal dilatation (Fig. 11). The bile ducts, instead of tapering toward the periphery, may show a premature narrowing or a beaded appearance with dilatations distal to the strictures. The disease may be considered to be primary if there is no history of bile duct surgery, calculi, carcinoma, or inflammatory bowel disease (51). Many patients with secondary sclerosing cholangitis have ulcerative colitis. Of 43 patients with sclerosing cholangitis (52), 28% had ulcerative colitis, while among 1474 patients with ulcerative colitis, 0.8% had sclerosing cholangitis. Ulcerative colitis is the commonest disease to be associated with sclerosing cholangitis. Whereas Whelton (53) claimed that the activity of the bowel disease did not appear to bear any relationship to the development of duct sclerosis, Kern (54) found the associated colitis to be usually severe and chronic. Resection of bowel does not affect the progress of the biliary disease (54).

Ulcerative colitis is also related to cirrhosis. Holdsworth et al. (55) found ulcerative colitis in 5% of 519 cirrhotics and Golding et al. (21) found that 4.6% of their patients with active chronic hepatitis, primary biliary cirrhosis, or cryptogenic cirrhosis had ulcerative colitis. The incidence of ulcerative colitis in the general population is 0.1%. Liver disease presenting at the same time as the colitis is usually an active cryptogenic cirrhosis, whereas when it presents after a long history of chronic relapsing colitis it is usually a postnecrotic type of cirrhosis. Progression from an active to a postnecrotic cirrhosis has been demonstrated and it is possible that the same etiological factor can precipitate both the colitis and the cirrhosis, but that one or the other may be clinically dominant at the start. One patient has been reported who had Crohn's ileitis 3 years before the onset of active chronic hepatitis (21).

Peptic Ulceration

The increasing use of endoscopy in gastrointestinal hemorrhage has revealed that many patients with cirrhosis bleed not from varices but from peptic ulcers. While patients with cirrhosis and portal hypertension frequently bleed from esophageal and gastric varices,

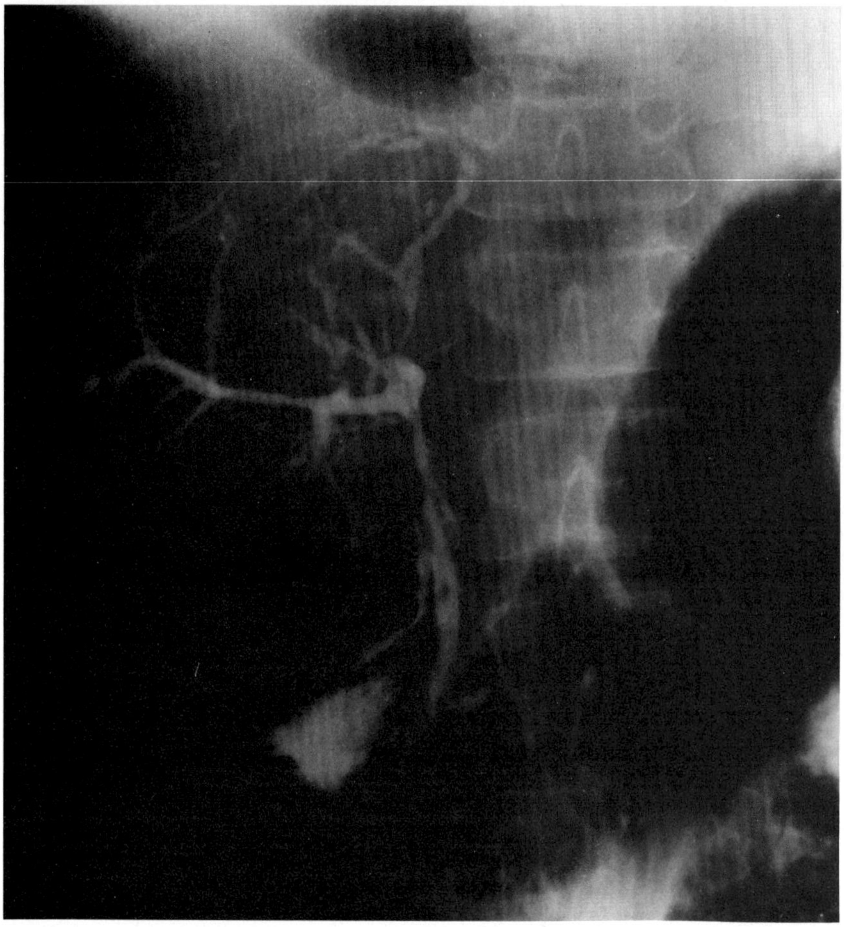

Figure 11 Male, 40 years. Sclerosing cholangitis with ulcerative colitis. Endoscopic canulation of pancreatic and common bile duct. Multiple intra- and extrahepatic strictures of the bile ducts with intervening dilatation of mild degree.

there is in this group an increased incidence of peptic ulceration. Waldram et al. (56), in a series of 50 patients with portal hypertension and hematemesis or melena, have found that in 16% the bleeding had been from ulceration of the esophagus, stomach, or duodenum. In a cirrhotic patient bleeding should not be assumed to have arisen from varices unless other causes have been excluded by endoscopy.

References

1. Chalmers AH and Laws JW: Extrahepatic manifestations of liver disease. In *Recent Advances in Radiology and Medical Imaging*, Lodge T and Steiner RE (Eds). Churchill, Livingstone, London, 1979.
2. McKinney B: *Pathology of the Cardiomyopathies*. Butterworths, London, 1974.

3. Oram S: *Clinical Heart Disease*. Heinemann, London, 1971.
4. Martini GA: Extrahepatic manifestations of cirrhosis. *Clin Gastroenterol 4*:439, 1975.
5. Loyke HF: Reduction of hypertension after liver disease. *Arch Intern Med 110*:45, 1962.
6. Berthelot P, Walker IG, Sherlock S, Reid L: Arterial changes in the lungs in cirrhosis of the liver. Lung spider naevi. *N Engl J Med 274*:291, 1966.
7. Hutchison DCS: Alpha$_1$-antitrypsin deficiency and pulmonary emphysema: the role of proteolytic enzymes and their inhibitors. *Br J Dis Chest 45*:139, 1973.
8. Kravath RE, Scarpelli EM, Bernstein J: Hepatogenic cyanosis: arteriovenous shunts in chronic active hepatitis. *J Pediatr 78*:238, 1971.
9. Martini GA, Baltzer G, Arndt H: Some aspects of circulatory disturbances in cirrhosis of the liver. *Prog Liver Dis 4*:231, 1972.
10. Doyle FH, Read AE, Evans KT: The mediastinum in portal hypertension. *Clin Radiol 12*:114, 1961.
11. Felson B: *Chest Roentgenology*, 1st ed. W. B. Saunders, Philadelphia, 1973.
12. Warren R, Trewby PN, Laws JW, Williams, R: Pulmonary complications in fulminant hepatic failure. Analysis of serial radiographs from 100 consecutive patients. *Clin Radiol 29*:363, 1978.
13. Trewby PN, Warren R, Contini S, Crosbie WA, Wilkinson SP, Laws JW, Williams R: The incidence and pathophysiology of pulmonary edema in fulminant hepatic failure. *Gastroenterology 74*:859, 1978.
14. Hansoti RC and Shah NJ: Cirrhosis of liver simulating congenital cyanotic heart disease. *Circulation 33*:71, 1966.
15. Hutchinson DCS, Sapru RP, Sumerling MD, Donaldson GWK, Richmond J.: Cirrhosis, cyanosis and polycythemia: multiple pulmonary arteriovenous anastomoses. *Am J Med 45*:139, 1968.
16. Bashour FA, McConnell T, Miller WF: Circulatory and respiratory changes in patients with Laennecs cirrhosis of the liver. *Am Heart J 74*:569, 1967.
17. Cohen C: Liver pathology in alpha$_1$-antitrypsin deficiency. A review. *S Afr Med J 49*:849, 1975.
18. Berg NO and Eriksson S: Liver disease in adults with alpha$_1$-antitrypsin deficiency. *N Engl J Med 287*:1264, 1972.
19. Chrispin AR and Lessof L: The chest radiograph in juvenile cirrhosis (active chronic hepatitis). *Br J Radiol 38*:685, 1965.
20. Turner-Warwick M: Fibrosing alveolitis and chronic liver disease. *Q J Med 37*:133, 1968.
21. Golding PL, Smith M, Williams R: Multisystem involvement in chronic liver disease. Studies on the incidence and pathogenesis. *Am J Med 55*:772, 1973.
22. Metz RJ and Tompkins RK: The hepato-renal syndrome. *Surg Gynecol Obstet 143*:297, 1976.
23. Epstein M, Berk DP, Hollenberg NK, Adams DF, Chalmers TC, Abrams HL, Merrill JP: Renal failure in the patient with cirrhosis. *Am J Med 49*:175, 1970.
24. Bloodworth JMB and Summers SC: Renal glomerulosclerosis associated with cirrhosis of the liver: cirrhotic glomerulosclerosis. *Fed Proc 17*:429, 1958.
25. Koppel MH, Coburn JW, Mims MM, Goldstein H, Boyle JD, Rubini ME: Transplantation of cadaveric kidneys from patients with hepatorenal syndrome. *N Engl J Med 280*:1367, 1969.
26. Barnardo DE, Baldus WP, Maher FT: Effects of dopamine on renal function in patients with cirrhosis. *Gastroenterology 58*:524, 1970.
27. Lieberman E, Salinas-Madrigal L, Gwinn JL, Brennan LP, Fine RN, Landing BH: Infantile polycystic disease of the kidneys and liver: clinical, pathological and radiological correlations and comparison with congenital hepatic fibrosis. *Medicine (Baltimore) 50*:277, 1971.
28. Gleason DC, McAlister WH, Kissane J: Cystic disease of the kidneys in children. *Am J Roentgenol 100*:135, 1967.
29. Caroli J: Diseases of the intrahepatic biliary tree. *Clin. Gastroenterol 2*:147, 1973.
30. Hatfield PM and Pfister RC: Adult polycystic disease of the kidneys and liver (Potter Type II). *JAMA 222*:1527, 1972.

31. Anderson D and Tannen RL: Tuberous sclerosis and chronic renal failure. Potential confusion with polycystic kidney disease. *Am J Med 47*:163, 1969.
32. Hatfield PM, Scholz FJ, Wise RE: Congenital diseases of the gallbladder and bile duct. *Semin Roentgenol 11*:235, 1976.
33. Blyth H and Ockendon B: Polycystic disease of the kidneys and liver presenting in childhood. *J Med Genet 8*:257, 1971.
34. Bosniak MA and Ambos MA: Polycystic kidney disease. *Semin Roentgenol 10*:133, 1975.
35. Lang EK: Roentgenologic assessment of medullary cysts. *Semin Roentgenol 10*:145, 1975.
36. Schumacher HR: Hemochromatosis and arthritis. *Arthritis Rheum 7*:41, 1964.
37. Delbarre H: Les manifestations ostéo-articulaires de l'hémochromatose. *Presse Med 72*:2973, 1964.
38. Wardle EN and Patton HT: Bone and joint changes in hemochromatosis. *Ann Rheum Dis 28*:15, 1969.
39. Daymock IW, Hamilton EBD, Laws JW, Williams R: Arthropathy of hemochromatosis. *Ann Rheum Dis 29*:469, 1970.
40. Morgan DB, Spiers FW, Pulvertaft CN, Fourman P: The amount of bone in the metacarpal and phalanx according to age and sex. *Clin Radiol 18*:101, 1967.
41. Bywaters EGL, Hamilton EBD, Williams R: The spine in idiopathic hemochromatosis. *Ann Rheum Dis 30*:453, 1971.
42. Sheldon JH: *Haemochromatosis*. Oxford University Press, London, 1935.
43. Walker RJ, Dymock IW, Ansell ID, Hamilton EBD, Williams R: Synovial biopsy in hemochromatosis arthropathy. *Ann Rheum Dis 31*:98, 1972.
44. Hamilton EBD, Bomford A, Laws JW, Williams R: The natural history of arthritis in idiopathic hemochromatosis—progression of the clinical and radiological features over ten years. *Q J Med 50*:199, 1981.
45. Clarke AK, Galbraith RM, Hamilton EBD, Williams R: Rheumatic disorders in primary biliary cirrhosis. *Ann Rheum Dis 37*:42, 1978.
46. Ansell BM and Bywaters EGL: Histiocytic bone and joint disease. *Ann Rheum Dis 16*:503, 1957.
47. Lawrence JS: Prevalence of rheumatoid arthritis. *Ann Rheum Dis 20*:11, 1961.
48. Jackson DC and Simon G: Unusual bone and lung changes in a case of Gaucher's disease. *Br Med J 38*:698, 1965.
49. Wood RE, Boat TF, Doershuk CF: Cystic fibrosis. *Am Rev Respir Dis 113*:833, 1976.
50. Schwachman H: Gastrointestinal manifestations of cystic fibrosis. *Pediatr Clin North Am 22*:787, 1975.
51. Larsen CR, Scholz FJ, Wise RE: Disease of the biliary ducts. *Semin Roentgenol 11*:259, 1976.
52. Warren KW, Athanassiades S, Monge JI: Primary sclerosing cholangitis. A study of 42 cases. *Am J Surg 111*:23, 1966.
53. Whelton MJ: Sclerosing cholangitis. *Clin Gastroenterol 2*:163, 1973.
54. Kern F Jr: Hepatobiliary disorders in inflammatory bowel diseases. *Prog Liver Dis 5*:575, 1976.
55. Holdsworth CD, Hall EW, Dawson AM, Sherlock S: Ulcerative colitis in chronic liver disease. *Q J Med 34*:211, 1965.
56. Waldram R, Davis M, Nunnerley H, Williams R: Emergency endoscopy after gastrointestinal hemorrhage in 50 patients with portal hypertension. *Br Med J 4*:94, 1974.

33

Ascites and Peritoneal Fluid

Louis Kreel*
London Hospital Medical College
London, England

Introduction

Whereas the plain film of the abdomen will show only large amounts of fluid with any accuracy and requires considerable skill in interpretation, the newer imaging modalities, particularly computed tomography (CT), are capable of displaying small amounts of peritoneal fluid and even localized peritoneal thickening. It is nevertheless important and interesting to review the classical radiological signs of ascites, to assess their rationale and reliability, and to consider radiological management in the context of modern imaging methods.

Although radiology has developed and changed with great rapidity, the pathology, the relevant anatomy, and the concepts of fluid formation have progressed but slowly. The clinical associations of ascites, theories of formation, and the anatomy of the peritoneal cavity have been under review for centuries with the erudite studies of Von Recklinghausen, Schmidt, and Starling in the last century as outstanding examples. Von Recklinghausen (1,2) was concerned with the microanatomy of the peritoneum and described direct communications between the peritoneum and the lymphatics, which he called stomata and stigmata. Schmidt (3) examined the composition of pathological fluid collections in the peritoneum, and Starling (4,5) considered the relationship between osmotic and hydrostatic pressures in the formation of lymph.

Similar aspects have been investigated more recently (6–8). The mechanisms and pathways of fluid absorption from the peritoneum have become clearer with emphasis on

**Present affiliation:* Queen Mary's Hospital for the East End, London, England

both the mechanical and complex biochemical factors concerned in the formation of ascites.

The peritoneal cavity is not a simple large space but is subdivided into well defined compartments, fluid flowing from one area to another often preferentially and influenced by a number of factors. This dynamic aspect of peritoneal anatomy has been emphasized by Meyers (9). The importance of the retroperitoneal adipose tissue in the recognition of abdominal pathology has been made clear by Whalen et al. (10,11). Over the years, there has been controversy as to the value and mechanism of the radiological signs of abdominal fluid; with the help of numerous contributors (12–16), this has now been resolved.

The modern radiologist using ultrasonography (US) and CT can diagnose abdominal fluid collections with confidence, where only in the last decade his colleagues were groping among the shadows. Yet, overconfidence is still fraught with hazards, for there are a number of conditions that can simulate fluid collections, even on computed tomography. The new knowledge must be carefully integrated with the old, due cognizance being given to the physiology, anatomy, and pathology of peritoneal fluids.

Types of Peritoneal Fluid

Traditionally, peritoneal fluid has been described as transudates, exudates, pus, hemorrhagic, or chylous.

Transudates are clear and colorless with a protein content of less than 3.0 g per 100 ml and a density of less than 1.016 (17,18). Ascitic transudates are produced in long-standing heart failure, constrictive pericarditis, chronic renal failure, hypoproteinemic anasarca, and of course in hepatic cirrhosis and the Budd-Chiari syndrome.

Exudates have a high density (greater than 1.016) with a higher total protein content (greater than 3.0 g per 100 ml), are often yellowish, but may be hemorrhagic. Metastatic infiltrations of the peritoneum and chronic inflammatory disease such as tuberculosis are the commonest causes. Metastatic malignancy may also produce exudates or chylous ascites by obstruction to the draining vascular and lymphatic pathways. The ascites of chronic pancreatitis usually has a total protein content of about 3.0 g per 100 ml, often much more and may be serous, sanguinous, or chylous (19,20).

Pus in the peritoneal cavity is found in acute peritonitis, the commonest primary condition being pneumococcal and hemolytic streptococcal peritonitis occurring in young children (21). In secondary peritonitis due to perforation of a hollow viscus or from adjacent acute inflammation, particularly of the appendix or ischemic bowel, the responsible organism is usually *Escherichia coli*. The amount of peritoneal fluid is relatively small, while the local abdominal signs and symptoms are a prominent feature.

Hemorrhage into the peritoneal cavity is usually caused by trauma to the liver or spleen, whether from a surgical or radiological procedure or an accident. In acute hemorrhage, blood replacement and localization of the site of bleeding are the prime concern, with the radiological signs of peritoneal fluid of minor importance. In subacute or chronic hemorrhage, it is crucial to distinguish extraperitoneal, especially retroperitoneal, from peritoneal fluid, and computed tomography becomes invaluable. However, the tissue attenuation of blood in the peritoneal cavity alters with time and therefore produces variable radiological signs. Initially, blood has relatively high values similar to those of the liver or spleen and will become visible in the upper abdomen only after contrast enhancement of the liver. Blood is then shown as a curvilinear zone interposed between liver and inner margin of the upper abdominal wall. After 2–3 days the blood absorbs water and is then clearly delineated as a localized fluid collection if loculated, or with appearances similar to free ascites. The liver and spleen are usually uniformly displaced from the inner margin of the upper abdomen by a lower-density zone. Extraperitoneal hemorrhage develops similar attenuation characteristics and can be localized on anatomical criteria.

Sanguinous ascites can occur with malignancy, tuberculosis, and chronic pancreatitis. The quantity of blood is variable and the ascitic fluid may be bright reddish or dark, the appearances being similar on computed tomography or ultrasonography.

Chylous ascites is relatively uncommon compared with the other fluid accumulations in the peritoneal cavity. Almost 100 years ago the condition had been described as fluid of yellowish white color with a milky appearance, with delicate elementary particles and only very few cells shown on microscopy and with a threefold increase of fat particles after a fatty meal (22). Causes include trauma to the cysterna chyli and thoracic duct; infiltration by malignancy, especially from pancreatic carcinoma; thrombus in the left subclavian vein; and tuberculous lymphadenitis. In theory the low density of chylous ascites should produce characteristically low attenuation features on computed tomography.

Ascites is thus the accumulation of fluid in the peritoneal cavity. It may be confined to it, or may be associated with hydrothorax or with generalized anasarca. The fluid may be serous, sanguinous, or chylous and may be an exudate or transudate.

Anatomy of the Peritoneal Cavity

The peritoneal cavity, bounded by the mesothelial lined peritoneum, is divided into two major compartments, the upper abdominal cavity and the lower pelvic cavity. The abdominal cavity is further subdivided into five intercommunicating but nevertheless distinct spaces, this by the mesocolon above, the root of the mesentery below, and the ascending and descending colon on each side.

The *supramesocolic space* lies above the mesocolon and contains the main bulk of the liver, the spleen, and the stomach. It is further subdivided into the right and left subhepatic spaces and into the right and left subphrenic spaces, the latter by the falciform ligament.

The *lesser peritoneal sac* lies behind the stomach and communicates with the greater peritoneal cavity by the foramen of Winslow, which lies just above the duodenal bulb anterior to the portal vein.

The *inframesocolic space* is divided by the root of the mesentery, which passes craniocaudally from left of the midline to the right iliac fossa, separating a larger left compartment from a smaller right. Each inframesocolic space is thus bounded by the colon above and laterally, the mesentery medially, and the brim of the pelvis below.

The *right and left paracolic gutters* lie lateral to the ascending and descending colon, respectively, the right being larger and deeper than the left. The right paracolic gutter may have folds across (23), the hepatorenal and cecal folds, which can impede the flow of fluid. On the left side the phrenicocolic ligament acts as an even more effective impediment between the supramesocolic space above and the left paracolic gutter below.

The *pelvic cavity* is separated from the abdominal cavity by the brim of the pelvis posteriorly and the line of the iliac arteries laterally.

Movement of Fluid

Experimental studies and clinical observations (9) support the contention that there is a natural pathway for the flow of fluid in the abdomen. Gravity will inevitably lead to accumulation in the pelvis. With sufficient fluid in the pelvis or when the patient is horizontal, fluid will preferentially pass upward along the larger right paracolic gutter to the supramesocolic space and around the lateral margin of the liver. Fluid is most likely to become locculated in the posterior extension of the right subhepatic space (Morison's pouch). In the left paracolic gutter the fluid is usually confined below the phrenicocolic ligament.

Other factors also operate in the movement of fluid within the abdomen. Changes in upper abdominal pressure with respiration were noted more than a century ago (24) and substantiated more recently (25). The pressure in the lower abdomen was found to be three times that in the upper abdomen in the upright position (17). Other factors influencing the distribution of abdominal fluid include the site of origin of the fluid, the rapidity of its formation, presence of adhesions, position of intra-abdominal organs and their attachments, and the amount of fluid present. There is no doubt, for instance, that with marked ascites, fluid is clearly visible in the lesser sac on CT.

Ultrasonography has shown that in the supine patient, fluid first collects around the tip of the liver and later along the flank and lateral liver margin (17). With considerable ascites, fluid is found throughout the abdomen except posteriorly, where the liver rests on the anterior pararenal fascia. In only 1 of 14 cases did US show fluid around the spleen, although with CT the finding of perisplenic fluid is much more frequent.

Goldberg et al. (26), using US by the A mode in cadaver experiments, could detect as little as 100 ml of fluid introduced into the peritoneal cavity. With position change in patients with larger amounts of ascites, altered patterns could be shown whenever free fluid was present. The smallest amount of ascitic fluid seen by CT to date was in a patient with cirrhosis complicated by a hepatoma in the left lobe of the liver. The fluid lay along the posterolateral wall of the liver and was associated with thickening of the right pararenal fascia and the left paracolic peritoneum (Fig. 1).*

The other important application of anatomy of the abdomen relates to detection of fluid on plain films (13,15,27). The properitoneal or extraperitoneal fat line lies between the internal oblique abdominal muscle and the lateral outer wall of the colon, the "flank stripe." When fluid accumulates in the paracolic space lateral to the colon, the distance between the flank stripe and the intraluminal cecal gas increases (Fig. 2).

*The following codes will be used in figures throughout this chapter and is listed here for easy reference. A, aorta; B, bladder; C, colon; D, duodenum; GB, gallbladder; H, hemorrhage; I, inferior vena cava; J, jejunum; K, kidney; L, liver; M, mesentery; P, pancreas; Ps, psoas muscle; St, stomach; Sp, spleen; Ut, uterus; V, vertebral body.

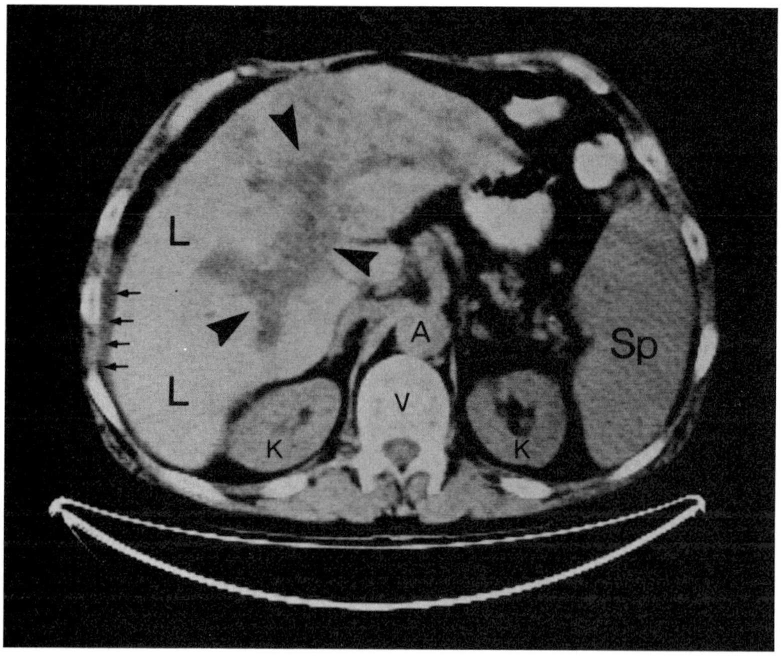

Figure 1A Minimal ascites. Cirrhosis with hepatoma and widening of the porta hepatis (arrowheads). The fluid is visible adjacent to the posterior margin of the liver (short arrows).

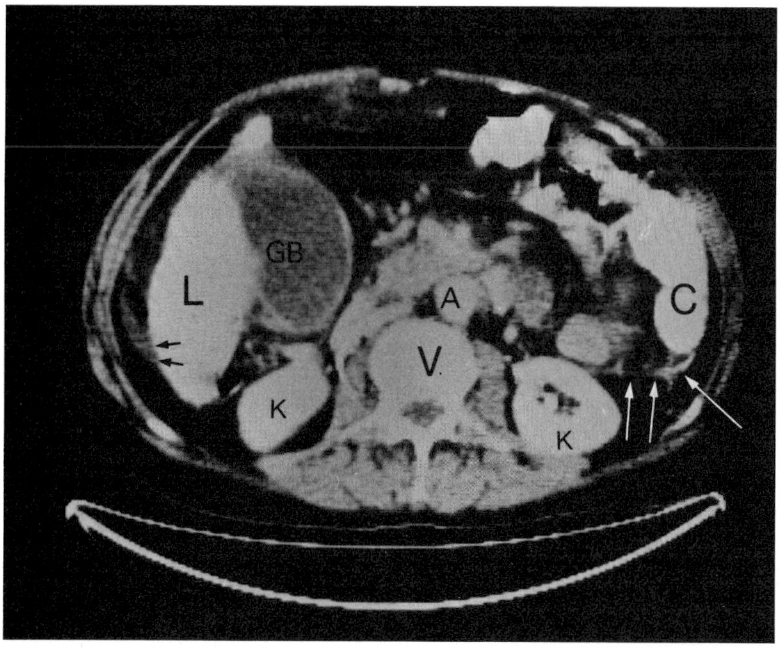

Figure 1B In addition to the minimal ascites (black arrows), there is slight thickening of the left pararenal space (white arrows).

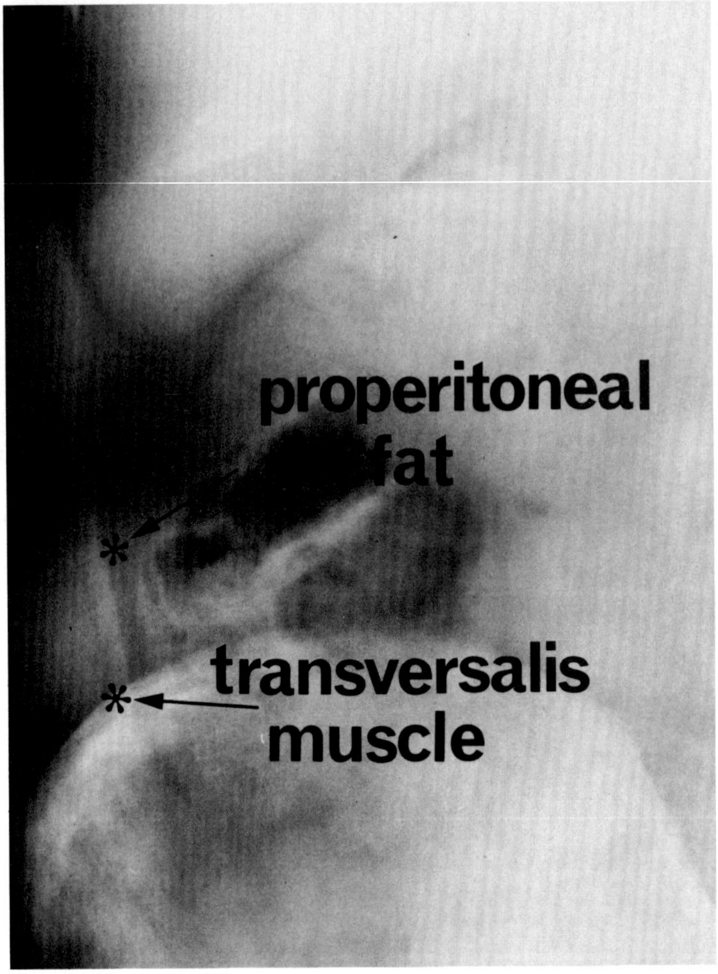

Figure 2 The properitoneal (extraperitoneal) fat layer is seen medial to the soft tissue density of the transversalis muscle.

Aspects of Physiology

An admirable summary of the important concepts concerning the accumulation of fluid in the peritoneal cavity and of possible transport mechanisms is given by Rusznyyak et al. (28).

Cavities lined with serous membranes are *not* part of the lymphatic system and the minimal amount of fluid normally present, less than 20 ml, differs significantly from that of lymph extracellular fluid. No direct communications between lymphatics and the peritoneal cavity have been demonstrated and the stomata and stigmata of Von Recklinghausen (1) are now considered to be artifacts. More credence is given to the presence of microscopic holes—the suctorial organs described in 1878 (29)—on the diaphragmatic aspect of the peritoneum. When the diaphragm contracts in inspiration, these holes become wider and longer, decreasing the pressure in them and aspirating fluid.

On expiration the holes are compressed, squeezing the substances in them through the mesothelial layer into the lymphatics.

A number of different elements are to be considered in describing absorption from the peritoneal cavity, including red blood cells, protein and colloid molecules, and water and crystalloids.

Absorption of corpuscular elements from the peritoneum proceeds slowly. It has been shown that only about one-sixteenth of infused blood is absorbed in 6 hr (30). Absorption is promoted by a high intra-abdominal pressure, vigorous respiration, and good muscle tone. In infants most red cells were found to be absorbed from the peritoneal cavity in 7–8 days (31).

Corpuscular elements are absorbed almost entirely from the peritoneal surface of the diaphragm, hence the increased absorption in animal experiments when they are held in the head-down position. Neither the parietal peritoneum nor the mesentery play a significant part in corpuscular absorption (32). It is also of considerable interest that the lymph originating from the lymphatics of the diaphragm is transported by the right lymphatic trunks and not the thoracic duct (33), bearing in mind that the right lymphatic trunks are inconstant, independent of each other, and empty separately into the large veins of the neck.

Absorption of colloids and protein molecules occurs through the lymphatics. It would appear that protein from blood plasma continually diffuses into the peritoneal cavity, to be removed by the lymphatics. The protein level in the peritoneum thus reflects a dynamic equilibrium and has been estimated at nearly 80 g, or about 75% of the circulating albumin per day.

Absorption of crystalloids and water is mainly by blood capillaries. Hypertonic and hypotonic solutions infused into the peritoneal cavity are rapidly rendered isotopic by the water diffusing into or out of the peritoneal cavity, with equilibrium being established on both sides of the peritoneal membrane. Glucose diffuses more slowly, so that equilibration is a slower process. It is interesting that radioactive crystalloids infused into the peritoneal cavity appeared more quickly in the urine than in the thoracic duct (34).

Ascites Formation in Cirrhosis

It has been shown repeatedly that large amounts of fluids injected into the peritoneal cavity can be rapidly absorbed by the peritoneal lymphatics, yet in hepatic cirrhosis there can be a large accumulation of ascites. The factors influencing the formation of ascites include those acting locally in the peritoneal cavity and the more general factors associated with an overall increase in water of the body, largely through renal mechanisms.

The *local factors* operate by upsetting the equilibrium between the hydrostatic and osmotic pressures, as propounded by Starling in 1894 (5). Intravascular osmotic pressure is reduced by the low serum albumin of hepatic cirrhosis and associated increase in plasma volume, while the hydrostatic pressure is increased largely by a postsinusoidal obstruction of the portal circulation. Experimentally, the most effective method of producing ascites is by suprahepatic constriction of the inferior vena cava and is its cause in the Budd-Chiari syndrome. With the increased portal pressure, fluid weeps through the surface of the liver and through the serosal surface of the intestine.

Lymph drainage acts as an important pathway for the removal of ascitic fluid and its accumulation implies a decompensation of this mechanism. It has been suggested (35) that the thoracic duct inflow into the left subclavian vein can act as a relative stenosis and may be a critical factor in the formation of ascites.

Retention of body water can be due to a number of renal factors. Blood flow through the kidneys can be diminished because of internal shunting of blood; glomerular filtration rate is then reduced and sodium reabsorption increased. Sodium reabsorption is further increased by a stimulation of aldosterone excretion in cirrhosis, through a renin-angiotensin mechanism.

The formation of ascites, particularly in liver disease, is therefore complex and depends on local factors—increasing hydrostatic pressure and a relative incompetence of the drainage mechanism—as well as a generalized retention of fluid through hormonal action and altered renal function.

Causes of Ascites

A wide variety of conditions can be associated with ascites, including hepatic cirrhosis and the Budd-Chiari syndrome. Constrictive pericarditis and chronic congestive cardiac failure are also notable causes. In these conditions blood flow through the suprahepatic portion of the inferior vena cava is impeded. In renal failure, nephrosis, and nutritional hypoalbuminemia, dilution of plasma proteins occurs. In Meigs' syndrome, ovarian tumors such as fibroma, granulosa cell tumor, and theca cell tumor are associated with ascites and a hydrothorax. In recent years, chronic pancreatic ascites has become a recognized entity (the ascitic amylase remaining high even though the serum amylase is normal), and it is noteworthy that this condition responds to a small dose of radiotherapy, 400–500 rad given to the pancreas (36). Other causes include mesothelioma, peritoneal metastases, and tuberculosis, chylous ascites having been mentioned previously. Rare causes include those found in children, such as in galactosemia and neonatal obstruction of the urethra caused by valves.

Conventional Radiology of Ascites

Chest Film

It is now almost mandatory to start radiological investigations of the abdomen with a chest film. Although not many previously undiagnosed conditions will be uncovered by the chest film in the investigation of ascites, important information may be missed without it. A large pleural effusion, especially on the right side, may be a feature of chronic cardiac failure, liver disease, or the Meigs' syndrome. More important, pulmonary or bone metastases may be present or a bronchial carcinoma may be visible. An absent breast shadow would have similar implications.

In chylous effusions a superior mediastinal mass with tracheal displacement, usually to the left, may be visible and be due to lymph nodes or a goiter. Other common findings are a raised right hemidiaphragm from an enlarged liver or the upwardly displaced diaphragm due to the ascites itself. Pericardial calcification associated with constrictive pericarditis or a large pericardial effusion are other possible conditions to be detected, and very rarely the pleural plaques of asbestosis, an indication of possible peritoneal mesothelioma. Occasionally, mediastinal lymphadenopathy, whether due to lymphoma, carcinoma, or tuberculosis, may become the vital clue to the etiology of the ascites.

Most or all of these conditions will involve the liver either indirectly through congestion or directly by metastases.

Plain Abdominal Films

The diagnosis of fluid in the peritoneal cavity by plain film radiography is difficult, unreliable, and usually possible only after at least 400 ml of fluid have accumulated. Traditionally, the plain film features of ascites are divided into direct and direct signs.

The *indirect signs* depend on the increased bulk of the abdomen or the effects of displacement and, in practice, seem to be more imaginary than real. On statistical analysis (15,37) most of the indirect signs were found to be unhelpful or were valid only when the volume of ascite fluid exceeded 800–1000 ml.

1. *Diffuse haziness* implies poor visualization of the abdominal tissue planes with a low overall contrast or underexposure. In most cases these appearances are due to the large size of the patient or a poor radiographic technique.
2. *Bulging of the flank* certainly does occur with gross ascites but also with meteorism and adiposity. The main criticisms of this sign are its unreliability and the gross ascites required to produce it.
3. *Indistinct psoas margins*, blurred or nonvisualized, signify retroperitoneal fluid and not ascites (38). Absence of the left psoas margin is not too uncommon in normal individuals.
4. *Poor definition* of intra-abdominal organs is most frequently seen with poor or deficient fat planes, especially in children, rather than with ascites or may be produced by poor radiographic technique, such as movement blurring.
5. *Erect position density increase* compared with the supine film should, on a priori grounds, be a correct sign. Yet, in practice, it is more likely to occur with a pendulous anterior abdominal wall or from technical causes.
6. *Separation of small-bowel loops* is yet another sign that owes more to the powers of imagination than to reality and is not borne out by statistical analysis (39).
7. *Gas-containing small bowel* is said to float, while fluid-filled bowel should sink in the supine position of a patient with ascites. This earlier observation could not be substantiated by CT.

To dismiss the indirect radiographic signs of ascites in such cavalier fashion requires justification which has been based on careful observations in a number of reliable studies (15,37–39), and more recently on CT, which displays ascites, fat planes, bowel loops, and abdominal contours with exceptional clarity. It thus became clear that the indirect plain film signs of ascites cannot be substantiated. The direct signs, although not unequivocal, are less prone to observor error and considerably more reliable.

The *direct signs* of intraperitoneal fluid on plain abdominal radiographs include medial displacement of the lateral liver border (12), linear soft tissue density between the properitoneal fat and the margin of the colon (40), obliteration of the hepatic angle (14,38), and the "dog-ears" sign in the pelvis (16,37).

1. *Medial displacement of the lateral liver border* was called Hellmer's sign by Frimman-Dahl (13). Although its validity has been questioned by some authors, it is entirely vindicated by experimental and clinical study (17) and by the unequivocal appearances on CT. Ascitic fluid ascends preferentially via the right paracolic gutter, accumulating in the superior mesocolic space around the margins of the liver (9). Normally, the liver has tissue attenuation values higher than the other abdominal organs and some 60–80 Hounsfield units greater than ascitic fluid. The displacement of the lateral liver edge from the upper abdominal wall can thus be imaged, confirming Hellmer's sign, which is positive in about 80% of cases with ascites.
2. The *hepatic angle* is normally visible in approximately 80% of patients (15) and obliterated in ascites (14). There has been considerable discussion as to exactly why the hepatic angle is seen. Whalen et al. (10) maintain that the liver indents the

posterior retroperitoneal adipose tissue, thus causing the hepatic angle to become visble. Whatever the true explanation, it has now been confirmed by many studies that the loss of this angle is a valid sign of ascites on the plain film of the abdomen, in adults as well as in children (37,41).

3. *Medial displacement of the cecum and ascending colon* with lateral displacement of the properitoneal fat line has produced a useful sign of ascites (16). The ascent of fluid in the paracolic gutters leads to increased separation of the properitoneal fat line from the air-outlined colonic lumen and is seen as a band of soft tissue density more than 2 mm wide; it was present in over 90% of patients with ascites (15). Both Hellmer's sign and the displacement of the lateral wall of the ascending or descending colon can be brought out by total body opacification, especially if combined with conventional tomography. The increased density of the liver and the wall of the colon in the parenchymal phase of contrast enhancement allows their clear demonstration within a fluid collection (Fig. 3).

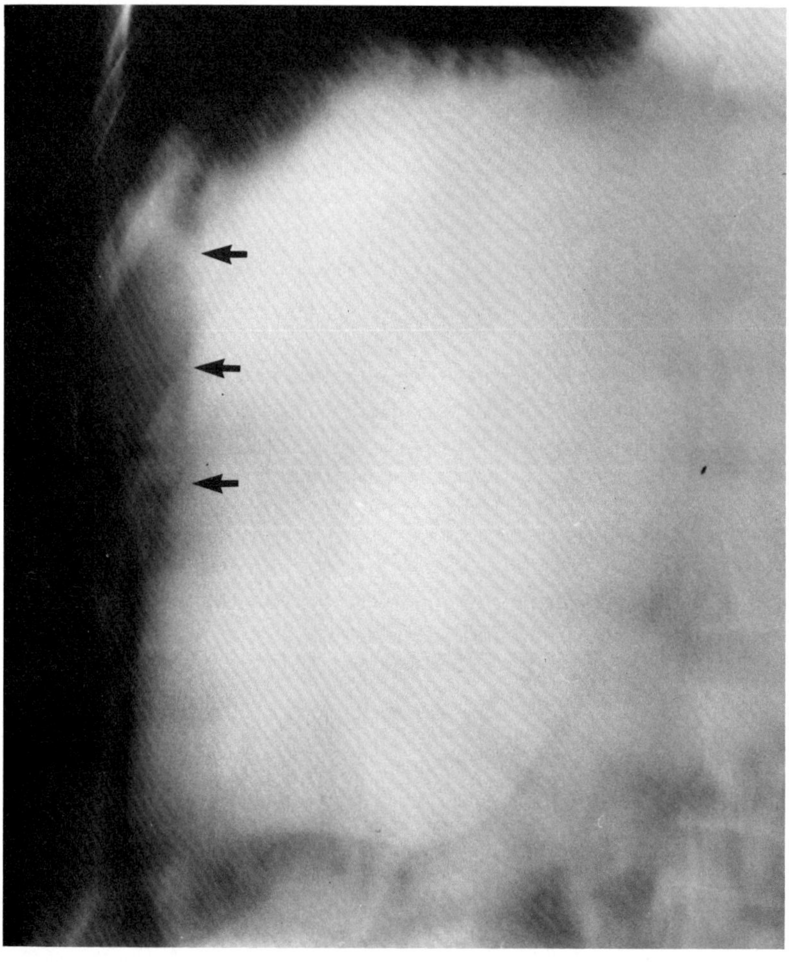

Figure 3 Hellmer's sign (arrows) brought out in the parenchymal phase of "total body opacification."

4. *Fluid in the pelvis*. Because the pelvis is the lowest part of the peritoneal cavity, fluid may be discerned there down to the level of the peritoneal line (40). It was McCort (38) who drew attention to the appearance of earlike protrusions extending laterally above the bladder shadow, caused by fluid in the retrovesical, pararectal space. He called this the "dog-ears sign."

Ultrasonographic Diagnosis of Ascitic Fluid

Even for the experienced radiologist the plain film diagnosis with lesser amounts of ascites is difficult or even illusory. With US and CT, interpretation and subjective opinion have largely been removed, these modalities providing a reliable objective assessment of the presence and quantity of ascites (Fig. 4). A number of interesting observations could be made with US (17). In cadavers after an injection of 40 ml into the peritoneum, fluid could be shown around the tip of the liver; with 800 ml, fluid was present around the lateral liver margin; and with 1600 ml, it was found anterior to the liver as well. Posteriorly, where the liver lies on and above the right kidney, fluid is usually absent. Further observed was the relative paucity of fluid around the spleen. A distinction between a transudate and exudate can often be made by US (Fig. 5).

Computed Tomography

The overall sensitivity of CT far surpasses the other imaging modalities. Given adequate perirenal and properitoneal adipose tissue, even the normal lateroconal fascia can be demonstrated (42). The lateroconal fascia extends forward from the line of fusion of the two renal fasciae to merge into the parietal peritoneum anterolateral to the ascending or descending colon (9) (Fig. 6). Fascial thickening is easily visible, particularly in chronic pancreatitis, lymphoma, peritonitis, and aortic dissections.

A personal review of 30 cases of ascites in a variety of conditions, including hepatic cirrhosis, abdominal malignancy, and renal failure have led to the following conclusions. In the supine position ascitic fluid, even in small amounts, is most easily seen along the lateral margin of the liver (Fig. 7). It shows up clearly because of the large difference in tissue attenuation between fluid and liver. With slightly more fluid it is also seen toward the anterior aspect of the liver and can also appear in the left pararenal space (Fig. 8), at the angle between the parietal peritoneum and the lateroconal fascia. With some conditions, such as pancreatic carcinoma, the fluid may initially be more prominent on the left side than around the liver (Fig. 9). The porta hepatis may become prominent at an early stage (Fig. 10) and later, as accumulated fluid displaces the liver from the abdominal wall, the fluid is also seen in the lesser sac anterior to the pancreas (Fig. 11). As the ascites becomes more massive, fluid is seen surrounding the liver and spleen, but its quantity around the spleen and behind the liver remains relatively small (Fig. 12).

Gross ascites produces a remarkable appearance, contrasting with the denser liver and spleen and filling the periphery of the upper abdomen to produce a gap between the quadrate and right lobes, the portal vein being clearly visible (Fig. 13). With CT there is no doubt about ascitic fluid commonly accumulating between the spleen and the lateral abdominal wall, influenced by the relative size of the liver and spleen. With a small liver fluid surrounds it entirely, and when associated with splenomegaly is obvious on the left side as well (Fig. 14). With a normal or enlarged liver and small spleen the fluid accumulation is usually more prominent around the liver than the spleen but by no means

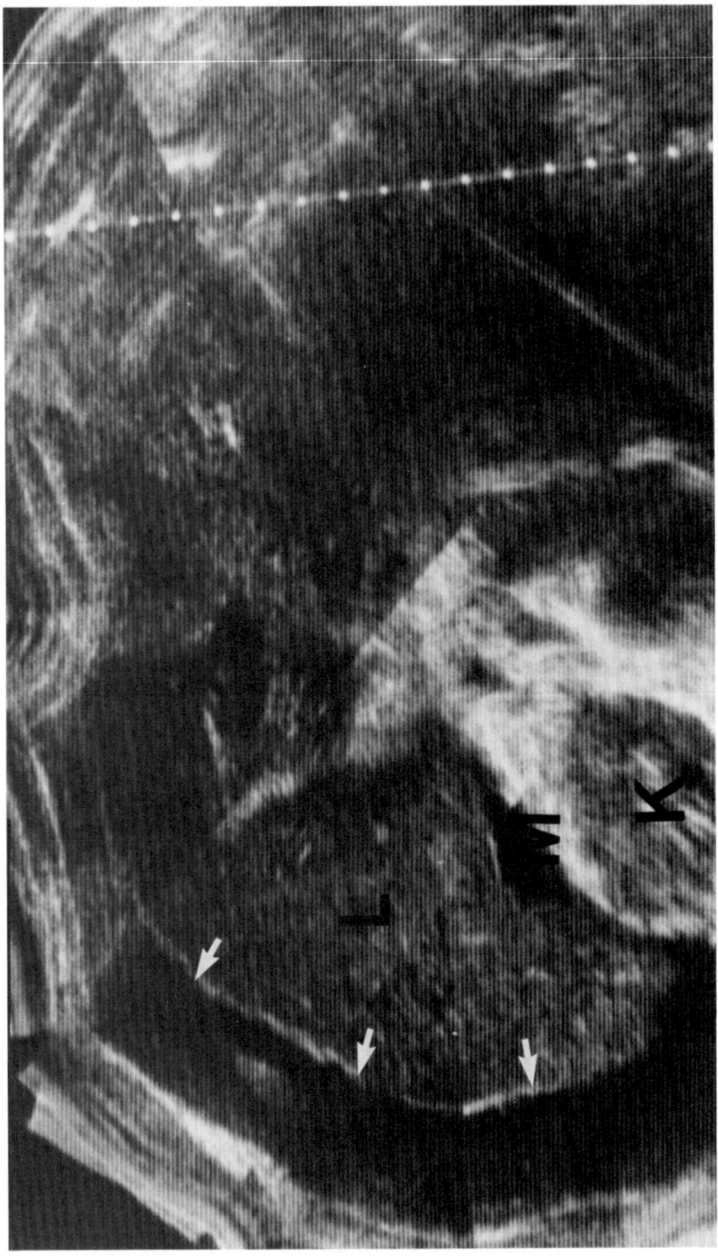

Figure 4
(A)

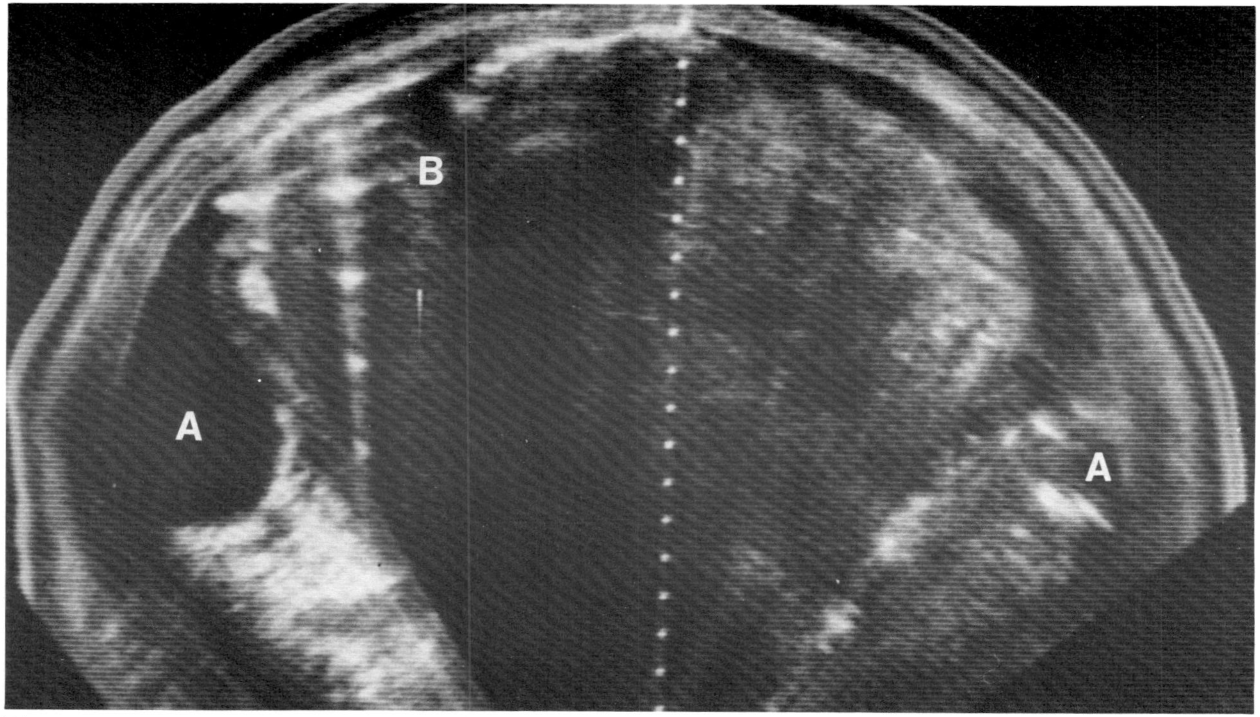

(B)

Figure 4 US shown transudate in cirrhosis. (A) Transverse section, liver (L) surrounded by ascites (arrows). Fluid in Morrison's pouch (M) above right kidney (K). (B) Lower transverse section. Ascites (A) in paracolic gutters. Bowel (B) shows fanlike arrangement, as seen with transudates. (From Gefter WB, Arger PH, Edell SL: Sonographic patterns of ascites. *Semin. Ultrasound*, 1981.)

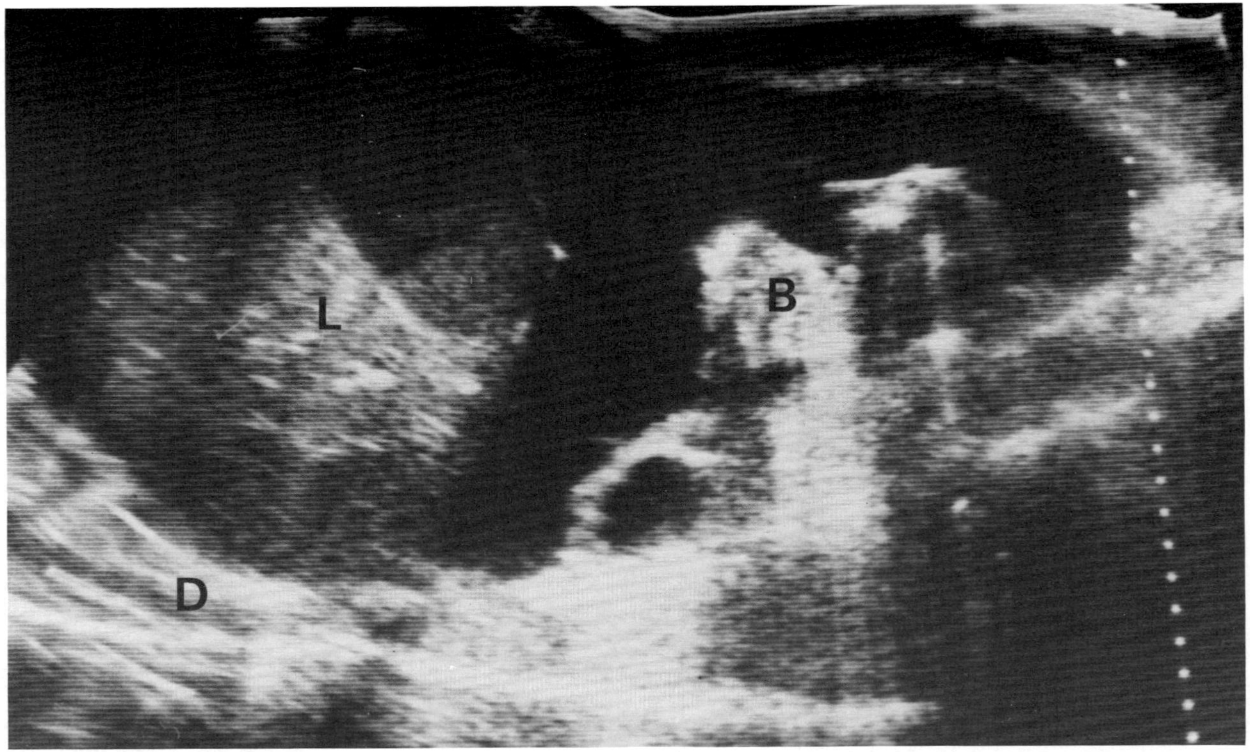

(A)

Figure 5 Exudate with ovarian carcinoma. (A) Sagittal section 9 cm right of midline shows massive ascites. Posteriorly the liver (L) adheres to the diaphragm (D). Matted bowel loops (B).

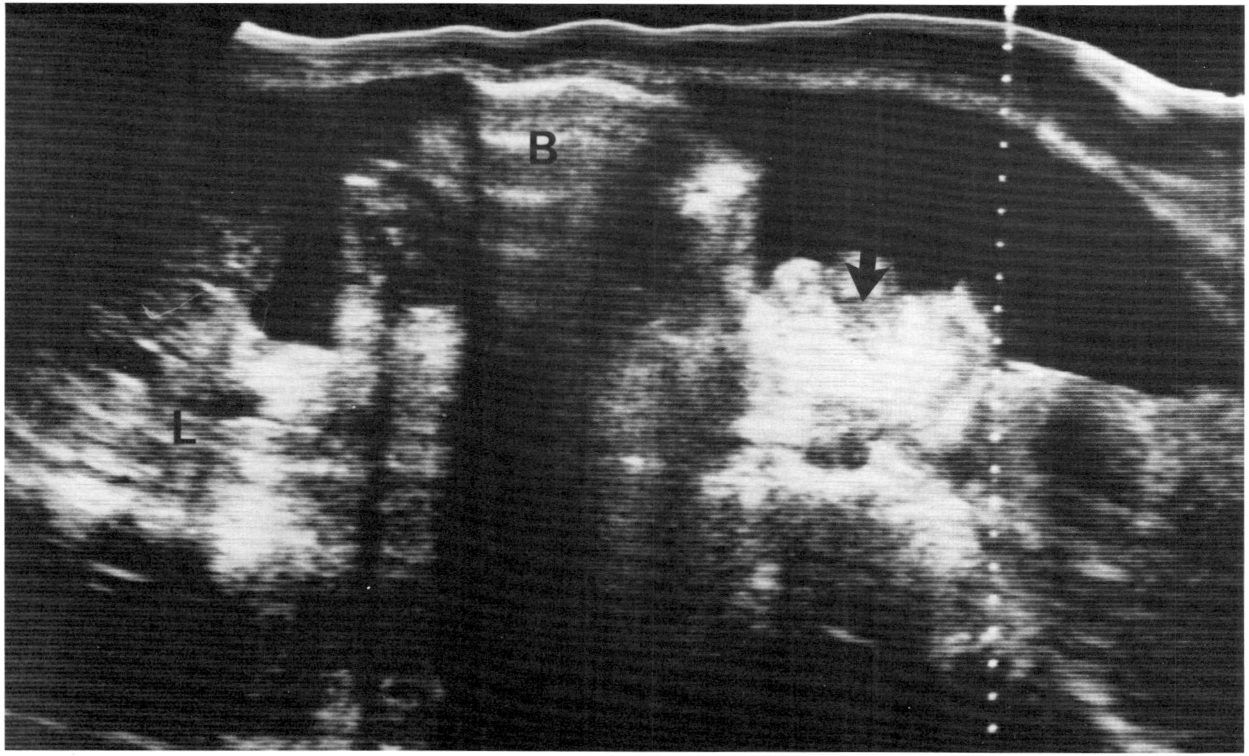

(B)

Figure 5 (continued)

(B) Sagittal section nearer the midline shows floating bowel (B) superiorly and matted, probably tumor-involved bowel (arrow) inferiorly, behind the ascites. (From Gefter WB, Arger PH, Edell SL: Sonographic patterns of ascites. *Semin. Ultrasound*, 1981.)

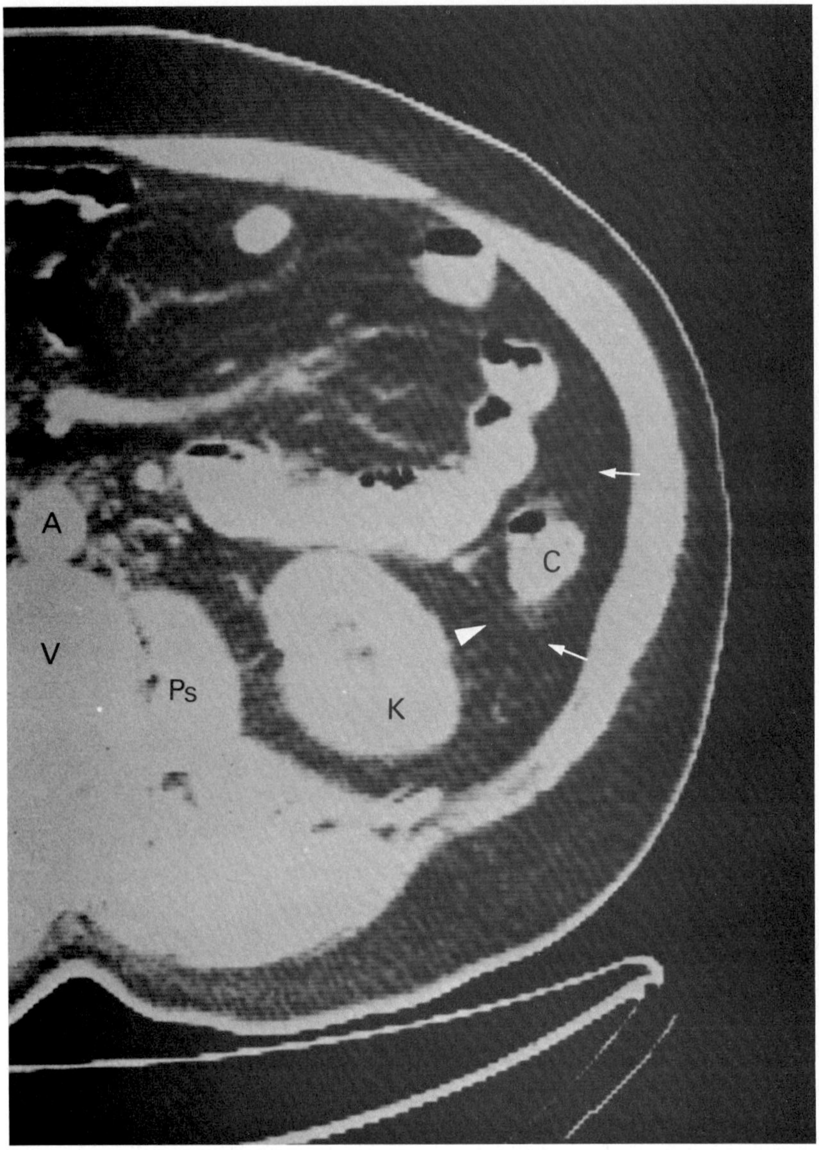

Figure 6 Normal lateroconal (white arrows) and anterior pararenal fascia (arrowhead) visible on CT in an individual with well-developed fat planes.

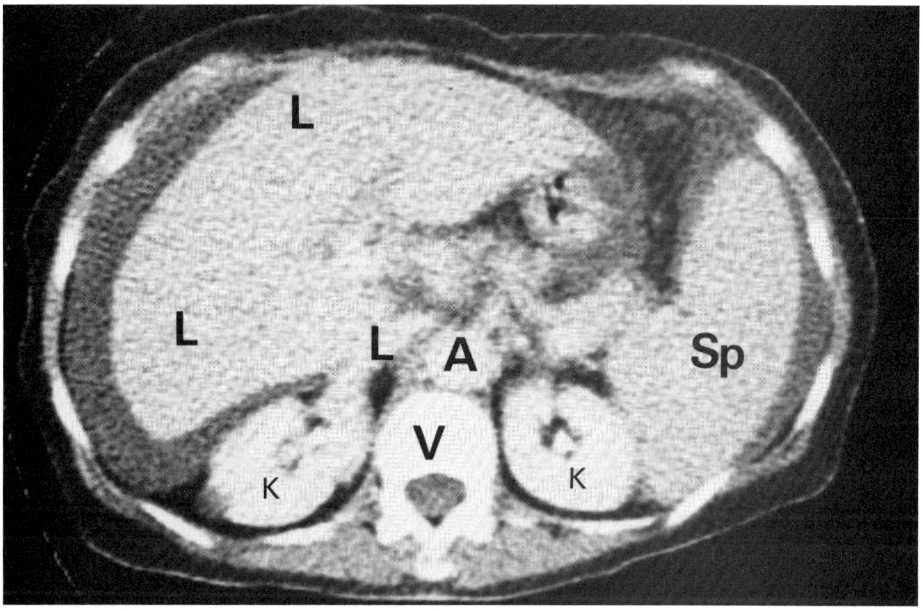

Figure 7 Ascitic fluid is clearly visible on CT because the liver usually has higher attenuation values than other abdominal organs and considerably more than ascitic fluid (liver 6–80 Hounsfield units, ascitic fluid 1–2 H units). A small cyst is shown on the right kidney.

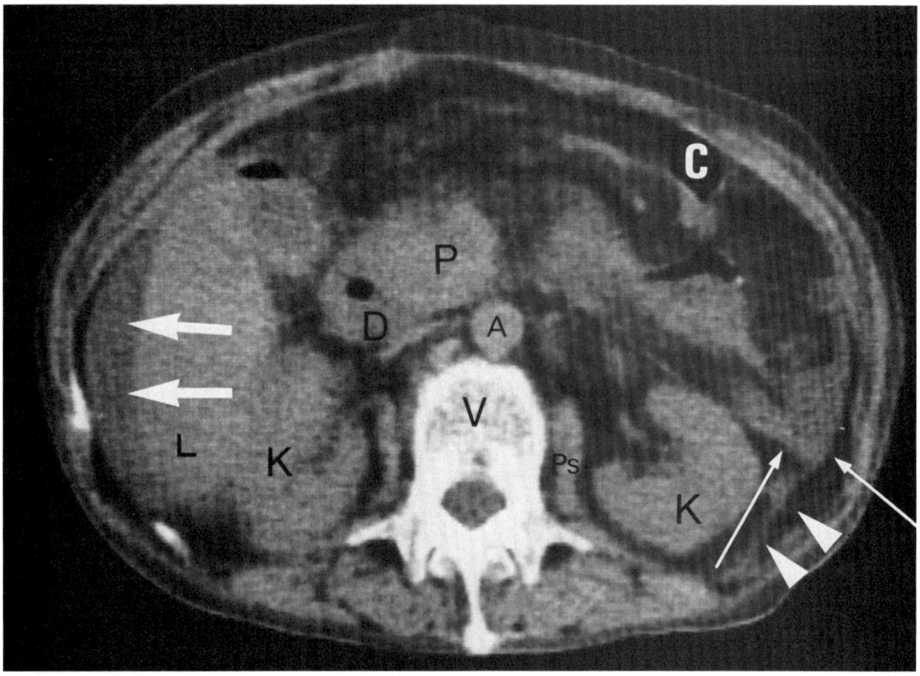

Figure 8 Case of carcinoma of the pancreas. Fluid accumulates lateral to the liver (large arrows) and is often also seen anterior to the left pararenal space (small arrows). The left posterior pararenal fascial plane (arrowheads) is thickened.

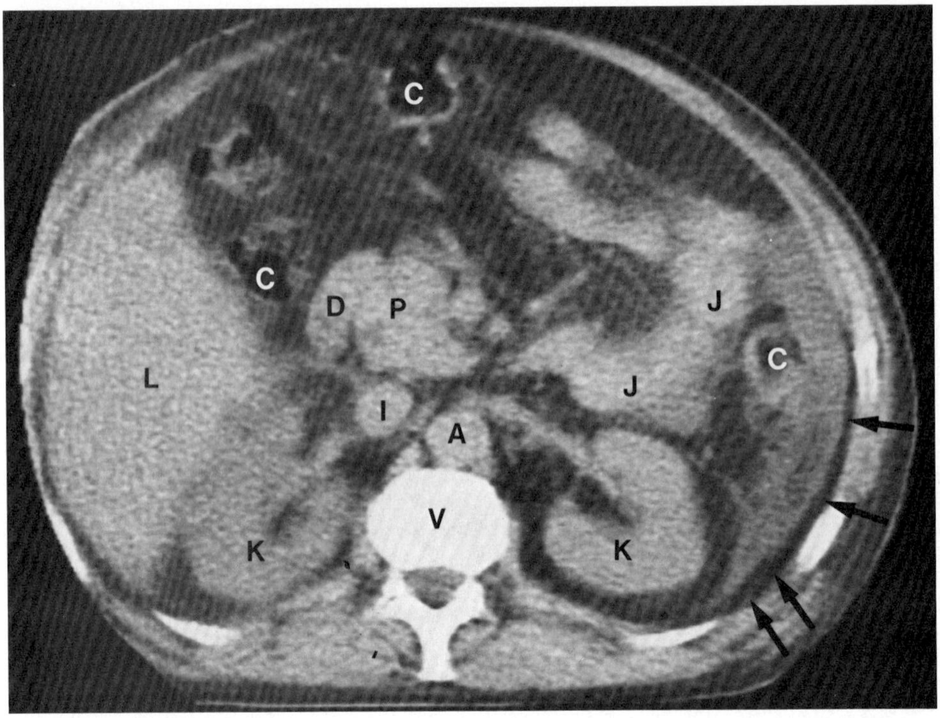

Figure 9 In some conditions, such as pancreatic carcinoma, the ascites may appear more prominently on the left, anterior and lateral to the perirenal fascia (arrows) than around the liver.

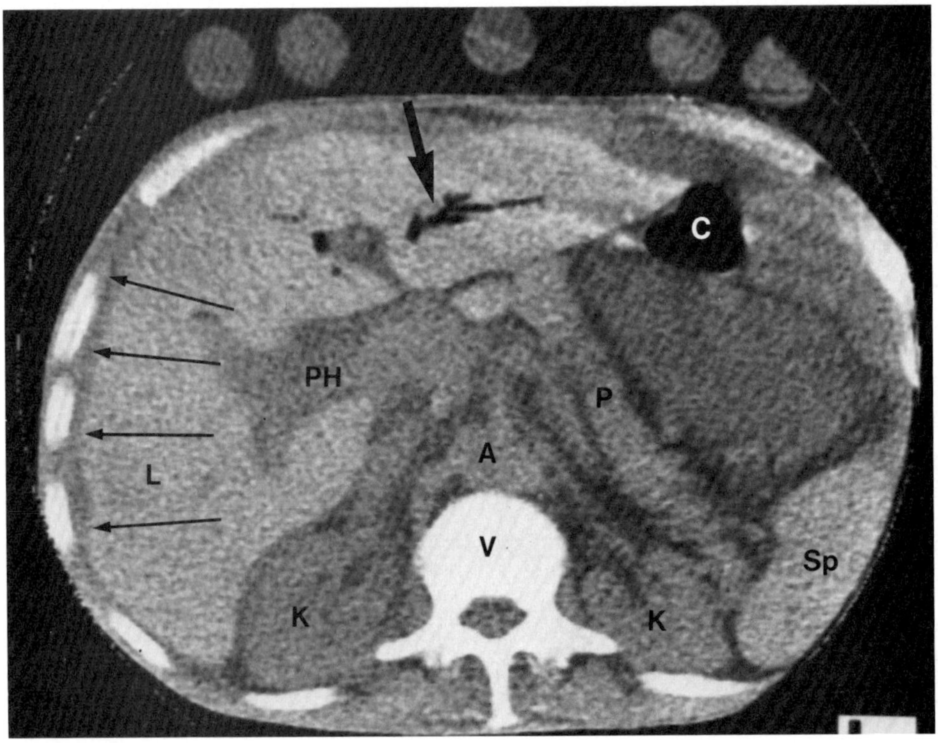

Figure 10 The porta hepatis (PH) is prominent even though there is only a small amount of fluid around the liver (small arrows). Gas is present in bile ducts (arrow) because of a choledochojejunostomy.

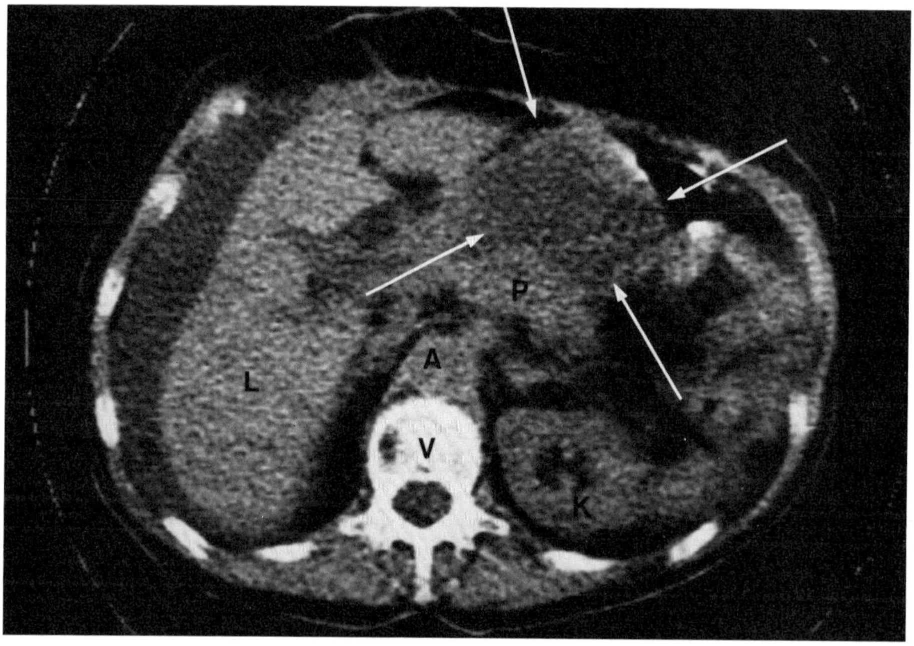

Figure 11 The ascitic fluid is most marked around the liver, which is displaced away from the abdominal wall but is also visible in the subhepatic space anterior to the pancreas (arrows).

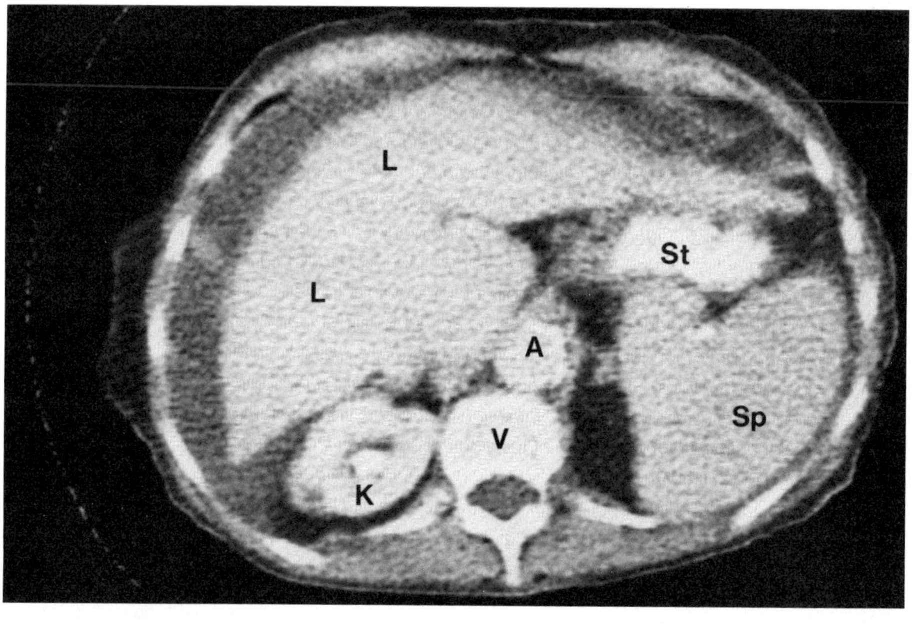

Figure 12 Marked ascites with more fluid around the liver than around the spleen but very little behind the liver, where the posterior margin is still in contact with the right kidney.

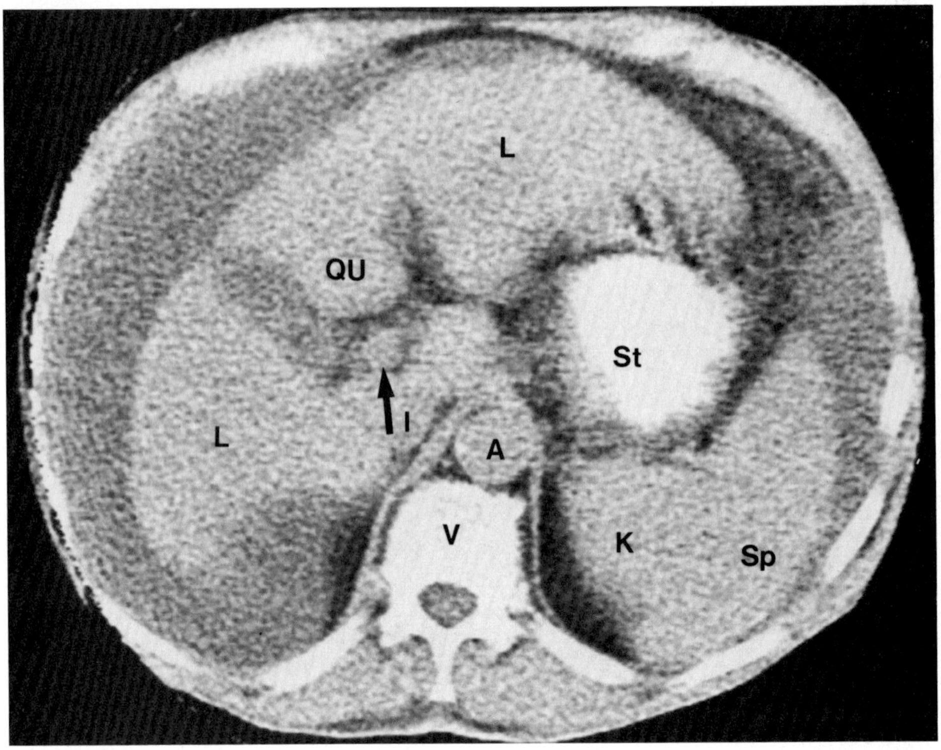

Figure 13A Gross ascites in a patient with liver cirrhosis. Small right lobe, an enlarged quadrate lobe (Qu), and prominence of the porta hepatis, with the portal vein clearly visible (arrow). Considerable fluid is also present between the spleen and lateral abdominal wall.

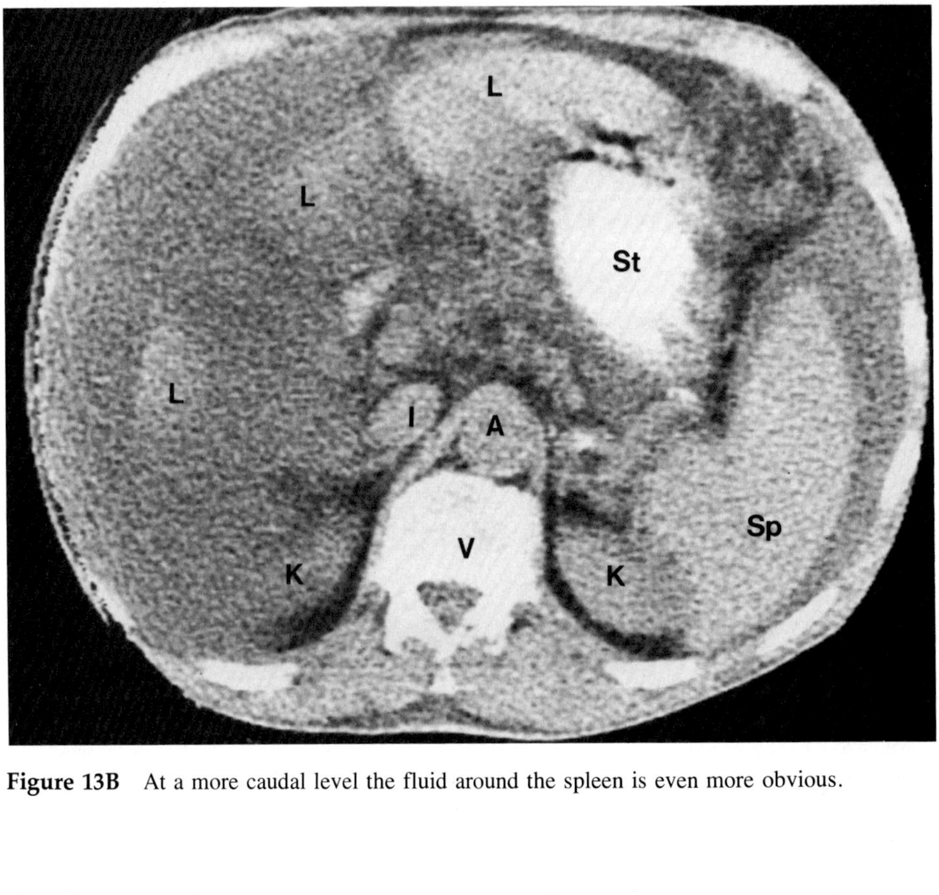

Figure 13B At a more caudal level the fluid around the spleen is even more obvious.

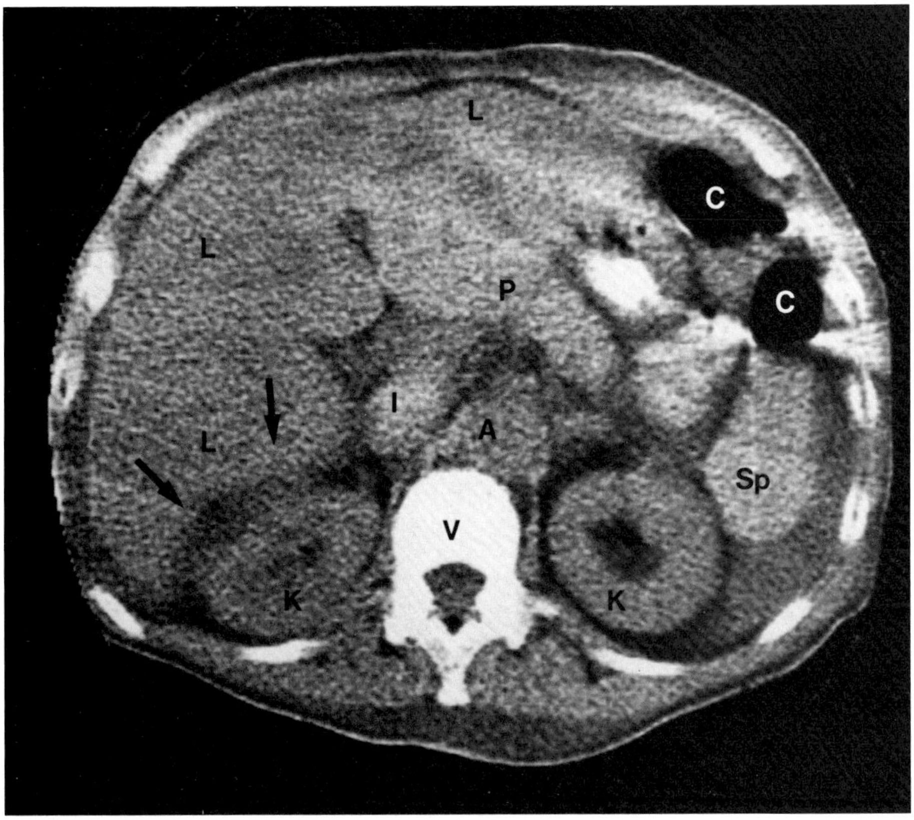

Figure 14 The ascitic fluid in this case is more marked posteriorly behind the liver and spleen and on the right side is interposed between the liver and kidney (arrows).

invariably so, and the ascites may at times be more marked posteriorly (Fig. 14), or at other times more marked anteriorly (Fig. 15).

CT makes it possible to check on some of the signs used in the plain film diagnosis of ascites. Small-bowel loops are compressed into the center of the abdominal cavity, lying more anteriorly with the mesentery forming a striking fanlike low-density pattern which stretches forward and to the left out of the mesenteric root (Fig. 16). Small-bowel loops with gas or with contrast may be found "floating" or "sinking," and this may vary between the upper and lower abdomen (Fig. 17).

Ascites does not interfere with the visualization of the solid abdominal organs and, if anything, the pancreas (Fig. 18), the liver, spleen, and uterus (Fig. 19) are more clearly defined and retroperitoneal tumors readily diagnosed. The peritoneal seeding in malignant

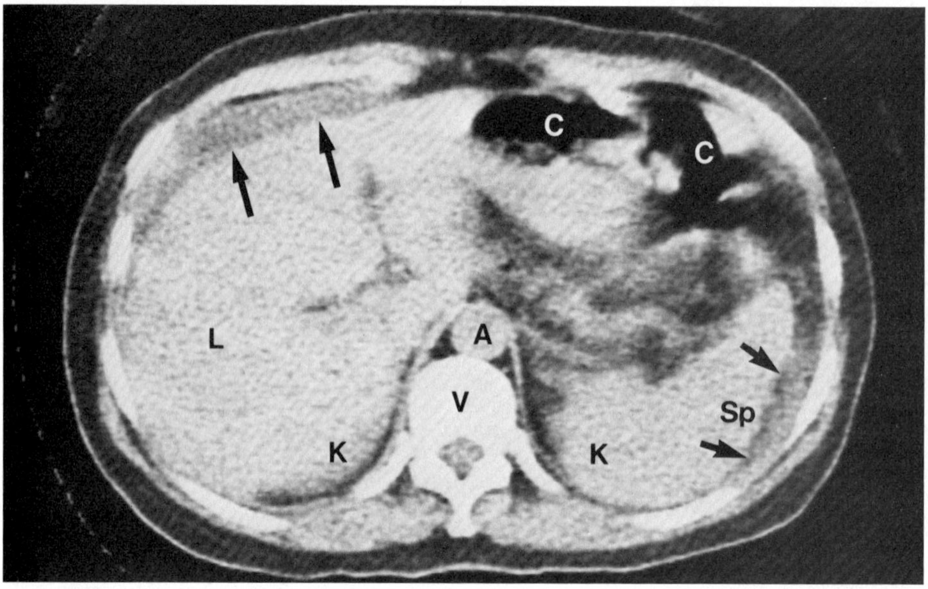

Figure 15 The fluid is most marked anterior to the liver (long arrows), with no fluid between the posterior margin and the right kidney; some fluid lateral to the spleen (arrows).

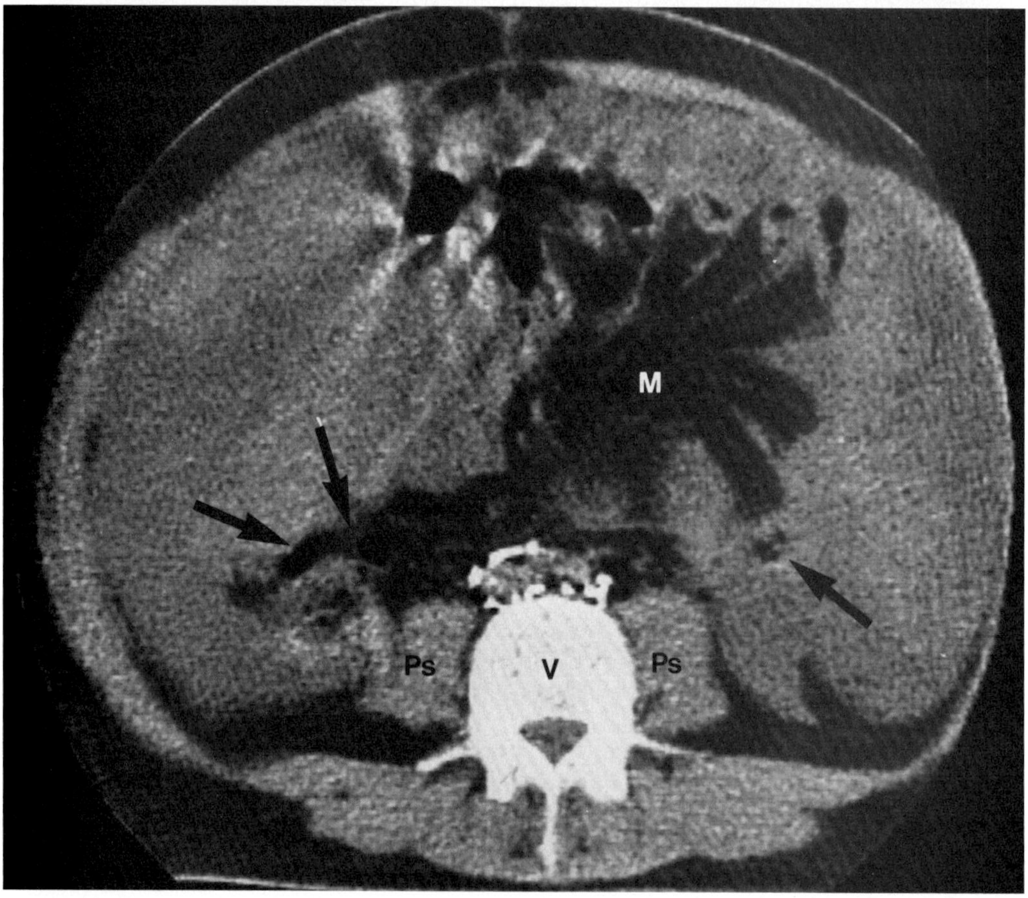

Figure 16 Gross ascites with the mesentery (M) clearly visible as a fan-shaped low-density region. Most gas-filled bowel loops lie anteriorly, but there are also gas-filled loops lying posteriorly on both the right and left sides (arrows).

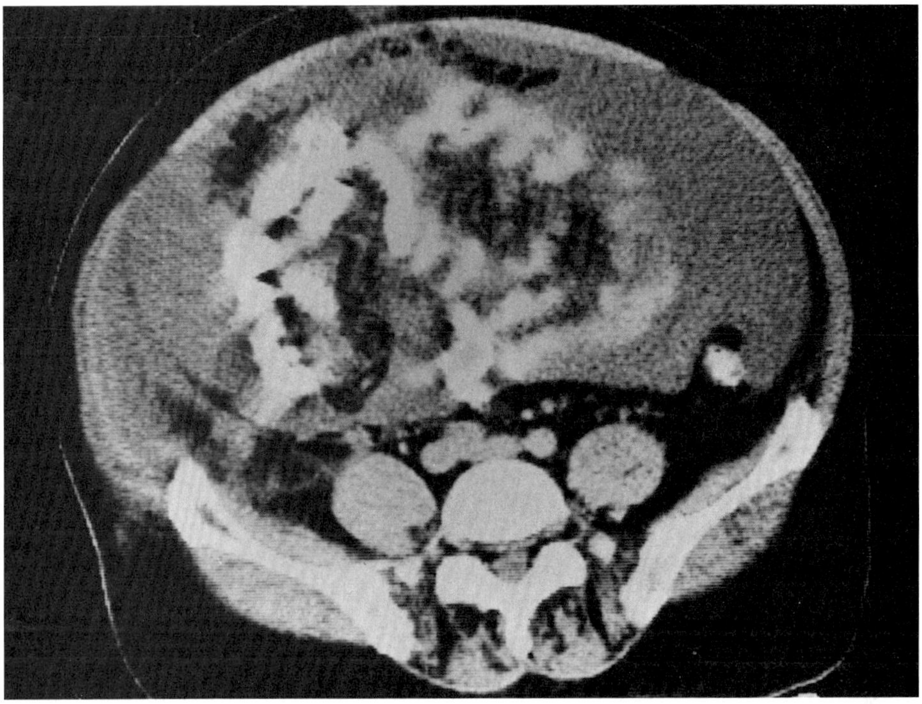

Figure 17 Contrast and gas-filled small bowel lying both anteriorly and posteriorly in a case of gross ascites. CT shows clearly that the plain film sign of gas-filled loops floating and fluid-filled loops sinking in ascitic fluid is unreliable.

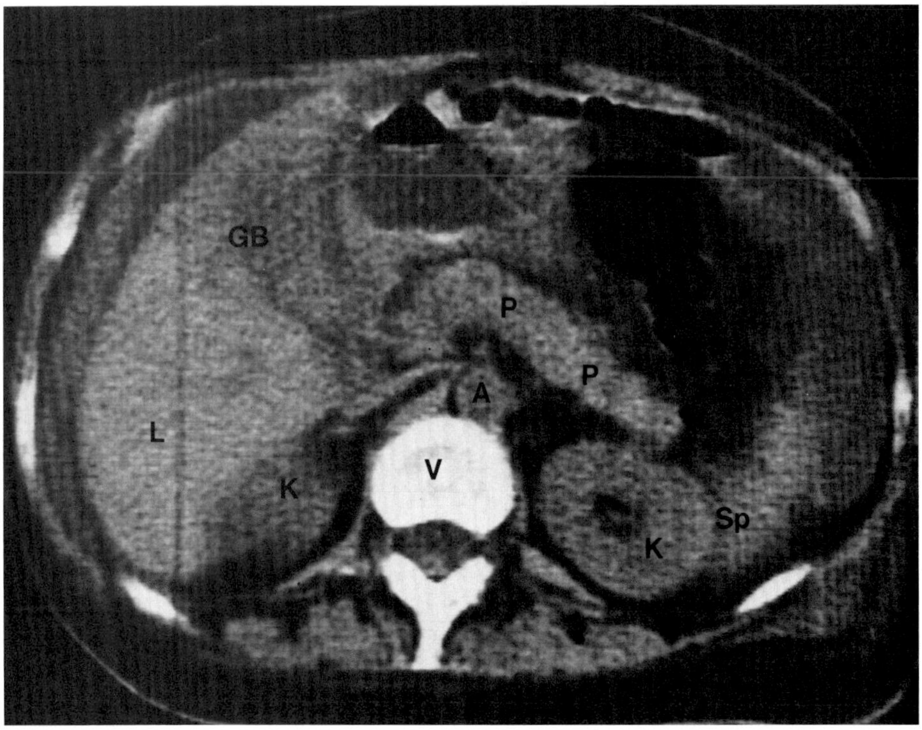

Figure 18 The normal pancreas (P) is well shown and its visualization is enhanced rather than impeded by the ascitic fluid.

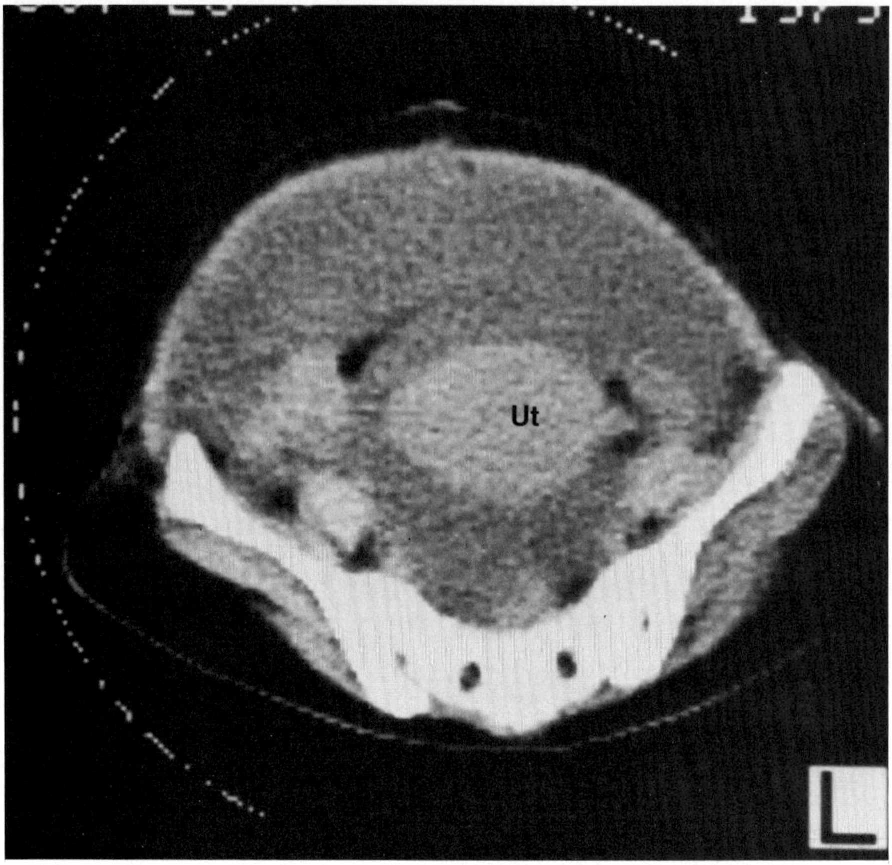

Figure 19 Gross pelvic ascites outlining the uterus (Ut), which is clearly visible.

ascites is, however, rarely demonstrated by CT but may produce a localized peritoneal effusion, particularly adjacent to the liver (Fig. 20).

Differential Diagnosis of Ascites with CT

Localized Collections

These can be easily distinguished from free ascites by observing the distribution of the fluid (Fig. 21). Thus subphrenic or subhepatic abscesses, mesenteric cysts, loculated peritoneal effusions, and pancreatic pseudocysts appear as localized accumulations, often causing local indentation of adjacent organs; they do not encircle the liver or spleen.

Fresh Blood

Its higher attenuation values make it relatively easy to distinguish fresh peritoneal blood (Fig. 22) or fresh localized blood (Fig. 23) from exudates, transudates, or pus. There may be difficulties in its recognition around the liver unless contrast enhancement is used. The increased attenuation of the contrast-enhanced liver then allows visualization of the adjacent blood.

Colloid Infiltration

A real difficulty arises on CT examination in distinguishing colloid carcinomatous infiltration (Fig. 24) or pseudomyxoma peritonei (Fig. 25) from ascites or a localized fluid collection (Fig. 26). On palpation these infiltrating conditions feel solid, and on CT there is a greater local displacement of abdominal organs. When in doubt, needle aspiration of an obvious low-density area would be diagnostic for fluid but would yield no aspirate in colloid carcinoma or pseudomyxoma peritonei.

Difficult Areas

In the pelvis and immediately beneath the diaphragm the recognition of ascites may be more difficult. In the pelvis the urine in the bladder may not be distinguishable from ascites (Fig. 27) unless there is contrast medium in the bladder (Fig. 28). A pleural effusion may also interpose posteriorly between the liver and the posterolateral margin but will lie behind the crus of the diaphragm and in front of the posterior rib and will not be seen on more caudal scan sections (Fig. 29).

Causes of Ascites

The other important aspect of diagnosis with CT is the recognition of a possible cause. A pericardial effusion or calcification can be identified on the lower thoracic sections. Abdominal mass lesions such as a pancreatic carcinoma or para-aortic lymphadenopathy may be uncovered or a liver lesion, such as hepatoma, shown. In the vast majority of cases, however, the primary diagnosis is already known and CT or other investigations to elucidate the etiology of the ascites will be required only rarely.

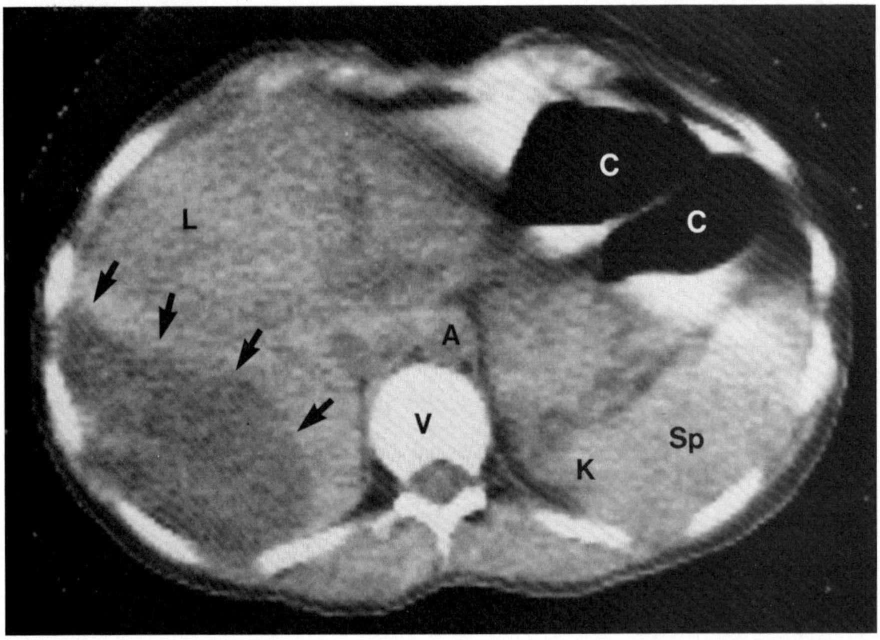

(A)

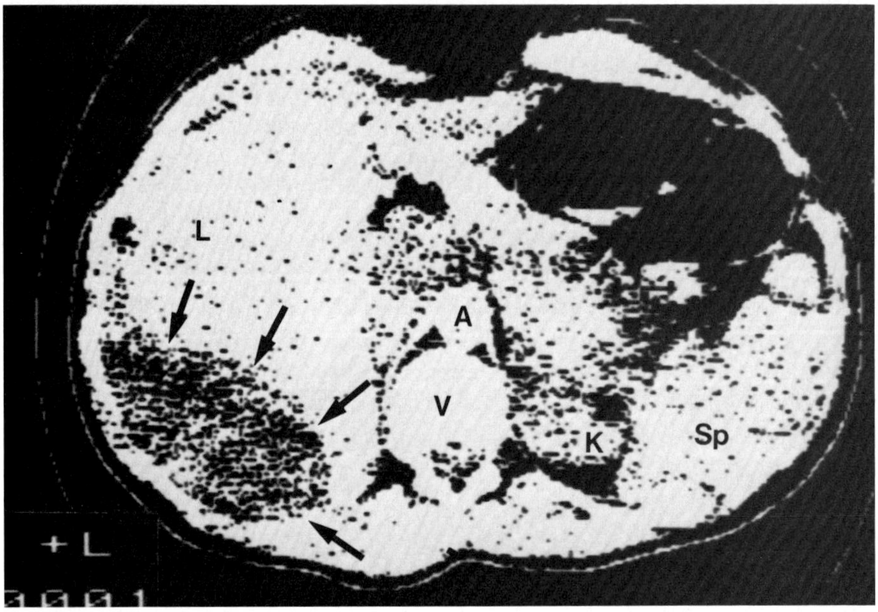

(B)

Figure 20 Patient with peritoneal metastases. (A) Associated localized peritoneal effusion (arrows), metastases not demonstrable. (B) With window level and window width reduced to 1, attenuation of the fluid collection is shown to be that of water.

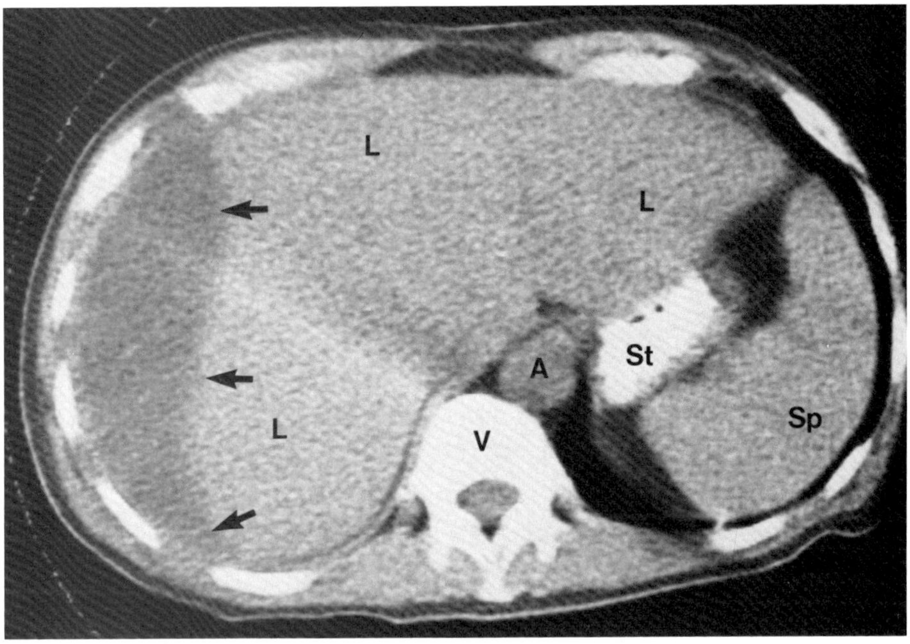

Figure 21 Local fluid collection such as a subphrenic abscess are easily distinguished from ascites. The indentation of the liver is often quite marked (arrows).

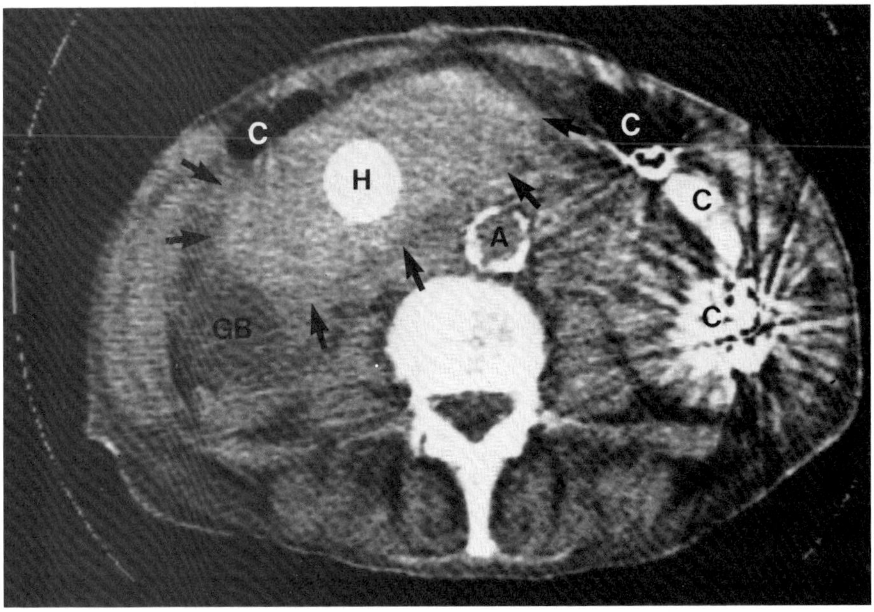

Figure 22 Fresh peritoneal blood shows as an area of higher attenuation (arrows), as designated by the white "region of interest" circle (H, hemorrhage). Artifacts around the colon due to barium.

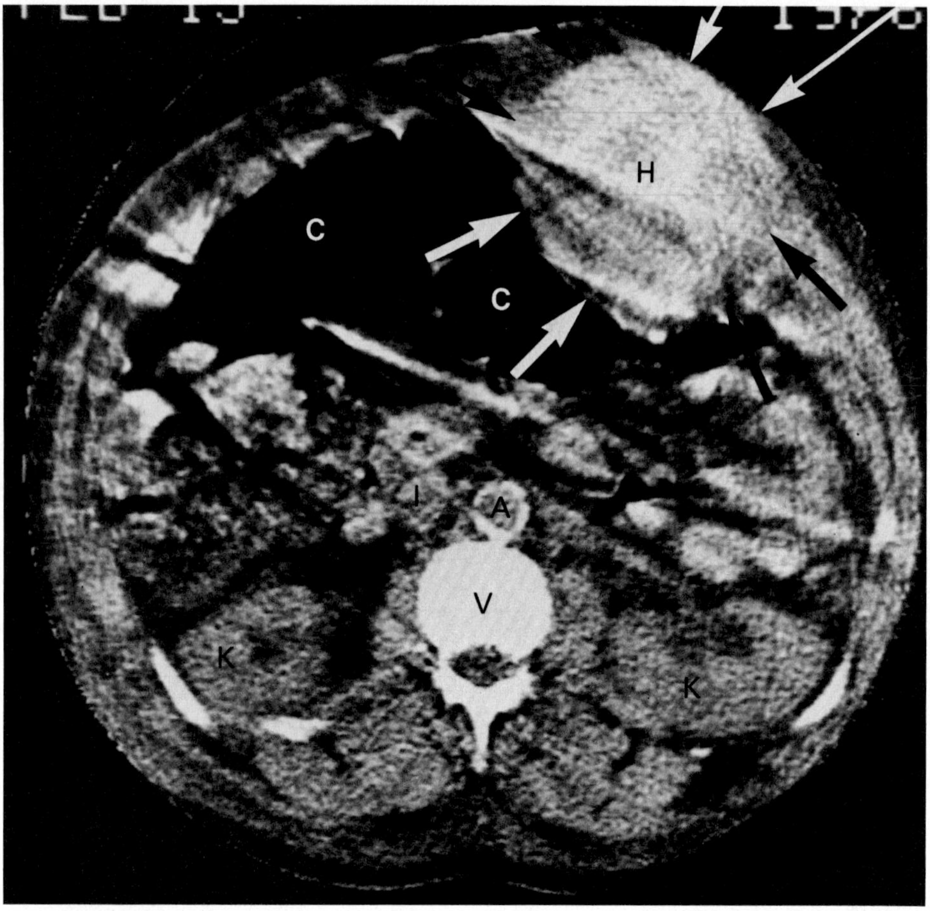

Figure 23 Hemorrhage into the anterior abdominal muscles in a patient with liver cirrhosis. The extraperitoneal location of the fluid collection is obvious in spite of the movement streak artifacts.

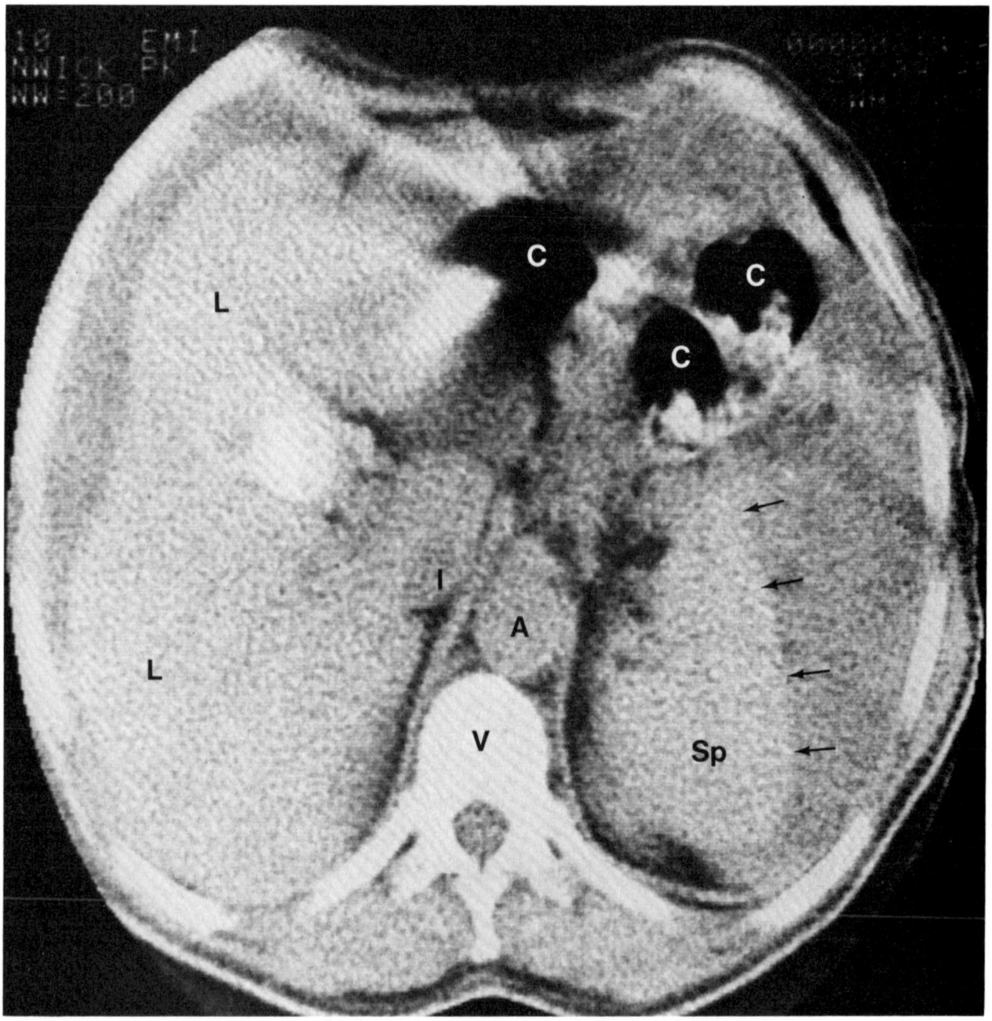

Figure 24 Colloid carcinoma infiltrating the peritoneum resembles ascites, but the indentation of the liver and straightening of the outer splenic margin (arrows) is not a feature of ascites.

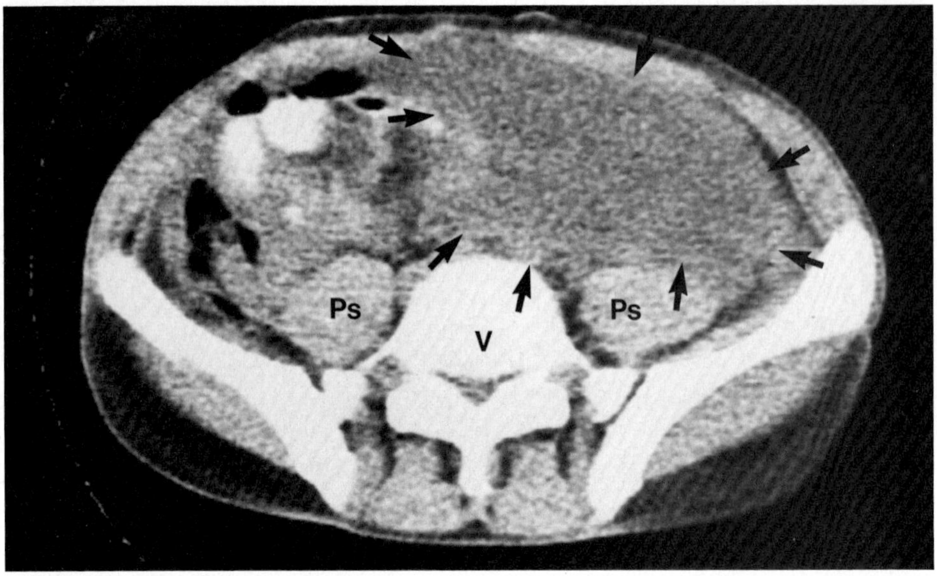

Figure 25 Pseudomyxoma peritonei (arrows) resembles ascites, but on abdominal palpation feels solid and on tapping no fluid can be aspirated.

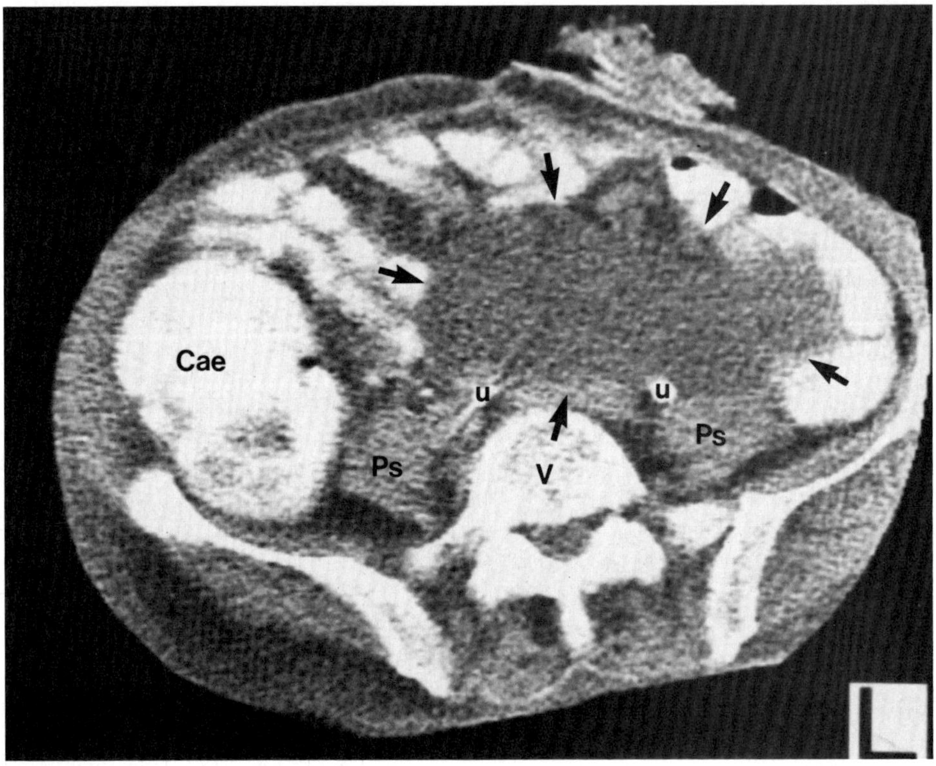

Figure 26 Loculated postoperative fluid in the left iliac fossa (arrows) (Cae, Cecum; U, ureter; Ps, psoas).

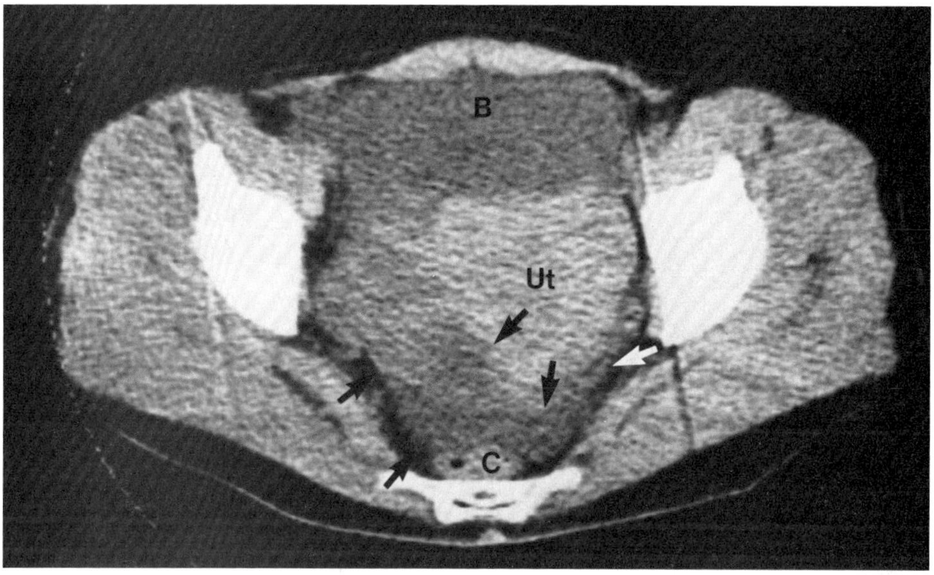

Figure 27 Pelvic ascites (arrows) has the same CT attenuation as urine in the bladder (B).

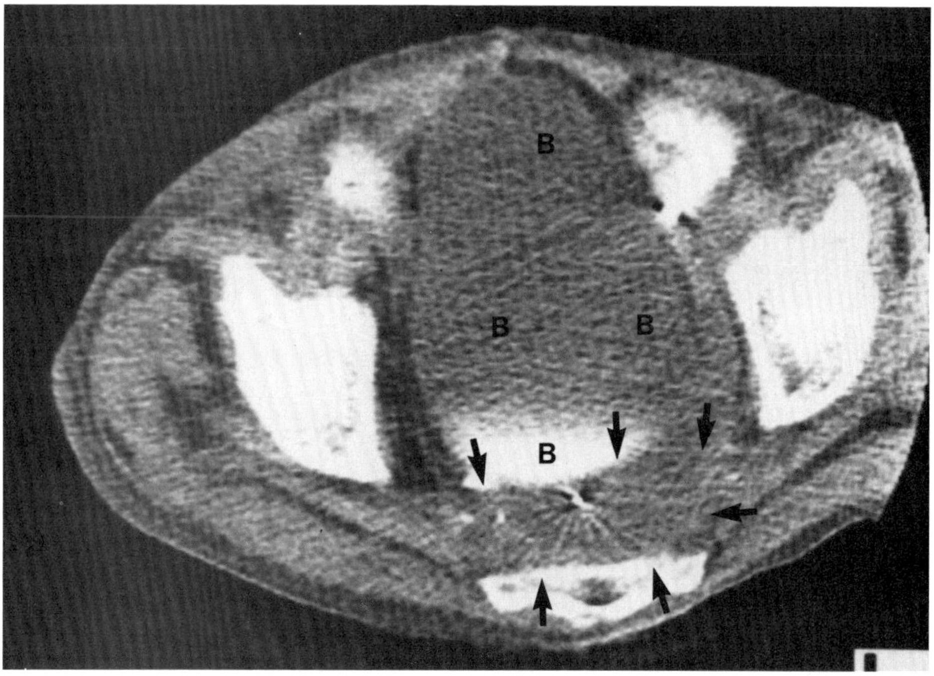

Figure 28 To be sure of the margin of the bladder posteriorly, contrast medium can be given intravenously and the presacral ascites is then delineated (arrows).

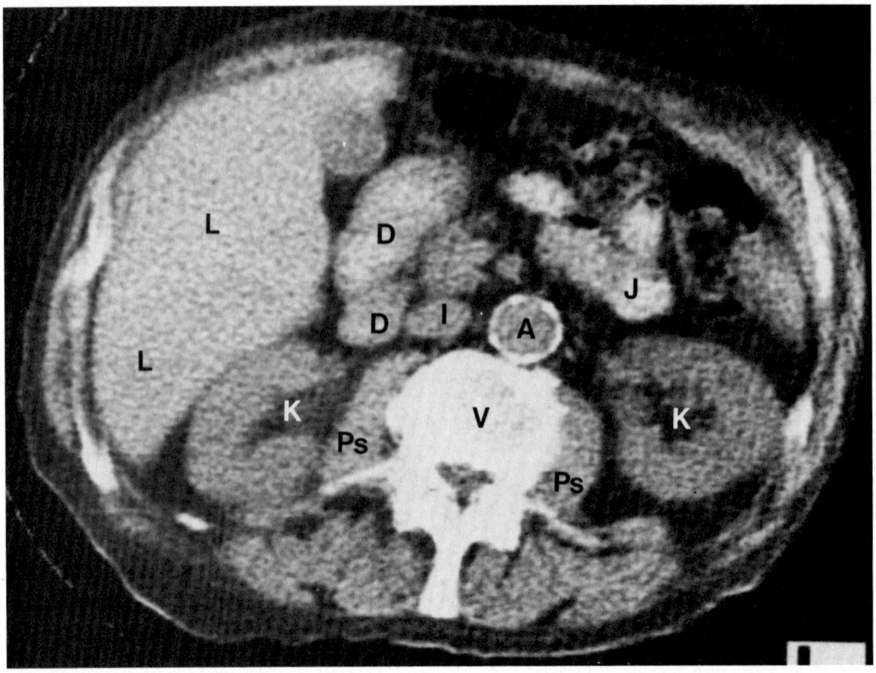

(A)

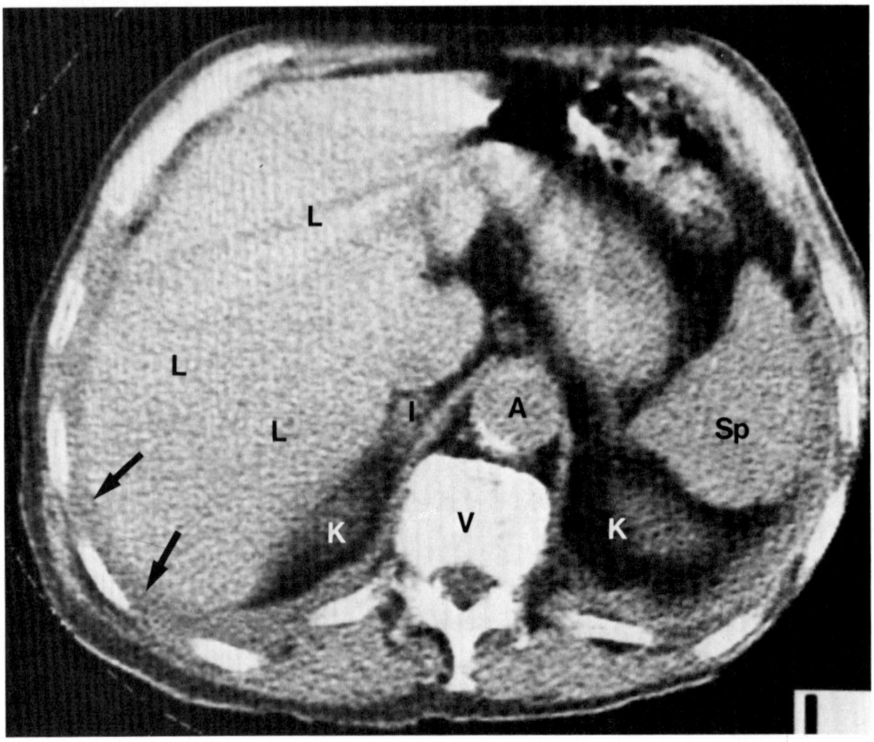

(B)

Figure 29 (A) No fluid is visible around the liver. (B) On the more cranial section fluid is demonstrated posterolaterally (arrows). This fluid lies behind the crus of the diaphragm, indicating that it is a pleural effusion.

References

1. Von Recklinghausen: *Die Lymphgefässe und ihre Beziehungen zum Bindegewebe*. Hirschwald, Berlin, 1862.
2. Von Recklinghausen: Zur Fettresorption. *Virchows Arch 26*:172, 1863.
3. Schmidt C: *Charakteristik der epidemischen Cholera gegenüber verwandten Transsudationsanomalien*. A. Reyher, Leipzig, 1850.
4. Starling EH: Contribution of the physiology of lymph secretion. *J Physiol 14*:131, 1893.
5. Starling EH: The influence of mechanical factors on lymph production. *J Physiol 16*:224, 1894.
6. Zhdanov DA: *General Anatomy and Physiology of the Lymphatic System*. "Medgigiz," Leningrad, 1952.
7. Szabó G, Rév J, Solti: Über die Rolle humoraler Faktoren bei den durch Veränderungen des effektiven kreisenden Blutvolumens Zustandekommenden Abweichungen in der Wasser und Salzausscheidung. *Acta Med Hung 10*:15, 1956.
8. Courtice FC: Pulmonary edema. Clinical implications of laboratory experiments. *Aust NZ J Surg 22*:177, 1953.
9. Meyers MA: The spread and localization of acute intraperitoneal effusions. *Radiology 95*:547, 1970.
10. Whalen JP, Berne AS, Riemenschmeider PA: The extraperitoneal perivisceral fat pad. I. Its role in the roentgenological visualization of abdominal organs. *Radiology 92*:466, 1969.
11. Whalen JP and Berne AS: The extraperitoneal perivisceral fat pad. II. Roentgen interpretation of pathological alterations. *Radiology 92*:473, 1969.
12. Hellmer H: Die Konturen des rechten Leber Lappens beim Ascites. *Acta Radiol 23*:533, 1942.
13. Frimann-Dahl J: *Roentgen Examinations in Acute Abdominal Diseases*. Blackwell, Oxford, 1960.
14. Margulies M and Stoane L: Hepatic angle in roentgen evaluation of peritoneal fluid. *Radiology 88*:51, 1967.
15. Keefe EJ, Gagliardi RA, Pfister RC: The roentgenographic evaluation of ascites. *Am J Roentgenol 101*:388, 1967.
16. McCort JJ: *Radiographic Examination in Blunt Abdominal Trauma*. W. B. Saunders, Philadelphia, 1966.
17. Proto AV, Lane EJ, Marangola JP: A new concept of ascites fluid distribution. *Am J Roentgenol 126*:974, 1976.
18. Page LB and Culver PJ: *A Syllabus of Laboratory Examinations in Clinical Diagnosis*. Harvard University Press, Cambridge, Mass., 1966.
19. Davis RE and Graham DY: Pancreatic ascites: the role of endoscopic pancreatography. *Am J Dig Dis 20*:977, 1975.
20. Donowitz M, Kerstein MD, Spior HM: Pancreatic ascites. *Medicine (Baltimore) 53*:183, 1974.
21. Santulli TV: In *Pediatrics*, 16th ed, Rudolph AM, Barnett HL, Einhorn AH (Eds). Appleton-Century-Crofts, New York, 1977.
22. Hirschler A and Buday K: Toyabbi Ielentes a Chylous Ascitesrol (New Contribution to Chylous Ascites). *Orv Hetil 33*:107, 1899.
23. Mitchell GAG: The spread of acute intraperitoneal effusions. *Br J Surg 28*:291, 1940.
24. Wegner G: Chirurgische Bemerkungen über die Peritonealhöhle mit besonderer Berücksichtigung der Ovariotomie. *Arch Khn Chir 20*:51, 1877.
25. Proto AV, Lane EJ, Marangola JP: A new concept of ascitic fluid distribution. *Am J Roentgenol 126*:974, 1976.
26. Goldberg BB, Goodman GA, Clearfield HR: Evaluation of ascites by ultrasound. *Radiology 96*:631, 1970.

27. Laurell H: A contribution to roentgenological differential diagnosis in the presence of free fluid in the abdomen. *Acta Radiol 16*:42, 1935.
28. Rusznyak I, Foldi M, Szabo G: *Lymphatics and Lymph Circulation, Physiology and Pathology*. Pergamon Press, Oxford, 1960.
29. Bizzozero G and Salvioli G: Studii sulla struttura e sui linfactici delle serose umane. *Arch Sci Med 2*:247, 1976.
30. Florey H and Witts LJ: Absorption of blood from the peritoneal cavity. *Lancet 1*:1323, 1928.
31. Hedenstedt S: Elliptocyte transfusions as method in studies on blood destruction, blood volume and peritoneal resorption. *Acta Chir Scand 95*:1, 1947.
32. Courtice FC and Simmons WJ: Physiological significance of lymph drainage of the serous cavities and lungs. *Physiol Rev 34*:419, 1954.
33. Courtice FC and Steinbeck AW: Absorption of protein from peritoneal cavity. *J Physiol 114*:336, 1951.
34. Notkin JA: Die Aufsaugung in den serosen Höhlen (Die Bedeutung der Lymphgefässe). *Virchows Arch 225*:471, 1925.
35. Witte MH, Witte CL, Dumont AE: Progress in liver disease: physiological factors involved in the causation of cirrhotic ascites. *Gastroenterology 61*:742, 1971.
36. Morton RE, Deluca R, Reisman TN, et al.: Pancreatic ascites: successful treatment with pancreatic radiation. *Am J Dig Dis 21*:333, 1976.
37. Franken EA: Ascites in infants and children. *Radiology 102*:393, 1972.
38. McCort JJ: Rupture or laceration of the liver by nonpenetrating trauma. *Radiology 78*:49, 1962.
39. Hoffman RB, Wankmuller R, Rigler LG: Pseudoseparation of bowel loops: fallacious sign of intraperitoneal fluid. *Radiology 88*:51, 1966.
40. Frimann-Dahl J: *Roentgen Examinations in Acute Abdominal Diseases*. Charles C Thomas, Springfield, Ill, 1951.
41. Bai KI, Ramamohan C, Subrhmanyam MVG: Radiographic evaluation of ascites in 25 children. *Indian Pediatr 12*:1001, 1925.
42. Kreel L: Computerized tomography of the pancreas. *Comput Axial Tomogr 1*:287, 1976.

34

Radiology of Liver Transplantation

John W. Laws, Heather B. Nunnerley
King's College Hospital
London, England

Introduction

Liver transplantation is currently reserved for patients with liver disease not amenable to other forms of treatment. These patients fall into two main groups:

1. Those with end-stage hepatic cell failure
2. Those with a primary liver tumor not suitable for resection

The liver failure is usually due to such conditions as primary biliary cirrhosis, prolonged active chronic hepatitis, sclerosing cholangitis, or the Budd-Chiari syndrome. The most common primary hepatic tumor to undergo treatment by transplantation is the hepatoma, which has not spread outside the liver, yet is not suitable for resection, either because of its situation within the liver or because of some feature of its blood supply. Patients with bile duct tumors are rarely considered suitable, as these tumors have a particularly poor prognosis following transplantation (1,2).

Our experience of radiology in hepatic transplantation has been confined to adults (3). Although in some centers bile duct atresia is treated by hepatic transplantation (2), at King's College Hospital the Kasai operation is preferred (4–6).

Preoperative Assessment

When any patient is considered for orthotopic liver transplantation, for whatever reason, it is important at an early stage to know whether the portal vein and inferior vena cava are patent and to have detailed knowledge of the varied arterial anatomy of the liver in the individual patient. In addition, if the transplant is being considered because of the presence of a liver tumor, it is essential to exclude, as far as possible, the presence of metastatic disease. If the tumor is found to be confined to the liver, it is important to assess whether or not there is any possibility of a resection of the tumor by hepatic lobectomy. The sequence of events is illustrated in the flowchart, Table 1.

In the pretransplantation radiological assessment, therefore, an attempt is made to answer the following questions, the precise method used depending in part on the resources and expertise available.

Has There Been Metastatic Spread?

To the Lymph Nodes?

Lymphangiography is an unreliable method of demonstrating metastatic spread to lymph nodes either in the porta hepatis or in the para-aortic region since a normal lymphangiogram will in no way exclude the presence of metastatic disease in lymph

Table 1 Flowchart for Preoperative Assessment

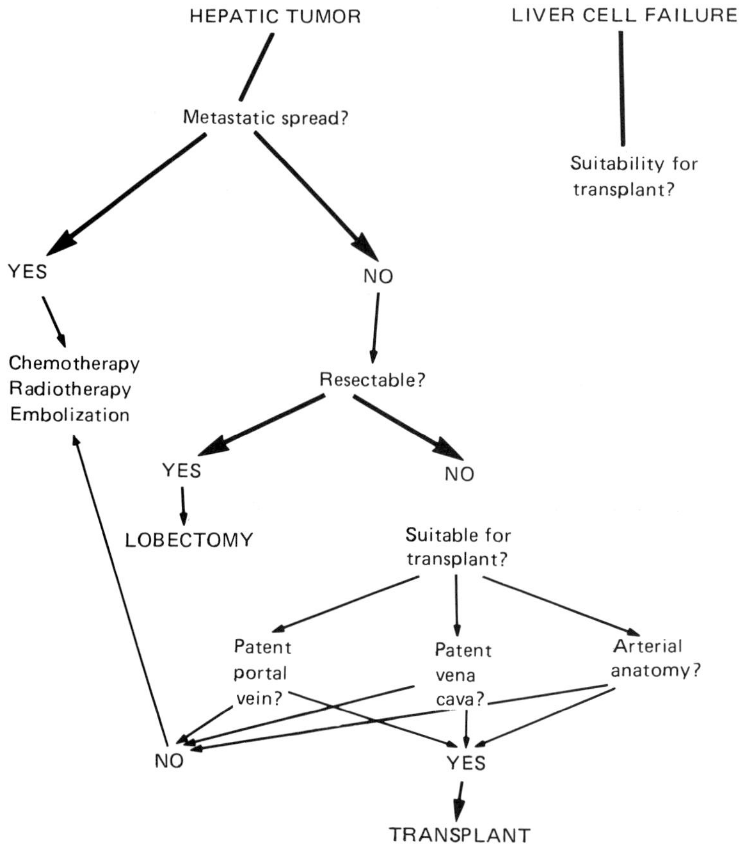

nodes. Many of the relevant lymph nodes do not fill with contrast medium even in the normal individual. Thus false negative examinations are very common and false positives occur occasionally. *Ultrasound* may show enlarged lymph nodes either in the porta hepatis or in the para-aortic region, but occasionally, because of technical difficulties such as the presence of excess gas, ultrasound may not prove satisfactory. *Computerized tomography (CT)* is, however, a very good method of demonstrating enlargement of the lymph nodes and, if available, is the method of choice (Fig. 1).

To the Lungs?

It is fairly common for hepatomas in the late stage to metastasize to the lungs. Anterior and lateral *chest films* should, therefore, be taken together with whole *lung tomograms,* if any suspicious lesions are seen. *Computerized tomography* may show lesions not demonstrable by other methods, particularly in the periphery of the lungs and around the hila.

To Bone?

It is uncommon for a hepatoma to metastasize to bone and even less common for a cholangiocarcinoma to do so. Even so, an *isotope scan* of the skeleton followed by localized radiographs of any suspicious area should be carried out (Fig. 2). Tomography may be necessary. In case of doubt, *percutaneous biopsy* to obtain cells for histological sections or cytology may be important.

Is the Tumor Resectable?

If the tumor is confined to one lobe, and lobectomy is possible, this must be preferred to a hepatic transplant. It will be necessary to show the blood supply of the tumor and its relationship to the liver fissures and to exclude, as far as possible, lesions in other parts of the liver remote from the main tumor.

The main tumor may well be demonstrated by *ultrasound* and may appear to be confined to one lobe (Fig. 3). It is, however, difficult to exclude the presence of small lesions elsewhere in the liver by means of ultrasound, although lesions about 2 cm in diameter may be shown. *Computerized tomography,* best with contrast enhancement, will usually delineate the tumor clearly and will show its relationship to the major fissures within the liver. If there has been spread of tumor across the fissures or if there are metastatic lesions in the liver remote from the main tumor mass, this will be shown in most instances.

Arteriography is capable of showing small vascular metastatic tumors not visible by any other method. It has the added advantage of demonstrating the arterial anatomy, relevant when partial resection of the tumor is being considered. Oblique views may be required to identify the segmental distribution within the liver of the various major branches of the hepatic artery (Fig. 4). Large tumors can distort the liver to such a degree that the optimal obliquity for angiography can be found only by trial and error. In these cases, the normal liver may form only a relatively small addendum to the huge tumor mass. A vascular tumor may ''steal'' blood from the rest of the liver so that demonstration of the normal part of the liver may be difficult. For this reason, selective injection into the right, middle, and left hepatic arteries is frequently necessary in order to exclude small lesions within lobes not involved by the main mass of the tumor.

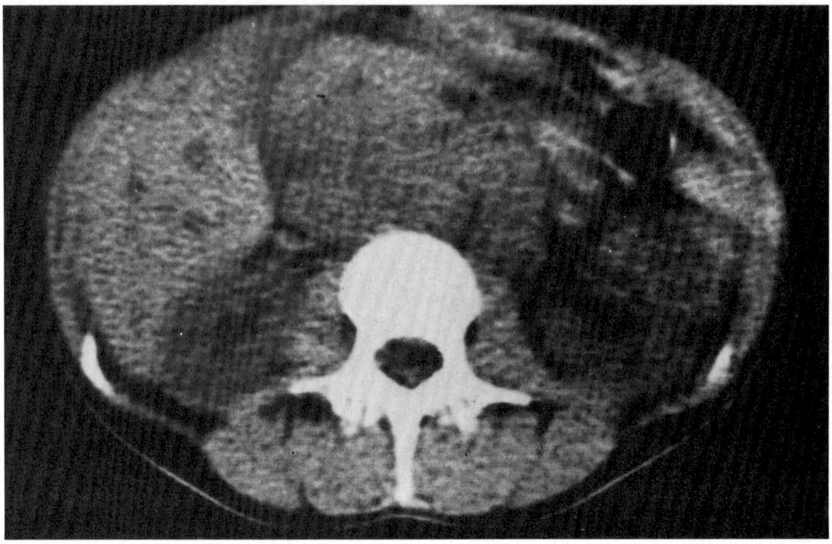

Figure 1A Female, 28 years. Hepatoma. CT section through the liver and kidney shows a low-density tumor involving the left lobe of the liver predominantly. The loss of outline of the aorta and inferior vena cava was due to tumor spread to paraaortic lymph nodes.

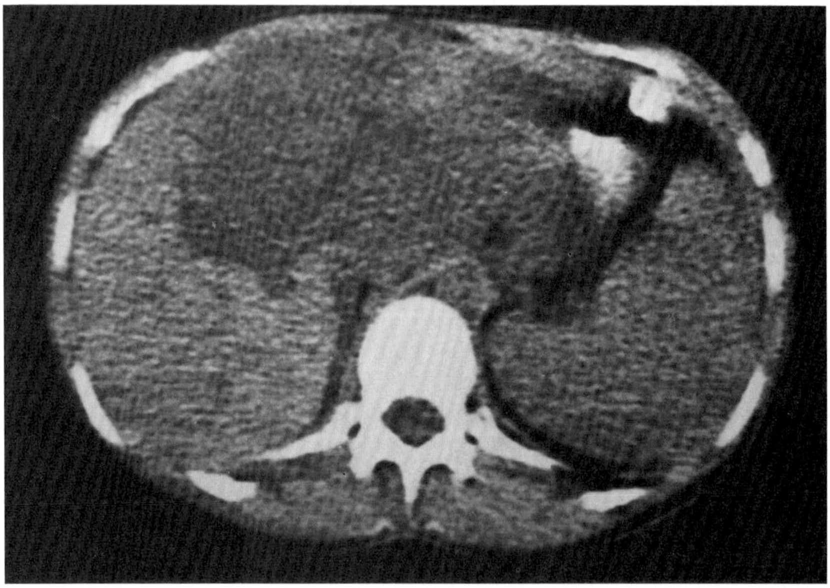

Figure 1B In another patient, section through the liver and spleen shows a low-density tumor involving the left lobe and the anterior medial aspect of the right lobe of the liver.

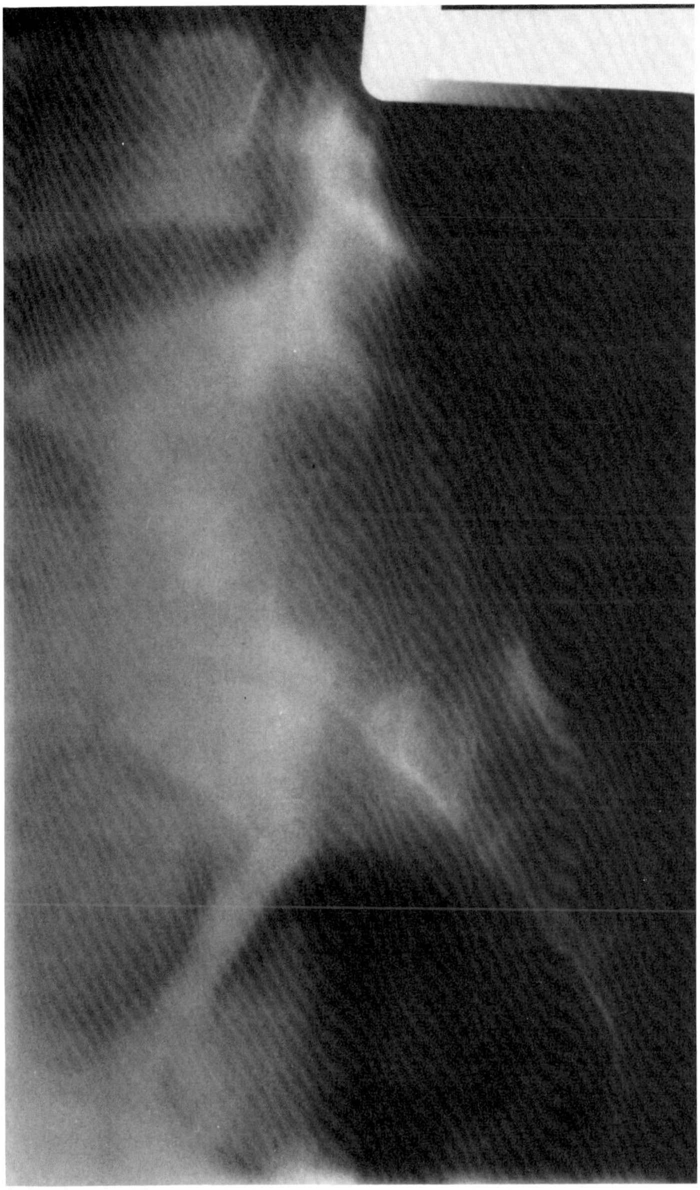

Figure 2 Male, 50 years. Metastatic hepatoma. Lateral tomogram of the sacrum showing a lytic metastatic deposit from the hepatoma.

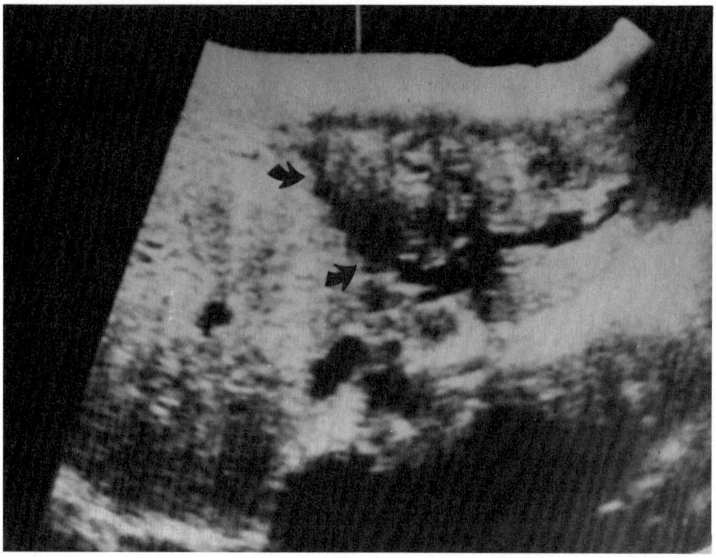

Figure 3 Female, 28 years. Large cholangiocarcinoma. Ultrasound examination, transverse abdominal scan showing tumor extension across the midline from the left into the right lobe (arrows). Dilated bile ducts are visible.

Is the Portal Vein Patent?

It is necessary to demonstrate the patency of the portal vein since its occlusion, whether by tumor or as a result of portal hypertension, will prevent liver transplantation. This is best done by an *arterioportogram,* following selective injection into the superior mesenteric artery and the celiac or splenic artery. In patients with portal hypertension and massive collateral circulation, the diversion of blood from the portal vein into these collaterals may prevent demonstration of the portal vein. *Direct transhepatic portal venography* may then be necessary to ensure that the main portal vein is still patent and suitable for anastomosis (Fig. 5). Although ultrasound may demonstrate a normal superior mesenteric vein and portal vein, in our experience it is less reliable than arteriography in demonstrating occlusion of these vessels.

Is the Inferior Vena Cava Patent?

Pressure on the inferior vena cava by a large tumor may occlude it, hepatic vein thrombosis can extend into the inferior vena cava, or the tumor can cause occlusion by direct invasion. If caval thrombosis is suspected, an inferior venacavogram in the anterior and lateral projections is essential.

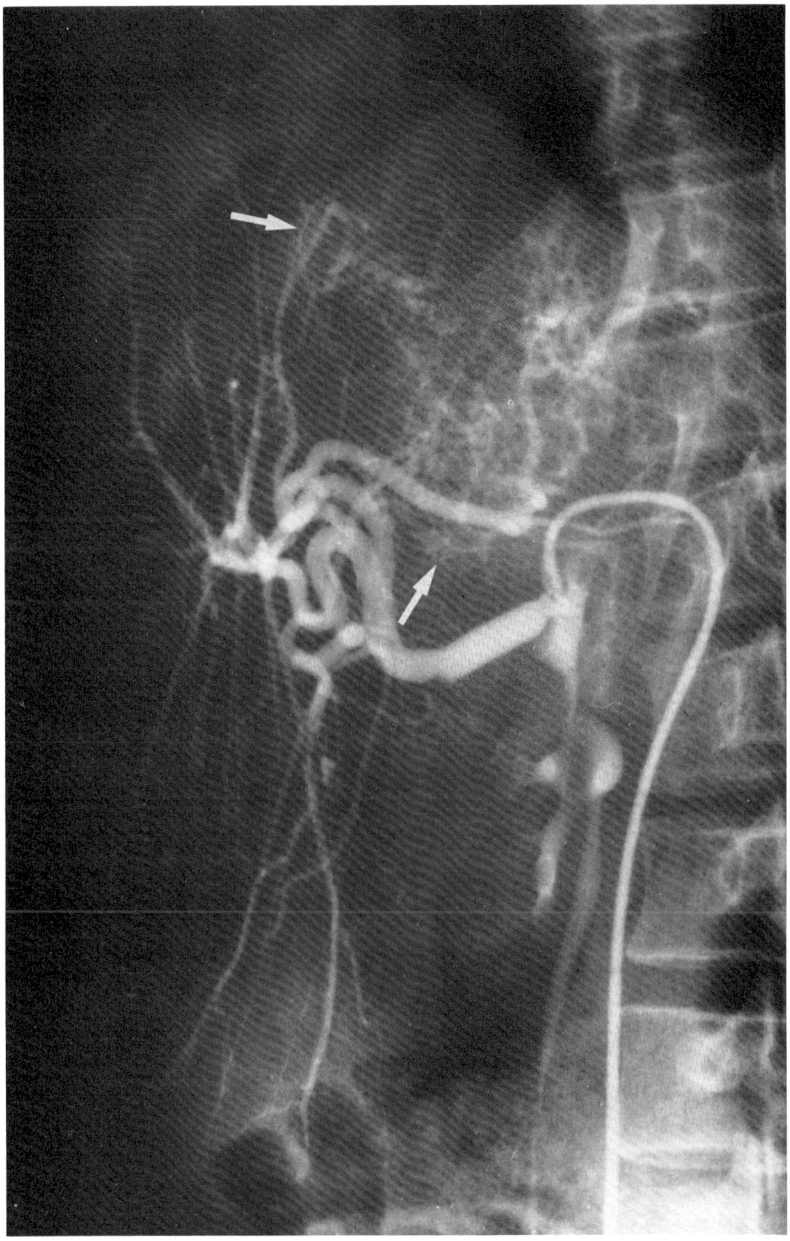

Figure 4A Female, 30 years. Hepatoma. Oblique view hepatic arteriogram showing hepatoma confined to the left lobe (arrows). Left lobectomy was undertaken.

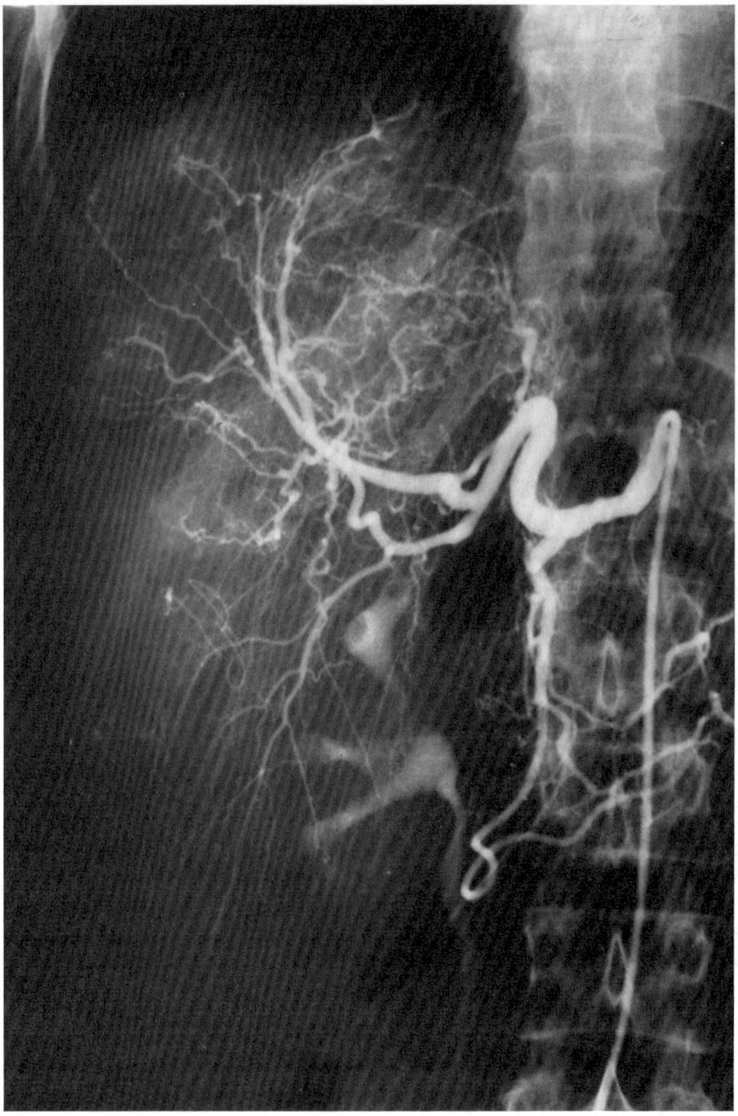

Figure 4B Oblique hepatic arteriogram showing recurrence of hepatoma in the remaining right lobe.

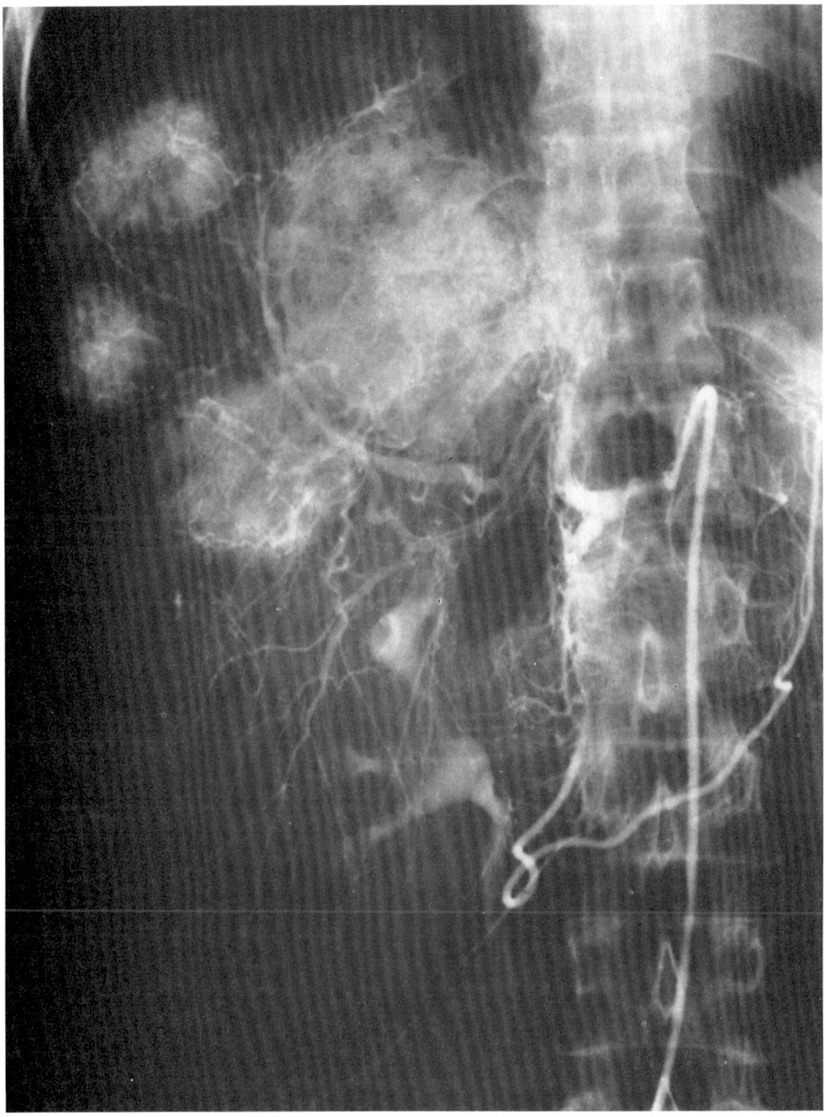

Figure 4C The late hepatogram phase demonstrates extensive tumor masses. At this stage, the patient had an hepatic transplant.

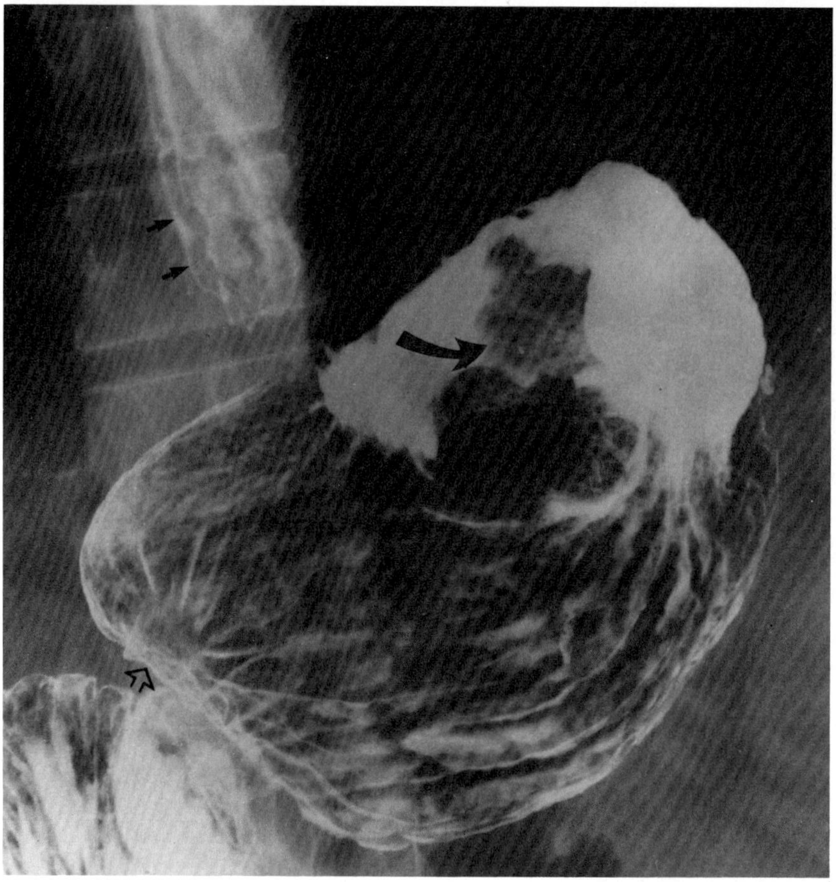

Figure 5 Male, 40 years. Hepatic failure due to cirrhosis. Barium examination outlines esophageal varices (arrows), large gastric varices (curved arrow), and the scar of a chronic gastric ulcer (open arrow) near the gastrojejunal anastomosis. Confirmation by endoscopy. An arterioportogram showed massive collaterals but did not opacify the portal vein. Transhepatic portography demonstrated portal vein patency. The patient is awaiting liver transplantation.

What Is the Arterial Anatomy?

The arterial anatomy of the liver is very variable and should be known before transplantation is undertaken. Arteriography is important not only to demonstrate the arterial supply of the tumor but also because it may demonstrate encasement of major branches of the hepatic artery outside the liver, which may render transplantation difficult or impossible.

Postoperative Management

Immediate Postoperative Period

In the immediate postoperative period the radiological changes that are found are those common to any upper abdominal surgery. For example, *chest films* may well show evidence of fluid overload, collapse, consolidation, or evidence of an inhalation pneumonia. As many of these patients have been in end-stage liver failure before surgery, these complications are even more common than after the average abdominal operation.

Abdominal films may give evidence of prolonged ileus, as shown by distention of large and small bowel, and the presence of fluid levels on films taken with a horizontal ray. Slightly later there may be evidence of subhepatic or subphrenic abscess formation, the latter being shown in the usual way by elevation of the right dome of the diaphragm, gas/fluid levels beneath the right diaphragm, and a right basal pleural reaction.

Biliary Complications

Of the many surgical anastomoses necessary for an orthotopic hepatic transplantation, the biliary anastomoses are the ones that produce the most common and troublesome complications. These can occur immediately after surgery, after a short delay, or in the long-term follow-up of the patient.

In the early days of liver transplantation, mechanical biliary complications were frequent and troublesome, with the leakage of bile, fistulae, sinuses, and strictures. Debris frequently collected above a stricture. However, the design of the anastomosis between the donor gallbladder and the recipient common bile duct has now been modified in a number of ways in order to overcome these complications. The most satisfactory method is still a matter of dispute (7). An anastomosis in which the donor gallbladder acts as a conduit between the donor common bile duct and a short segment of the recipient common bile duct has significantly reduced the frequency of biliary complications (8).

A T tube is left in place until satisfactory bile drainage into the gut has become established and cholangiography has shown that the anastomosis is satisfactory, that intrahepatic bile ducts are not dilated, and that no debris is present within the biliary tree (Fig. 6).

At a later stage, after the T tube has been removed, ultrasound may provide useful evidence about the caliber of the intrahepatic bile ducts. If dilatation of the bile ducts is shown either by ultrasound or by isotope scanning, it may be necessary to carry out a fine needle transhepatic percutaneous cholangiogram in order to demonstrate the underlying cause (Fig. 7). Cholangitis with intrahepatic abscess formation may occur if there is any obstruction to the biliary drainage; this can be demonstrated by cholangiography.

Immunosuppression

Patients, after liver transplantation, suffer from the side effects of immunosuppressive therapy in the same way as those following renal transplantation. In particular, these patients are susceptible to infections, sometimes by organisms not usually pathological in humans. *Klebsiella* and tuberculous infections are seen with prolonged treatment. Significant osteoporosis and vertebral collapse may occur with long-term steroid therapy.

Tumor Recurrence

Patients may develop a recurrence of their malignant tumor within their transplanted liver (Fig. 8) or may develop metastases elsewhere. An increase in the level of α-fetoprotein in the serum usually indicates recurrence of a hepatoma. *Serial isotope scans* and *ultrasound* examinations are usually the earliest methods of demonstrating the involvement of the donor liver in a recurrence of the tumor. *Arteriography* may be necessary to confirm this

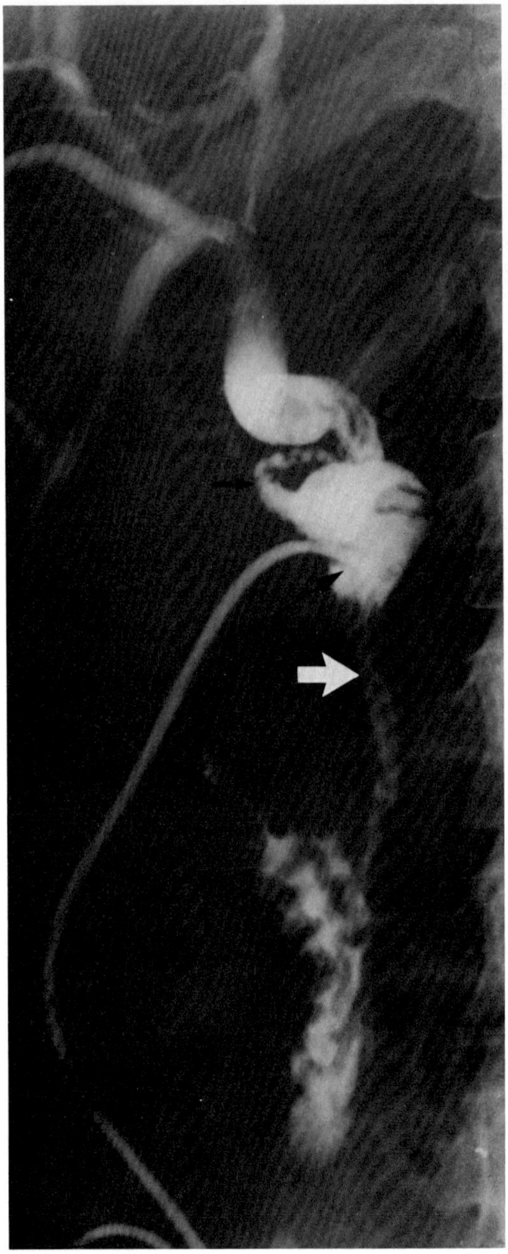

Figure 6 Female, 26 years. Budd-Chiari syndrome. Post-transplantation T tube cholangiogram. The donor hepatic duct (open arrow), cystic duct (small arrow), and gallbladder (long arrow) act as conduit to be joined to the recipient lower end of common bile duct (white arrow).

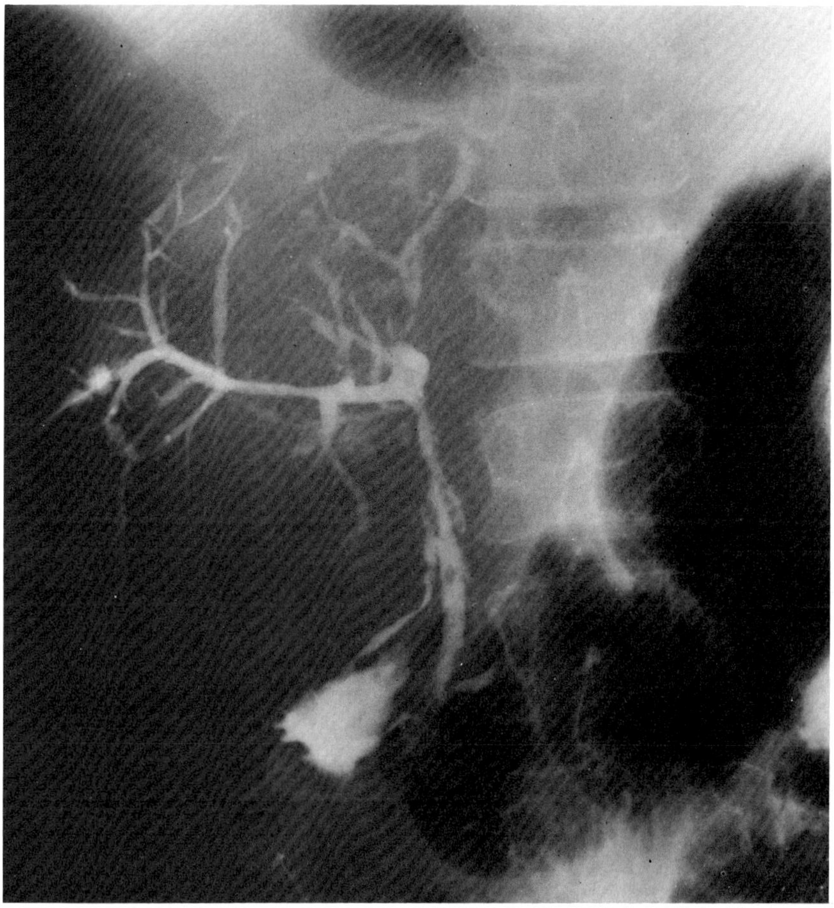

(A)

Figure 7 Male, 37 years. Sclerosing cholangitis. (A) Percutaneous cholangiogram before transplantation. (B) Percutaneous cholangiogram after transplantation showing debris in a dilated donor common bile duct above a stricture.

and will be essential if further surgery or treatment by arterial embolization is being considered.

Recurrence of Other Primary Hepatic Conditions

It is now known that, besides a recurrence of tumor, other primary conditions may recur in the transplanted liver. For example, primary biliary cirrhosis and sclerosing cholangitis have been seen to reappear in transplanted livers.

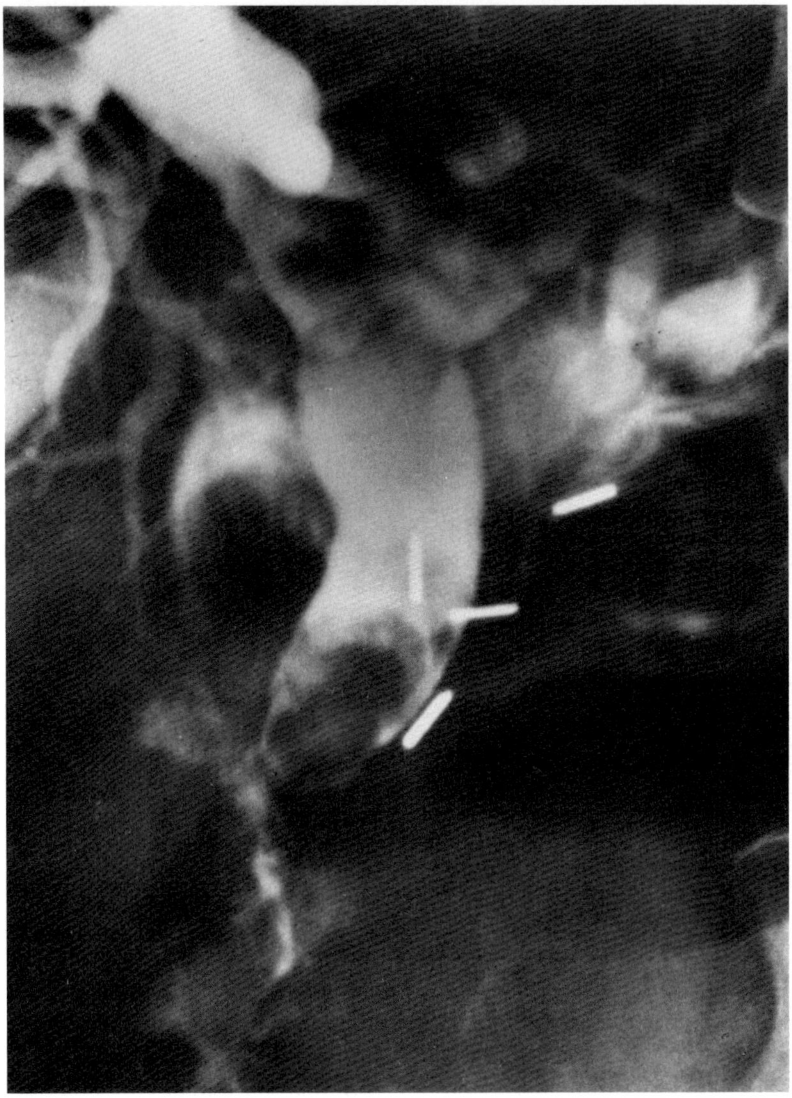

(B)

Figure 7 (continued)

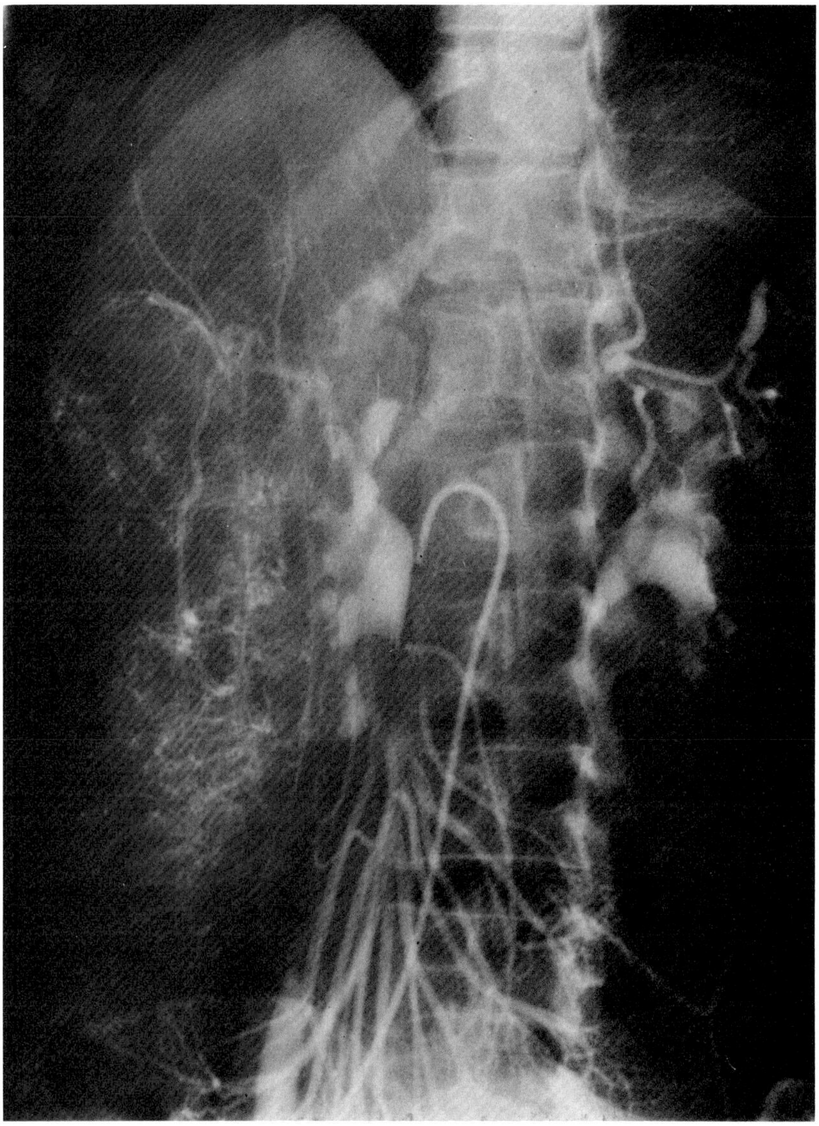

Figure 8A Female, 38 years. Hepatoma. Oblique arteriogram showing a vascular hepatoma mainly in the right lobe of the liver. The patient had an hepatic transplant.

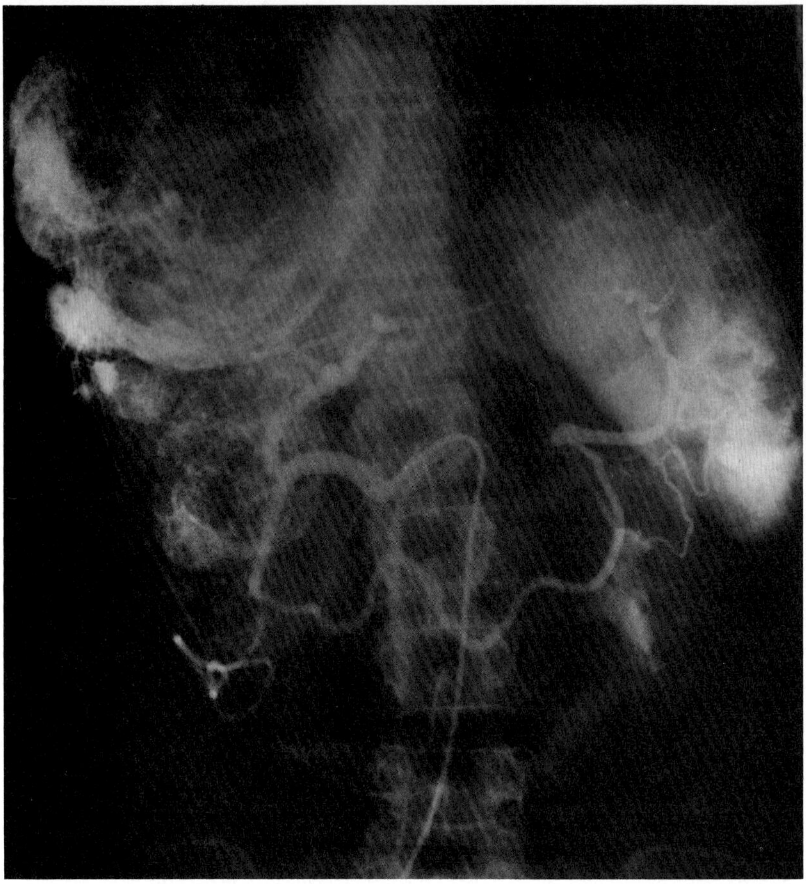

Figure 8B Six years later — arteriogram shows a recurrence of hepatoma in the transplanted liver.

Conclusion

Radiological techniques have a very important role in the preoperative assessment and postoperative management of patients undergoing orthotopic liver transplantation. Full and accurate information can be obtained only by the use of all radiological modalities, including plain radiography, ultrasound, contrast studies, and computerized tomography, each of which makes a complementary contribution.

References

1. Williams R, Smith M, Shilkin KB, Herbertson B, Jaysey B, Calne RY: Liver transplantation in men; the frequency of rejection, biliary tract complications, and recurrence of malignancy based on an analysis of 26 cases. *Gastroenterology 64*:1026, 1973.
2. Starzl TE, Koep LJ, Halgrimson CG, Hood J, Schroter CPJ, Porter KA, Weill R: Fifteen years of clinical liver transplantation. *Gastroenterology* 77:375, 1979.

3. Galne RY, Williams R, Lindop M, Farman JV, Tolley ME, Rolles K, MacDougall B, Neuberger J, Wyke RJ, Raffery AT, Duffy TJ, Wight DD, White DJG: Improved survival after orthotopic liver grafting. *Br Med J 283*:115, 1981.
4. Kasai M, Suzuki H, Osashi E, Ohi R, Chiba T, Okamoto A: Technique and results of operative management in biliary atresia. *World J Surg 2*:571, 1978.
5. Howard ER and Mowat AP: Extra hepatic biliary atresia. Recent developments in management. *Arch Dis Child 52*:825, 1977.
6. Psacharopoulos HT, Howard ER, Portman B, Mowat AP: Extrahepatic biliary atresia; preoperative assessment and surgical results in 47 consecutive cases. *Arch Dis Child 55*:851, 1980.
7. Calne RY, McMaster P, Portman B, Wall WJ, Williams R: Observations on preservation, bile drainage and rejection in 64 human orthoptic liver allographs. *Ann Surg 186*:282, 1977.
8. Calne RY: A new technique for biliary drainage in orthotopic liver transplantation utilizing the gall bladder as a pedicle graft conduit between the donor and recipient common bile ducts. *Ann Surg 184*:605, 1976.

35

Recent Developments

Herbert Y. Kressel
Hospital of the University of Pennsylvania
Philadelphia, Pennsylvania

Introduction

The rapid development of medical imaging instrumentation and applications challenges the physician both in understanding the new technology and in integrating the new developments within the existing approaches to the diagnosis of disease. In this chapter we will briefly review some recent advances in imaging of the liver, both in terms of technical development and potential clincial applications. We will briefly consider several recent developments: (1) dynamic or rapid sequence CT scanning; (2) newer contrast materials for CT examination of the liver; (3) nuclear magnetic resonance scanning; (4) endoscopic cholangiography and placement of biliary prostheses; and (5) digital subtraction angiography.

Rapid Sequence CT Scanning

Since its clinical introduction, CT scanning has proved to be an effective tool for examining the liver. With this modality, focal liver lesions may be detected, the presence and etiology of bile duct obstruction identified, and gross changes in the composition of the liver such as fatty infiltration of iron deposition noted. While abnormalities may be easily identified, characterization of the lesions on the basis of morphology or density alone is often difficult.

The introduction of 3rd and 4th generation CT scanners with larger numbers of detectors and higher heat capacity x-ray tubes has permitted the development of dynamic or rapid sequence CT scanning. With this modification, a series of CT images may be obtained consecutively without the need for significant interscan delay. The serial scanning sequence may be performed at the same scan plane, thus permitting assessment of regional contrast enhancement over time as a means of aiding tissue characterization, or in different scan planes by table incrementation, thus permitting evaluation of a large volume of tissue during peak enhancement. The latter form of dynamic scanning may be of value in providing improved detection of focal lesions or in yielding increased anatomic information by identifying the contrast enhanced vascular anatomy over a larger volume of tissue.

The specifications of rapid sequence scanning modifications vary by manufacturers. In general, hardware modifications permit "to and fro" gantry motion rather than initiating all scans at the same point with unidirectional gantry motion. Software modifications permitting table incrementation between scans may be available, as is preprogramming of scan timing sequence. At the University of Pennsylvania we have evaluated the rapid sequence scanning capability of a modified Philips T-300 CT scanner. With this unit a 360° gantry motion can be completed in 4.2 seconds and a new scan may be initiated every seven seconds. Images may be obtained from the full 360° data or from three partial reconstructions obtained during this time period. In addition, software is provided which permits graphic display and analysis of time density data. Both the sequence of scans and the method of contrast administration may vary depending on the purpose of the examination.

Two types of applications are commonly employed in rapid sequence scanning. The first may be termed CT angiography and attempts to image the vascular structures immediately adjacent to the target organ and to obtain peak parenchymal contrast enhancement in an effort to optimize visualization of focal liver lesions. In this application time density analysis for tissue characterization is generally not performed and incremented CT scanning during sustained intravascular and parenchymal content enhancement is attempted.

Enhancement of the arterial and venous structures in and about the vascular structures in the porta hepatis may be helpful in identifying mass lesions in this region (1,2). In addition, vascular enhancement may be useful in defining the extent of tumors.

Nonincremental Scanning: Bolus Enhancement Patterns

Tissue characterization through the analysis of contrast uptake in a variety of liver lesions has been a subject of considerable interest (3–9). This approach requires delivery of a single large 60–100 ml bolus of iodinated contrast material through a large bore intravenous catheter.

Performing rapid serial scans in the same plane presents some technical problems. Sustained breath holding is not feasible during the entire scanning period. Thus, it may be difficult to maintain the same scan plane throughout the entire examination. Failure to do so will surely affect the resultant time-density curve. In addition to problems in maintaining the scan plane, renal and cardiac function will affect the characteristics of a contrast bolus as it passes through a target organ. In patients with low output cardiac states such as congestive heart failure or cardiomyopathy, a poor input function to the bolus will be observed which will broaden the enhancement pattern. In patients with poor renal function, delayed contrast excretion will also affect the observed enhancement pattern.

There has been great disparity in the enthusiasm with which different investigators describe their experience with rapid-sequence scanning and the interpretation of vascular

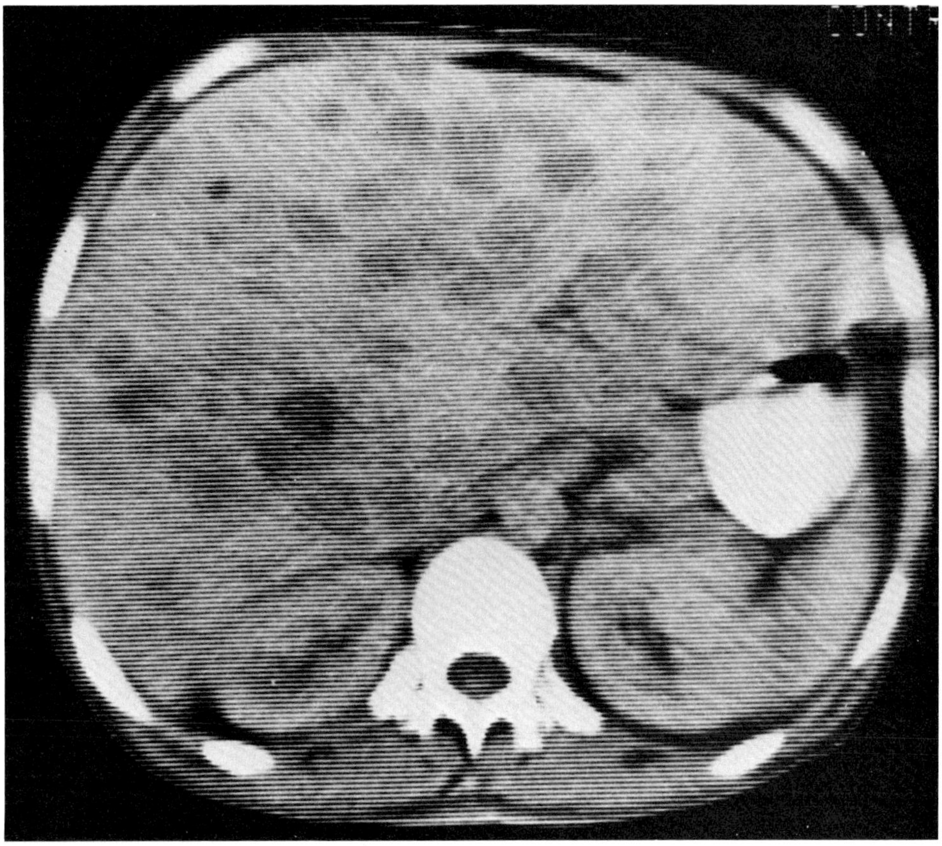

(A)

Figure 1 Variable enhancement patterns in a patient with multifocal hepatoma. (A) Precontrast scan. Multiple ill-defined lucencies are present throughout the liver. (B) Arterial phase. Note multifocal rim and parenchymal enhancement as well as persistent nonenhancing region in right lobe (arrow). (C) Late parenchymal phase. The rim enhancement is no longer apparent. The parenchymal lucencies are once again more prominent.

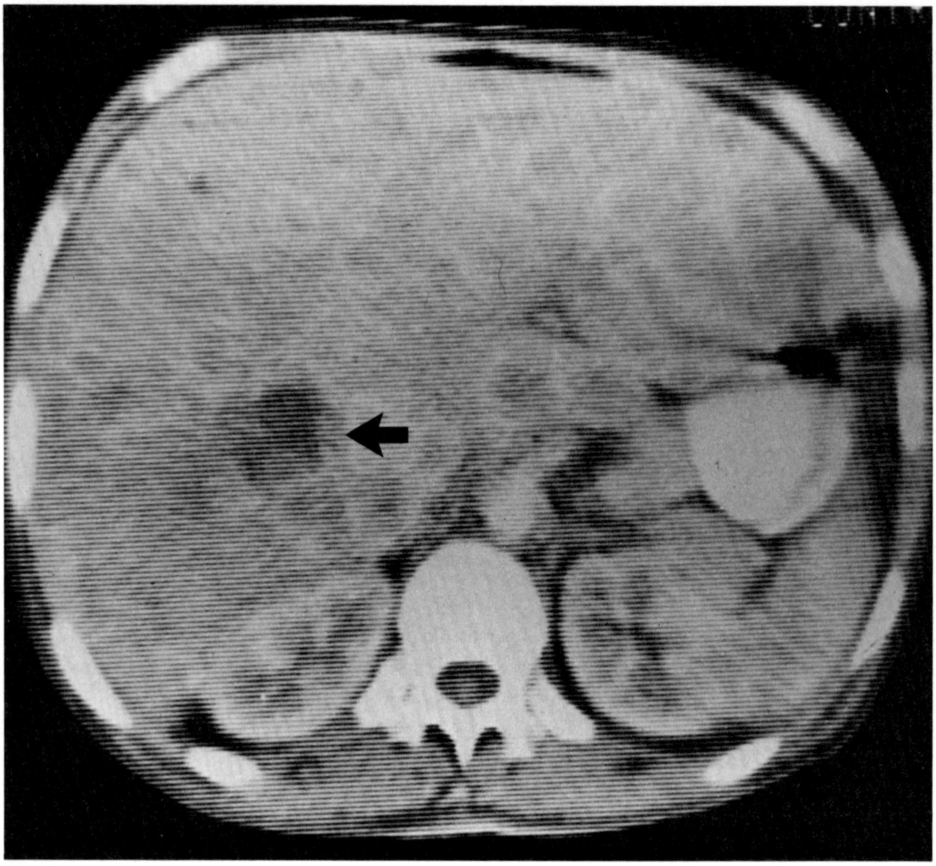

(B)
Figure 1 (continued)

enhancement patterns. Moss et al. (8) could not identify characteristic enhancement patterns in a variety of hepatic neoplasms. They noted that lesions of the same histology can exhibit different enhancement patterns in the same patient. In addition, the apparent pattern of enhancement was extremely variable in the first minute, and the times chosen for data collection could greatly affect the apparent enhancement patterns identified.

Araki, Itai, (5,7) and others have reported on the enhancement patterns of hepatic neoplasms during dynamic scanning, following bolus injection. In their series, serial scans were obtained at 15 seconds, 1 minute, 2 minutes, and 5 minutes. They reported *hepatocellular carcinoma* to be typically associated with rapid enhancement which was diffuse and cleared rather rapidly. There was considerable variability: a few hepatomas appeared hypovascular (Fig. 1). Metastatic tumors tended to show a slight and transient ring enhancement with bolus injection and appeared to have a slight decrease in attenuation toward the center on precontrast scans. Nodular margins were noted (Fig. 2).

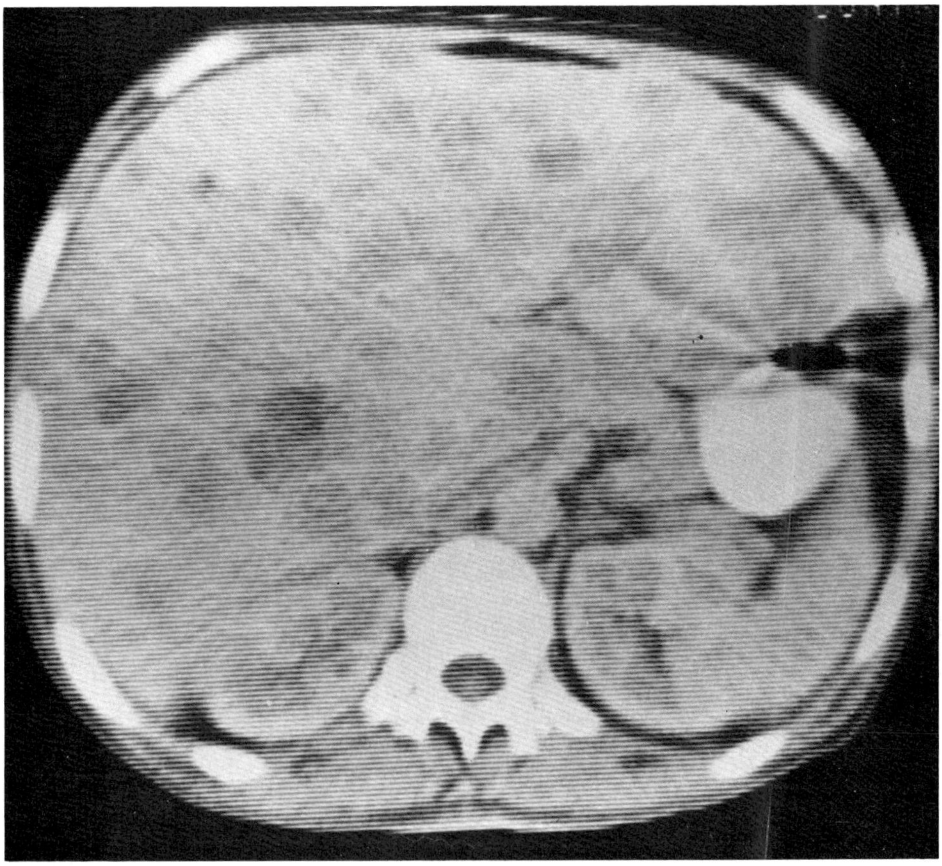

(C)

Benign tumors can be characterized by rapid-sequence CT scans. *Hemangiomas* (9,10) display characteristic enhancement patterns. They tend to be characterized by dense accumulation of contrast material which occurs near the periphery of the lesion, and spreads centrally to the regions of low density. This results in a marked decrease in lesion size on late, postcontrast scans (Fig. 3). *Focal nodular hyperplasia* of the liver typically demonstrates prompt uniform hypervascularity, and subsequently becomes isodense with the remainder of the liver on delayed scans (11).

The significance of the various enhancement patterns remains somewhat uncertain. The lack of uniformity in the techniques employed may account for some of the reported discrepancies. Nonetheless, when identified, characteristic patterns for enhancement, particularly with hemagiomas and metastatic disease, may be helpful in differential diagnosis.

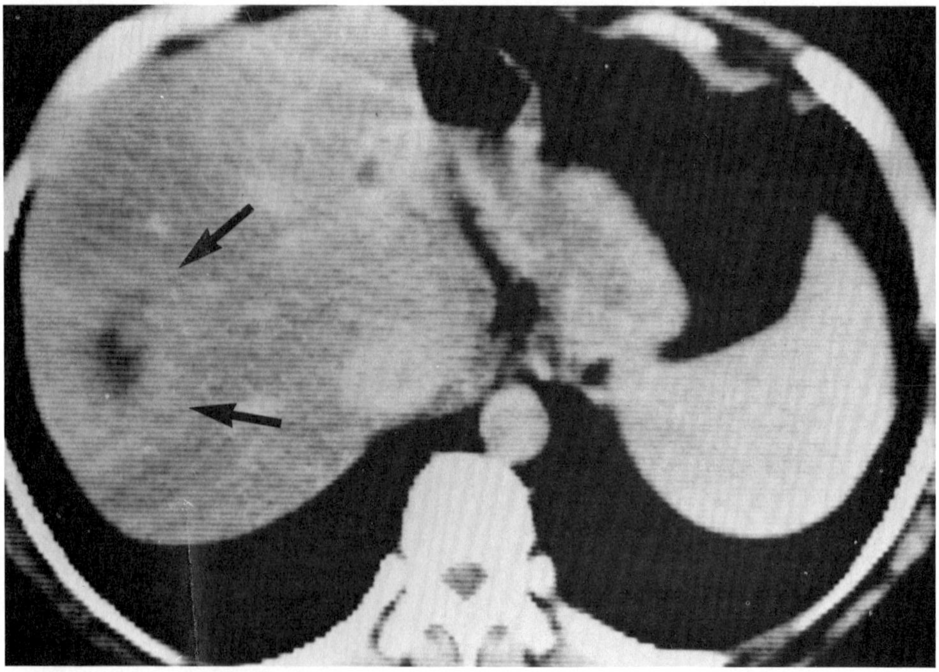

Figure 2 Metastasis. Rapid sequence scan in patient with metastatic breast carcinoma. Note rim enhancement with nodular margins in the right lobe (arrows).

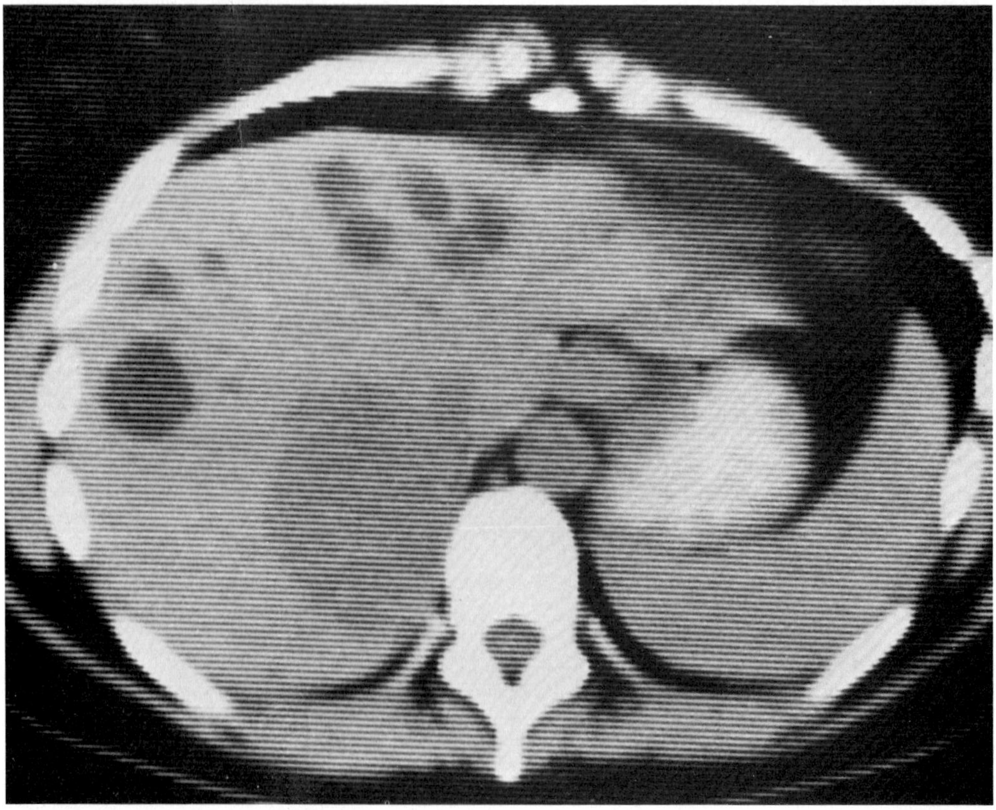

Figure 3A

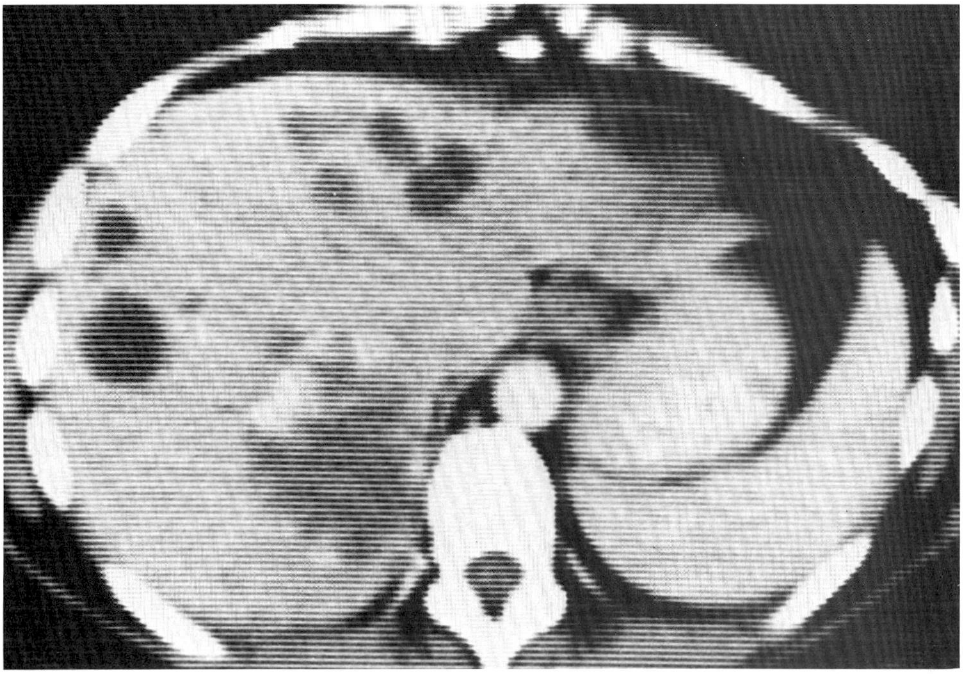

(B)

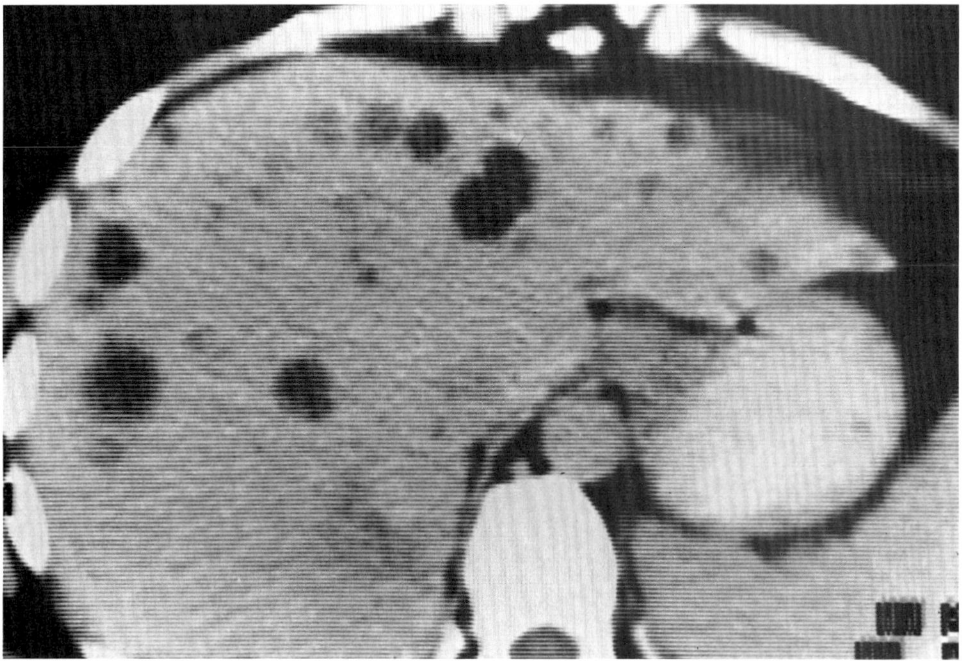

(C)

Figure 3 Thirty-eight-year-old female with hemangioma of the liver and multiple hepatic cysts. (A) Precontrast scan demonstrates multiple 1-2 cm low density lesions in the right and left lobes of the liver (cysts) and a larger somewhat higher density lesion posteriorly in the right lobe. (B) Rapid sequence scan, arterial phase. Note the dense contrast accumulation peripherally in the larger lesion (hemangioma). The smaller lesions (cysts) do not demonstrate any enhancement within the lesion or the periperhy. (C) Late parenchymal phase. The hepatic cysts are unchanged. Note the marked diminution in apparent size of the enhanced hemangioma.

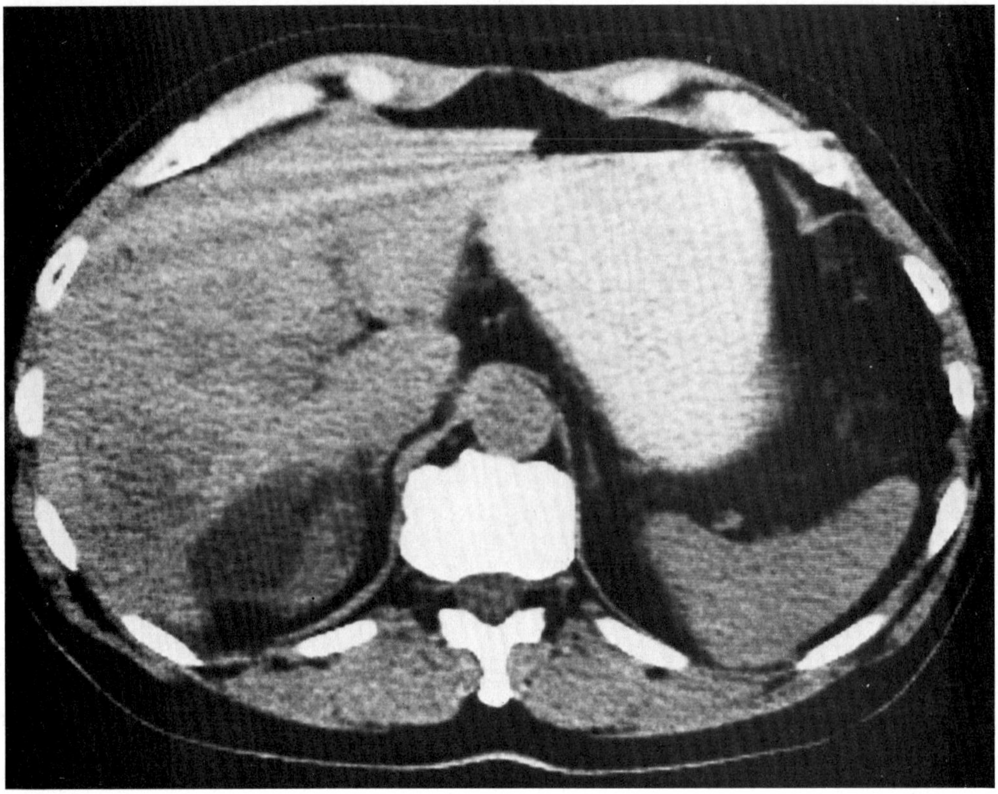

(A)

Figure 4 (EOE 13) Contrast enhancement in metastatic disease. Patient with metastatic colon carcinoma. (A) Precontrast CT scan through the liver. A vague lucency is identified posteriorly in the right lobe of the liver (an upper pole right renal cyst is also present). (B) Postcontrast (ethiodized oil emulsion 13). The metastasis is easily noted (arrow). Portal venous structures are also apparent.

Newer Contrast Agents

Although incremental dynamic CT scanning through a volume may afford increased contrast between functioning parenchyma and space occupying lesions, the transient nature of this means of contrast enhancement has led others to develop new contrast agents to aid in CT evaluations of the liver.

In 1979 Vermess et al. (12) reported the development of an ethiodized oil emulsion (EOE 13), for use in CT scanning of the liver and spleen. This compound contains 53% of iodinated ester of poppyseed in an emulsion. As the ester enhances only functioning parenchymal reticuloendothelial cells but not tumor or vessels, marked improvement in tumor visualization may occur. More recently, the experience in 60 examinations has been reported (13). The authors confirmed the marked improvement in visualization of hepatic space occupying lesions with this new agent (Fig. 4). In addition, they reported that

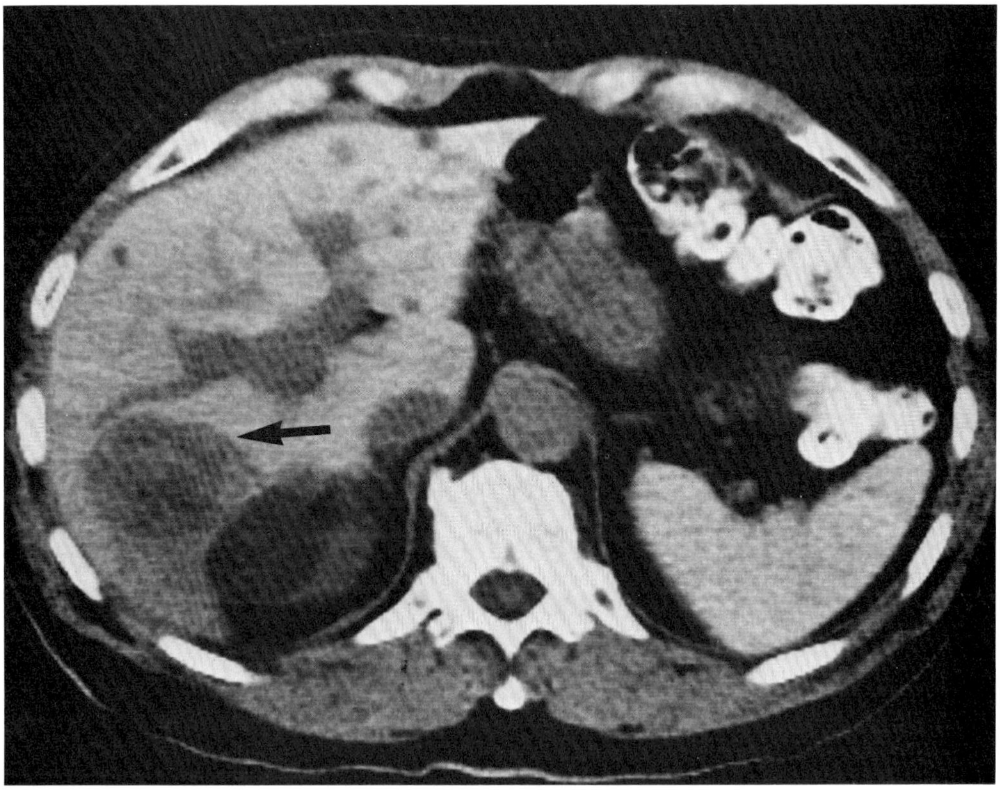

(B)
Figure 4

pretreatment with hydrocortisone reduced the incidence of associated side effects, including fever, chills, and rigors that had been problematic initially.

Nuclear Magnetic Resonance

Principles

Nuclear magnetic resonance (NMR) is a phenomenon which has been widely employed as a tool in biochemical and chemical analysis. Atomic nuclei with an unequal number of protons and neutrons have intrinsic magnetic properties. When subjected to a strong steady magnetic field, the nuclear spins of these atoms align and precess parallel to the field (Fig. 5a). The precession occurs at a specific frequency, the Larmor frequency, which is determined by the inherent properties of the nucleus of a given atom, the gyromagnetic ratio, and is directly proportional to the magnetic field strength. The precessional frequency is, in general, in the radiofrequency range.

Once aligned, the vector of the nuclear spins may be displaced by application of a pulsed radio frequency (RF) wave, which is applied at or near the natual Larmor frequency (Fig. 5b). By varying the duration of the RF pulse, the magnitude of the

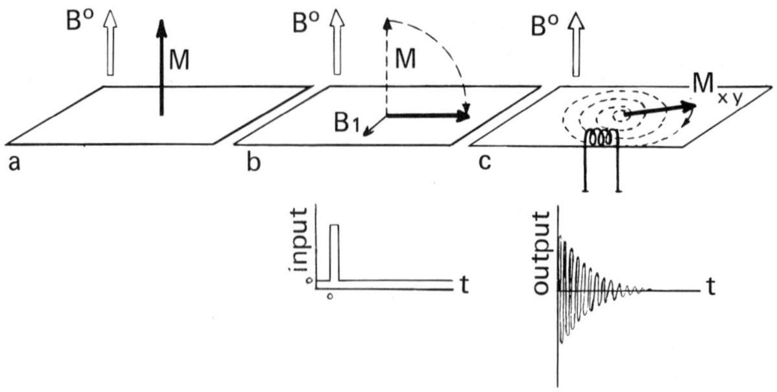

Figure 5 Nuclear magnetic resonance. (a) When subjected to a magnetic field B°, the nuclear spins of hydrogen nuclei align with the magnetic field producing a net magnetization vector M. (b) The vector of align spins is displaced 90° by a radio frequency pulse B, at the Larmor frequency. (c) Once the RF is discontinued, a RF signal is emitted (output) as the spins once again realign along the main magnetic field.

displacement may be varied. Typically, spins are rotated 90° or 180° by the applied RF pulse. Once the RF is discontinued the spins revert to their original orientation along the magnetic field and in so doing emit an RF signal at the same Larmor frequency (Fig. 5c).

The emitted signal decays as the spins once again realign along the main magnetic field. Two time constants describe the signal decay, or magnetic relaxation. T_2 is termed the spin–spin, or transverse relaxation time and describes the time required for the nuclear spins to get out of phase with each other while spinning at approximately right angles to the constant magnetic field. The total time required for the vector of spins to revert to their original orientation along the magnetic field is T_1, or the spin–lattice or longitudinal relaxation time.

The relaxation time for a given atom relates directly to its local chemical environment. In pure water the proton spin–lattice relaxation time (T_1) at room temperature is approximately 3 seconds, while in biologic tissue it varies from several hundred milliseconds to 2 seconds.

The relaxation times for tissues in the body may vary greatly in health and disease. In 1971 Damadian (14) reported that proton relaxation times were longer in neoplastic tissue than in normal tissue. No doubt, this discovery stimulated interest and activity in biochemical imaging with nuclear magnetic resonance.

In 1973 Lauterbur (15) showed that spatial localization of the emitted signal could be achieved by spatially encoding the signal through the use of magnetic field gradients. If a gradient magnetic field is applied across the object to be imaged, the net magnetic field will be stronger on one side of the object than the other, and as a result the resonant frequency of the nuclei will be higher on the side with the stronger field. The net signal received will be a commposite consisting of many different frequencies corresponding to different spatial locations. By means of a Fourier transform, a mathematical analysis performed by a digital computer, a plot of the frequency distribution or a projection of the signal is made. If a number of such projections are obtained in different directions by changing the orientation of the gradient fields the image may be generated by use of reconstruction techniques much as in CT.

NMR Imaging: Potential Advantages

Due to its abundance in biological systems H' has been the nucleus from which medical images have been obtained. By controlling the sequence and timing of the radio frequency pulses, images can be obtained in which the contrast is a function at proton density, T_1 or T_2 or a combination of these variables. In addition, in many of the data acquisition schemes (pulse sequences) flowing blood does not give a signal and vascular lumen of large vessels may easily be identified.

The anatomic detail present on the images produced is excellent, and approaches that of existing CT units. In addition, in the abdomen, respiratory and bowel gas motion appear to provide less artifact than normally seen in CT despite long data acquisition times (Fig. 6).

In most units available, the plane of data collection may be varied electronically, and direct data collection is possible in the cross axial, coronal, and sagittal plane. The

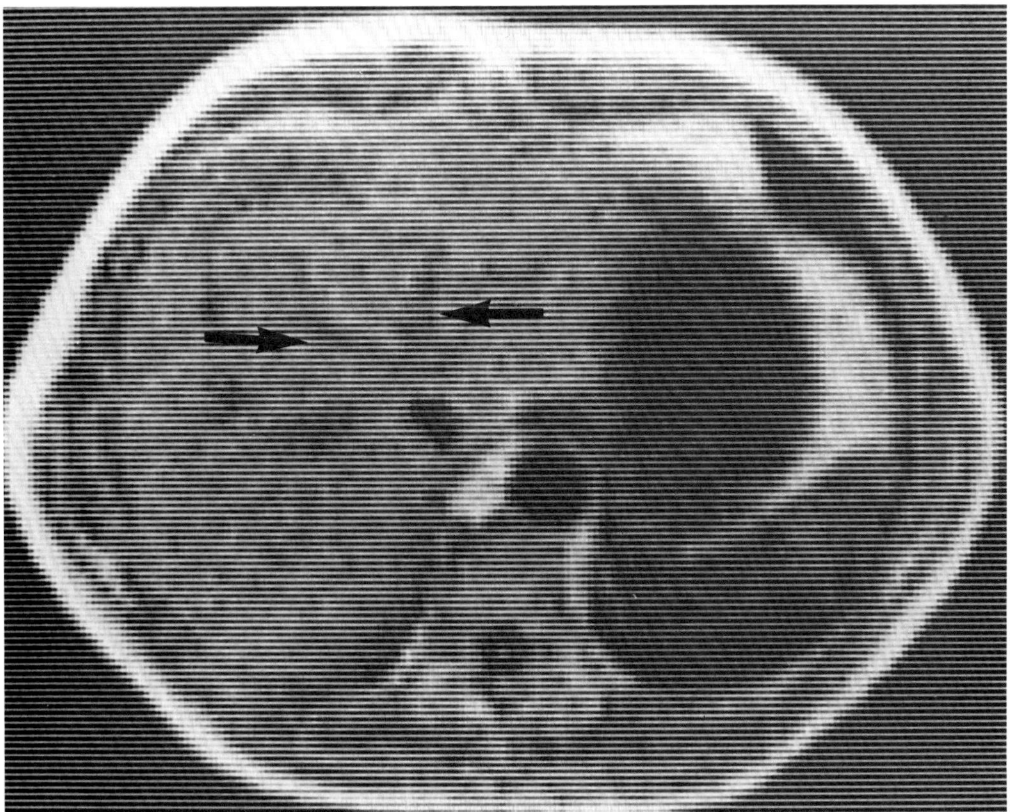

Figure 6 NMR scan of the liver. Normal liver. Note the vascular lucencies (arrows) and the absence of artifact around the stomach.

coronal and sagittal images produced are superior to those obtained by reformatting cross axial computed tomographic images. Thus the ability to obtain high quality images in any axis may be helpful in defining the extent of disease.

The early work on in vitro specimens suggested that NMR parameters such as T_1 might prove to be excellent discriminators of disease. Although early workers (14,16) had reported that the T_1 of tumors was prolonged when compared to normal tissue, others had subsequently demonstrated an overlap between malignant tumors and other, non-neoplastic disease processes. Davis *et al.* (17) working with implanted hepatomas in rats noted that relaxation times in 70 percent of their cases were unique enough to allow classification as tumors although the remaining 30 percent overlapped those found in abscesses and hematomas. In addition to T_1 in different disease processes, there appear to be differences in the T_1 observed on imaging units and those obtained at in vitro spectroscopy, and some apparent difference exists between relaxation times derived from different NMR scanning units.

The reports available clearly demonstrate that a wide spectrum of disease processes involving the liver may be identified at NMR scanning (18,19). Drawing conclusions or comparing the results from different centers at this time is difficult as the images and their significance vary widely, depending on the pulse sequence and interpulse intervals used, which may vary significantly from unit to unit.

A wide variety of disease processes involving the liver may be readily identified. Space occupying lesions, such as metastatic disease or tumors, can be identified, comparably to other imaging modalities such as nuclear medicine, ultrasound or computed tomography. Vascular tumors show very high contrast. Some diffuse hepatocellular disease does clearly appear to be more readily identified with NMR. Specifically, cirrhosis with its markedly prolonged relaxation time, and liver atrophy. Other parenchymal liver diseases such as hepatitis or infarct may be more readily identified on NMR scans than at computed tomographic examination. Surprisingly, fatty liver may be difficult to detect.

The NMR relaxation times have not proved to be as specific indicators of disease as was initially hoped. In the human studies to date, a variety of diffuse liver diseases show considerable overlap, as do neoplasms. Although NMR represents an exciting development in imaging, additional work is needed to find the optimal NMR imaging method for liver disease as well as to precisely define its role in the diagnostic armamentarium.

Endoscopic Cholangiography and Placement of Biliary Endoprostheses

An advantage hitherto claimed for percutaneous transhepatic cholangiography (PTC) over endoscopic retrograde cholangiopancretography (ERCP) has been the ability of the former method to follow diagnostic imaging by transhepatic biliary drainage procedures. Increasingly, endoscopists have developed methods which may now equal or even surpass the range of diagnostic/interventional possibilities offered by PTC.

A 3F-balloon catheter is now available and can be employed to increase the injection pressure of contrast medium into the common duct sufficiently to overcome the obsructing effect of very tight, unduly long or multiple strictures. In this way, the full extent of such strictures as well as the intrahepatic bile duct system above them can be opacified without increasing bile duct pressure within the liver substance (20). The same balloon catheter can be used to bring common duct stones into the duodenum after papillotomy.

Endoprostheses of a caliber sufficient to provide long-term biliary drainage (9F) can now be introduced through a duodenoscope, as yet available as a prototype only. When

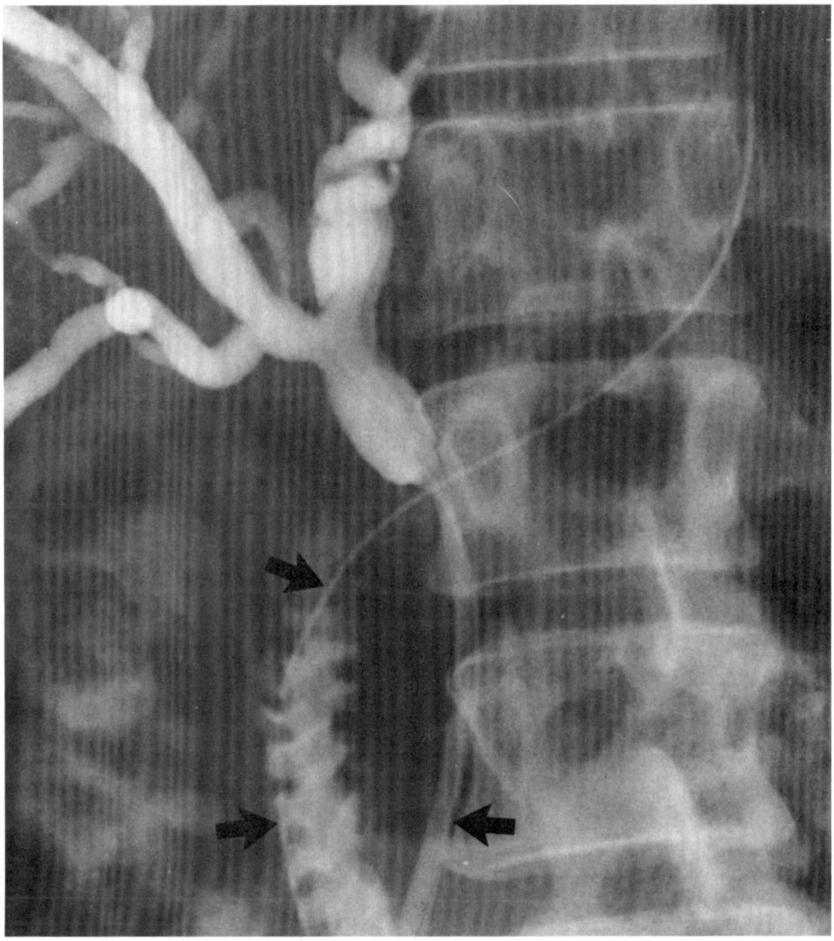

Figure 7 Endoscopic placement of biliary drainage catheter in a patient with malignant stricture of the common bile duct. Note the nasobiliary catheter (arrows) used for flushing and debridement. (Courtesy of M. Cremer and L. Engelholm, Erasmus Hospital, Brussels, Belgium).

considered indicated after cholangiography, a wire guide is introduced through the diagnositc catheter and advanced through the stricture into the right hepatic duct. A 9F drainage stent is then taken through the stricture, using another catheter as "pusher". The stent has a sigma-shaped tip to anchor it above the stricture, with its numerous sideholes at the concave aspects of the curves (21). If patient survival is considered to be less than 4-6 months, the stent is cut so that its distal termination should not reach the papilla. In patients with a more favorable survival outlook, a distally curved catheter is used with the curve extending into the duodenum. In this way, should the catheter become obstructed by biliary sludge after a few months, it can readily be exchanged by endoscopic means. It is considered advisable to perform a limited papillotomy before such stent placement to avoid pancreatic duct blockage by the 9F endoprosthesis (23).

A fine nasobiliary catheter is frequently introduced alongside the stent to reach a hepatic duct above the stricture and is used for temporary flushing and debridement (Fig. 7). It is only rarely possible to intubate the left hepatic duct through the endoscope.

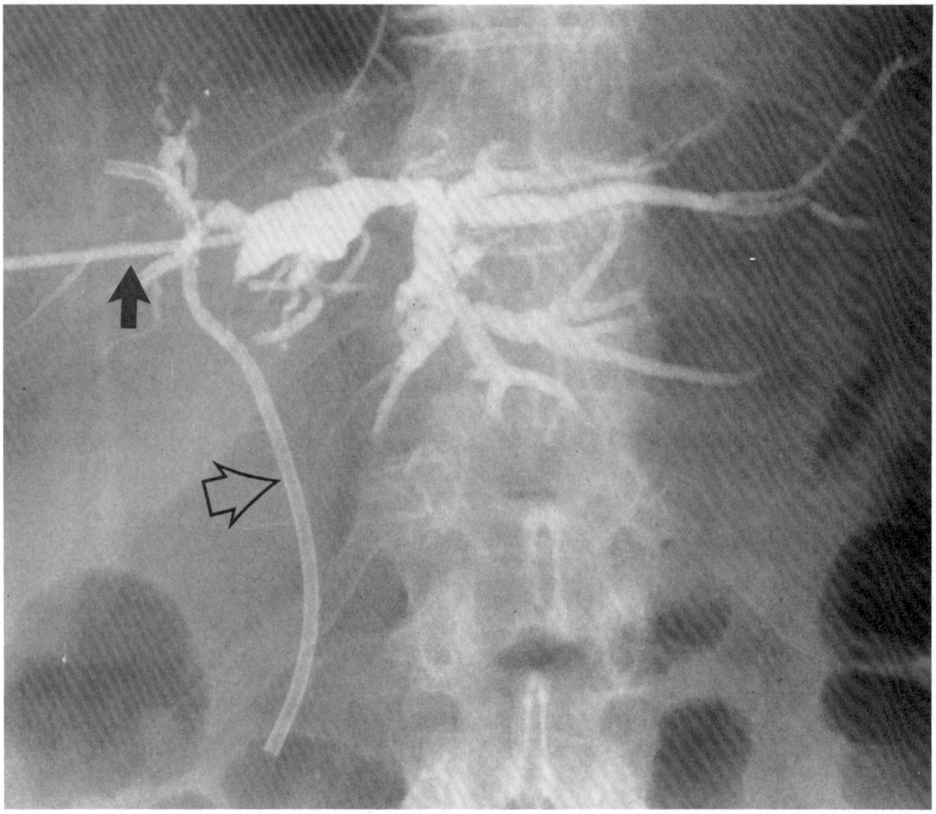

Figure 8 Biliary endoprosthesis in a patient with a Klatskin tumor. The endoscopically placed endoprosthesis (open arrow) drains the right lobe. A percutaneous transhepatic catheter (arrow) drains the left lobe of the liver. (Courtesy of M. Cremer and L. Engelholm, Erasmus Hospital, Brussels, Belgium.)

In the case of a Klatskin tumor, the left lobe would therefore have to decompressed transhepatically (Fig. 8)

Digital Subtraction Angiography

Methods of digital image processing have made a significant impact in radiology. Intravenous arteriography has become an established method, mostly with regard to imaging of the carotid, renal, and peripheral vasculature. Significant further improvement of equipment is likely.

At the present state of the art the systemic venous administration of contrast medium cannot produce levels of density in the portal vein sufficient for digital subtraction imaging. It is possible, however, to combine this new technique with arterioportography either to obtain improved portal venous detail at conventional rates of contrast injection or to produce acceptable portal venous images with significantly-reduced rates and amounts of injected contrast (Fig. 9).

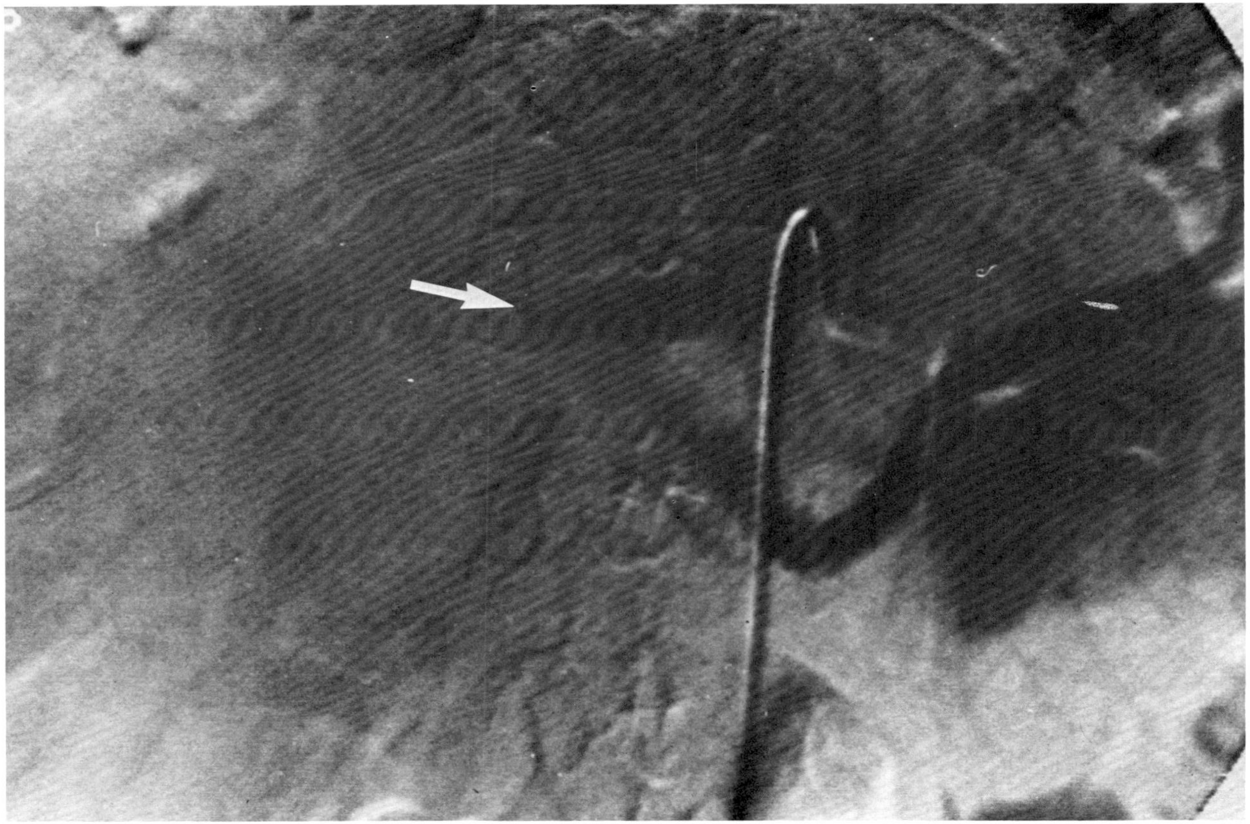

Figure 9
Digital venous portography in a patient with hepatoma. Digital portogram following a 10cc contrast injection at 3 ml/sec into the celiac artery. There is occlusion of the right portal vein (arrow) due to the right lobar hepatoma. (Courtesy of Kyung Cho, Department of Radiology, University Hospital, Ann Arbor, Michigan.)

References

1. Korobkin M, Kressel HY, Moss AA, Koeheler RE: Computed tomographic angiography of the Body CT. *Radiology 126:* 807, 1978.
2. Hacker H, Becker H: Time controlled computed tomographic angiograph. *JCAT 1:* 405, 1977.
3. Marchal GJ, Baert AL, Wilms GE: CT of non-cystic liver lesions. *Am J Radiol 135:* 57, 1980.
4. Tada S, Dukuda K, Aoyagi Y, Harada: CT of abdominal malignancies: dynamic approach. *Am J Radiol 135:* 455, 1980.
5. Araki I, Itai Y, Furui S, Tasaka A: Dynamic CT densitometry of hepatic Tumors. *Am J Radiol 135:* 1037, 1980.
6. Kunstlinger G, Federle MP, Moss AA, Marks W: Computed tomography of hepatocellular carcinoma. *Am J Radiol 134:* 431, 1980.
7. Itai Y, Araki T, Furui S, Akira T: Differential diagnosis of hepatic masses on computed tomography, with particular reference to hepatocellular carcinoma. *JCAT 5:* 834, 1981.
8. Moss AA, Dean PB, Axel L, Goldberg HI, Glazer GM, Friedman MA: Dynamic CT of hepatic masses with intravenous and intraarterial contrast materialj. *Am J Radiol 138:* 847, 1982.
9. Itai Y, Furui S, Arabi T, Yashiro N, Tasaka A: Computed tomography of cavernous hemangioma of the liver. *Radiology 137:* 149, 1980.
10. Freeny PC, Vimont R, Barnett DC: Cavernous hemangioma of the liver: ultrasonography arteriography and computed tomography. *Radiology 132:* 143, 1979.
11. Rogers JV, Mack LA, Freeny PC, Johnson ML, Sones PJ: Hepatic focal nodular hyperplasia angiography, CT, sonography, scintigraphy. *Am J Radiol 137:* 983, 1981.
12. Vermess M, Chatterji DC, Doppman JL, Grimes G, Adamson RH. Development and experimental evaluation of a contrast medium for computed tomographic examination of the liver and spleen *JCAT* 3: 25, 1979.
13. Vermess M, Doppman JL, Sugarbaker PH, Fisher RI, O'Leary TJ, Chatterji DC, Grimes G, Adamson RH, Willis M, Edwards BK: Computed tomography of the liver and spleen with intravenous lipoid contrast material: review of 60 examinations. *Am J Radiol 138:* 1063, 1982.
14. Damadian R: Tumor detection by nuclear magnetic resonance. *Science 171:* 1151, 1971.
15. Lauterbur PC: Image formation by induced local interactions: examples employing nuclear magnetic resonance. *Nature 243:* 190, 1973.
16. Damadian R, Zaner K, Hor D, DiMaio T: Human tumors detected by NMR. *Proc Nat Acad Sci USA 7:* 1471, 1974.
17. Davis PL, Kaufman L, Crooks LE, Miller TR: Detectability of hepatomas in rat livers by nuclear magnetic resonance imaging. *Invest Radiol 16:* 354, 1981.
18. Smith FW, Mallard JR, Reid A, McDonnell MJ, Bydder GM, Steiner RE, Young IR, Clarke GJ, Pasmore T, Gilderdale DJ: Nuclear magnetic imaging in liver disease. *Lancet 1:* 963, 1981.
19. Doyle FH, Rennak JM, Banks LM: Nuclear magnetic resonance imaging of the liver: initial experience. *Am J Radiol 138:* 193. 1982.
20. Cremer M, Adler M, Dunham F, De Toeuf J, Lambilliotte JP: Intubation non operatoire des stenoses neoplastiques des voies bilaires. In *Actualites Digestives Medico Chirurgicales,* Mouiel, J (Ed). Masson, Paris, 1982, pp. 103–110.
21. Cremer M, personal communication, 1982.
22. Engelholm L, personal communication, 1982.

Index

Part A —pages 1–577
Part B —pages 579–1138

Part A —pages 1–577
Part B —pages 579–1138

About The Editors

HANS HERLINGER is Professor of Radiology at the University of Pennsylvania, Philadelphia and Honorary Consultant Radiologist, St. James's University Hospital, Leeds, England. In addition, Dr. Herlinger is the Organizing Chairman for the Annual Leeds Course in Gastroenterology for Radiologists. He has written over 50 papers, concentrating on arteriography and gastroenterology, and serves on the editorial boards of three journals in this field—*Journal of Gastrointestinal Radiology*, *Digestive Diseases and Sciences*, and the *Italian Journal of Gastroenterology*. Dr. Herlinger is a member of numerous professional societies and is a Fellow of the Royal College of Radiologists.

ANDERS LUNDERQUIST is Professor of Radiology and Head of the angiographic and gastrointestinal radiology sections of the University Hospital, Lund, Sweden. He has conducted extensive research in urology, vascular, and gastrointestinal radiology that has resulted in over 120 publications. Dr. Lunderquist is a member of the Swedish Society of Radiology, Scandinavian Society of Radiology, American Society of Gastro-Intestinal Radiology, and the European College of Angiography.

SIDNEY WALLACE is Professor of Radiology and the Deputy Head of the Department of Diagnostic Radiology at the University of Texas System Cancer Center, M. D. Anderson Hospital and Tumor Institute, Houston, Texas. His special research interests include the evaluation of new materials and techniques for percutaneous transcatheter intra-arterial approaches in occlusion therapy, chemotherapy, and immunotherapy. He has published more than 200 articles, many of them communicating promising results in the area of interventional radiology.